DIVERTICULAR DISEASE

MANAGEMENT OF THE DIFFICULT SURGICAL CA

DIVERTICULAR DISEASE
MANAGEMENT OF THE DIFFICULT SURGICAL CASE

John P. Welch, MD
Connecticut Surgical Group, Hartford, Connecticut
Clinical Professor of Surgery
University of Connecticut School of Medicine, Farmington, Connecticut
Adjunct Professor of Surgery
Dartmouth Medical School, Hanover, New Hampshire

Jeffrey I. Cohen, MD
Connecticut Surgical Group, Hartford, Connecticut
Associate Clinical Professor of Surgery
University of Connecticut
Attending Surgeon, Hartford Hospital and Connecticut Children's Medical Center
Hartford, Connecticut

William V. Sardella, MD
Connecticut Surgical Group, Hartford, Connecticut
Assistant Professor, Department of Surgery
Hartford Hospital, Hartford, Connecticut
Associate Professor of Surgery
University of Connecticut, Farmington, Connecticut
Adjunct Assistant Professor of Surgery
Dartmouth Medical School, Hanover, New Hampshire

Paul V. Vignati, MD
Connecticut Surgical Group, Hartford, Connecticut
Assistant Clinical Professor of Surgery
University of Connecticut School of Medicine
Attending Surgeon, Connecticut Children's Medical Center and John Dempsey Hospital
Farmington, Connecticut
Attending Surgeon, Hartford Hospital, Hartford, Connecticut

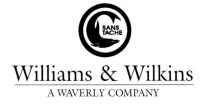

Williams & Wilkins
A WAVERLY COMPANY

BALTIMORE • PHILADELPHIA • LONDON • PARIS • BANGKOK
BUENOS AIRES • HONG KONG • MUNICH • SYDNEY • TOKYO • WROCLAW

Editor: Carroll C. Cann
Managing Editor: Paula Brown
Marketing Manager: Diane M. Harnish
Production Coordinator: Danielle Hagan
Project Editor: Robert D. Magee
Text/Cover Designer: Artech Graphics II
Illustration Planner: Wayne Hubbel
Typesetter: Graphic World, Inc.
Printer/Binder: RR Donnelley & Sons Company

351 West Camden Street
Baltimore, Maryland 21201-2436 USA

Rose Tree Corporate Center
1400 North Providence Road
Building II, Suite 5025
Media, Pennsylvania 19063-2043 USA

Accurate indications, adverse reactions and dosage schedules for drugs are provided in this book, but it is possible that they may change. The reader is urged to review the package information data of the manufacturers of the medications mentioned.

Printed in the United States of America

Library of Congress Cataloging-in-Publication Data

Diverticular disease : management of the difficult surgical case / [edited by] John P.
    Welch . . . [et al.]. — 1st ed.
        p.   cm.
    Includes bibliographical references and index.
    ISBN 0-683-08881-5
    1. Diverticulitis. 2. Diverticulitis—Surgery. I. Welch, John P. (John Paton), 1942-   .
        [DNLM: 1. Diverticulosis, Colonic—surgery. 2. Diverticulitis—surgery. 3. Di-
        verticulosis, Colonic—diagnosis. 4. Diverticulitis—diagnosis. 5. Diagnosis,
        Differential.   WI 425   D617 1998]
    RC862.D6D58   1998
    617.5'54—dc21   97-30348
                                                                            CIP

The publishers have made every effort to trace the copyright holders for borrowed material. If they have inadvertently overlooked any, they will be pleased to make the necessary arrangements at the first opportunity.

To purchase additional copies of this book, call our customer service department at **(800) 638-0672** or fax orders to **(800) 447-8438.** For other book services, including chapter reprints and large quantity sales, ask for the Special Sales department.

Canadian customers should call **(800) 665-1148,** or fax **(800) 665-0103.** For all other calls originating outside of the United States, please call **(410) 528-4223** or fax us at **(410) 528-8550.**

Visit Williams & Wilkins on the Internet: **http://www.wwilkins.com** or contact our customer service department at **custserv@wwilkins.com**. Williams & Wilkins customer service representatives are available from 8:30 am to 6:00 pm, EST, Monday through Friday, for telephone access.

98 99 00 01 02
1 2 3 4 5 6 7 8 9 10

DEDICATION

*This book is dedicated to Claude E. Welch, MD, a scholar surgeon
and passionate clinician who exercised uncanny judgment in
tough surgical situations for the benefit of his patients.*

FOREWORD

It is a distinct honor to be asked to write a foreword for a book, suggesting that the honoree may actually know something about the subject at hand and have something worthwhile to convey about the book and its editors. Drs. Welch, Cohen, Sardella, and Vignati are all experienced practicing clinical surgeons who are to be congratulated for assembling a number of experienced clinicians as authors for a unique text that is devoted exclusively to diverticular disease with its protean manifestations.

Although the text is focused predominantly on colonic diverticulosis, the editors have included small-bowel diverticula as well, making this the first comprehensive reference to congenital and acquired diverticular disease of both the small and large bowel.

A review of the table of contents immediately indicates the thrust of the book; that is, the topics are organized as clinical scenarios encountered in practice. The first section deals with diagnostic dilemmas in an attempt to refine the differential diagnosis. Section II presents challenging technical problems resulting from diverticulitis and the surgical therapeutic options with their respective complications. Section III presents particularly unusual subsets of patients with diverticulitis, whereas Section IV deals with unusual problems, including giant colonic diverticula and small-bowel diverticular disease.

In a successful attempt to make the book more readable and useful, there are a number of editorial additions, beginning with a summary of "Key Points" at the beginning of each chapter. Sentences are italicized within the text, thus providing a visual outline of each chapter. Editorial comments at the end of each chapter provide an opportunity to focus on the more controversial aspects of each topic. Finally, the references are annotated, with a summary sentence after each citation. All of these additions significantly enhance the value of the book.

Accomplishment of this ambitious undertaking, with a comprehensive presentation of all aspects of the surgical management of diverticular disease, is a feat for which the editors should be thoroughly congratulated. This book will be a unique reference for all specialists who are involved in the treatment of these common and uncommon disorders.

David J. Schoetz, MD
Chairman, Department of Colon-Rectal Surgery
Lahey Hitchcock Clinic
Burlington, Massachusetts

PREFACE

Why a book on diverticular disease? The subject is covered in a number of textbooks and in some monographs, but usually in general terms without reference to specific patients. We believe that the collection of topics in the following pages examines problems of particular interest to surgeons in a more detailed and specific manner than is otherwise available. We try to provide a practical approach to situations that can prove complex from the standpoint of both medical and surgical management.

We have arbitrarily divided the text into four sections. The section on Diagnostic Dilemmas pays particular attention to other intestinal diseases that can be confused with diverticular complications. One chapter is devoted to a discussion of radiologic diagnostic techniques. The section on Technical Problems concentrates on operative approaches to specific complications of diverticular disease. In the portion allotted to Selected Populations, we look at the impact of diverticular disease on certain groups such as young or immunosuppressed patients. Finally, the section on Unusual Problems looks at rare manifestations such as hepatic abscess, diverticulitis of the transverse colon, and bleeding jejunal diverticulosis.

There is a standard format for most of the chapters. Key points that are raised are listed at the beginning of each chapter. Illustrative cases are presented that are specifically related to the chapter topic, and comments follow each case. Major points in the text are italicized. At the end of each chapter, the editors have added comments on the text, as well as additional information in some instances. Nearly all of the references are annotated to simplify the task of studying other relevant sources of information.

In essence, we hope that this monograph will provide succinct, practical approaches to many of the vexing complications of diverticular disease to interested surgeons and physicians.

ACKNOWLEDGMENTS

The Hartford Hospital Department of Surgery, under the directorship of H. David Crombie, MD, has been very helpful to the authors by providing encouragement as well as funds to pay for transcription and audiovisual costs. As part of this arrangement, a number of surgical residents at Hartford Hospital were involved in writing chapters. The endowed Pyrtek Fund, established in honor of our esteemed colleague and mentor, Ludwig J. Pyrtek, M.D., was the source of funding for these educational expenses.

We would also like to thank the transcriptionists, in particular Nancy McCabe, who did the bulk of the work. In the medical library, Lisa Carter was extremely helpful in obtaining references and Shirley Gronholm provided a number of literature searches.

During the time-consuming organization of the manuscript, the personnel at Williams & Wilkins, particularly Carroll Cann, Susan Hunsberger, and Paula Brown, have provided support and answers to all of our questions

CONTRIBUTORS

Herand Abcarian, MD
Turi Josefsen Professor and Head,
    Department of Surgery
University of Illinois—Chicago
Chicago, Illinois

Cameron Akbari, MD
Instructor in Surgery
Harvard Medical School
Attending Surgeon
Beth Israel Deaconess Medical Center
Boston, Massachusetts

H. Randolph Bailey, MD
Clinical Professor of Surgery
Chief, Division of Colon and Rectal
    Surgery
University of Texas Medical School at
    Houston
Houston, Texas

Robert W. Beart, Jr., MD
Professor of Surgery, Department of
    Surgery
University of Southern California
Center for Colorectal Diseases
Los Angeles, California

Steven H. Brown, MD
Resident, Department of Surgery
Hartford Hospital
Hartford, Connecticut

Philip F. Caushaj, MD
Clinical Professor of Surgery
Yale University School of Medicine
New Haven, Connecticut
Chairman, Department of Surgery
Bridgeport Hospital
Yale New Haven Health
Bridgeport, Connecticut

Charles W. Chappius, MD
Clinical Assistant Professor of Surgery
Louisiana State University School of
    Medicine
New Orleans, Louisiana

Bertram T. Chinn, MD
Clinical Assistant Professor of Surgery
University of Medicine and Dentistry
    New Jersey, Robert Woods Johnson
    Medical School
Attending Surgeon, Muhlenberg Regional
    Medical Center
Plainfield, New Jersey
Attending Surgeon, John F. Kennedy
    Medical Center
Edison, New Jersey

Jeffrey L. Cohen, MD
Connecticut Surgical Group
Hartford Connecticut
Associate Clinical Professor of Surgery
University of Connecticut
Farmington, Connecticut
Attending Surgeon
Hartford Hospital
Attending Surgeon
Connecticut Children's Medical Center
Hartford, Connecticut

Isidore Cohn, Jr., MD, DSc
Professor of Surgery
Louisiana State University
New Orleans, Louisiana

Timothy C. Counihan, MD
Colon and Rectal Surgery Fellow
University of Minnesota, Division of
    Colon and Rectal Surgery
Minneapolis, Minnesota

Nilto Carias De Oliveira, MD
Senior Resident in Surgery
Hartford Hospital
Hartford, Connecticut
University of Connecticut School of
    Medicine
Farmington, Connecticut

Albert Del Pino, MD
Attending Surgeon, Department of Colon-
    Rectal Surgery
Cook County Hospital
Chicago, Illinois

Peter S. Edelstein, MD
Assistant Professor of Surgery
Stanford University
Stanford, California

Glen Egrie, MD
Surgical Resident, Department of Surgery
University of Connecticut School of
    Medicine
Farmington, Connecticut

Theodore E. Eisenstat, MD
Clinical Professor of Surgery
University of Medicine and Dentistry
    New Jersey
Robert Woods Johnson Medical School
Director, Colon and Rectal Surgery
    Residency
Muhlenberg Regional Medical Center
Attending Surgeon
John F. Kennedy Medical Center
Edison, New Jersey

Andrew Feldman, MD
Surgical Resident, Department of Surgery
University of Connecticut School of
    Medicine
Farmington, Connecticut

Lori L. Fritts, MD
Assistant Clinical Professor, Department
    of Surgery
University of Connecticut School of
    Medicine
Farmington, Connecticut
Attending Surgeon
Associate Director, Surgical Critical Care
    Division
Hartford Hospital
Hartford, Connecticut

F.A. Frizelle, MBChB, MmedSci
Colorectal Surgeon
Christchurch Hospital
Senior Lecturer in Surgery
Otago Medical School
Christchurch, New Zealand

Stanley M. Goldberg, MD, FACS, Hron.
    FRACS, Hron. FRCSEng
Clinical Professor of Surgery, Department
    of Surgery
Division of Colon and Rectal Surgery
University of Minnesota
Minneapolis, Minnesota

Michael J. Hallisey, MD
Assistant Clinical Professor
University of Connecticut School of
    Medicine
Farmington, Connecticut
Department of Radiology
Hartford Hospital
Hartford, Connecticut

Tadaaki Hiruki, MD, FRCPC
Assistant Professor, Department of
    Pathology
University of Toronto
Toronto, Ontario
Canada

Anthony L. Imbembo, MD
Professor of Surgery
Associate Dean for Academic
    Administration
University of Maryland School of
    Medicine
Baltimore, Maryland

Faek Jamali, MD
Surgical Resident, Department of Surgery
University of Connecticut School of
    Medicine
Farmington, Connecticut

Wanda Kirejczyk, MD
Attending Radiologist
St. Francis Hospital and Medical Center
Hartford, Connecticut

Edward C. Lee, MD
Assistant Professor of Surgery
Albany Medical College
Albany, New York

Walter E. Longo, MD
Associate Professor of Surgery
Director, Colorectal Research
Associate Professor of Anatomy
St. Louis University School of Medicine
St. Louis, Missouri

Stuart K. Markowitz, MD
Chairman, Department of Radiology
Section Chief, Gastrointestinal Imaging
Hartford Hospital
Hartford, Connecticut

Robin S. McLeod, MD, FRCS(C)
Associate Professor of Surgery
Head, Colorectal Surgery Program
University of Toronto
Toronto, Ontario
Canada

Frank B. Miller, MD
Professor of Surgery, Department of
   Surgery
University of Louisville
Louisville, Kentucky

Leon Morgenstern, MD
Emeritus Director of Surgery
Cedars-Sinai Medical Center
Emeritus Professor of Surgery
UCLA School of Medicine
Los Angeles, California

John J. Murray, MD
Staff Surgeon, Department of Colon and
   Rectal Surgery
Lahey Hitchcock Clinic
Burlington, Massachusetts

David L. Nahrwold, MD
Loyal and Edith Davis Professor and
   Chairman
Department of Surgery
Northwestern University Medical School
Surgeon-in-Chief
Northwestern Memorial Hospital
Chicago, Illinois

Richard L. Nelson, MD
Associate Professor of Surgery
University of Illinois College of Medicine
Assistant Professor of Epidemiology and
   Biostatistics
University of Illinois, Department of
   Public Health
Chicago, Illinois

Lucia Oliveira, MD
Chief, Department of Colon and Rectal
   Surgery
Hospital Mario Kroeff
Rio de Janeiro, Brazil

Rocco Orlando, III, MD
Associate Professor of Clinical Surgery
University of Connecticut School of
   Medicine
Farmington, Connecticut
Associate Director, Surgical Intensive
   Care Unit
Hartford Hospital
Hartford, Connecticut

Adrian E. Ortega, MD
Assistant Professor of Surgery
Center for Colorectal Diseases
University of Southern California
Los Angeles, California

William Pennoyer, MD
Surgical Resident, Department of Surgery
University of Connecticut School of
   Medicine
Farmington, Connecticut

George Perdrizet, MD, PhD
EMS Trauma Division
Department of Surgery
Hartford Hospital
University of Connecticut Medical Center
Hartford, Connecticut

James Pingpank, MD
Surgical Resident, Department of Surgery
University of Connecticut School of
   Medicine
Farmington, Connecticut

Hiram C. Polk, Jr., MD
Ben A. Reid, Sr. Professor and Chairman
Department of Surgery
University of Louisville
Louisville, Kentucky

Jay B. Prystowsky, MD
Assistant Professor of Surgery,
    Department of Surgery
Northwestern University Medical School
Chicago, Illinois

Carole S. Richard, MD, FRCS(C)
Mount Sinai Hospital
Toronto, Ontario
Canada

Grant V. Rodkey, MD
Associate Clinical Professor of Surgery
Harvard Medical School
Senior Surgeon
Massachusetts General Hospital
Staff Physician, Surgery
Boston Veterans Affairs Medical Center
Boston, Massachusetts

Lawrence Rusin, MD
Senior Staff, Department of Colon and
    Rectal Surgery
Lahey Clinic
Burlington, Massachusetts

John A. Ryan, Jr., MD
Chief of Surgery
Virginia Mason Medical Center
Seattle, Washington

Marilyn B. Sanford, MD
Chief Resident, Surgery
Virginia Mason Medical Center
Seattle, Washington

William V. Sardella, MD
Connecticut Surgical Group
Hartford, Connecticut
Assistant Professor, Department of
    Surgery
Hartford Hospital
Hartford, Connecticut
Associate Professor of Surgery
University of Connecticut
Farmington, Connecticut
Adjunct Assistant Professor of Surgery
Dartmouth Medical School
Hanover, New Hampshire

Larry S. Sasaki, MD
Associate Clinical Professor, Department
    of Surgery
Louisiana State University Medical Center
    at Shreveport
Shreveport, Louisiana

Stephanie L. Schmitt, MD
Department of Surgery
Medical Center of Central Massachusetts
Worcester, Massachusetts

Thomas Stahl, MD
Assistant Professor of Surgery
Department of Surgery
Georgetown University Medical Center
Washington, DC

Glenn W. Stambo, MD
Resident, Department of Radiology
Hartford, Hospital
Hartford, Connecticut

Charles A. Ternent, MD
Fellow, Department of Surgery, Section of
    Colon and Rectal Surgery
Creighton University School of Medicine
Omaha, Nebraska

Alan G. Thorsen, MD
Associate Professor of Surgery
Program Director, Section of Colon and
    Rectal Surgery
Creighton University School of
    Medicine
Clinical Associate Professor of Surgery
University of Nebraska College of
    Medicine
Omaha, Nebraska

Wayne B. Tuckson, MD
Assistant Professor, Department of
    Surgery
University of Louisville
Louisville, Kentucky

Juan P. Umana, MD
Surgery Resident
Columbia Presbyterian Medical
    Center
New York, New York

Anthony M. Vernava, MD
Chief of General Surgery
St. Mary's Health Center
Chief, Section of Colon and Rectal
    Surgery
Director, Colon and Rectal Surgery
    Residency Training Program
Associate Professor of Surgery
Director, Anorectal Physiology Lab
St. Louis University School of
    Medicine
St. Louis, Missouri

Paul V. Vignati, MD
Connecticut Surgical Group
Hartford, Connecticut
Assistant Clinical Professor of Surgery
University of Connecticut School of
    Medicine

Attending Surgeon
Connecticut Children's Medical
    Center
John Dempsey Hospital
Farmington, Connecticut
Attending Surgeon
Hartford Hospital
Hartford, Connecticut

John P. Welch, MD
Connecticut Surgical Group
Hartford, Connecticut
Clinical Professor of Surgery
University of Connecticut School of
    Medicine
Farmington, Connecticut
Adjunct Professor of Surgery
Dartmouth Medical School
Hanover, New Hampshire

Steven D. Wexner, MD
Chairman and Residency Program
    Director
Department of Colorectal
    Surgery
Cleveland Clinic Florida
Fort Lauderdale, Florida

Richard L. Whelan, MD
Assistant Professor of Surgery
Columbia University College of
    Physicians and Surgeons
New York, New York

Bruce G. Wolff, MD
Professor of Surgery
Mayo Clinic and Mayo
    Foundation
Rochester, Minnesota

CONTENTS

Chapter 1   An Overview
             Grant V. Rodkey, MD, John P. Welch, MD 1

SECTION 1:   Diagnostic Dilemmas

Chapter 2   **Abdominal Pain and Diverticulosis**
             Lucia Oliveira, MD, Steven D. Wexner, MD 33

Chapter 3   **Ischemic Colitis or Diverticulitis: A Challenging
             Diagnostic Dilemma**
             Walter E. Longo, MD, Anthony M. Vernava, MD 44

Chapter 4   **Colon Cancer Versus Diverticulitis**
             Richard L. Whelan, MD, Juan P. Umana, MD 55

Chapter 5   **Differentiation of Inflammatory Bowel Disease from
             Diverticulitis**
             Carole S. Richard, MD, Tadaaki Hiruki, MD, Robin S.
             McLeod, MD 67

Chapter 6   **Diverticular Hemorrhage**
             William Pennoyer, MD, Jeffrey Cohen, MD 76

Chapter 7   **Recurrent Sigmoid Diverticulitis**
             Charles W. Chappuis, MD, Isidore Cohn, Jr., MD 95

Chapter 8   **Radiologic Evaluation of Diverticular Disease of the
             Small and Large Intestines**
             Stuart K. Markowitz, MD, Wanda Kirejczyk, MD 102

Chapter 9   **Small Bowel Obstruction Complicating Colonic
             Diverticular Disease**
             Richard L. Nelson, MD 138

SECTION 2:   Technical Problems

Chapter 10   Colovesical Fistulas
Albert Del Pino, MD, Herand Abcarian, MD 151

Chapter 11   Colovaginal Fistulas
Bertram T. Chinn, MD, Theodore E. Eisenstat, MD .. 167

Chapter 12   Management of Coincident Diverticular Disease
Thomas Stahl, MD 174

Chapter 13   "Malignant" Diverticulitis
Leon Morgenstern, MD 181

Chapter 14   Diverticular Stricture
Andrew Feldman, MD, John P. Welch, MD 194

Chapter 15   Diverticular Abscess
Steven H. Brown, MD, Paul V. Vignati, MD, Glenn W.
Stambo, MD, Michael J. Hallisey, MD 206

Chapter 16   The Proper Surgical Treatment of Perforated
Sigmoid Diverticulitis with Generalized
Peritonitis
Marilyn B. Sanford, MD, John A. Ryan, Jr., MD 223

Chapter 17   Subacute Diverticulitis
William V. Sardella, MD, James Pingpank, MD 242

Chapter 18   Laparoscopic Operations for Diverticular Disease
Adrian E. Ortega, MD, Robert W. Beart, Jr., MD 251

Chapter 19   Reanastomosis Following the Hartmann Procedure
Larry S. Sasaki, MD, H. Randolph Bailey, MD,
FACS 262

Chapter 20   Intraoperative Colonic Lavage
An Option for Permitting Single-Stage Resection
John J. Murray, MD, Edward C. Lee, MD 274

Chapter 21   Complications of Surgery for Diverticulitis
Jeffrey L. Cohen, MD, Glen Egrie, MD,
William V. Sardella, MD, Paul V. Vignati, MD,
John P. Welch, MD 285

SECTION 3:   Selected Patient Populations

Chapter 22   Diverticular Disease in the Immunocompromised
Patient
George Perdrizet, MD, Cameron Akbari, MD 309

Chapter 23   Diverticular Disease and the Younger Patient
Peter S. Edelstein, MD, Stanley M. Goldberg, MD ... 319

Chapter 24   Critical Illness Arising From Diverticular Disease
Rocco Orlando, III, MD, Lori L. Fritts, MD 329

SECTION 4:   Unusual Problems

Chapter 25   Recurrent Diverticulitis Following Resection
Bruce G. Wolff, MD, F. A. Frizelle, MD 343

Chapter 26   Complications of Duodenal Diverticula
David L. Nahrwold, MD, Jay B. Prystowsky, MD ... 352

Chapter 27   Meckel's Diverticulum
Lawrence Rusin, MD 370

Chapter 28   The Atypical Presentations of Diverticulitis
Hiram C. Polk, Jr. MD, Wayne B. Tuckson, MD,
Frank B. Miller, MD 384

Chapter 29   Acquired Diverticula of the Small Bowel and
Appendix
Anthony L. Imbembo, MD 394

Chapter 30   Giant Diverticula of the Colon
Nilto Carias de Oliveira, MD, John P. Welch, MD ... 410

Chapter 31   Diverticulitis of the Transverse Colon
Faek Jamali, MD, John P. Welch, MD 419

Chapter 32   Cecal Diverticulitis
Alan G. Thorsen, MD, Charles A. Ternent, MD 428

Chapter 33   Hepatic Abscess Complicating Diverticulitis
Timothy C. Counihan, MD, Stephanie L. Schmitt, MD,
Philip F. Caushaj, MD 442

Index   453

1 An Overview

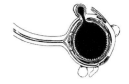

Grant V. Rodkey, MD
John P. Welch, MD

KEY POINTS
• Diverticular disease is a twentieth century malady
• Population of hospitalized patients is changing
• Pathophysiology may involve high-pressure zones in colon
• Elastosis and taenial shortening may cause bowel thickening
• CT scan and angiography major diagnostic advances
• Surgical trends: Aggressive resection One-stage (elective resection) One- or two-stage (emergent resection)
• Uncomplicated diverticulitis: medical treatment unless recurrent attacks or immunosuppressed patient
• Complicated diverticular disease: surgical management in most cases

HISTORICAL PERSPECTIVES

Diverticular disease is a malady of the twentieth century that probably is related to decreases in fiber content of the daily diet and to aging of the population. There were a few references to the disorder in the nineteenth century from authors such as Cruveilhier and Graser (1). Early in this century, descriptions of small numbers of cases came from centers such as the Mayo Clinic, and as the decades passed, many reports appeared, especially in the surgical literature. Currently, a high percentage of senior citizens have diverticular disease.

This portion of the chapter will examine developments in pathophysiology, diagnosis, and medical and surgical management of diverticular disease, as well as changes in the composition of the hospitalized patients.

Patient Populations

As diverticular disease was barely touched upon in the medical and surgical literature until the beginning of this century, the numbers of reported cases increased over time (2). However, in recent years, this trend may have started to reverse itself. With increasing expense of hospitalization, and more recently the strong emergence of managed care, there has been a tendency to hospitalize only patients with complicated disease. Patients with uncomplicated diverticulitis who may have been treated as inpatients with intravenous

Table 1.1.   Evolution of Patient Populations

More immunosuppressed patients
    Transplant recipients
    Individuals on chemotherapy
    AIDS
    Diabetes mellitus
    Chronic alcoholics
    Older patients
More advanced complications of diverticulitis
    Septic patients in intensive care unit

antibiotics now may be managed at home with oral or intravenous antibiotics. Education of the population at large about the benefits of a high-fiber diet also may have repercussions. Incidences in various populations are also changing, based on diet and migration: Japanese in Hawaii or blacks in the United States provide examples.

With advances in medical care and development of immunosuppressive drugs, the composition of the population of patients with diverticulitis has changed (see Table 1.1). *Patients have become increasingly older, more are immunosuppressed (3,4), and a higher percentage, at least in referral hospitals reporting their results, have advanced septic complications (5).* In series of patients with acquired immunodeficiency syndrome (AIDS) undergoing emergent abdominal surgery, diverticulitis is not mentioned, however, and a more likely cause of colonic pathology would be lymphoma or disseminated *Mycobacterium avium intracellulare* (6,7).

Natural History (8)

It has been well established that the risk of diverticular disease increases with age. There also may be an association with factors such as hiatus hernia, gallstones, varicose veins, and hemorrhoids, but not obesity, hypertension, or emotional factors (9,10). There is some controversy about the risk of polyps or carcinoma, but the diseases probably are coincidental (11,12). Acute diverticulitis even has been reported during the postoperative period after various surgical procedures (13). The risk of uncomplicated diverticulosis progressing to acute diverticulitis was estimated as 25% by Boles and Jordan in 1958 (14). Horner followed 503 patients in the office for a number of years and found that the overall incidence of diverticulitis was 17% and that the incidence of diverticulitis increased when patients were followed for increasing periods of time (15). This risk of developing diverticulitis may vary in different parts of the world. In a retrospective study from Japan, Kubo et al found diverticulitis in only 2.4% of 1124 cases of diverticular disease over 15 years (16). There also are different levels of risk in different populations. A prospective study suggested that patients admitted with diverticular disease have a high incidence of intake of nonsteroidal anti-inflammatory drugs (NSAIDs) and that intake of NSAIDs is associated with a more severe form of the disease (17). *Unfortunately, patients frequently present with significant complications despite few premonitory symptoms (18).*

What is the prognosis of patients hospitalized with diverticular disease? These data are hard to come by for a number of reasons: the paucity of prospective studies (19), the inadequacy of follow-up, the assumption that abdominal symptoms are related to diverticula (20), and the lack of clear definitions about the nature of recurrence. It has been estimated that there are 131,000 admissions annually for diverticulitis in the United States (21). In 1971, Parks and Connell reported a study of 455 patients hospitalized with diverticular disease: two-thirds of the population group were successfully managed medically (22); the remainder needed surgery. Others have estimated the risk of diverticulitis needing surgery to be 20% (23). In another review, it was believed that at least one-quarter of patients would need further hospitalization for recurrent inflammation (more than 70% of this group would continue to have symptoms). Ninety percent of these patients are readmitted within 5 years, and 50% are readmitted within 1 year (12). Larson et al (24) followed 132 patients who had been hospitalized with documented acute diverticulitis for an average of 9.2 years; 73% of the medically treated patients had no further symptoms or hospitalizations (compared with 79% of the surgical group). Nine percent of the medical group had later operations for diverticulitis. The authors also noted that 47–84% of patients in the literature remained asymptomatic after an attack of diverticulitis, and more contemporary reports report some recurrent symptoms after medical or surgical treatment (21). *It seems that the patient of reasonable risk who has recovered from an episode of uncomplicated acute diverticulitis need not undergo an operation to prevent a further complication and to improve the quality of life.*

The outcome of complicated diverticular disease, however, may be different. In one of the few prospective studies, Farmakis et al (25) followed 120 patients 5 years after hospital admission for complicated diverticular disease. Two of 77 patients who had been operated on (sigmoid resection) developed recurrent symptoms, compared with 37 of 43 patients managed conservatively. Many of the complications were the same as those of the index admission. Ten patients died of recurrent diverticular disease (nine had never been operated on) (25). These data argue for interval colectomy for patients who present with initially complicated diverticular disease. On the other hand, Sarin and Boulos also reported the prospective follow-up of 164 patients with complicated diverticular disease over a 4-year period. The recurrence rate of the 86 patients managed medically was 2% per patient year (5% per patient year for bleeding) of follow-up with a mortality of 1.3%; 52 patients having surgical treatment had no further admissions with recurrent disease (26).

In 1971, Painter and Burkitt also posed a hypothesis that diverticulosis is a deficiency disease caused by refining of carbohydrates (27,28). They believed that a low-residue diet is contraindicated in the treatment of diverticular disease and pointed out that African villagers (who ate a high-roughage diet) had no diverticular disease. In contrast, patients in Westernized countries have a fiber-deficient diet (8,29), smaller, firmer stools, and a higher pressure within the sigmoid colon with associated areas of segmentation.

Anatomic and Pathologic Studies (Figs. 1.1 through 1.3)

Diverticular disease was first described in the late eighteenth century by Ballie (30). Little further investigation was published before the mid-nineteenth century; some of the highlights of the early development of knowledge is summarized in Table 1.2. Terrill (31) proposed the use of the terms "diverticulosis" and "diverticulitis" and urged surgeons to submit cases for pathologic and clinical analysis (31) (Table 1.3). Telling and Gruner (32) wrote a detailed review of the pathologic manifestations of diverticular disease: their classification of mechanical and inflammatory changes is of continuing relevance (Table 1.4). Hughes also analyzed the clinicopathologic types of diverticulitis and their appropriate treatment, pointing out the confusion that exists in the medical literature when these nuances are ignored (33). Other studies gave some insight into the relationship of

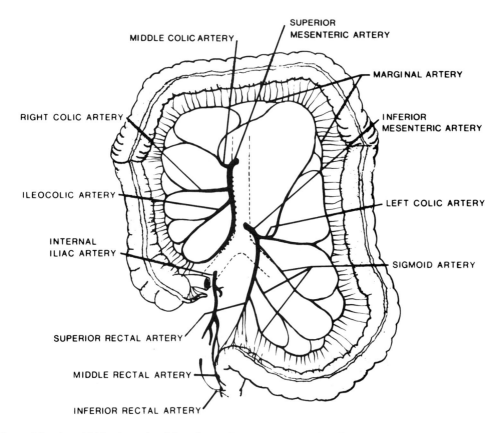

Figure 1.1. Arterial blood supply of the colon and rectum. (Reprinted with permission from Russell JC, Welch JP. Pathophysiology of bowel obstruction. In: Welch JP, ed. Bowel obstruction. Differential diagnosis and clinical management. Philadelphia: WB Saunders, 1990:28–58) [Ref. 148].

diverticulosis to lower gastrointestinal bleeding. The vasculature of the bowel wall containing diverticula was well defined following a series of injections of autopsy and surgical specimens with latex and with barium (30).

Berman et al countered the surgical tendency of increased use of one-stage elective resection for diverticular disease and stressed that a dysfunctional intestine was best managed medically (34). They classified diverticulitis into five pathologic types: acute edematous peridiverticulitis with local peritonitis (managed medically if possible), free perforation of a single diverticulum with generalized peritonitis, pericolic abscess, peridiverticulitis with fistula, and peridiverticulitis confused with carcinoma of the colon or ovary.

Much interest has been expressed with muscular changes in the colon that contains diverticula (35). Pathologic studies early in this century pointed out the characteristic thickening of the colonic wall involving the taeniae and smooth muscle (32). The thickening is not related to cellular hypertrophy or muscle cell hyperplasia (35). In a study of colons involved by uncomplicated diverticular disease and of controls, light and electron microscopic views showed a significant increase in the elastin content of the taeniae coli over controls (36). *It was believed that this elastosis might cause shortening of the taeniae, which in turn could cause corrugation of the circular muscle (which in itself had normal elastin content).*

The mechanism of formation of diverticula has been another area of interest. In anatomic studies, it was shown that elevated colonic pressures could cause mucosal herniation at points at which blood vessels penetrated the bowel wall (30). Usually, diverticula occur between the single mesenteric taenia and one of the antimesenteric taeniae (Fig. 1.4); blood vessels usually penetrate the colonic wall along the mesenteric border of the antimesenteric taeniae. Manometric studies led to the theory of segmentation, where the high pressures are generated in short segments of the colon (37) (see Chapter 2). The colonic wall in diverticular disease is also noncompliant, related to the thickened muscle and deranged collagen fibers (38). Studies of myoelectric activity and intraluminal pressures are conflicting and complex; the reader is referred elsewhere for further information (10).

Diagnostic Modalities

Early diagnostic studies were limited to radiographs, including plain films and contrast enemas — at first with bismuth. In 1914, Abbe discussed the use of bismuth to demonstrate diverticula. Later, studies with barium and gastrografin gained importance, as in the report of Spriggs and Marxer (39) in 1927, when the concept of the "prediverticular state" (a ragged radiologic appearance of the bowel wall believed to precede the development of

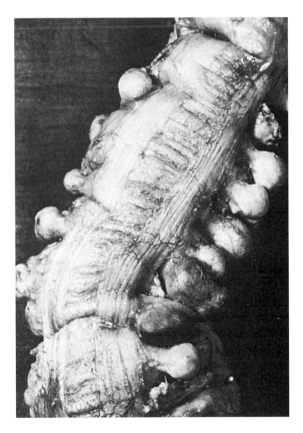

Figure 1.2.   A segment of sigmoid colon containing multiple diverticula. The taeniae are well seen. (Reprinted with permission from Goligher J. Surgery of the anus, rectum and colon. 5th ed. London: Bailliere Tindall, 1984:1087) [Ref. 149].

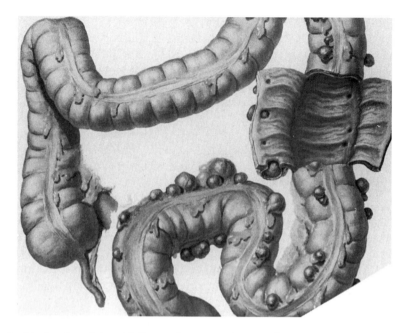

Figure 1.3. In this drawing of sigmoid diverticulosis extending into the descending colon, the appearance of diverticula from within the bowel is depicted as well. (Reprinted with permission from Oppenheimer E, ed. The CIBA collection of medical illustrations. Part II: Lower digestive tract. West Caldwell, NJ: CIBA Pharmaceutical Co., 1962;2:130) [Ref. 150].

diverticula) was raised (40). Unfortunately, barium studies were somewhat limited by interpretive variation between radiologists, and the poor correlation between the radiologic and clinical findings: e.g., it was difficult at times to differentiate diverticulosis from diverticulitis with barium alone. Rigid proctosigmoidoscopy did not play a major role in complicated diverticular disease, but with the introduction of colonoscopy and improved visualization of the sigmoid colon in the 1970s, the ability to differentiate cancer from diverticular disease improved (see Chapter 4).

Our diagnostic abilities have greatly improved since the early part of this century (41). *One of the greatest advances in diagnosis of complicated diverticular disease was the introduction of the computed tomography (CT) scan.* This test is extremely useful soon after the hospital admission, especially when the diagnosis is unclear, when further information is needed about the pericolonic anatomy and stratification of disease, or when contrast studies are not indicated (see Chapter 8) (42–44). At times, a contrast enema (45) is complementary to a CT scan or it is valuable in itself. There also has been some interest in the use of ultrasound, since the report of Parulekar in 1985 (41,46,47), especially in light of the expense and limited availability of CT scans. Obesity and gas, however, interfere with the effectiveness of ultrasonography and the examination is subjective. Some authors believe that its role should be examined further, because it is effective, inexpensive, and can be performed by nonspecialists; in prospective trials (in the hands of experts), the sensitivity is 84–98%, specificity is 80–96%, and overall accuracy is 82–98% (46).

Medical Treatment

A number of antibiotics effective in the treatment of diverticulitis have been introduced in recent years. Anaerobes and facultative gram-negative enteric organisms are most frequently responsible for pericolonic inflammation (48), and antibiotics should be given

Table 1.2.   Early Anatomic and Pathologic Studies[a]

1793	Mathew Baillie's *Morbid Anatomy* describes "scirrhus" of the sigmoid
1849	Cruveilhier makes first detailed account and notes fistulas
1899	Graser shows relation of diverticula to blood vessels
1904	Beer (115) summarizes clinical and pathologic aspects
1907	Terrill (31) proposes terms "diverticulosis" and "diverticulitis"
1908	Telling (116) collects 105 cases, with discussion of clinicopathologic aspects
1910	Keith (117) attributes diverticula to high intracolic pressures
1916	Drummond (118) describes pericolonic vessels and diverticula
1917	Telling and Gruner (32) publish detailed pathophysiologic and clinical studies
1961	Griffiths describes arterial blood supply of colon
1962	Slack defines position of colonic circumferential blood vessels to diverticula in autopsy-surgical specimens

[a]Includes data from Slack WW. The anatomy, pathology, and some clinical features of diverticulitis of the colon. Br J Surg 1962;50:185–190.

Table 1.3.   Basic Terminology Pertinent to Diverticular Disease

True diverticulum	Contains all layers of bowel wall
False diverticulum	Absence of muscular layer
Diverticulosis	Noninflamed diverticula
Diverticulitis	Inflamed diverticula
Diverticular disease	Entire disease spectrum
Uncomplicated diverticulitis	Includes phlegmon, peridiverticulitis
Complicated diverticulitis	Includes abscess, fistula, obstruction, or free perforation
One-stage procedure	Resection and anastomosis without a stoma
Two-stage procedure	Includes stoma and resection
Three-stage procedure	Stoma usually at first stage

Table 1.4.   Early Classification of Pathologic Changes[a]

A. Mechanical
    1. Formation of fecal concretions in the diverticula
    2. Torsion of the diverticulum
    3. Lodgment of foreign bodies within diverticula
B. Inflammatory
    1. Diverticulitis: gangrenous, acute, subacute, chronic, latent
    2. Passage of organisms without perforation
    3. Peridiverticulitis: chronic inflammation with tendency to stenosis
    4. Diverticular perforation leading to:
        Local abscess;
        Fistula, especially into the bladder;
        Suppuration in a hernial sac
    5. Adhesion formation, especially to small bowel, bladder, female reproductive tract
    6. Chronic peritonitis, local
    7. Chronic sigmoid mesenteritis
    8. Metastatic suppuration
    9. Development of carcinoma

[a]After Telling WH, Gruner OC. Acquired diverticula, diverticulitis, and peridiverticulitis of the large intestine. Br J Surg 1917;4:468–560.

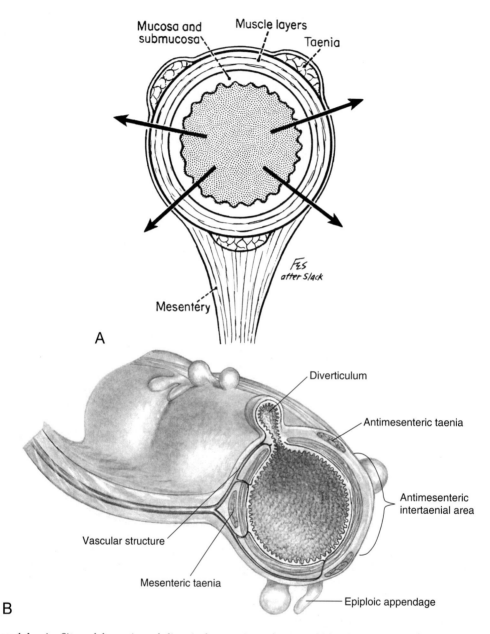

Figure 1.4. **A.,** Sites of formation of diverticula at points of entry of blood vessels into the colonic wall. (Reprinted with permission from Hackford AW, Veidenheimer MC: Diverticular disease of the colon. Current concepts and management. Surg Clin North Am 1985;65:347–363.) **B.,** Anatomy of the colon that contains diverticula.

for at least 10 days. In the presence of complicated problems such as abscesses or peritonitis, antibiotics should be continued for up to 4–6 weeks, and elective surgery can be performed when inflammation is controlled (48). Bowel rest and occasionally nasogastric suction are important until peristalsis and the overall patient condition improve. Initially, the diet is liquid and then low in residue as the edema involving the colon subsides.

Over the long term, a diet high in fiber and bran effectively decreases dyspeptic and colonic symptoms in patients with diverticulosis (28,49–51). This diet should be taken by the patient soon after recovering from an episode of acute diverticulitis. However, there may be other variables involved in the development of diverticular disease, such as the type of meat in the diet (52). Ornstein et al believe that dietary fiber may do little more than relieve constipation (53), although their study has been criticized in that there was too little difference in the daily fiber intake between the bran and the placebo periods (52).

Diverticular Bleeding

The current management of lower gastrointestinal bleeding as a consequence of diverticulosis is covered extensively in Chapter 6. Publications dealing with this complication were limited during the first part of the century. In 1953, Cate (54) reported the need for a subtotal colectomy in a case of massive diverticular bleeding. Using injection techniques, in 1955, Noer (55) emphasized the close relationship of diverticula to vessels in the colonic wall, and he showed the vessel in the wall of the diverticulum that was responsible for bleeding. He pointed out that macroscopic rectal bleeding was found in 11% of more than 2800 cases of diverticulosis.

Scarborough (56) emphasized the importance of ruling out a colorectal neoplasm in patients with diverticular disease who have rectal bleeding. Evidence grew that diverticulosis was the most common cause of severe rectal bleeding (57). Laparotomy was particularly important at the time and frequently was "blind" as far as the site of bleeding was concerned. Methods of localizing the bleeding site were numerous and crude, before the widespread use of techniques such as bleeding scans, selective angiography, and colonoscopy in the 1970s (58–63). Today, blind colectomy should be considered rarely, considering the diagnostic techniques at our disposal (64).

Surgical Treatment (Tables 1.5 through 1.10)

The surgical treatment of diverticular disease was initiated during the first decade of the twentieth century and was limited to patients who had severe complications. In a comprehensive early study, Mayo recommended drainage of abscesses and the treatment of obstruction by "artificial anus" (colostomy), with later resection of the obstructed segment. He also discussed the terms "diverticulitis" and "peridiverticulitis" (65).

During the next three decades, various surgical strategies were attempted, including permanent proximal colostomy without resection of the diseased segment; proximal colostomy and drainage followed by colostomy closure without resection (also invariably followed by recurrent diverticulitis); and increasingly, preliminary proximal colostomy followed by resection of the quiescent diseased segment and anastomosis and a subsequent

---

Table 1.5.   Important Developments in Surgery for Diverticular Disease

---

Improved anesthesia
Intensive care units
Antibiotics
Blood transfusions
Gastrointestinal tract decompression
Surgical staplers

Table 1.6.   Surgical Trends in Diverticular Disease

Abandonment of three-stage procedures
More aggressive use of resection
Longer lengths of resection
More accurate bleeding localization and resection
Use of on-table lavage
Use of CT scans for diagnosis
Percutaneous drainage of abscesses

Table 1.7.   Important Surgical Historical Trends

1940s	Three-stage procedures for complicated disease
1950s	One-stage resection/anastomosis for uncomplicated disease
1970s	Questioning of three-stage operations
	Aggressive primary resection of primary focus
	Popularity of Hartmann procedure
1980s	Use of percutaneous drainage for abscesses
	Selective anastomosis in presence of perforation
1990s	On-table lavage for obstruction, some cases of perforation
	Limited use of laparoscopic resection for elective resection

third operation for closure of the colostomy (three-stage procedure) (Fig. 1.5). Surgeons (66) demonstrated the relative safety of this planned approach, and mortality rates decreased from 17 to 6%.

With the widespread use of antibiotics, elective resection of uncomplicated diverticular disease increased in popularity by the 1950s (67–70). Mortality rates were low. The management of complicated diverticulitis was more complex and controversial (Fig. 1.6). *Evidence accumulated that the three-stage approach was associated in many instances with a significant cumulative morbidity and mortality, as well as a long period of hospitalization (71–73).* A significant number never had second- or third-stage operations, in part due to high mortality rates following colostomy and drainage (73,74). It became apparent that active sigmoid diverticulitis would persist in 8% of cases, even after the creation of a proximal defunctioning colostomy. *Persistent sepsis was a particular problem following transverse colostomy and drainage, because the column of stool in the left colon tended to leak at the site of sigmoid perforation (74).*

Interest gradually increased in early resection of diverticulitis to shorten the period of hospitalization (75). This tendency increased with time, especially in the acute setting (76).

As more data accumulated, *attempts were made to stratify patients according to certain criteria that defined patients at high risk of developing severe complications within a short period of time* (Table 1.9). This type of data was useful, especially in convincing patients and their referring physicians of the need for a major operation, and these criteria remain useful in evaluating patients for severity of disease.

Some surgeons attempted to extend the indications for one-stage resections in the presence of septic conditions (77–80) (Figs. 1.7 and 1.8). However, this approach was controversial, and not without risk (81,82), and was questioned by many others (83). *The*

Table 1.8.   Diverticular Disease: Representative Surgical Series

Year	Authors	Number of Patients	Mortality (%)
1930	Rankin/Brown (119)	48	
1940	Hayden (120)	49	33
1942	Smithwick (66)	75	
1944	Young/Young (121)	28	14
1947	Pemberton et al (122)	389	
1950	Mayo/Blunt (123)	202	3.5
1950	Fallis/Marshall (124)	33	6.1
1950	Boyden (125)	38	0
1953	Welch et al (67)	139	5.7
1955	Judd/Mears (126)	68	1.5
1957	Waugh/Walt (127)	320	3.1
1958	Colcock (68)	131	1.5
1960	Smithwick (128)	30	0
1960	Boyden/Neilson (129)	46	9
1964	Ponka/Shaalan (71)		
1942–1951	a)	32	7
1952–1961	b)	86	1
1965	Rodkey/Welch (130)	200	5.5
1969	Rodkey/Welch (131)	50	6
1969	Mitty et al (132)	377	3
1970	Ponka (72)	50	8
1971	Botsford et al (133)	252	8
1971	Byrne/Garick (134)	43	35
1972	MacGregor et al (135)	70	27
1974	Rodkey/Welch (75)	338	4
1975	Tolins (136)	71	22
1976	Classen et al (137)	208	11
1977	Eng et al (76)	46	0
1979	Nunes et al (91)	25	8
1982	Letwin (138)	46	4.4
1983	Alexander et al (112)	93	6.4
1983	Eisenstat et al (139)	182	3
1985	Hackford and Veidenheimer (1)	141	9
1986	Lambert et al (140)	105	30
1987	Gregg (141)	175	4
1988	Schein/Decker (89)	12	17
1990	Moreaux/Vons (142)	177	0
1991	Tyau et al (143)	23[a]	39
		55[b]	2
1991	Sarin/Boulos (26)	52	12
1994	Ambrosetti et al (144)	66	3
1995	Isbister/Prasad (90)	27	7
1996	Belmonte et al (145)	227	1
1996	Chua (146)	17	12
1997	Wedell et al (108)	224	6

See Table 16.2, Chapter 16 for a list of series dealing primarily with perforated diverticulitis with extensive peritonitis.
[a]Immunocompromised patients
[b]Nonimmunocompromised patients

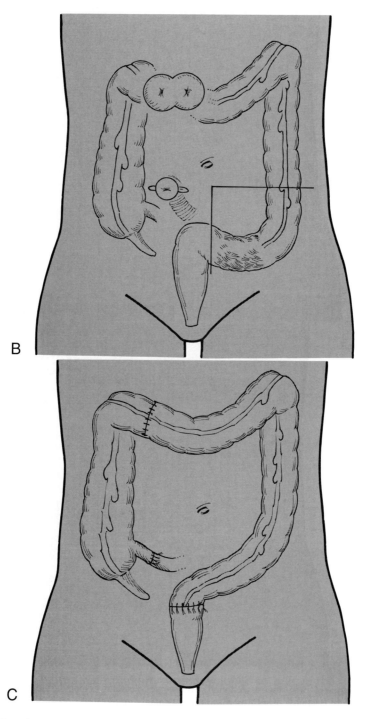

Figure 1.5.—*continued*

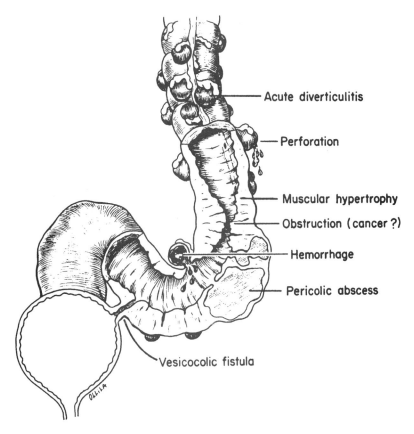

Figure 1.6. Complications of diverticular disease. (Reprinted with permission from Zollinger RW, Zollinger RM. Diverticular disease of the colon. Adv Surg 1971;5:255–280) [Ref. 151].

The intracolonic bypass has been proposed as an operation to protect against anastomotic leakage (102). It has some appeal when there is some concern about anastomotic integrity in the postoperative period, such as in the presence of an intraabdominal abscess or in an immunocompromised patient. This procedure also has not gained widespread popularity, perhaps because most surgeons would avoid performing an anastomosis if they feared it might leak.

Finally, laparoscopic colectomy has emerged, although this technique has been limited primarily to colorectal cancer at this time. There is evidence that laparoscopic procedures shorten hospitalization and lessen postoperative pain (Fig. 1.12); there are limited reports of its use for elective resection of diverticular disease (103,104). The technique seems to be particularly useful for closure of the colostomy following the Hartmann procedure, although pelvic adhesions involving the small bowel may interfere technically.

A number of considerations are necessary before the surgeon embarks on elective surgery today (for conditions such as recurrent diverticulitis, recovery following percutaneous abscess drainage, colonic stricture, colovesical fistula, or small mesenteric abscess, but not for uncomplicated diverticulosis) such as patient age, medical risk, and severity of the episode of diverticulitis (Table 1.11). Risk factors that are associated with the need for operation are summarized in Table 1.12 (105). Ideally, the acute inflammation is allowed to subside before the operation is performed; this usually occurs within 6–8

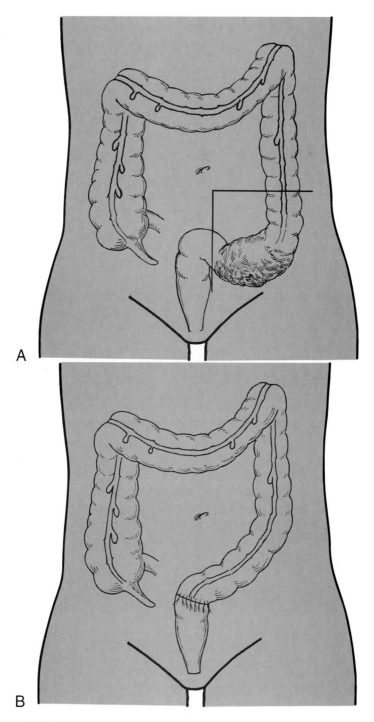

Figure 1.7.   Technique of one-stage resection and anastomosis.

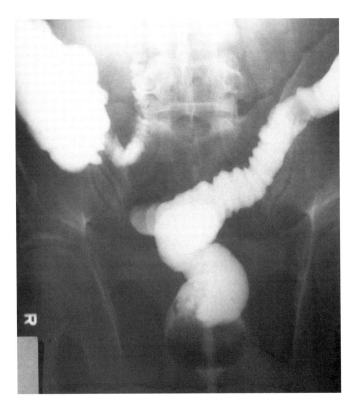

Figure 1.8. Radiologic appearance (barium enema) of a hand-sewn Baker anastomosis (side-to-end) of the sigmoid colon to the proximal rectum. This is a useful type of anastomosis if the surgeon elects to perform the procedure with standard suture technique.

Table 1.11.   Indications for Surgery with Diverticulitis[a]

Absolute
   Disease complication
      sepsis
      fistula
      obstruction
   Recurrent disease
   Failure to improve with medical therapy
   Clinical deterioration
   Failure to exclude carcinoma
Modifying Factors
   Chronic stricture
   Young age
   Immunocompromise
   Right-sided diverticulitis

[a]After Freeman SR, McNally PR. Diverticulitis. Med Clin North Am 1993;77:1149–1167.

weeks (106). An appropriate medical and antibiotic bowel prep is performed. Rectal and vaginal examinations or CT scans are useful in assessing the response to therapy. At the time of anastomosis, the splenic flexure must be mobilized approximately 10% of the time (106) (Fig. 1.13). The mortality should be low, although morbidity may be significant (107).

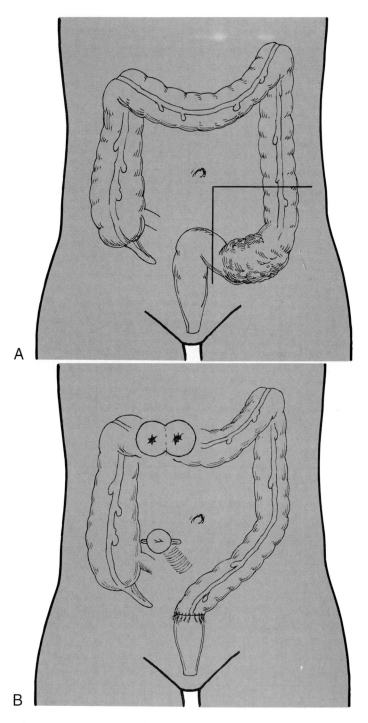

Figure 1.9. **A.,** In the two-stage operation, the Hartmann procedure usually is performed initially. This illustration shows the segment of sigmoid colon that is resected. **B.,** Alternatively, sigmoid resection and anastomosis is performed and protected with a diverting stoma. **C.,** In the second stage, the stoma is taken down and intestinal continuity is reestablished.

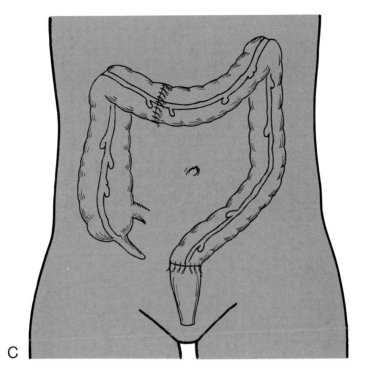

Figure 1.9.—*continued*

Table 1.12.   Risk Factors for Severe Complications of Diverticulitis[a]

Recurrent attacks of local inflammation
Persistent tender left lower quadrant mass
Dysuria associated with sigmoid diverticulosis
Diarrhea, constipation, or bloating associated with lower abdominal pain/diverticulosis
Rapid progression of symptoms from onset
Age younger than 50 years, especially males
Immunocompromised patients
Marked deformity or obstruction of sigmoid by contrast study
Clinical signs/radiographs equivocal in excluding carcinoma

[a]See Welch CE. Controversial problems association with diverticulitis. Proc R Soc Med 1970;63:57–61.

Today, the surgeon approaches the complex patient (with peritonitis or failure to respond to medical therapy) more aggressively than in the past (5), with primary resection of longer segments of colon either as part of a one- or two-stage procedure (Fig. 1.14). The three-stage procedure is virtually nonexistent (108) (Table 1.13). The Hartmann procedure is the most common approach for perforated diverticulitis, although alternatives such as primary anastomosis with transverse colostomy have been proposed because of the difficulty of later anastomosis of the colon to the rectal segment (109). In some cases, patients will be immunosuppressed or elderly; in others cases, a complex perforation may

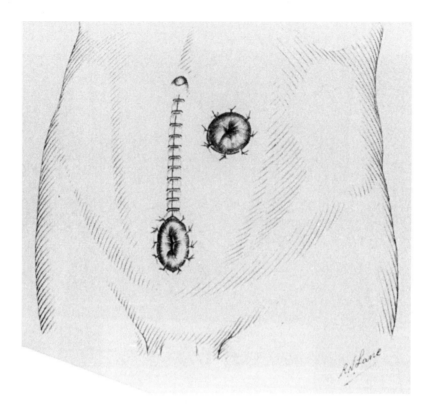

Figure 1.10.   Appearance of an end colostomy and mucous fistula; the latter can be brought through the inferior portion of the wound. (Reprinted with permission from Todd IP, Fielding LP, eds. Rob and Smith's operative surgery. Alimentary tract and abdominal wall. Part 3: Colon, rectum and anus. 4th ed. London: Butterworths, 1983) [Ref. 152].

Table 1.13.   Operations for Diverticular Disease

One-stage
  Resection and primary anastomosis
Two-stage
  Hartmann procedure
  Sigmoid resection, end colostomy, mucous fistula
  Resection and anastomosis, proximal colostomy
Three-stage
  Preliminary colostomy and drainage
  Later resection and anastomosis, colostomy closure

necessitate repeat laparotomies and wound care may become complex (110). If possible, these patients should be prepared for elective rather than urgent operation by appropriate control of sepsis and bowel preparation (111).

CURRENT APPROACHES

This section will provide a brief overview of our approaches to diverticular disease, which has been termed a "multifaceted disease process with no singular solution" (112).

The reader is directed to a statement on practice parameters prepared by the Standards Task Force of the American Society of Colon and Rectal Surgeons for a concise summary (113). A list of some of the important basic definitions used in this monograph are summarized in Table 1.3. Detailed discussions of the complex aspects of diverticular disease make up the bulk of this book and are not covered here.

Diverticular disease should be considered in any patient presenting with abdominal pain, distention suggestive of colonic obstruction, or lower gastrointestinal bleeding. The surgeon confronts diverticulitis most commonly and the myriad complications of this process must be handled in different ways. Typically, the patient with sigmoid diverticulitis has left lower quadrant pain and tenderness of varying degrees, fever, and irregular bowel habits. Urinary symptoms may occur, as well as symptoms of small bowel obstruction such as vomiting and periumbilical cramps.

Initial laboratory evaluation should include a complete blood count, sedimentation rate, urinalysis, and abdominal flat and upright films. Additional diagnostic tests are indicated if the diagnosis is unclear, because disorders such as inflammatory bowel disease, colon cancer, intestinal obstruction, ischemic colitis, or urinary disorders can be confused. We would consider a water-soluble contrast enema if obstruction was present and at times to

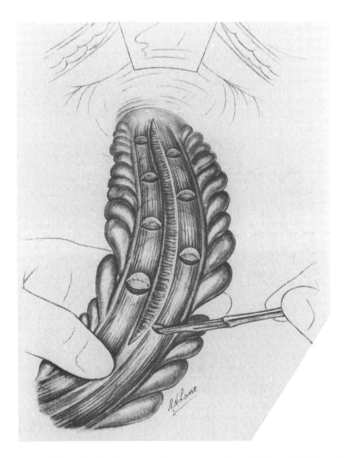

Figure 1.11. Transverse and longitudinal myotomies are operations of historical interest that are no longer done. (Reprinted with permission from Todd IP, Fielding LP, eds., Rob and Smith's operative surgery. Alimentary tract and abdominal wall. Part 3: Colon, rectum and anus. 4th ed. London: Butterworths, 1983) [Ref. 152].

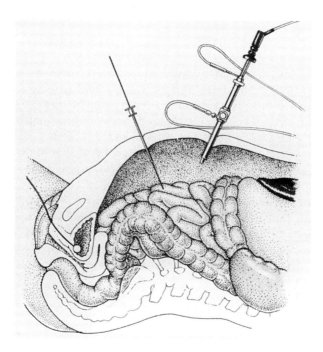

Figure 1.12.   Diverticulitis may be discovered at the time of laparoscopy performed to evaluate abdominal pain. (Reprinted with permission from Todd IP, Fielding LP, eds. Rob and Smith's operative surgery. Alimentary tract and abdominal wall. Part 3: Colon, rectum and anus. 4th ed. London: Butterworths, 1983) [Ref. 152].

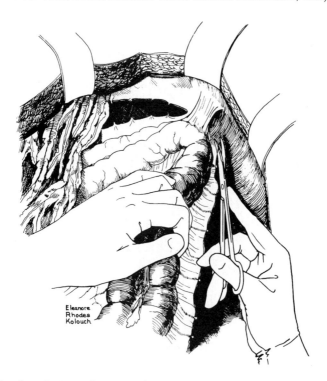

Figure 1.13.   Dividing the colonic attachments at the splenic flexure. (Reprinted with permission from Welch JP. Carcinoma of the colon. In: Welch JP, ed. Bowel obstruction. Differential diagnosis and clinical management. Philadelphia: WB Saunders, 1990:546–574) [Ref. 153].

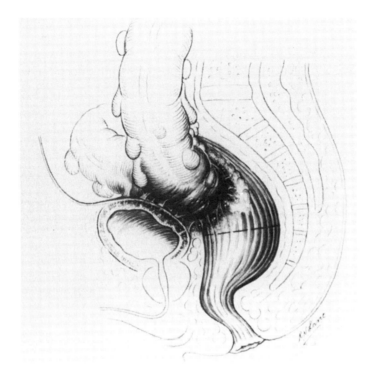

Figure 1.14. Dissection in a patient with a diverticular abscess involving the pelvis. (Reprinted with permission from Todd IP, Fielding LP, eds. Rob and Smith's operative surgery. Alimentary tract and abdominal wall. Part 3: Colon, rectum and anus. 4th ed. London: Butterworths, 1983) [Ref. 152].

confirm suspicion of free perforation that would necessitate urgent surgery. Our test of choice, however, usually is a CT scan, because this provides considerable information about the colon as well as extracolonic tissues, of special interest when complications of diverticulitis are considered. We have had little use for ultrasound, except as an adjunct to abscess drainage. Barium enema is avoided if there is any suspicion of diverticulitis because of the potential dangers of extravasated barium. Early endoscopy also risks perforation at a site of microperforation.

Uncomplicated diverticulitis is treated either on an outpatient or an inpatient basis. In the more complex case, the bowel is put at complete rest and wide-spectrum antibiotics that are effective against aerobes and anaerobes of the colon (such as a second-generation cephalosporin-metronidazole combination) are delivered intravenously. As the patient improves (most patients with uncomplicated diverticulitis do), clear liquids are given initially and the diet is advanced, sometimes following discharge from the hospital. Eventual resection may be indicated if the attack was recurrent or occurred in a young or immunocompromised patient (114). In the instance of a worsening physical examination or complaints of abdominal pain, additional diagnostic imaging is indicated. This could result in percutaneous drainage of an abscess, resection of a persistent phlegmon or fistula associated with diverticulitis, or a Hartmann procedure or possible on-table lavage with anastomosis for obstruction.

In each case of uncomplicated diverticulitis, outpatient treatment can be considered if the patient is reliable and in good health (as opposed to an immunosuppressed or frail patient). A liquid diet is given along with oral antibiotics. The individual should be warned of signs of worsening disease, such as increasing abdominal pain or fever and chills, and hospitalization should then be arranged.

Hemorrhage due to diverticular disease is managed within a hospital setting; the details of treatment appear in Chapter 6.

EDITORIAL COMMENTS

This chapter highlights major changes in the surgical approach to diverticular disease that have been made in the twentieth century. One- and two-stage procedures have emerged as the operations of choice, and in many instances, they have shortened periods of hospitalization in the managed-care era.

The great variety of clinical presentations and pathologic sequelae of diverticular disease are emphasized. Many studies in the literature fail to define these particular factors precisely in the patient populations, and comparing different series in the literature in a meaningful way is difficult. The exact pathogenesis of the disorder is still unknown, although the likely role of low-residue diets is suggested by epidemiologic studies of different populations and by changes in disease incidence with migration into Westernized countries.

Development of sophisticated diagnostic techniques, intensive care units, antibiotic regimens, and modern day anesthesia has led to an overall improved survival. However, successful management of complex cases will, without question, continue to challenge surgeons well into the twenty-first century.

REFERENCES

1. Hackford AW, Veidenheimer MC. Diverticular disease of the colon. Current concepts and management. Surg Clin North Am 1985;65:347–363. *This reference has some interesting historical notes, along with current concepts, and includes 64 references.*
2. Kyle J, Davidson AI. The changing pattern of hospital admissions for diverticular disease of the colon. Br J Surg 1975;62:537–541. *When hospital admissions for symptomatic diverticular disease were studied in Scotland, there was a significant increase of admissions from the early 1960s to the early 1970s.*
3. Weiner HL, Rezai AR, Cooper PR. Sigmoid diverticular perforation in neurosurgical patients receiving high-dose corticosteroids. Neurosurgery 1993;33:40–43. *Five patients with primary and metastatic central nervous system tumors developed freely perforated diverticulitis; four patients survived surgery. If possible, the dose of steroids should be decreased in patients with known diverticular disease.*
4. Mullykaugas-Luosujarvi R. Diverticulosis—a primary cause of life-threatening complications in rheumatoid arthritis. Clin Exp Rheumatol 1995;13:79–82. *The death rate from diverticular disease was five times as high in a rheumatoid arthritis population as in the Finnish population as a whole. NSAIDS may have played a major role.*
5. Rodkey GV, Welch CE. Changing patterns in the surgical treatment of diverticular disease. Ann Surg 1984;200:466–478. *This publication discusses the major trends seen in a group of 350 surgical patients from 1974 to 1983; other developments in surgery of the disease beginning in 1911 at the Massachusetts General Hospital are also discussed.*
6. Wyatt SH, Fishman EK. The acute abdomen in individuals with AIDS. Radiol Clin North Am 1994;32:1023–1042. *Severe abdominal pain may be seen in this population, even in the absence of true surgical complications such as perforation or abscess formation. CT is a valuable test, allowing assessment of the bowel, lymph nodes, and abdominal viscera.*
7. Whitney AM, Brunel W, Russell TR, et al. Emergent abdominal surgery in AIDS: experience in San Francisco. Am J Surg 1994;168:239–243. *A review of 57 AIDS patients who had 63 emergent laparotomies. Causes of colon bleeding, perforation, or obstruction included lymphoma, iatrogenic, toxic megacolon, and unknown, but diverticulitis is not mentioned.*
8. Almy TP, Howell DA. Diverticular disease of the colon. N Engl J Med 1980;302:324–331. *An excellent review of epidemiology, natural history, and pathogenesis, with 119 references.*
9. Brodribb AJ. Treatment of symptomatic diverticular disease with a high fiber diet. Lancet 1977;1:664–666. *The author compared the incidence of other conditions in 40 patients with diverticular disease and in 80 controls.*
10. Keighley MR, Williams NS. Surgery of the anus, rectum and colon. London: WB Saunders, 1993:1128–1211.
11. Eide TJ, Stalsberg H. Diverticular disease of the large intestine in Northern Norway. Gut 1979;20:609–615. *The authors showed no increase in the incidence of colorectal cancer or polyps in patients with diverticular disease.*

12. Parks TG. Natural history of diverticular disease of the colon. Clin Gastroenterol 1975;4:53–69. *The natural history is discussed in relation to many factors such as age, sex, number of diverticula, diet, irritable bowel syndrome, and cancer.*

13. Badi-Perez JM, Valverde-Sintas J, Franch-Arcas G, et al. Acute postoperative diverticulitis. Int J Colorectal Dis 1989;4:141–143. *Four cases of postoperative diverticulitis are reported after cardiac and noncardiac procedures. Possible etiologies included advanced age, morphine and steroid use, postoperative constipation, and mucosal ischemia.*

14. Boles RS, Jordan SM. The clinical significance of diverticulosis. Gastroenterology 1958;35:579–582. *Patients with uncomplicated diverticulosis followed for an average of 15 years developed hemorrhage, obstruction, or perforation due to diverticular disease in 15%. The association of diverticulosis with hiatus hernia and gallstones (Saint's triad) may be as high as 6%.*

15. Horner JL. Natural history of diverticulosis of the colon. Am J Dig Dis 1958;3:343–350. *A long-term office follow-up of 503 patients with diverticulosis. Only 0.4% were operated on. The author recommends surgery only for certain complications following consultation between the physician and surgeon.*

16. Kubo A, Kagaya T, Nakagawa H. Studies on complications of diverticular disease of the colon. Jpn J Med 1985;24:39–43. *During barium enema examinations, 1124 patients were found to have diverticular disease. Over 15 years, patients were followed for clinical symptoms and with possible barium enema or colonoscopic exams: 2.4% developed signs of diverticulitis.*

17. Wilson RG, Smith AN, Macintyre IM. Complications of diverticular disease and non-steroidal anti-inflammatory drugs: a prospective study. Br J Surg 1990;77:1103–1104. *Ninety-two patients were followed prospectively over 3 years: the incidence of NSAID intake was higher than controls (P < .001) and the risk of perforation or peritonitis was higher than in controls (P < .001).*

18. Parks TG. Prognosis in diverticular disease of the colon. Proc R Soc Med 1970;63:1262–1263. *This short paper includes discussions of duration of symptoms, acute exacerbations, and follow-up data.*

19. Krukowski ZH, Matheson NA. Emergency surgery for diverticular disease complicated by generalized and fecal peritonitis: a review. Br J Surg 1984;71:921–927. *In this extensive review, the authors note only one prospective study in the literature and the inaccurate categorization of patient groups.*

20. Hughes LE. Diverticular disease of colon (letter). BMJ 1970;1:496. *This letter complains that much of the data dealing with the natural history of diverticular disease is spurious: bowel symptoms are attributed to known diverticula when this may not be the case; barium contrast studies are assumed an accurate way of assessing the extent of disease and its complications when they are not; and surgery is indicated prophylactically for uncomplicated disease, when experience shows little difference in the outcome of surgically and medically treated groups.*

21. Munson KD, Hensien MA, Jacob LN, et al. Diverticulitis. A comprehensive follow-up. Dis Colon Rectum 1996;39:318–322. *Of 65 patients with diverticulitis reviewed retrospectively, 62% of the medical group (32 patients) and 27% of the surgical group (33 patients) had continuing symptoms.*

22. Parks TG, Connell AM. The outcome in 455 patients admitted for treatment of diverticular disease of the colon. Br J Surg 1970;57:775–778. *Forty-three percent of the medically treated patients had persistent symptoms.*

23. Chappuis CW, Cohn I Jr. Acute colonic diverticulitis. Surg Clin North Am 1988;68:301–313. *A general review with 78 references. Primary resection of the colon is advocated in all operative cases.*

24. Larson DM, Masters SS, Spiro HM. Medical and surgical therapy in diverticular disease. A comparative study. Gastroenterology 1976;71:734–737. *Ninety-nine patients were followed medically and 33 patients were treated surgically for an average of 9.2 years. Once recovered, 73% of the medical group and 79% of the surgical group had no further symptoms or hospital admissions due to diverticular disease.*

25. Farmakis N, Tudor RG, Keighley MR. The 5-year natural history of complicated diverticular disease. Br J Surg 1994;81:733–735. *One hundred twenty patients were followed prospectively 5 years following admission for complicated diverticular disease; 2 of 77 patients who had initial sigmoid resection developed complications of diverticular disease, compared with 37 of 43 patients managed conservatively.*

26. Sarin S, Boulos PB. Long-term outcome of patients presenting with acute complications of diverticular disease. Ann R Coll Surg Engl 1994;76:117–120. *One hundred sixty-four patients with complicated diverticular disease (excluding fistulas) were followed prospectively for a median of 4 years. The low risk of readmission (2% per patient year for diverticulitis, 5% for lower GI bleeding) did not justify elective operation in these patients.*

27. Painter NS, Burkitt DP. Diverticular disease of the colon: a deficiency disease of western civilization. BMJ 1971;2:450–454. *One hundred thirty-two hospitalized patients with documented diverticulitis were followed for an average of 9.2 years. Similar percentages (73% of medical group, 79% of surgical group) of patients remained free of further symptoms of diverticulitis during the follow-up period. The authors recommend medical treatment of patients with diverticulitis, except surgical management for those who develop complications.*

28. Painter NS. Diverticular disease of the colon. S Afr Med J 1982;61:1016–1020. *Of 70 patients receiving a bran diet for symptomatic diverticular disease, 87% had relief or elimination of symptoms.*

29. Mendelhoff AI. Thoughts on the epidemiology of diverticular disease. Clin Gastroenterol 1986;15:855–877. *The best epidemiologic evidence available associates total dietary fiber intake with the development of diverticular disease. A detailed review.*

30. Slack WW. The anatomy, pathology, and some clinical features of diverticulitis of the colon. Br J Surg 1962;50:185–190. *The author reviews the literature and examines a group of surgical and autopsy specimens following latex and barium injections.*

31. Terrill JJ. Diverticulosis and diverticulitis. Tex Med 1909;4:72–75. *This short publication by a pathologist contains a rudimentary classification of types of diverticular disease.*

32. Telling WH, Gruner OC. Acquired diverticula, diverticulitis, and peridiverticulitis of the large intestine. Br J Surg 1917;4:468–560. *A comprehensive summary of the pathologic, anatomic, and clinical aspects of diverticular disease with more than 200 references. Includes detailed pathologic findings in 90 individual clinical cases (many from the literature) and an algorithm relating pathologic changes and clinical symptoms.*

33. Hughes LE. Complications of diverticular disease: inflammation, obstruction and bleeding. Clin Gastro-enterol 1975;4:147–170. *A discussion of the pathologic variants of diverticular disease and their management.*
34. Berman LG, Burdick D, Heitzman ER, et al. A critical reappraisal of sigmoid peridiverticulitis. Surg Gynecol Obstet 1968;127:481–491. *The authors examine the pathology of diverticulitis and classify manifestations into five types. They feel that surgical treatment should be based on pathologic findings and that restraint should be used in managing the colon remote from the site of perforation surgically, especially in a prophylactic fashion.*
35. Morson BC. Pathology of diverticular disease of the colon. Clin Gastroenterol 1975;4:37–52. *This pathologist feels that increased tone of the taeniae causes shortening of the bowel and consequent muscle thickening.*
36. Whiteway J, Morson BC. Elastosis in diverticular disease of the sigmoid colon. Gut 1985;26:258–266. *A light and electron microscopic study of 25 specimens of uncomplicated diverticular disease and of 25 controls. An increase of elastin content of the taeniae coli of greater than 200% over controls was noted.*
37. Painter NS. The cause of diverticular disease of the colon, its symptoms and its complications. J R Coll Surg Edinb 1985;30:118–122. *A discussion of the development of diverticula and the role of segmentation.*
38. Thomson HJ, Busuttil A, Eastwood MA, et al. Submucosal collagen changes in the normal colon and in diverticular disease. Int J Colorectal Dis 1987;2:208–213. *Patients with diverticular disease had tightly packed collagen fibrils in the left colon.*
39. Spriggs EI, Marxer OA. Multiple diverticula of the colon. Lancet 1927;1:1067–1074. *An interesting account of the observation of 208 cases of diverticular disease followed over a number of years. Contains numerous drawings of findings in contrast studies.*
40. Marcus R, Watt J. The "pre-diverticular state." Its relationship to diverticula in the anti-mesenteric intertaenia area of the pelvic colon. Br J Surg 1964;51:676–682. *The authors review the literature and feel that little knowledge has been gained about the "pre-diverticular state" since it was described in 1925.*
41. McKee RF, Deignan RW, Krukowski ZH. Radiological studies in acute diverticulitis. Br J Surg 1994;81:560–565. *A useful illustrated review of the diagnostic modalities available today.*
42. Hulnick DH, Megibow AJ, Balthazar EJ, et al. Computed tomography in the evaluation of diverticulitis. Radiology 1984;152:491–495. *The authors recommend CT for the early study of suspected diverticulitis.*
43. Cho KC, Morehouse HT, Alterman DD, et al. Sigmoid diverticulitis: diagnostic role of CT—comparison with barium enema studies. Radiology 1990;176:111–115. *CT scan is recommended as the early study in the acutely ill patient, especially if the diagnosis is unclear.*
44. Hachigian MP, Honickman S, Eisenstat TE, et al. Computed tomography in the initial management of acute left-sided diverticulitis. Dis Colon Rectum 1992;35:1123–1129. *Following this study of 59 patients (32% had complicated diverticulitis), the authors concluded that the test was valuable and that it disclosed information about extracolonic disease and anatomy helpful to the surgeon and allowed early percutaneous drainage of abscesses.*
45. Wexner SD, Dailey TH. Initial management of left lower quadrant peritonitis. Dis Colon Rectum 1986;29:635–638. *The early use of a water-soluble contrast enema was accurate and cost-effective.*
46. Zielke A, Hasse C, Nies C, et al. Prospective evaluation of ultrasonography in acute colonic diverticulitis. Br J Surg 1997;84:385–388. *Seventy-four patients with acute colonic diverticulitis (excluding those with generalized peritonitis) were studied with ultrasound. There was a false-negative result in 12 patients and a false-positive reading in five patients. The procedure is recommended in the hands of "sonographically trained surgeons."*
47. Yacoe ME, Jeffrey RB Jr. Sonography of appendicitis and diverticulitis. Radiol Clin North Am 1994;5:899–912. *This discussion includes some illustrations of CT scans and ultrasonography of the same entities, such as gas or pericolonic abscess. Ultrasound has been used less for diverticulitis than appendicitis and is considered an adjunct to CT scanning.*
48. Duma RJ, Kellum JM. Colonic diverticulitis: microbiologic, diagnostic, and therapeutic considerations. Curr Clin Top Infect Dis 1991;11:218–247. *A well-illustrated discussion, including a table of pertinent bacteria and various antimicrobial agents. Includes 33 references.*
49. Leahy AL, Ellis RM, Quill DS, et al. High fiber diet in symptomatic diverticular disease of the colon. Ann R Coll Surg Engl 1985;67:173–174. *Patients with fiber supplements developed fewer complications and required less surgery (P < .05).*
50. Taylor I, Duthie HL: Bran tablets and diverticular disease. BMJ 1976;1:988–990. *Bran tablets served to significantly increase daily stool weight and decrease intestinal transit time.*
51. Hyland TM, Taylor I. Does a high fiber diet prevent the complications of diverticular disease? Br J Surg 1980;67:77–79. *75% of a group of 100 patients admitted to the hospital with acute diverticular disease were treated with a high-fiber diet; after 5–7 years, over 90% remained symptom-free.*
52. Heaton KW. Is bran useful in diverticular disease. BMJ 1981;283:1523–1526. *An editorial that comments on the controversial trial of Ornstein et al.; further studies are recommended.*
53. Ornstein MH, Littlewood ER, Baird IM, et al. Are fiber supplements really necessary in diverticular disease of the colon? A controlled clinical trial. BMJ 1981;282:1353–1356. *A double-blind controlled trial of 58 patients. Fiber supplements decreased constipation, but had no benefit on the pain score, lower bowel symptom score, and total symptom score.*
54. Cate WR Jr. Colectomy in the treatment of massive melena secondary to diverticulosis. Ann Surg 1953;137:558–560. *This patient survived an urgent subtotal colectomy. The author found only one similar case (reported by Stone in 1944) where laparotomy was performed to control blood loss from diverticulosis.*
55. Noer RJ. Hemorrhage as a complication of diverticulitis. Ann Surg 1955;141:674–685. *This series included 20 patients with diverticular disease who had rectal bleeding. Three patients operated on as emergencies died. The distribution of blood vessels within the diverticula made severe hemorrhage likely in the event of erosion or ulceration. He referred to a report by Smith in 1951 in which bleeding from diverticula was seen through a sigmoidoscope.*
56. Scarborough RA. The significance of rectal bleeding in diverticulosis and diverticulitis of the colon. Dis

Colon Rectum 1958;1:49–52. *The author reports 89 patients with malignant or premalignant tumors of the colorectum who had lower gastrointestinal bleeding presumed to be due to known diverticular disease.*

57. Noer RL, Hamilton JE, Williams DJ, et al. Rectal hemorrhage: moderate and severe. Ann Surg 1962;155:794–805. *In this study of 245 patients with gross rectal bleeding, diverticulosis was responsible for 71% of all massive rectal hemorrhage. About one-fourth of the bleeding from diverticulosis was termed as severe.*

58. Rosenberg IK, Rosenberg BF. Massive hemorrhage from diverticula of the colon, with demonstration of the source of bleeding. Ann Surg 1964;159:570–573. *The authors point out the difficulty at that time of identifying the actual site of bleeding in the colon. A colectomy specimen showed microscopic evidence of a vessel covered by a clot that otherwise communicated freely with the bowel lumen.*

59. Maynard EP III, Vorhees AB Jr. Arterial hemorrhage from a large bowel diverticulum. Gastroenterology 1956;31:210–211. *A bleeding diverticulum was isolated by emptying the colorectum of blood with a rectal tube, and applying rubber-shod clamps at 10-cm intervals along the colon wall until an isolated segment in the transverse colon filled with blood.*

60. Steer ML, Silen W. Diagnostic procedures in gastrointestinal hemorrhage. N Engl J Med 1983;309:646–649. *A brief summary of available procedures.*

61. Gennaro AR, Rosemon GP. Colonic diverticula and hemorrhage. Dis Colon Rectum 1973;16:409–415. *Seventeen percent of 500 patients with diverticular disease had hemorrhage from the colon. Selective angiography was useful in localizing the bleeding site in some of the patients.*

62. Baum S, Rosch J, Potter CT, et al. Selective mesenteric arterial infusion in the management of massive diverticular hemorrhage. N Engl J Med 1973;288:1269–1272. *Seven of 15 patients ceased to bleed following selective arterial infusion.*

63. Drapanas T, Pennington DG, Kappelman M, et al. Emergency subtotal colectomy: preferred approach to management of massively bleeding diverticular disease. Ann Surg 1973;177:519–526. *The authors point out the futile, hazardous nature of operative maneuvers used to identify the bleeding point.*

64. McGuire HH Jr. Bleeding colonic diverticula. A reappraisal of natural history and management. Ann Surg 1994;220:653–656. *In this study of 78 patients admitted with lower gastrointestinal tract bleeding from no other detectable cause than diverticula, bleeding continued in 25% and in most patients requiring 4 or more units of blood per day.*

65. Mayo WJ. Acquired diverticulitis of the large intestine. Surg Gynecol Obstet 1907;5:8–15. *One of the earliest surgical series; only 19 patients were reviewed from the literature.*

66. Smithwick RH. Experiences with the surgical management of diverticulitis of the sigmoid. Ann Surg 1942;115:969–985. *Resection is recommended if possible for complex forms of diverticulitis; preliminary transverse colostomy is desirable if resection is contemplated.*

67. Welch CE, Allen AW, Donaldson GA. An appraisal of resection of the colon for diverticulitis of the sigmoid. Ann Surg 1953;138:332–343. *A report of 114 colon resections; discusses the role of elective resection of uncomplicated diverticulitis.*

68. Colcock BP. Surgical management of complicated diverticulitis. N Engl J Med 1958;259:570–573. *Inadequate surgery is one cause of major complications with diverticulitis. Resection and anastomosis is recommended to avoid recurrent attacks and complications of diverticulitis.*

69. Waugh JM. Surgical management of diverticulitis of the colon. Mayo Clin Proc 1961;36:489–491. *Seventy-one percent of patients having resection were treated or to be treated with 1-stage procedures.*

70. Moore RM, Kirksey OT Jr. One-stage resection in selected cases of sigmoid diverticulitis. Ann Surg 1954;139:826–832. *The authors found that primary resection and anastomosis could be used more widely in properly selected patients.*

71. Ponka JL, Shaalan K. Changing aspects in surgery of diverticulitis. Arch Surg 1964;89:31–42. *In the 1940s, three-stage procedures were used in more than one-half of the patients; in the next decade, one-stage procedures were used in nearly one-half of the patients. The duration of hospitalization for one-stage, two-stage, and three-stage procedures was 22, 41, and 63 days, respectively.*

72. Ponka JL. Emergency surgical operations for diverticular disease. Dis Colon Rectum 1970;13:235–242. *In elderly, poor-risk patients, the three-stage procedure was preferred in 26 of 42 individuals with diverticulitis or bleeding.*

73. Rugtiv GM. Diverticulitis: selective surgical management. Am J Surg 1975;130:219–225. *An analysis of 115 operations done over a 20-year period. Three-stage procedures were associated with considerable morbidity, and aggressive 2-stage resections are promoted.*

74. Wara P, Sorensen K, Berg V, et al. The outcome of staged management of complicated diverticular disease of the sigmoid colon. Acta Chir Scand 1981;147:209–214. *A retrospective study of 83 consecutive patients having staged procedures. Many transverse colostomies turned out to be permanent, and serious anastomotic complications occurred despite the presence of a colostomy.*

75. Rodkey GV, Welch CE. Colonic diverticular disease with surgical treatment. A study of 338 cases. Surg Clin North Am 1974;54:655–674. *Recognizes the surgical advances, but also points out the serious problems including rapid-onset complications, high rates of anastomotic leaks, high mortality for emergency operations, high complication rates, and long, costly hospitalizations. With 117 references.*

76. Eng K, Ranson JH, Localio SA. Resection of the perforated segment. A significant advance in treatment of diverticulitis with free perforation or abscess. Am J Surg 1977;133:67–72. *Primary resection with or without anastomosis is recommended for perforated diverticulitis.*

77. Ryan P. Emergency resection and anastomosis for perforated sigmoid diverticulitis. Br J Surg 1958;45:611–616. *The author recommends immediate resection; an anastomosis is done unless there is extensive diffusing peritonitis.*

78. Ryan P. The effect of surrounding infection upon leaking of colonic wounds: experimental studies and clinical experience. Dis Colon Rectum 1970;13:124–126. *Includes experimental work evaluating anastomotic healing in dogs; the author is in support of primary anastomosis.*

79. Madden JL, Tan PY. Primary resection and anastomosis in the treatment of perforated lesions of the colon with abscess or diffusing peritonitis. Surg Gynecol Obstet 1961;113:646–650. *The authors favor primary anastomosis, even in the presence of peritonitis.*

80. Farkouh E, Hellou G, Allard M, et al. Resection and primary anastomosis for diverticulitis with perforation and peritonitis. Can J Surg 1982;25:314–316. *Fifteen patients with perforated diverticulitis and diffuse peritonitis had resection and primary anastomosis after meeting a number of criteria including reasonably good patient health, no fecal contamination and the distal segment of colon lying above the peritoneal reflection.*

81. Schrock TR, Deveney CW, Dunphy TE. Factors contributing to leakage of colonic anastomoses. Ann Surg 1973;177:513–518. *Included in this review of 1703 colonic anastomoses were 216 anastomoses for diverticular disease, with a 3.7% anastomotic leak rate. Elective resection of diverticular disease was associated with a 0.6% leak rate (when no infection was present).*

82. Garnjobst W, Hardwick C. Further criteria for anastomosis in diverticulitis of the sigmoid colon. Am J Surg 1970;120:264–269. *In a review of 98 sigmoid resections for diverticulitis, anastomotic complications were most frequent when the resection was at or below the rectosigmoid junction.*

83. Welch CE, Welch JP. Resection and anastomosis of the colon in the presence of peritonitis. In: Delaney JP, Varco RL, eds. Controversies in surgery II. Philadelphia: WB Saunders, 1983:342–349. *A discussion of the risks of carrying out an anastomosis in the presence of peritonitis.*

84. Bell GA. Closure of colostomy following sigmoid colon resection for perforated diverticulitis. Surg Gynecol Obstet 1980;150:85–90. *A retrospective analysis of 70 patients. Use of a distal mucous fistula diminished the length of hospital stay and the number of complications.*

85. Boyden AM. Two-stage (obstructive) resection of the sigmoid in selected cases of complicated diverticulitis. Ann Surg 1961;154(Suppl):210–214. *Selective use of the two-stage resection for complicated diverticulitis is advocated, rather than routine use of three-stage procedures.*

86. Haas PA, Haas GP: A critical evaluation of the Hartmann's procedures. Am Surg 1988;54:380–385. *Seventy-six cases were performed for diverticulitis. In 42 patients, the colostomy was not closed because of patient age or medical and surgical risks.*

87. Pain J, Cahill J. Surgical options for left-sided large bowel emergencies. Ann R Coll Surg Engl 1991;73:394–397. *The Hartmann procedure was the most accepted operation for different forms of perforated diverticulitis in this questionnaire answered by 200 consulting surgeons.*

88. Tudor RG, Farmakis N, Keighley MR. National audit of complicated diverticular disease: analysis of index cases. Br J Surg 1994;481:730–732. *This paper analyzes the management of 300 patients with complex diverticular disease treated at 30 hospitals in the United Kingdom between 1985 and 1988.*

89. Schein M, Decker G. The Hartmann procedure. Extended indications in severe intra-abdominal infection. Dis Colon Rectum 1988;31:126–129. *The authors prefer a Hartmann closure to a mucous fistula, especially if repeated laparotomies are necessary.*

90. Isbister WH, Prasad J. Hartmann's operation: a personal experience. Aust N Z J Surg 1995;65:98–100. *The authors tended to do hand-sewn anastomoses when reestablishing gastrointestinal continuity and the leak rate was low.*

91. Nunes GC, Robnett AH, Kremer RM, et al. The Hartmann procedure for complications of diverticulitis. Arch Surg 1979;114:425–429. *Based on experience with 25 patients, the authors recommend wider use of the Hartmann procedure. The average total hospitalization for both stages was 23 days.*

92. Saini S, Meuller PR, Wittenberg J, et al. Percutaneous drainage of diverticular abscess: an adjunct to surgical therapy. Arch Surg 1986;121:475–478. *An experience with 17 patients, including follow-up data.*

93. Reilly M. Sigmoid myotomy. Br J Surg 1966;53:859–863. *The author describes the experience in 28 cases, most of which were carried out for uncomplicated diverticular disease.*

94. Reilly MC. The place of sigmoid myotomy in diverticular disease. Acta Chir Belg 1979;78:387–390. *Seventy-five percent of a series of 104 patients involved chronic uncomplicated "troublesome" diverticular disease; the rest involved resolved complicated diverticulitis, provided that all signs of pus or peritonitis had disappeared.*

95. Hodgson J. Transverse taeniamyotomy for diverticular disease. Dis Colon Rectum 1973;16:283–289. *An early experience with 6 patients. The author believed that there was less morbidity and mortality than longitudinal myotomy.*

96. Landi E, Fianchini A, Landa L, et al. Multiple transverse taeniamyotomy for diverticular disease. Surg Gynecol Obstet 1979;148:221–226. *There was a significant decrease of the mean motility index after natural and pharmacologic stimuli in 11 patients 1 year following the operation.*

97. Kettlewell MG, Maloney GE. Combined horizontal and longitudinal colomyotomy for diverticular disease: preliminary report. Dis Colon Rectum 1977;20:24–28. *A description of the operation in six patients. The authors felt that this operation added a more complete myotomy than Reilly's operation and that there was less risk of mucosal perforation since the circular muscle was not completely divided.*

98. Correnti FS, Pappalardo G, Mobarhan S, et al. Follow-up results of a new colomyotomy in the treatment of diverticulosis. Surg Gynecol Obstet 1983;156:181–186. *A report of a new form of myotomy with simultaneous incision of longitudinal and circular muscle fibers applied in 10 patients with advanced symptomatic diverticulosis.*

99. Veidenheimer MC, Lawrence DC. Anastomotic myotomy: an adjunct to resection for diverticular disease. Dis Colon Rectum 1976;19:310–313. *Twenty-three patients had anastomotic myotomy with the theoretical advantages of making the anastomosis at a more proximal level and of enlarging the luminal diameter of the anastomosis. There were no major complications, although two patients may have had anastomotic leaks.*

100. Smith AN, Attisha RP, Balfour T. Clinical and manometric results one year after sigmoid myotomy for diverticular disease. Br J Surg 1969;56:895–899. *A series of 14 patients with no active inflammation underwent this operation with considerable initial morbidity. An additional patient died after developing medication-related ileus and colonic dehiscence.*

101. Mayefsky E, Sicular A, Hodgson WJ. Recurrent diverticulitis after conservative surgery. Mt Sinai J Med 1979;46:556–558. *Two patients developed diverticulitis after transverse taeniamyotomy; one had inflammation proximal to the site of the previous myotomy.*

102. Ravo B, Ger R. Temporary colostomy—an outmoded procedure? A report on the intracolonic bypass. Dis Colon Rectum 1985;28:904–907. *The intracolonic bypass was used in 29 patients (including 10 with perforated diverticulitis), and temporary colostomy was avoided in all.*

103. Bruce CJ, Coller JA, Murray JJ, et al. Laparoscopic resection for diverticular disease. Dis Colon Rectum 1996;39:S1–S6. *A retrospective comparison of laparoscopic and open resections. The laparoscopic procedures were associated with overall higher costs, but less postoperative pain and shorter hospital stays.*

104. Liberman MA, Phillips EH, Carroll BJ, et al. Laparoscopic colectomy vs. traditional colectomy for diverticulitis. Outcome and costs. Surg Endosc 1996;10:15–18. *The total hospital charges were less in the laparoscopic group of patients.*

105. Welch CE. Controversial problems associated with diverticulitis. Proc R Soc Med 1970;63:57–61. *A concise discussion on indications for operation and types of procedures of choice.*

106. Roberts PL. Alternatives in surgery for diverticulitis. Semin Colon Rectal Surg 1990;1:69–73. *A concise discussion of the operative alternatives used today.*

107. Bokey EL, Chapuis PH, Pheils MT. Elective resection for diverticular disease and carcinoma: comparison of postoperative morbidity and mortality. Dis Colon Rectum 1981;24:181–182. *Morbidity was higher in the diverticular disease group; 17 of 47 patients needed proximal colostomy.*

108. Wedell J, Banzhaf G, Chaoui R, et al. Surgical management of complicated colonic diverticulitis. Br J Surg 1997;84:380–383. *The Hartmann procedure is the most popular, but resection and primary anastomosis are the safest procedures for all stages of complicated diverticulitis. The latter also diminishes costs.*

109. Maddern GJ, Nejjari Y, Dennison A, et al. Primary anastomosis with transverse colostomy as an alternative to Hartmann's procedure. Br J Surg 1995;82:170–171. *Six of 40 patients having primary anastomosis and a transverse colostomy died. In 20 patients having colostomy closure, there was no morbidity or mortality.*

110. Dumanian GA, Llull R, Ramasastry SS, et al. Postoperative abdominal wall defects with enterocutaneous fistulae. Am J Surg 1996;172:332–334. *A discussion of 10 patients with postoperative wound dehiscence and enterocutaneous fistulas managed with early skin grafting onto the granulated abdominal viscera.*

111. Rothenberger DA, Wiltz O. Surgery for complicated diverticulitis. Surg Clin North Am 1993;73:975–992. *This review concentrates on the appropriate surgical procedures and includes a complex algorithm for treatment of acute diverticulitis.*

112. Alexander J, Karl RC, Skinner DB. Results of changing trends in the surgical management of complications of diverticular disease. Surgery 1983;94:683–690. *Ninety-three patients underwent surgery, usually for serious complications. Complications were more numerous in patients not having primary resection of the diseased segment and time of hospitalization was prolonged as well.*

113. Roberts P, Abel M, Rosen L, et al. Practice parameters for sigmoid diverticulitis—supporting documentation. Dis Colon Rectum 1995;38:125–132. *An excellent summary of current guidelines in the diagnosis and management of sigmoid diverticulitis and its complications prepared by the Standards Task Force of the American Society of Colon and Rectal Surgeons. Sixty-nine references are alluded to.*

114. Schoetz DJ Jr. Uncomplicated diverticulitis. Indications for surgery and surgical management. Surg Clin North Am 1993;73:965–974. *The indications for elective resection are discussed, with emphasis on the safety of elective rather than emergency resection.*

115. Beer E. Some pathological and clinical aspects of acquired (false) diverticula of the intestine. Am J Med Sci 1904;128:135–145. *A summary of experimental studies concerned with the etiology of diverticular disease; the author also examines clinical reports discussing stenosis, pericolic abscess, and colovesical fistulas, primarily from the German literature.*

116. Telling WH. Acquired diverticula of the sigmoid flexure. Lancet 1908;1:843–850, 928–931. *A study of pathologic and clinical aspects, including 105 case studies.*

117. Keith A. A demonstration on diverticula of the alimentary tract of congenital or of obscure origin. BMJ 1910;1:376–381. *A discussion of the anatomy of various diverticula with a list of specimens in London museums at the time.*

118. Drummond H. Sacculi of the large intestine, with special reference to their relations to the blood vessels of the bowel wall. Br J Surg 1916;4:407–413. *Includes a number of microscopic views of the colon. The author believed that the diverticula were related to a general deficiency of nonstriated muscle of the individual.*

119. Rankin FW, Brown PW. Diverticulitis of the colon. Surg Gynecol Obstet 1930;50:836–847. *A good early description of the major manifestations of diverticulitis, although the data in the series of patients from the Mayo Clinic is limited.*

120. Hayden EP. Surgical problems in diverticulitis. N Engl J Med 1940;222:340–343. *An early surgical series from the Massachusetts General Hospital.*

121. Young EL, Young EL III. Diverticulitis of the colon. A review of the literature and an analysis of 91 cases. N Engl J Med 1944;230:33–38. *A review of 84 patients, including 28 who were operated on for complications of acute and chronic diverticulitis.*

122. Pemberton J, Black BM, Maino CR. Progress in the surgical management of diverticulitis of the sigmoid colon. Surg Gynecol Obstet 1947;85:523–534. *A large series from the Mayo Clinic, including 389 patients. In approximately 25% of patients, carcinoma could not be ruled out preoperatively. Results were poor when a stoma was closed without previous resection of disease. Approximately 80% were cured following primary resection or following resection done after establishing a colonic stoma.*

123. Mayo CW, Blunt CP. The surgical management of the complications of diverticulitis of the large intestine. Surg Clin North Am 1950;30:1005–1012. *In this analysis of complicated cases, only one patient did not have resection.*

124. Fallis LS, Marshall MR. Acute diverticulitis of the large bowel. Am J Surg 1950;80:198–203. *Transverse colostomy was recommended by the authors for surgical cases.*

125. Boyden AM. The surgical treatment of diverticulitis of the colon. Ann Surg 1950;132:94–109. *The author noted a significant decrease of morbidity compared to other reports. The average total duration of colostomy was only 9 weeks. In many cases, preliminary colostomy is unnecessary and even contraindicated.*

126. Judd ES Jr, Mears TW. Diverticulitis. Progress toward wider application of single-stage resection. Arch Surg 1955;70:818–825. *The authors advocate one-stage resection in carefully selected cases.*

127. Waugh JM, Walt AJ. An appraisal of one stage anterior resection in diverticulitis of the sigmoid colon. Surg Gynecol Obstet 1957;104:690–698. *The authors note the trend toward increased use of resection and anastomosis without colostomy.*

128. Smithwick RH. Surgical treatment of diverticulitis of the sigmoid. Am J Surg 1960;99:192–205. *With selective use of different procedures, no patients died following surgery in this series. The greatest danger is anastomotic leak.*

129. Boyden AM, Neilson RO. Reappraisal of the surgical treatment of diverticulitis of the sigmoid colon. Am J Surg 1960;100:206–216. *Morbidity was reduced by the frequent selection of primary resection and a shortened duration of colostomy before definitive resection.*

130. Rodkey GV, Welch CE. Diverticulitis of the colon: evolution in concept and therapy. Surg Clin North Am 1965;45:1231–1243. *An interesting history of surgical advances in the treatment of diverticular disease, including treatment at the Massachusetts General Hospital. Includes 85 references.*

131. Rodkey GV, Welch CE. Surgical management of colonic diverticulitis with free perforation or abscess formation. Am J Surg 1969;117:265–269. *A study of 50 patients that critically examines the cost of three-stage procedures and recommends primary excision in patients presenting with abscess or free perforation.*

132. Mitty WF, Befeler D, Grossi C, et al. Surgical management of complications of diverticulitis in patients over seventy years of age. Am J Surg 1969;117:270–276. *Morbidity and mortality rates were greater for patients over 70 years of age; the mortality rate was 0 for patients older than 70 years of age who had elective three-stage procedures.*

133. Botsford TW, Zollinger RM Jr, Hicks R. Mortality of the surgical treatment of diverticulitis. Am J Surg 1971;121:702–705. *Most deaths were due to sepsis, and anastomotic leaks were the major preventable cause of death, especially after one-stage resection.*

134. Byrne JJ, Garick EI. Surgical treatment of diverticulitis. Am J Surg 1971;121:379–384. *This series of 43 patients includes a good discussion of treatment trends in the surgical literature.*

135. MacGregor AB, Abernathy BC, Thomson JW. The role of surgery in diverticular disease of the colon. J R Coll Surg Edinb 1972;15:137–144. *Examines 204 consecutive admissions for diverticular disease: 70 were treated with initial operation and the remainder were treated medically. The authors believe it is difficult to predict which patients will develop severe complications.*

136. Tolins SH. Surgical treatment of diverticulitis. Experience at a large municipal hospital. JAMA 1975;232:830–832. *The major reasons for mortality included delayed diagnosis, inadequate surgery, and high incidence of associated disease.*

137. Classen JN, Bonardi R, O'Mara CS, et al. Surgical treatment of acute diverticulitis by staged procedures. Ann Surg 1976;184:582–586. *A retrospective review of 208 patients. The overall mortality of three-stage resections was 11%; 8.5% died after the first stage.*

138. Letwin ER. Diverticulitis of the colon. Clinical review of acute presentations and management. Am J Surg 1982;143:579–581. *A study of 46 patients, 17 of whom had staged procedures. The mortality rate was 4.4%.*

139. Eisenstat TE, Rubin RJ, Salvati EP. Surgical management of diverticulitis: the role of the Hartmann procedure. Dis Colon Rectum 1983;26:429–432. *The Hartmann procedure is recommended for complex diverticulitis and one-stage resection and anastomosis in the elective setting.*

140. Lambert ME, Knox RA, Schofield PF, et al. Management of the septic complications of diverticular disease. Br J Surg 1986;73:576–579. *The authors prefer resection but colostomy and drainage is acceptable when the perforation is not "communicating."*

141. Gregg RO. An ideal operation for diverticulitis of the colon. Am J Surg 1987;153:285–290. *All deaths occurred in the group of 140 who underwent emergency procedures.*

142. Moreaux J, Vons C. Elective resection for diverticular disease of the sigmoid colon. Br J Surg 1990;77:1036–1038. *A consecutive series of patients that had elective resection of diverticular disease. Five of 72 patients operated on for chronic symptoms had an unexpected abscess. There were no anastomotic leaks.*

143. Tyau ES, Prystowsky JB, Joehl RJ, et al. Acute diverticulitis. A complicated problem in the immunocompromised patient. Arch Surg 1991;126:855–859. *Forty immunocompromised patients are compared to 169 nonimmunocompromised patients; all patients had acute diverticulitis. The risk of free perforation, need for surgery, and postoperative mortality were higher in the immunocompromised group.*

144. Ambrosetti P, Robert JH, Witzig J-A, et al. Acute left colonic diverticulitis: a prospective analysis of 226 consecutive cases. Surgery 1994;115:546–550. *An analysis of the immediate outcome and follow-up of acute left colonic diverticulitis, with special attention to patient age, gender, and initial CT findings.*

145. Belmonte C, Klas JV, Perez JJ, et al. The Hartmann procedure. First choice or last resort in diverticular disease? Arch Surg 1996;131:612–617. *The authors point out that the morbidity of closure of the bowel following the Hartmann procedure is high. They prefer ileostomy if fecal diversion is desired following resection and anastomosis.*

SECTI

2

146. Chua CL. Surgical considerations in the Hartmann's procedure. Aust N Z J Surg 1996;66:676–679. *This review of 105 patients includes 17 patients with diverticular abscesses. A good current literature review is included.*
147. Freeman SR, McNally PR. Diverticulitis. Med Clin North Am 1993;77:1149–1167. *A useful basic summary, including a table of useful antibiotics and a practical approach to diagnosis; 64 references are included.*
148. Russell JC, Welch JP. Pathophysiology of bowel obstruction. In: Welch JP, ed. Bowel obstruction. Differential diagnosis and clinical management. Philadelphia: WB Saunders, 1990:28–58.
149. Goligher J. Surgery of the anus, rectum and colon. 5th ed. London: Bailliere Tindall, 1984:1087.
150. Oppenheimer E, ed. The CIBA collection of medical illustrations. Part II: Lower digestive tract. West Caldwell, NJ: CIBA Pharmaceutical Co., 1962;2:130.
151. Zollinger RW, Zollinger RM. Diverticular disease of the colon. Adv Surg 1971;5:255–280.
152. Todd IP, Fielding LP, eds. Rob and Smith's operative surgery. Alimentary tract and abdominal wall. Part 3: Colon, rectum and anus. 4th ed. London: Butterworths, 1983.
153. Welch JP. Carcinoma of the colon. In: Welch JP, ed. Bowel obstruction. Differential diagnosis and clinical management. Philadelphia: WB Saunders, 1990:546–574.

-
-
-
-

ILLUST

A 60-
distentic
nature.
spontan
afebrile.
lower q
included
the pati
oral cep
underw
losis wi

Six n
examina
within i
tomogra

CASE

*Desp
fact, the
findings
during
a CT ex

episode. If acute inflammation is shown on the CT examination, a more aggressive approach can be undertaken with a potential longer course of antibiotics followed by strict dietary recommendations. If this course of action fails with resultant recurrent symptoms, surgical intervention can be considered. However, if a CT examination is normal during the acute phase, treatment should be limited to conservative medical management.

DISCUSSION

Since its first description by Cruveilhier in 1849, the incidence and treatment of diverticular disease has changed. Initially, it was regarded as a medical curiosity. Today, however, with the advancing age of the population, diverticular disease of the colon is increasing in incidence. Moreover, younger patients are more commonly developing symptomatic diverticular disease (1,2). It is estimated that 5–10% of persons older than 45 years of age have acquired diverticula of the colon with an increased incidence of up to 60% after the age of 80 years (3). The condition is characterized by the presence of acquired herniations of the mucosal layers that protrude through the bowel wall.

The pathogenesis of these pseudodiverticular formations probably is related to alterations in colonic pressures due to fiber-deficient diets (4). Supportive evidence for this hypothesis includes the myriad demographic studies that show high incidences of diverticulosis in Western countries. Conversely, diverticulosis is virtually absent in countries in which a low-fat high-fiber diet is consumed. Parks, in a detailed review of the natural history of diverticular disease, pointed out important aspects such as the incidence of the disease among younger and elderly individuals, the relation of the diet, and the correlation between symptoms and pathologic findings (5). In 80% of the cases, the pseudodiverticula are asymptomatic—a condition known as diverticulosis. However, in approximately 20% of cases, the patients will experience various symptoms, the most common being abdominal pain (6).

Abdominal pain is undoubtedly the most frequent complaint resulting from disorders that involve the gastrointestinal tract. Therefore, location, intensity, duration, and type of abdominal pain are all important aspects of differential diagnosis. Other important factors to consider include urinary and gynecologic symptoms. To better understand the mechanism of abdominal pain in diverticular disease, considerations regarding the pathophysiology of pain are necessary.

Painful stimuli are basically transmitted by type-A-delta and type-C fibers. The former are distributed mainly to muscle and skin and mediate acute, well-localized pain. The latter fibers can be found in muscle, periosteum, parietal peritoneum, and viscera and mediate poorly localized and nonacute pain. Both types of fibers are triggered by strong mechanical stimulation and variations of temperature. Haupt et al believe that substances such as bradykinin and KCl also may activate pain receptors, either directly or by decreasing their thresholds to other noxious stimuli (7).

The visceral afferent fibers that mediate pain travel with the sympathetic or parasympathetic nerves. Stimuli from the colon, appendix, and pelvic viscera enter the tenth and eleventh thoracic segments by sympathetic nerves (mesenteric plexus and lesser splanchnic nerves), whereas the sigmoid colon and rectum are innervated by fibers that enter the eleventh thoracic segment and the first lumbar segment through the lowest splanchnic nerve. The algisensitive fibers reach the medulla through the dorsal root ganglia, run cranially or caudally for some segments through Lissauer's tract, and end in the neurons localized in the posterior horn. These neurons generate fibers that cross to the other side of the medulla and terminate cranially in the spinothalamic and spinoreticu-

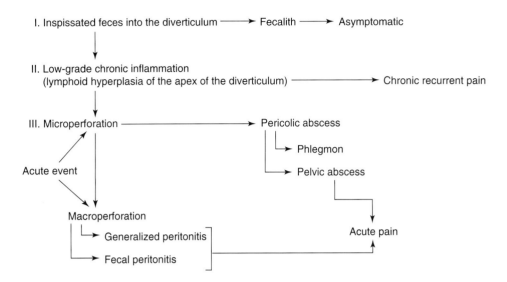

Figure 2.1. Sequence of events in acute inflammation of a diverticulum.

lothalamic tracts. In either case, cerebral terminations receive fibers from both sides of the body. The spinothalamic and spinoreticular tract neurons synapse within the thalamus with third-order neurons that run to the somatosensory cortex (sensory and discriminative aspects of pain) or synapse within the pons and medulla with third-order neurons that run predominantly to the limbic system and frontal lobe ("motivational affective aspects of pain"), respectively (8,9).

Despite all of these complex neuronal pathways that mediate abdominal visceral pain sensation, the paucity of visceral afferent nerves is responsible for the difficulty in localizing the pain. *General rules for localizing abdominal pain are related to the embryologic origin of the organ.* The distal one-third of the transverse, descending, and rectosigmoid colon are derived from the hindgut. Pain radiating from these organs usually is felt between the umbilicus and the pelvis. Also, because of its bilateral innervation, the pain may have a predominance to one side. Unlike the skin and other parts of the body, abdominal viscera and the visceral peritoneum are insensitive to many stimuli. *The main mechanism of initiating pain to the abdominal viscera is stretching or tension in the wall of the gut.* The nerve endings of pain fibers in the colon and small bowel are located in the muscular wall, and distention from forceful muscular contraction can cause pain. Other known stimuli for abdominal pain include inflammation (bacterial or chemical), ischemia, or the effects of sensory nerve involvement with tumor.

Visceral pain can be described as colic, cramping, burning, or gnawing and usually is followed by nausea, vomiting, sweating, pallor, and other vagal symptoms (6).

The pathogenesis of diverticular disease involves increased intraluminal pressures and exaggerated segmentation contractions especially seen after meals, both related to lack of sufficient bulk in the stool. The mild, recurrent colic or crampy postprandial pain, usually felt in the left lower quadrant, is therefore a logical symptom constellation.

Alternatively, inflammation of the small diverticular pouches is responsible for more acute, steady, and severe abdominal pain (Fig. 2.1).

As mentioned previously, diverticulosis is the mere presence of diverticula in the colon. Nevertheless, *mild clinical symptoms such as postprandial colicky cramps or episodic abdominal*

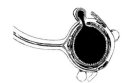

3 Ischemic Colitis or Diverticulitis: A Challenging Diagnostic Dilemma

Walter E. Longo, MD
Anthony M. Vernava, MD

KEY POINTS

- Abdominal pain common in both entities
- Suspect ischemic colitis if bloody diarrhea
- Empiric treatment (bed rest, antibiotics) appropriate for either illness
- CT scan early diagnostic test of choice if diagnosis unclear
- Colonoscopy—excellent diagnostic test when ischemia suspected

INTRODUCTION

Bowel ischemia should always be suspected in any patient with abdominal pain. It may be caused by arterial occlusive disease, venous occlusive disease, and nonocclusive ischemia resulting from low-flow states. *Ischemic colitis is the most common form of gastrointestinal ischemia. Nevertheless, it is a rare entity and accounts for only 1–2% of colonic pathology.* Most episodes are not associated with major vascular occlusion, and it is now recognized that most cases result from impaired colonic perfusion. It usually presents as an acute abdominal illness with abdominal pain and rectal bleeding. The correct diagnosis often is confirmed after the ischemic episode has taken place and has been verified either endoscopically or in the operating room. The disease is often segmental in nature, involving either the splenic flexure or the sigmoid colon; however, total colonic ischemia may occur. Therapy and outcome of ischemic colitis are entirely dependent on the severity of disease. Most cases do not warrant surgical exploration and respond favorably to simple conservative measures such as bowel rest, hydration, and antibiotics. Surgery is indicated for severe forms of disease, either those that have failed conservative therapy or when peritoneal signs are present and full-thickness necrosis is suspected. Symptoms of colonic ischemia often mimic those of acute colonic diverticulitis. Often, they are indistinguishable short of laparotomy or laparoscopy. This review attempts to differentiate their subtleties.

ILLUSTRATIVE CASES

Case 1

A 68-year-old female with a history of hypertension and stable angina presented to the emergency room with a 24-hour history of left lower quadrant pain and bloody diarrhea. She had been hospitalized 4 years previously with diverticulitis and had responded to intravenous antibiotics.

pain ma
of dive
Howev
lower
change
Tabl
manife
sympto
The
in diffe
believe
conditi
colonic
acute i
diverti
Physica
(Table
mechar
abscess
occurre
If fever
rate wi
Whe
other co
ischem
radicul
syndro
be bet
conside
most o
Beca
quantit
these p
process
inflami
diagno
entire
process
tumors
Oth
gastroi
care m
radiolog
of a pe
signific
colonic
Epis
by objec
medical
as well

F
d

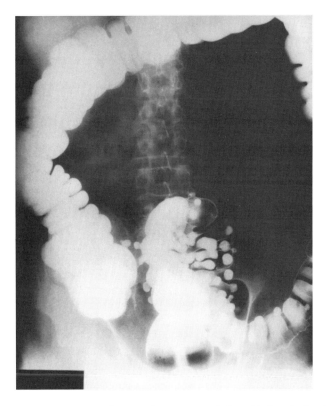

Figure 2.4. Barium enema showing the presence of sigmoid diverticular disease.

symptoms will tend to recur, probably due to an underlying motility disorder and high intestinal wall tension. It is unlikely that sigmoid resection will benefit these patients and may only lead to an increased intensity of the patient's symptoms. Although it is tempting to remove the "diverticular disease," in the absence of objective evidence for diverticulitis, the option of surgical intervention should not be offered.

CONCLUSIONS

In summary, we make the following considerations when assessing abdominal pain in patients with diverticulosis of the colon.

1. Differentiate abdominal pain caused by symptomatic diverticulosis or that produced by acute diverticulitis, for which prompt antibiotic therapy is required.
2. For patients with "benign" symptomatic diverticulosis, dietary orientation, fiber supplements, antispasmodics, and analgesics are all viable treatment options (6).
3. Exclude all conditions that may mimic symptomatic diverticular disease, particularly colorectal neoplasia and inflammatory bowel disease.
4. Consider the coexistence of irritable bowel disease in patients with a chronic history of mild abdominal pain and associated complaints for whom dietary and other conservative measures may relieve the symptoms.

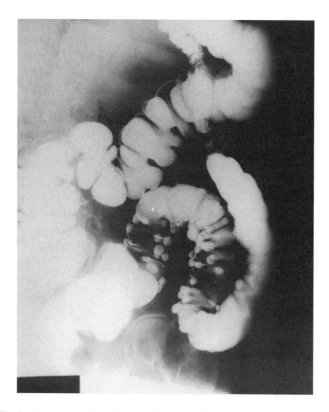

Figure 2.5. Barium enema, lateral view, of diverticular disease restricted to the sigmoid.

5. Despite the most sophisticated methods of diagnosis, meticulous clinical history and careful physical examination are of paramount importance in understanding abdominal pain and diverticulosis.

EDITORIAL COMMENTS

The authors touch on a very complex subject in this chapter: abdominal pain. In many cases, abdominal pain is difficult to quantify, and it can be highly subjective. Our understanding of such symptoms is by no means complete. Another confusing issue is the relationship of abdominal pain and bowel dysfunction to diverticulosis and other disorders, such as the frequently encountered irritable bowel syndrome. Suffice it to say that a number of illnesses associated with these symptoms can resemble each other; the differential diagnosis is outlined in Table 2.2. The irritable bowel syndrome and symptomatic diverticulosis may even occur together in some patients (13,14).

Patients with diverticulosis of the colon are, in most cases, asymptomatic; others develop episodes of abdominal pain and irregular bowel habits ("painful diverticulosis"). The pathogenesis of diverticular formation is related to two factors: the strength of the colon wall and the pressure difference between the lumen and the serosa (15). Findings associated with diverticular disease, beyond the scope of this discussion, are thickening of the colon wall (16,17) (myochosis) that can precede the development of diverticula (15); aging; a low-fiber diet (15,18,19); deterioration of elastin in the colon wall and foreshortening of the taeniae (20); motility disturbances (in symptomatic diverticulosis) (15); altered myoelectric patterns (21); and increased intraluminal pressure (22), with "segmentation" of the colon into pressure compartments (23) (Figs. 2.6 and 2.7).

What is the treatment of recurring abdominal pain associated with diverticulosis but without any history of inflammation? Treatment of painful diverticulosis (24) and irritable bowel is similar, involving a high-fiber diet, significant fluid intake, and in the case of abdominal pain, possible antispasmodics (25–28). Although it is tempting to remove the "diverticular disease" because of ongoing pain, we strongly agree that in the absence of objective evidence for diverticulitis, the option of surgical intervention should not be offered. It is unlikely that sigmoid resection would result in a resolution of such a problem; an intensification of the patient's symptoms could result instead.

Table 2.2.   Differential Diagnosis of Chronic/Recurrent Bowel Dysfunction[a]

Irritable bowel syndrome
Diverticular disease of the colon
Lactase deficiency
Drugs (laxatives)
Infections (bacterial, parasitic)
Colorectal/endocrine tumors
Malabsorption
Inflammatory bowel disease
Psychiatric causes
Metabolic disorders

[a]Bowel dysfunction is defined as diarrhea or constipation with or without abdominal pain. (After Drossman DA. Irritable bowel syndrome. In: Kirshner JB, Shorter RG, eds. Diseases of the colon, rectum and anal canal. Baltimore: Williams & Wilkins, 1988:131–139.)

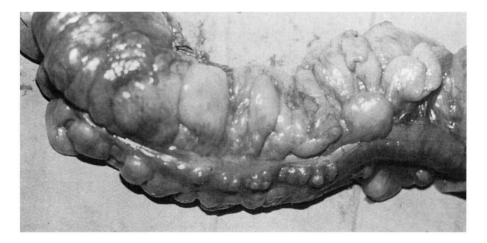

Figure 2.6.   Inflamed, thickened sigmoid colon with diverticular disease (phlegmon) [Ref. 30].

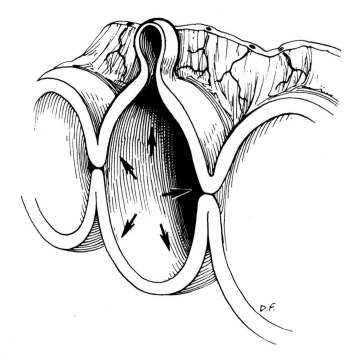

Figure 2.7. A schematic representation of "segmentation" in the colon; compartments of high pressure lead to development of diverticula at points of weakness in the colonic wall. (Reprinted with permission from Pemberton JH, Armstrong DN, Dietzen CD. Diverticulitis. In: Yamada T, ed. Textbook of gastroenterology. 2nd ed. Philadelphia: JB Lippincott, 1995:1879) [Ref. 29].

REFERENCES

1. Morson BC. Pathology of diverticular disease of the colon. Clin Gastroenterol 1975;4:37–52. *This and ref. no. 5 are part of a 223-page monograph on diverticular disease of the colon.*
2. Painter NS. Diverticular disease of the colon: the first of the western diseases shown to be due to a deficiency of dietary fibre. S Afr Med J 1982;61:1016–1020. *An interesting account of the changes in diet in late nineteenth-century England with the later appearance of diverticular disease. Documents relief of symptoms in a group of patients with diverticular disease taking bran in the diet.*
3. Schoetz DY. Uncomplicated diverticulitis. Surg Clin North Am 1993;73:965–974. *One of the major goals is to define the patients who will benefit from surgical therapy. Patients with repeated attacks, of young age, or in an immunocompromised state are surgical candidates.*
4. Mazier WP. Diverticulitis. In: Mazier WP, Levien DH, Luchtefeld MA, et al, eds. Surgery of the colon, rectum and anus. Philadelphia: WB Saunders, 1995:617–656.
5. Parks TG. Natural history of diverticular disease of the colon. Clin Gastroenterol 1975;4:53–69. *An increase in the number and size of diverticula is not seen with aging in all patients. Patients with total colonic involvement are, in many cases, younger than those with isolated sigmoid involvement. There is a poor correlation of clinical features and pathologic findings.*
6. Naitove A, Smith RE. Diverticular disease of the colon. In: Sleisinger MH, Fortran JS, eds. Gastrointestinal disease. 5th ed. Philadelphia: WB Saunders, 1993:1347–1363.
7. Haupt P, Janig W, Kohler W. Response pattern of visceral afferent fibres, supplying the colon, upon chemical and mechanical stimuli. Eur J Physiol 1983;398:41–47. *In the cat, visceral afferent fibers may encode noxious stimuli applied to the colon.*
8. White JC, Sweet WH. Pain in abdominal visceral disease. In: Thomas CC, ed. Pain and the neurosurgeon. Springfield, IL: Charles C. Thomas, 1969:560.
9. Klein KB, Mellinkoff SM. Approach to the patient with abdominal pain. In: Yamada T, ed. Textbook of gastroenterology. Philadelphia: JB Lippincott, 1991:660–681.
10. Connell AM, Jones FA, Rowlands EN. Motility of the pelvic colon. Abdominal pain associated with colonic hypermotility after meals. Gut 1965;6:105. *Describes a group of patients who developed very high pressures in the sigmoid colon after meals.*

11. Rothenberger DA, Wiltz O. Surgery for the complicated diverticulitis. Surg Clin North Am 1993;73:975–992. *In the absence of free perforation, most patients can be operated on a semiurgent or elective basis, leaving the option of primary anastomosis open.*
12. Haiart DC, Stevenson P, Hantley RC. Leg pain: an uncommon presentation of perforated diverticular disease. Ann R Coll Surg Edinb 1989;34:17–20. *Reports five patients with perforated diverticulitis who had thigh or leg pain as a predominant symptom. Three ultimately developed thigh emphysema.*
13. Thompson WG. Do colonic diverticula cause symptoms? Am J Gastroenterol 1986;81:613–614. *The author proposes that a fiber-deficient diet could predispose to both colonic diverticulosis and the irritable bowel syndrome, which may or may not coexist in an individual.*
14. Goy JA, Eastwood MA, Mitchell WD, et al. Fecal characteristics contrasted in the irritable bowel syndrome and diverticular disease. Am J Clin Nutr 1976;29:1480–1484. *No detectable difference was found in fecal wet weight, dry weight, and total bile acid excretions; the changes suggested a common etiology for these disorders.*
15. Almy TP, Howell DA. Diverticular disease of the colon. N Engl J Med 1980;302:324–331. *An excellent discussion, with an emphasis on nonsurgical aspects, including pathogenesis, with 119 references.*
16. Thomson HJ, Busuttil A, Eastwood MA, et al. Submucosal collagen changes in the normal colon and in diverticular disease. Int J Colorectal Dis 1987;2:208–213. *Collagen fibrils become smaller and more tightly packed in the left colon than in the right with advancing age, especially in the presence of diverticular disease.*
17. Watters DA, Smith AN. Strength of the colon wall in diverticular disease. Br J Surg 1990;77:257–259. *A review of the evidence that the mechanical properties of the bowel are key factors in the development of diverticular disease. The tensile strength and the elasticity of the colon (especially the left side) decline with age.*
18. Painter NS, Burkitt DP. Diverticular disease of the colon: a deficiency disease of western civilization. Br Med J 1971;2:450–454. *A well-publicized geographic study pointing to the relationship of dietary fiber to diverticular disease.*
19. Medeloff AI. Thoughts on the epidemiology of diverticular disease. Clin Gastroenterol 1986;15:855–877. *The author notes that fiber intake by individuals is three to five times greater in some underdeveloped companies than in westernized populations. Describes experimental studies, hospital discharge data, and associated diseases, and proposes future studies.*
20. Whiteway J, Morson BC. Pathology of the ageing—diverticular disease. Clin Gastroenterol 1985;14:829–846. *The authors feel that the muscular thickening in diverticular disease reflects elastosis and contracture of the taenia coli in the presence of normal muscle cells.*
21. Taylor I, Duthie HL. Bran tablets and diverticular disease. Br Med J 1976;1:988–990. *An abnormal rapid electrical rhythm in colonic smooth muscle was found in 80% of a group of 20 patients with symptomatic diverticular disease initially; the rhythm remained in only 40% of patients after treatment for 1 month with bran tablets.*
22. Arfwidsson S. Pathogenesis of multiple diverticula of the sigmoid colon in diverticular disease. Acta Chir Scand 1964;342(Suppl):1–68. *High intrasigmoid pressures were found in patients with diverticular disease; the pressure changes may have been related to increased sigmoid motor activity.*
23. Painter NS, Truelove SC, Ardran GM, et al. Segmentation and the localization of intraluminal pressures in the human colon, with special reference to the pathogenesis of colonic diverticula. Gastroenterology 1965;49:169–177. *A widely quoted study of intracolonic measurements in normal subjects and in patients with diverticulosis. The authors conclude that contraction of the colonic wall, together with segmentation of the colon, allows increases in intraluminal pressure and formation of diverticula at the weak points in the colonic wall.*
24. Cheskin LJ, Bohlman M, Schuster MM. Diverticular disease in the elderly. Gastroenterol Clin North Am 1990;19:391–403. *Symptomatic or painful diverticulosis refers to diverticulosis with clinical symptoms but no evidence of inflammation. If the patient has a life-long history of similar episodes of left lower quadrant pain, the diagnosis of irritable bowel should be considered; a first attack in the elderly suggests other illnesses such as colon cancer.*
25. Horner JT. Natural history of diverticulosis of the colon. Am J Dig Dis 1958;3:343–350. *A study of 503 patients followed in an office setting from 1 to 18 years. Only two patients (0.4%) required surgery.*
26. Hyland JM, Taylor I. Does a high fiber diet prevent the complications of diverticular disease? Br J Surg 1980;67:77–79. *More than 90% of patients with diverticular disease taking a high-fiber diet remained symptom-free on a high-fiber diet.*
27. Littlewood ER, Ornstein MH, McLean Baird I, et al. Doubts about diverticular disease. BMJ 1981;283:1524–1526. *Combination treatment with fiber, antispasmodics, and anxiolytic agents tends to be effective in treatment of irritable bowel syndrome; the same may be effective for symptomatic diverticular disease.*
28. Francis CY, Whorwell PJ. The irritable bowel syndrome. Postgrad Med J 1997;73:1–7. *An excellent review with 41 references. This disorder varies from trivial to incapacitating and affects 15–20% of the Western population. Noncolonic symptoms are common. The authors emphasize the importance of patient education as well as diet and drug therapy.*
29. Pemberton JH, Armstrong DN, Dietzen CD. Diverticulitis. In: Yamada T, ed. Textbook of gastroenterology. 2nd ed. Philadelphia: JB Lippincott, 1995:1879.
30. Drossman DA. Irritable bowel syndrome. In: Kirshner JB, Shorter RG, eds. Diseases of the colon, rectum and anal canal. Baltimore: Williams & Wilkins, 1988:131–139.

3 Ischemic Colitis or Diverticulitis: A Challenging Diagnostic Dilemma

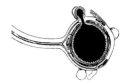

Walter E. Longo, MD
Anthony M. Vernava, MD

KEY POINTS

- Abdominal pain common in both entities
- Suspect ischemic colitis if bloody diarrhea
- Empiric treatment (bed rest, antibiotics) appropriate for either illness
- CT scan early diagnostic test of choice if diagnosis unclear
- Colonoscopy—excellent diagnostic test when ischemia suspected

INTRODUCTION

Bowel ischemia should always be suspected in any patient with abdominal pain. It may be caused by arterial occlusive disease, venous occlusive disease, and nonocclusive ischemia resulting from low-flow states. *Ischemic colitis is the most common form of gastrointestinal ischemia. Nevertheless, it is a rare entity and accounts for only 1–2% of colonic pathology.* Most episodes are not associated with major vascular occlusion, and it is now recognized that most cases result from impaired colonic perfusion. It usually presents as an acute abdominal illness with abdominal pain and rectal bleeding. The correct diagnosis often is confirmed after the ischemic episode has taken place and has been verified either endoscopically or in the operating room. The disease is often segmental in nature, involving either the splenic flexure or the sigmoid colon; however, total colonic ischemia may occur. Therapy and outcome of ischemic colitis are entirely dependent on the severity of disease. Most cases do not warrant surgical exploration and respond favorably to simple conservative measures such as bowel rest, hydration, and antibiotics. Surgery is indicated for severe forms of disease, either those that have failed conservative therapy or when peritoneal signs are present and full-thickness necrosis is suspected. Symptoms of colonic ischemia often mimic those of acute colonic diverticulitis. Often, they are indistinguishable short of laparotomy or laparoscopy. This review attempts to differentiate their subtleties.

ILLUSTRATIVE CASES

Case 1

A 68-year-old female with a history of hypertension and stable angina presented to the emergency room with a 24-hour history of left lower quadrant pain and bloody diarrhea. She had been hospitalized 4 years previously with diverticulitis and had responded to intravenous antibiotics.

She appeared ill and diaphoretic with a blood pressure of 160/90, pulse of 110, and temperature of 101.6°F. She had marked localized left lower quadrant tenderness to light palpitation, as well as guarding and rebound tenderness. No masses were appreciable. Rectal and pelvic examinations were unremarkable, except for melanotic stool. The white blood cell count was 18,000 with a left shift. The hematocrit was 36%, blood gases and lactate level were normal, and abdominal films were negative.

Treatment included vigorous intravenous fluid resuscitation and broad-spectrum antibiotic coverage. A computed tomography (CT) scan performed with oral and rectal contrast demonstrated a marked thickening of the sigmoid colon with streaking in the paracolic mesenteric fat. Diverticula were noted. The CT findings were most consistent with a segmental colitis, presumably ischemic. With several days of treatment, the fever and abdominal tenderness resolved. A subsequent colonoscopy showed segmental mucosal ulcerations with edema of the surrounding mucosa and submucosal hemorrhage, consistent with ischemic colitis. Biopsies of the sigmoid colon were confirmatory.

CASE COMMENTS

This case illustrates the similar clinical presentation of acute diverticulitis and ischemic colitis. Bloody diarrhea is a hallmark of ischemic colitis and, in the presence of acute onset abdominal pain, the diagnosis should be suspected. The initial treatment of both ischemic colitis and diverticulitis is essentially the same (bowel rest, intravenous antibiotics).

CT is of particular value early because it is noninvasive and, in some cases, it can distinguish ischemic colitis from diverticulitis. One should avoid colonoscopy or barium enema because of the risk of perforation in the presence of acute diverticulitis. If the CT scan suggests ischemic colitis, medical treatment is continued, and colonoscopy or barium enema is completed as the illness resolves.

The differential diagnosis of segmental colitis includes Crohn's colitis, infectious colitis, and pseudomembranous colitis. Endoscopy and biopsy are preferred as a diagnostic procedure if stool cultures are negative.

Case 2

A 70-year-old white female admitted 2 weeks previously for an exacerbation of chronic obstructive pulmonary disease (COPD), and who subsequently developed a bilobar pneumonia, ventilator dependency, and renal failure requiring dialysis, suddenly was found to be in shock, with a distended abdomen and generalized peritonitis. The white blood cell count was 42,000 with 60% bands.

CASE COMMENTS

This immunocompromised patient developed shock, presumably related to an abdominal catastrophe. Perforated diverticulitis would be less likely in this setting than ischemic colitis with transmural involvement of the colon wall leading to septicemia. Laparotomy would represent the only chance of salvaging this patient, and the chance of survival with any form of therapy would be slim.

Case 3

A 61-year-old white male with a medical history significant for two previous admissions for diverticulitis treated medically underwent an uncomplicated repair of an abdominal aortic aneurysm. On postoperative day 7, the patient was eating a regular diet, but on the morning of discharge, he developed sharp left lower quadrant abdominal pain and fever to 101°F. He subsequently passed a diarrheal stool and vomited.

CASE COMMENTS

This patient developed an abrupt change on the seventh postoperative day after being advanced to a regular diet. Acute diverticulitis would have to be considered, especially considering the previous admissions with this diagnosis. Ischemic colitis is possible as well, because this complication can occur as late as 1–2 weeks postoperatively, although one would have expected to have seen diarrhea develop sooner after the aortic surgery. If the stools were grossly bloody, ischemic colitis would be more likely; an abdominal mass would suggest diverticulitis or a postoperative hematoma.

Case 4

A 60-year-old white male developed abdominal pain, nausea, and vomiting at home and was brought to the hospital by his son. He was otherwise healthy except for an unexplained 30-pound weight loss over the past 3 months and 3 days of persistent diarrhea. His vital signs were unremarkable and physical examination revealed mild abdominal tenderness in the right lower quadrant. He was prepped gently for colonoscopy, and at endoscopy the next morning, a diffuse colitis manifest by contact bleeding and linear ulcers were noted contiguously from his rectosigmoid to his cecum. The diagnosis of Crohn's colitis was made. That night, the patient became acutely hypotensive and was in excruciating abdominal pain, and a 10-cm-diameter transverse colon was noted on an abdominal radiograph. He was taken emergently to the operating room.

CASE COMMENTS

This patient developed an acute abdomen soon after a colonoscopy showing widespread colitis. Diverticula were not mentioned in the colonoscopy report and, thus, diverticular perforation would be unlikely. A colonoscopic perforation would be expected to cause pneumoperitoneum, which should be demonstrable on upright films. This clinical picture of a toxic colitis can be a sign of pancolonic ischemic colitis in rare instances.

PATHOGENESIS AND SPECTRUM OF COLONIC ISCHEMIA

The presentation of this disease is variable and the diagnosis and management of patients remain challenging. It frequently occurs in elderly and debilitated patients with a variety of underlying medical problems. The original insult precipitating the ischemic event usually cannot be established. The outcome of colonic ischemia rests on numerous factors, including the severity, extent, and rapidity of the ischemic insult, in addition to the therapy given.

Colonic ischemia may result from numerous causes, such as occlusion of the blood supply to the colon or diffuse, small-vessel disease, such as in diabetes mellitus, rheumatoid arthritis, or amyloidosis. Systemic vascular disorders may also be present. "Spontaneous" episodes of ischemic colitis generally are viewed as localized forms of nonocclusive ischemia, perhaps in association with small-vessel disease. Profound systemic insults leading to clinical shock, including cardiac failure, sepsis, hypovolemia, and neurogenic injury, precipitate intense vasoconstriction and arteriovenous shunting. A variety of medications also have been implicated in ischemic colitis. In most cases, there is no identifiable cause, no iatrogenic injury, no preceding problem, and no precipitating episode delineated. These symptoms often are consistent with acute diverticulitis. *Attention to previous attacks of diverticulitis and the presence of a mass in the lower abdomen may help in its differential.*

There are two principal forms of ischemic colitis based on clinical findings: *(a)* a *nongangrenous* type subdivided into a transient reversible form and a chronic form and *(b)* a *gangrenous* type. The nongangrenous transient form involves the mucosa or submucosa and is characterized by edema, submucosal hemorrhage, and possible partial mucosal necrosis. In general, transient ischemic colitis is followed by a complete structural and functional recovery over the course of time. The damaged muscularis is replaced by fibrous tissue over a recovery period of weeks to months and frequently results in a colonic stricture (2,3). Finally, gangrenous ischemic colitis involves a transmural necrotizing injury.

Any part of the colon may be involved, but the splenic flexure, descending colon, and sigmoid are most commonly involved. Localized, nonocclusive ischemia classically involves watershed areas of the colon such as the splenic flexure (Griffiths' point) and the junction of the sigmoid and rectum (Sudek's point). However, recent reports have demonstrated an increased incidence of right colon ischemia (3). Rectal ischemia is rare. Diverticulitis most commonly involves the sigmoid colon. Tenderness often can be in the right lower quadrant, where the sigmoid may either be redundant or fixed to the right side of the pelvis. *Lower abdominal tenderness away from the left lower quadrant is not a reliable way to differentiate between the two disease entities.*

CLINICAL PRESENTATION

The clinical presentation varies according to the severity, extent, and rapidity of the ischemic insult, the resistance of the bowel wall to hypoxia, and its intrinsic ability to protect itself against bacterial invasion. Ischemic colitis generally develops as an acute abdominal illness in patients older than 60 years of age who have had no previous colonic problems (4). The most constant signs and symptoms include abdominal pain, diarrhea, alteration in bowel function, and hematochezia. The blood loss in these patients usually is minimal. The character of the pain is sudden in onset, crampy, and often localized to the left side of the lower abdomen. An urgent desire to defecate frequently accompanies the pain. Anorexia, nausea, and vomiting, secondary to an associated ileus, may be present. The abdominal examination often is significant for mild distention and tenderness that usually corresponds to the site of the ischemic colon. Significant fever is not common. Rectal examination reveals heme-positive stool. Cardiovascular examination usually is unremarkable. Laboratory evaluation often reveals a moderate leukocytosis with a left shift.

For comparison, patients with acute diverticulitis usually present with abdominal pain that is localized to the left lower quadrant; it may be related to a recent bowel movement. Up to 25% of patients will have had a previous attack. Physical examination reveals localized peritonitis in the left lower quadrant. A mass may be present. Free perforation will produce generalized peritoneal signs. Contrast enemas and CT scan may reveal diverticulitis and an abscess or phlegmon.

DIAGNOSIS

The diagnosis of colonic ischemia depends on early and repeated clinical evaluations of the patient and serial roentgenographic or endoscopic studies of the colon. *The clinician must retain a high index of suspicion.*

In a patient with suspected colonic ischemia who has no signs of peritonitis and normal or nonspecific abdominal plain films, colonoscopy should be performed. A plain radiograph that demonstrates free intra-abdominal air secondary to perforation, air within the bowel wall, or portal venous air signifies advanced ischemia or colon infarction and must be succeeded by immediate exploratory laparotomy. Although enzyme determinations are used routinely in the assessment of cardiac and hepatic necrosis, there currently is no specific serum marker of intestinal viability. Certain findings such as a thickened bowel wall may be present on CT, but these are not specific. Colonoscopy is the preferred diagnostic study over barium enema because it is considerably more sensitive in diagnosing mucosal abnormalities, and biopsies of both normal and abnormal-appearing tissue may be obtained. The precise endoscopic and histologic picture of ischemic colitis depends on the rate of the ischemic insult and when in the natural history of the disease the diagnostic studies are completed. Focal areas of pale and edematous mucosa with interspersed areas of confluent hyperemia or punctate ulceration are indicative of the beginning stages of ischemia. Histologic evidence of mucosal infarction is pathognomonic for ischemia. Most common changes are vascular congestion and damage in the superficial half of the mucosa.

DIFFERENTIAL DIAGNOSIS

Acute colonic ischemia may be quite difficult to differentiate from other colonic conditions. Most commonly these include diverticulitis, ulcerative colitis, Crohn's colitis, and infectious colitis. Due to the frequent location of acute colonic ischemia in the sigmoid colon, it frequently may be difficult to differentiate this condition from acute diverticulitis. Often, the history and physical examination will fail to differentiate between these two disease entities. Although a previous history of documented attacks of diverticulitis may sway the physician to suspect recurrent diverticulitis, the authors have seen the new onset of acute sigmoid ischemia in patients with previous sigmoid diverticulitis. Clearly, *patients with either ischemic colitis or diverticulitis complain primarily of abdominal pain. However, unlike colonic ischemia, the pain with diverticulitis often is associated with urinary symptoms* such as dysuria, frequency, urgency, or nocturia secondary to an inflammatory reaction near the bladder. Furthermore, unlike diverticulitis, the pain of colonic ischemia often is associated with gastrointestinal symptoms such as nausea, vomiting, or diarrhea. Rectal bleeding is common in diverticulosis and highly unlikely in acute colonic diverticulitis. *The presence of bloody diarrhea should sway one to suspect colonic ischemia.*

Physical examination is similar in both conditions. Low-grade fever and abdominal distention, secondary to ileus, is seen commonly in either disease. The abdominal examination ranges from mild tenderness and voluntary guarding to the presence of peritonitis with a boardlike abdomen and all of the signs of an acute abdominal catastrophe. However, *an abdominal mass may suggest a diverticular phlegmon or abscess rather than colonic ischemia.* Plain films of the abdomen may reveal characteristic "thumbprinting" in patients with colonic ischemia. Similarly, if a barium enema is performed, this thumbprinting pattern and edema of the bowel wall will be present.

Colonoscopy has been responsible largely for the increasing awareness of ischemic colitis. Direct *visualization of the colonic mucosa is the best method to differentiate colonic ischemia from acute diverticulitis.* One can obtain mucosal biopsies and exclude other pathologies. Colonoscopy demonstrates mucosal edema, contact bleeding, friable mucosa, and necrotic ulcers.

MANAGEMENT

After the diagnosis has been established and the clinical examination does not suggest intestinal gangrene or perforation, the patient is treated expectantly (5,6). Generally, if the patient has abdominal pain, parenteral fluids are administered, empiric broad-spectrum antibiotics are given systematically to cover aerobic and anaerobic colonic bacteria, and the bowel is placed at rest. Cardiac function and oxygen delivery are optimized, and medications that may contribute to mesenteric vasoconstriction or colonic ischemia are withdrawn as soon as possible. Appropriate management of patients seen acutely, during or soon after the ischemic episode, requires serial roentgenographic or endoscopic evaluations of the colon and continued monitoring of pertinent serum chemistries, at least including the hemoglobin, white blood cell count, and electrolytes. There should be no attempt to prepare the bowel for surgery because this may precipitate a colonic perforation or toxic dilation of the colon. If partial-thickness ischemia is identified, the therapy will be similar. In most cases of colonic ischemia, signs and symptoms of the illness subside within 24–48 hours and there is a virtual complete clinical and roentgenographic resolution within 1–2 weeks.

Clinical deterioration despite conservative therapy, manifest as signs and symptoms of sepsis, peritoneal irritation, free intra-abdominal air, or extensive gangrene visualized at endoscopy, *indicates colonic infarction and mandates expeditious laparotomy and segmental colon resection.* Persistent concerns about remaining or ongoing ischemia mandate a planned second-look laparotomy as well. Published reviews of surgical therapy indicate that all patients with colonic gangrene should have a colostomy or ileostomy and a primary anastomosis should not be attempted. If the ileum and transverse colon is viable and well vascularized, gross contamination is limited, and the patient has experienced no recent hemodynamic instability, we would perform an ileocolostomy in patients with right-sided ischemic colitis. Approximately 75% of patients with spontaneous ischemic colitis have left-sided colonic involvement, and these patients almost invariably should undergo colon resection with a proximal stoma and distal mucous fistula or Hartmann pouch.

Certain patients will present late with full-thickness gangrene involving variable amounts of colon with signs and symptoms of a catastrophic abdominal illness including sepsis and shock. Shock-associated ischemic colitis initially may be a much more subtle process and frequently will be diagnosed only at the time of exploratory laparotomy. Many of these patients are already hospitalized for a concomitant critical illness and may not manifest abdominal pain because of their associated debilitated state. In addition to abdominal pain, the findings of marked abdominal distention, radiographic evidence of a nonresolving ileus, and clinical deterioration with fever and leukocytosis should augment suspicion that ischemic colitis is present. A number of patients have concurrent medical conditions, such as cardiovascular disease, diabetes mellitus, renal insufficiency, and hematologic disorders, present alone or in combination.

Ischemic colitis after aortic surgery is a potentially lethal complication. A high index of suspicion, early recognition with endoscopy, and urgent operative intervention, when indicated, are essential to decrease the accompanying high morbidity and mortality rates associated with this disease process. The overall incidence of clinically evident ischemic colitis, determined retrospectively, has been between 1 and 2% after elective aortic reconstruction (7). *Intestinal ischemia may occur after abdominal aortic reconstruction for occlusive disease but is more likely to occur after repair of aneurysmal disease,* presumably related to the status of the mesenteric collateral circulation. Morbidity and mortality rates parallel the degree of severity of bowel ischemia. Transmural involvement portends a 50–100%

mortality rate (8). When ischemia is limited to the muscularis mucosa, mortality is reduced but morbidity from late stricture of the colon may result.

Signs and symptoms may be difficult to detect in the patient who has undergone recent major abdominal surgery, with altered abdominal findings and cardiovascular physiology and an altered mental status caused by recent general anesthesia. Elicitation of abdominal findings may be difficult. Grossly bloody or guaiac-positive diarrhea is the most common early manifestation of ischemic colitis and usually occurs within 1–2 days after aortic surgery, although it may occur as late as 2 weeks postoperatively. Diarrhea is estimated to occur in approximately two-thirds to three-fourths of those patients with ischemic colitis after aortic reconstruction and is bloody in approximately one-half of these individuals (9). Metabolic acidosis, leukocytosis, progressive oliguria, tachycardia, and hypotension also can develop with particularly aggressive forms of ischemic colitis. Various radiologic studies have been used in the past but provide little additional information compared with direct inspection of the colonic mucosa.

The aggressiveness of treatment required to resolve this often fatal complication of aortic reconstruction is directly proportional to the severity of the ischemic colitis. For early, mild ischemic colitis, nonoperative therapy, as described previously, incorporating intravenous fluids, bowel rest, and broad-spectrum antibiotic treatment, is continued until the ischemic injury heals. Ischemic colitis that progresses, despite supportive measures, is evidenced by the persistence of diarrhea, which may become bloody, deterioration of vital signs, worsening of abdominal signs and symptoms, and progressive deterioration by serial endoscopic examinations. This scenario requires immediate operative treatment with resection of the involved colon. Primary anastomosis is contraindicated because of the potential danger of leak.

A rare fulminating form of colonic ischemia, referred to as total colonic ischemia involving all or most of the colon and rectum, has been identified in a few patients (10). These patients experience the sudden onset of toxic universal colitis portrayed by bleeding, fever, severe diarrhea, abdominal pain, and tenderness, often with signs of peritonitis. They uniformly have sustained deleterious systemic insults that may render the entire colon susceptible to ischemia. *The clinical course typically accelerates rapidly.* The management of this condition, similar to that for other forms of fulminating colitis, necessitates total abdominal colectomy with an ileostomy. Further clinical deterioration mandates proctoscopy to evaluate any ischemia that may progress to involve the rectum. *A second-stage proctectomy has been required for some patients,* within 1 month of the original surgery. The histologic appearance is a combination of ischemic changes and severe colitis.

CONCLUSIONS

Despite the fact that ischemic colitis is the most common form of gastrointestinal ischemia, it still remains largely underdiagnosed. It occurs most frequently in individuals with no antecedent medical illnesses. It also represents one of the many disorders that is a consequence of shock and must be suspected appropriately in these patients. *The most significant factors related to improved outcome in the therapy of colonic ischemia are prompt recognition and aggressive management.* Early diagnosis by colonoscopy and interval clinical and endoscopic evaluation, to ascertain progression or regression of the ischemic process, should promote earlier successful diagnosis of full-thickness necrosis warranting expeditious surgical intervention. The operative therapy for ischemic colitis, whether associated with stricture or gangrene, includes colon resection. In the evaluation of patients with abdominal pain and tenderness, the history often will not allow differentiation between ischemia and diverticulitis. Pain associated with urinary symptoms or pneumaturia should sway one toward diverticulitis. Physical examination often is misleading. However, patients with diverticulitis rarely have bleeding and patients with ischemia rarely have a palpable mass. Imaging may be helpful. An abscess or phlegmon points toward diverticulitis. Thumb-printing and transverse ridging suggests ischemia. Colonoscopy is valuable in differentiating colitis (ischemic or inflammatory bowel disease); however, diagnosis may be limited due to poor bowel preparation. Laparoscopy as a diagnostic tool may be misleading unless full-thickness infarction secondary to gangrenous ischemic colitis occurs. All too often, the diagnosis is dictated by the success of nonoperative therapy, findings at laparotomy, or the occurrence of a delayed stricture. Due to many patients presenting with abdominal pain and tenderness who are successfully treated nonoperatively, and with the high incidence of diverticulosis in the advancing age population, it is difficult to know exactly the number of patients who are diagnosed accurately with either ischemic colitis or diverticulitis.

EDITORIAL COMMENTS

We have tended to see two characteristic populations of patients with ischemic colitis, broadly associated with outpatient or inpatient status. Patients "coming off the street" commonly present with a picture reminiscent of Marston's (11) classic descriptions: they have symptoms of self-limited abdominal pain, rectal bleeding, and mild left-sided abdominal tenderness, without evidence of significant peritonitis. These patients could include middle-aged females on hormone replacement without a history of vascular disease (12); radiographs classically demonstrate thumbprinting in the splenic flexure, and symptoms resolve quickly without the use of antibiotics or hospitalization (Fig. 3.1). Their presentation resembles that of patients with uncomplicated diverticulitis, who typically have left lower quadrant tenderness, leukocytosis, and at least a several-day history of irregular bowel habits, but without rectal bleeding. Inflammatory bowel disease also must be considered (13,14). A CT scan often is diagnostic. We are not prone to perform colonoscopy initially for these patients because the procedure is not recommended for acute diverticulitis and probably would add little to the initial treatment of ischemic colitis. On the other hand, if the CT scan is normal, later colonoscopy could be performed to rule out other segmental colonic disorders.

Much less frequently, patients present to the emergency room with a catastrophic illness, including generalized abdominal pain, tenderness, and heme-positive stools. Ischemic colitis with transmural changes in this group necessitates urgent abdominal colectomy. These patients should have stomas because they are at risk of anastomotic leaks.

The most problematic population, encountered more frequently by colorectal and general surgeons, are the sick, hospitalized patients (15,16) in intensive care units or on medical floors at times recovering from aortic aneurysmectomy (17–19) or other major cardiovascular procedures. These patients are unlikely to have diverticulitis, especially when rectal bleeding accompanies abdominal pain. Abdominal examination is difficult because of the recent incision and a variable mental status, perhaps involving a ventilator. Patchy or confluent ischemia of the left colon precipitated by hypotension, division of the inferior mesenteric artery, a previous history of peripheral vascular surgery, and other factors is best detected by sigmoidoscopy/colonoscopy at the bedside (Fig. 3.2) (20). Any segment of the colon can be involved; if the diagnosis is encountered in the operating room, stomas in general are favored over attempts at anastomosis.

CT examination also can add valuable information in the inpatient population, especially if there is some suspicion of complicated diverticulitis or of perforation (Figs. 3.3 and 3.4). In such cases, endoscopy should not be performed unless the CT scan is nondiagnostic or raises suspicion of

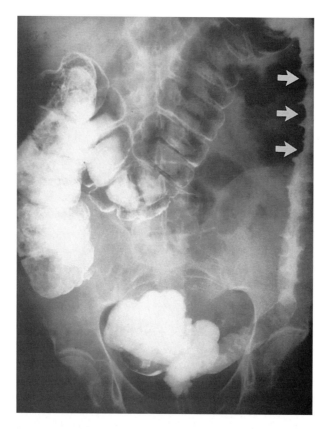

Figure 3.1.   A postevacuation view after a barium enema in a patient with ischemic colitis involving the left colon. Marked thumbprinting (arrows) is present.

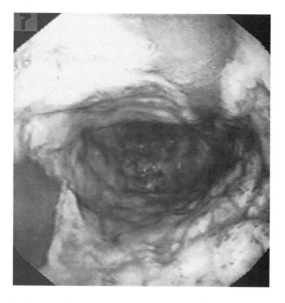

Figure 3.2.   This endoscopic picture of a patient after aortic aneurysmectomy demonstrates patchy necrosis of the mucosa.

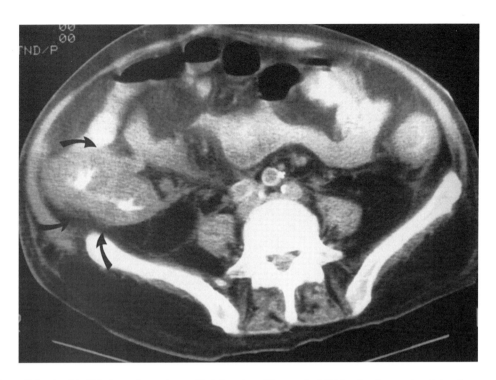

Figure 3.3. In this CT view of a patient with ischemic colitis, marked thickening is seen involving the cecum (arrows). The patient had arterial disease, and a prosthetic graft is seen.

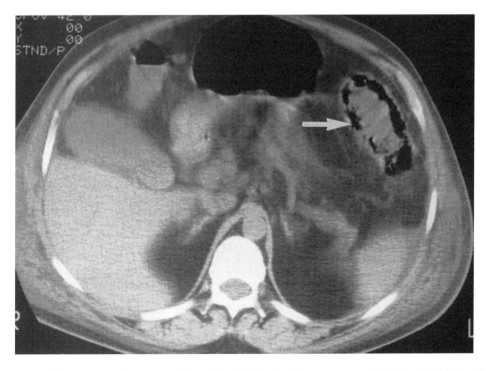

Figure 3.4. This CT view of a patient with an infarcted left colon shows pneumatosis in the wall of the involved colon (arrow).

possible ischemic colitis. We would urgently perform endoscopy after aortic surgery at the slightest hint of ischemia.

We have seen some cases of rectal ischemia as well, especially in patients who have had previous peripheral vascular procedures. In this situation, it may be valuable to leave a Hartmann rectal segment open with transrectal drainage rather than attempt abdominoperipheral resection in these septic patients.

REFERENCES

1. Trinh TD, Jones B, Fishman EK. Amyloidosis of the colon presenting as ischemic colitis: a case report and review of the literature. Gastrointest Radiol 1991;16:133–136. *Describes 21 cases of abnormal barium enemas in patients with amyloidosis of the colon. Luminal narrowing and loss of haustrations were the most common findings; these changes may have been ischemic, at least in part.*
2. Brandt LJ, Boley SJ. Colonic ischemia. Surg Clin North Am 1992;72:203–229. *The number of patients with ischemic colitis will increase with aging of the population. Wider use of colonoscopy will lead to earlier diagnosis. Efforts should be made to identify high-risk groups for the illness.*
3. Landreneau RJ, Fry WJ. The right colon as a target organ of nonocclusive mesenteric ischemia. Arch Surg 1990;125:591–594. *The authors speculate that a proximal mesenteric steal involving more proximal branches of the SMA circulation may occur during periods of hypotension.*
4. Longo WE, Ballantyne GH, Gusberg RJ. Ischemic colitis: patterns and prognosis. Dis Colon Rectum 1992;35:726–730. *Elderly and diabetic patients and individuals with ischemia following aortic surgery or hypotension have a poor prognosis.*
5. Fitzgerald SF, Kaminski DL. Ischemic colitis. Semin Colon Rectal Surg 1993;4:222–228. *Ischemic colitis is one of many disorders that can be precipitated by shock and reperfusion. Early diagnosis, frequently by colonoscopy, is a significant factor in improving outcome.*
6. Kaleya RN, Boley SJ. Colonic ischemia. Perspect Colon Rectal Surg 1990;3:62–81. *A succinct review with 20 references.*
7. Barnett MG, Longo WE. Intestinal ischemia after aortic surgery. Semin Colon Rectal Surg 1993;4:229–234. *This review details the colonoscopic findings and the potential lethality of this illness.*
8. Stamos JM. Colonic ischemia. In: Mazier WP, Luchtefeld MA, Levine DH, et al, eds. Surgery of the colon, rectum, and anus. Philadelphia: WB Saunders, 1995:705–713.
9. Maupin GE, Rimar SD, Villalba M. Ischemic colitis following abdominal aortic reconstruction for ruptured aneurysm. A 10-year experience. Am Surg 1989;55:378–380. *Twenty-seven percent of 71 patients surviving operation for ruptured abdominal aortic aneurysms developed ischemic colitis, with a mortality of 58%. Routine flexible sigmoidoscopy is recommended early in the postoperative course before clinical sepsis occurs.*
10. Welch GH, Shearer MG, Imrie CW, et al. Total colonic ischemia. Dis Colon Rectum 1986;29:410–412. *Describes three cases of total colonic ischemia; two of the onsets were insidious.*
11. Marston A, Pheilss MY, Thomas ML, et al. Ischemic colitis. Gut 1966;7:1–15. *A useful clinical description of 16 cases of spontaneous colonic ischemia. The cases are graded by severity.*
12. Barcewicz PA, Welch JP. Ischemic colitis in young adult patients. Dis Colon Rectum 1980;23:109–114. *Examines the clinical course of a group of young adults. A possible association of ischemic colitis with hormone intake is mentioned.*
13. Marston A. Ischemia. Clin Gastroenterol 1985;14:847–862. *In the acute phase, ischemic colitis must be differentiated from acute diverticulitis; in the chronic stages, it can be confused with ulcerative colitis or Crohn's disease.*
14. Eisenberg RL, Montgomery CK, Margulis AR. Colitis in the elderly: ischemic colitis mimicking ulcerative and granulomatous colitis. Am J Roentgenol 1979;133:1113–1118. *A study of eight patients older than 60 years of age. The clinical history and response to treatment may be a more useful way to differentiate ischemic colitis from Crohn's disease and ulcerative colitis than pathologic sections or radiographs.*
15. Boerner RM, Fried DB, Warshauer DM, et al. Pneumatosis intestinalis. Two case reports and a retrospective review of the literature from 1985 to 1995. Dig Dis Sci 1996;41:2272–2285. *An excellent clinical description of the differential diagnosis and etiologies of this curious entity; with 131 references.*
16. Carr ND, Wells S, Haboubi NY, et al. Ischemic dilation of the colon. Ann R Coll Surg Engl 1986;68:264–266. *Nine patients with spontaneous ischemic colitis developed colonic dilation and presented difficult diagnostic problems.*
17. Welling RE, Roedersheimer R, Arbaugh JJ, et al. Ischemic colitis following repair of ruptured abdominal aortic aneurysm. Arch Surg 1985;120:1368–1370. *Six of seven patients died; all had resection of necrotic colon within the first postoperative week.*
18. Hagihara PF, Ernst CB, Griffen WO Jr. Incidence of ischemic colitis following abdominal aortic reconstruction. Surg Gynecol Obstet 1979;149:571–573. *One hundred sixty-three patients had colonoscopy following elective or urgent reconstruction of the abdominal aorta; 11 had ischemic colitis.*
19. Fiddian-Green RG, Amelin PM, Herrmann JB, et al. Prediction of the development of sigmoid ischemia on the day of aortic operations. Arch Surg 1986;121:654–660. *The duration of an abnormally low intramural pH on the day of operation was the best predictor for symptoms and signs of ischemic colitis and for postoperative mortality.*
20. Siegenthaler M, Vignati P, Rosson R. Lower endoscopy in the critically ill. Presented at Society of American Gastrointestinal Endoscopic Surgeons (SAGES), San Diego, CA, March 1997. *Eighty-eight colonoscopies were performed over a 4-year period. The clinical indications were possible ischemia in 41% and lower gastrointestinal bleeding in 39%. The diagnostic yield for ischemia was 86%.*

4 Colon Cancer Versus Diverticulitis

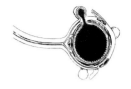

Richard L. Whelan, MD
Juan P. Umana, MD

KEY POINTS

- Diverticulitis and colon cancer may coexist in the same patient
- Rectal bleeding with diverticular disease should be evaluated with endoscopy
- CT imaging is the most likely test to distinguish between diverticulitis and perforated cancer; however, many of the inflammatory changes can be seen in both
- Only evaluate sigmoid and left colon if doing contrast study in acute setting
- Barium enema less sensitive than colonoscopy in detecting neoplasms
- Endoscopy has limited value in the acute setting; however, it is the procedure of choice to visualize the sigmoid 6–8 weeks after acute attack has resolved
- Surgery may be needed if colonoscopy cannot traverse diseased segment

ILLUSTRATIVE CASE

A 68-year-old man presented to the emergency room with a 3-day history of left lower quadrant abdominal pain and discomfort associated with diarrheal bowel movements. He had no previous history of similar symptoms and no other recent change in bowel habits. In the emergency room, the patient was noted to have a temperature of 40°C, a tender left lower quadrant mass, and a hemoccult positive stool. Initial white blood count was 18,000, hematocrit was 36%, blood urea nitrogen was 44, and creatinine was 1.4. The patient was admitted to the hospital, hydrated, placed on bowel rest, and administered intravenous antibiotics. A computed tomography (CT) scan of the abdomen and pelvis was obtained, which demonstrated sigmoid diverticulitis with an associated phlegmon. Over the next 5 days, the patient improved, he became afebrile, and his abdominal pain and tenderness subsided. He was discharged on oral ciprofloxacin and Flagyl to complete a 14-day course of therapy.

Six weeks later, the patient felt fine but still suffered from intermittent diarrhea and had a vague fullness in the left lower quadrant on examination. Sigmoidoscopic examination was attempted but unsuccessful secondary to luminal narrowing and patient discomfort. Therefore, a barium enema was performed to evaluate the sigmoid mucosa. Extensive diverticulosis was noted with mild spasm. Unfortunately, the radiologist could not be sure whether a neoplastic lesion was present in the sigmoid colon. Considering the uncertainty of the patient's workup, as well as the persistent change in bowel habits, heme-positive stool, and mild anemia, the patient underwent an exploration with sigmoid resection. At the time of surgery, the patient did have a 3-cm perforated carcinoma in the midsigmoid colon.

DISCUSSION

The differential diagnosis in previously uninvestigated patients with left lower quadrant tenderness and an abdominal mass includes diverticulitis with abscess or phlegmon and perforated colon cancer. Because the treatment of these two disorders is considerably different, it is important to establish a diagnosis early in the course of illness. Many patients with complicated diverticular disease can be managed conservatively using antibiotics and interventional techniques to percutaneously drain localized collections. After the inflammation has resolved, often several months later, a more thorough elective evaluation can be performed. At that time, a decision can be made regarding surgery. However, a patient strongly suspected of harboring a perforated colon malignancy will, with few exceptions, come to surgery much earlier in the course of the illness. Most perforations that occur in patients with colon tumors are localized (1,2). If left untreated, these contained perforations may generalize. The survival rates following resection for patients with localized perforation in the absence of distant metastases is approximately 45%, whereas only 7% of patients with generalized perforations survive (2).

Therefore, it is important to make an early attempt to differentiate between diverticular disease and neoplasm in these patients. On purely clinical grounds, it is very difficult to make this distinction (3,4). The diagnostic tests at our disposal include: *(a)* plain abdominal radiographs, *(b)* contrast enemas, *(c)* CT, *(d)* sigmoidoscopy or colonoscopy, and *(e)* ultrasonography. Currently, contrast enemas and CT scans are the most commonly performed tests in this setting. Magnetic resonance imaging (MRI) and radionuclide imaging are not commonly used for this purpose. Following are a brief discussion and a review of the results of each test in this setting.

Plain Films

Plain films usually are obtained early in the evaluation and are useful because they may reveal a pneumoperitoneum, ileus, complete or partial bowel obstruction, or a mass effect. An erect chest film is the best means of detecting a pneumoperitoneum. However, plain radiographs are not useful in establishing the diagnosis of or differentiating between diverticulitis and carcinoma.

Contrast Enemas

Contrast studies, including both barium and water-soluble contrast enemas, are very useful in the setting of suspected diverticulitis and are performed without bowel preparation. In general, an inferior study with less mucosal detail is obtained when water-soluble contrast is used instead of barium. *However, extravasation of water-soluble contrast is far less dangerous than extravasated barium, and for this reason, the former is often used in this setting.* In the acute setting, air contrast is not used because of concerns that even low-pressure air insufflation may lead to perforation of a weakened diverticulum. Therefore, single contrast studies are performed most often.

It is not the goal of the study to examine the entire large bowel. The goal is to evaluate the sigmoid and possibly the descending colon for causes of left lower quadrant abdominal pain and suspected mass. The finding of sigmoid diverticula in such a patient suggests that the clinical diagnosis of diverticulitis is correct. The possible radiologic findings in a patient with diverticulitis include: *(a)* diverticulosis with or without spasm, *(b)* sigmoid irregularity, *(c)* pericolic inflammation or mass effect, *(d)* near complete or complete obstruction, or *(e)* extravasation of contrast via perforation. Possible radiologic findings in patients without diverticular disease include: *(a)* normal examination, *(b)* partially or fully obstructing lesions, *(c)* polyps, and *(d)* colitic changes(loss of haustral markings, ulcerations, etc.). *It is important for the radiologist to be aware of the suspected diagnosis.* The radiologist should instill the contrast under low pressure and should carefully watch for extravasation, which, if found, would lead to immediate termination of the examination.

How often is the clinical diagnosis of acute diverticulitis ultimately proved correct? Hiltunen et al reported that only 47% of their 53 study patients with the initial clinical diagnosis of acute diverticulitis actually had radiologic evidence supporting the diagnosis on early water-soluble contrast enemas (5). The findings in the remaining patients included: *(a)* normal colon, 24.5%; *(b)* diverticulosis without evidence of inflammation or mass, 19%; *(c)* cancer, 7.6%; *(d)* ischemic colitis, 1.9%. The most common findings in the acute diverticulitis group, beside the presence of diverticula, were a spastic segment of sigmoid (92%) and intramural spread of contrast (24%). Two of the three cancers were definitively diagnosed on the water-soluble contrast enema, whereas the third required endoscopy to confirm the diagnosis.

It can be very difficult to differentiate between carcinoma and diverticulitis. Luminal narrowing is seen commonly with both disorders. The finding of diverticula in a narrowed segment of colon suggests diverticular disease but does not rule out a malignancy. The following radiologic criteria are believed to be characteristic of diverticulitis and helpful in distinguishing diverticular disease from carcinoma: *(a)* intact mucosal lining throughout the narrowed segment; *(b)* a gradual transition from normal to diseased colon (tapered, not shouldered, borders); *(c)* an intramural mass deforming the colon lumen but with intact overlying mucosa; and *(d)* a lengthy diseased segment, 6 cm or longer. It is important that the full length of the narrowed segment be visualized to make an accurate diagnosis.

How accurate are contrast enemas in detecting neoplastic lesions in patients with concomitant diverticular disease? Not surprisingly, air-contrast barium enema is more sensitive in patients with less than 15 diverticula than for those with more numerous diverticula (6–8). Boulos et al reported that double contrast studies were inaccurate in 43% of patients with diverticular disease in regard to the detection of cancers and adenomas (8). Schnyder et al, looking at a similar population of patients, reported that associated neoplasms were correctly diagnosed in only 50% of patients (3). *Most errors were false-negative interpretations.* Dean and Newell found that the barium enema was correct in predicting associated carcinoma in 44% of patients (four of nine) with both diverticular and malignant disease (9) (Figs. 4.1 through 4.3).

Sigmoidoscopy and Colonoscopy

Early endoscopic evaluation of the colon in patients believed to have acute diverticulitis may be dangerous for several reasons. Firstly, it usually is very difficult to pass the scope through the sigmoid segment in question due to narrowing or fixation. To definitively rule out a carcinoma, it is necessary to fully traverse the area of concern (Fig. 4.4). There also is concern that the inflamed bowel may be perforated by the scope tip or the bowing shaft of the scope during insertion. Finally, insufflating the bowel to perform the examination may result in a pressure-related perforation of a weakened diverticulum. *Most authorities agree that, for these reasons, sigmoidoscopy in the setting of suspected acute diverticulitis is contraindicated.*

Patients whose acute infections are successfully treated medically should undergo either a flexible sigmoidoscopy, colonoscopy, or barium enema 6–8 weeks after the acute episode to fully evaluate the diseased segment. Numerous studies have demonstrated that barium enema in patients with diverticulosis is less sensitive than sigmoidoscopy in detecting neoplasms of the sigmoid and rectum (6,7,10) (Fig. 4.5). As mentioned, to exclude the possibility of a neoplasm, it is necessary to fully traverse the diverticular segment with the scope. Endoscopic examination can be very difficult in the setting of diverticular disease because of luminal narrowing and fixation of bowel loops. The failure rate of colonoscopy in the general population of patients with diverticular disease is 16–17% (6,11). The incompletion rate rises when the population is limited to patients with severe disease. Dean and Newell reported a colonoscopy failure rate of 47% in a group of 36 patients in whom barium enema raised the possibility of a cancer in a diverticular segment (9). *When it is not possible to fully traverse the diseased segment of bowel, a malignancy cannot be excluded and surgery must be considered.* Some have suggested that patients with severe diverticular disease should undergo both sigmoidoscopy and air-contrast barium enema to improve the neoplasm detection rate (6).

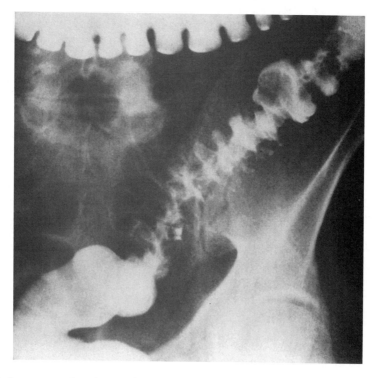

Figure 4.1. Barium enema view shows a long segment of diverticulitis. A polypoid mass is present, which proved to be a carcinoma. (Reprinted with permission from Schnyder P, Moss A A, Thoeni RF, et al. A double-blind study of radiologic accuracy in diverticulitis, diverticulosis, and carcinoma of the sigmoid colon. J Clin Gastroenterol 1979;1:55–66.)

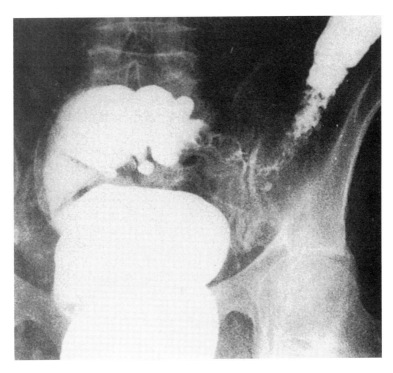

Figure 4.2. This patient had a carcinoma that created an irregular polypoid mass just distal to an area of sigmoid diverticulitis. (Reprinted with permission from Schnyder P, Moss AA, Thoeni RF, et al. A double-blind study of radiologic accuracy in diverticulitis, diverticulosis, and carcinoma of the sigmoid colon. J Clin Gastroenterol 1979;1:55–66.)

Computed Tomography

CT is widely used in the diagnosis of both simple and complicated diverticulitis. With one exception, there is a general consensus in the radiologic literature regarding the merits of CT in this setting. Many believe that CT is the radiologic procedure of choice for patients suspected of having diverticulitis (12–17). The CT criteria for the diagnosis of acute diverticulitis are: *(a)* the presence of diverticula, *(b)* localized colonic wall thickening (>4–5 mm), *(c)* adjacent pericolic fat inflammation, and *(d)* possibly an associated collection (16). Neff et al proposed a CT-based staging system (17). Cho et al in a prospective study found that CT was 93% sensitive in diagnosing patients with diverticulitis (16). In addition to providing information about the colonic lumen and wall, CT also provides information regarding the mesentery, adjacent structures, and other intra-abdominal organs. In the study by Cho et al, alternative diagnoses were offered in 69% of patients who were shown by CT not to have diverticular disease. For CT to be useful, the bowel must be well opacified with intraluminal contrast. *The best studies are obtained by giving gastrointestinal contrast orally and also by instilling contrast or air transrectally.* Is it possible to distinguish between diverticulitis with an abscess and a perforated colon cancer using CT? This can be an exceedingly difficult task using clinical criteria alone. Padidar et al recently proposed several CT criteria that they believe are helpful in differentiating colon cancers from diverticulitis (18). They performed a retrospective comparison of the CT scans of 69 patients with surgically proven diverticulitis to the scans of 29 patients with proven sigmoid colon carcinoma. They specifically looked for differences in the appearance of the mesentery. They found that fluid at the root of the mesentery was present in 36% of those with diverticulitis, whereas it was present in only 10% of the patients with cancer ($P < .001$). Likewise, mesenteric vascular engorgement was found in 29% of patients with diverticulitis and in none of the patients with cancer ($P < .001$). They suggest that the presence of one or both of these signs may help distinguish between the two diagnoses (Figs. 4.6 and 4.7). However, one major flaw of this study is the fact that only 3 of the 29 colon cancers used for comparison were perforated. The scans from these three perforated tumors were the only tumor scans that showed fluid at the root of the mesentery. Therefore, the proposed radiologic signs may be nonspecific signs of mesenteric inflammation. *By relying on these signs, radiologists might misdiagnose perforated cancers; unfortunately, this involves the group of patients most in need of prompt recognition.*

Hulnick et al have shown that it is possible to detect perforated tumors via CT (4). In a retrospective study of 39 patients with perforated colonic tumors, CT correctly diagnosed the problem in 95% of patients, whereas with contrast enema, the correct diagnosis was made in only 50% of patients. In 41% of patients, CT also diagnosed associated intra-abdominal metastases. Only in the detection of enteroenteric fistulas were contrast enemas superior to CT. Despite these encouraging results, it usually is difficult to distinguish between a perforated tumor and complex diverticular disease.

In conclusion, *a strong case can be made for using CT as the initial radiologic test for patients suspected of having complex diverticular disease.*

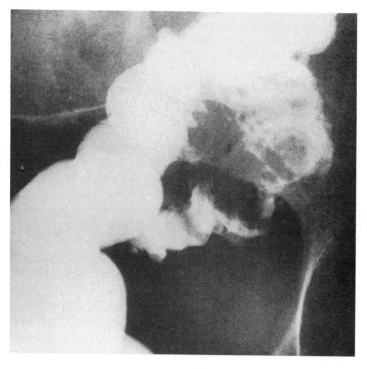

Figure 4.3. A polypoid mass lying within a short segment of sigmoid diverticulitis proved to be edematous mucosa; no malignancy was present. (Reprinted with permission from Schnyder P, Moss AA, Thoeni RF, et al. A double-blind study of radiologic accuracy in diverticulitis, diverticulosis, and carcinoma of the sigmoid colon. J Clin Gastroenterol 1979;1:55–66.)

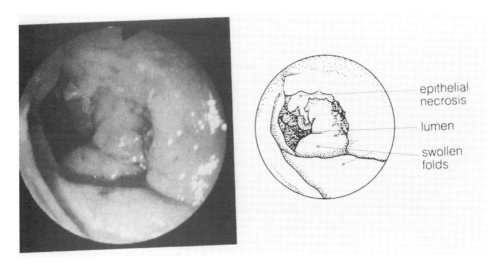

Figure 4.4. Endoscopic view of a colon with resolving acute diverticulitis. Some edema and epithelial destruction remain. (Reprinted with permission from Silverstein FE, Tytgat GN. Colon III: diverticular disease, vascular malformations, and other colonic abnormalities. In: Atlas of gastrointestinal endoscopy. J. B. Lippincott, Philadelphia, 1991:12.5) [Ref. 34].

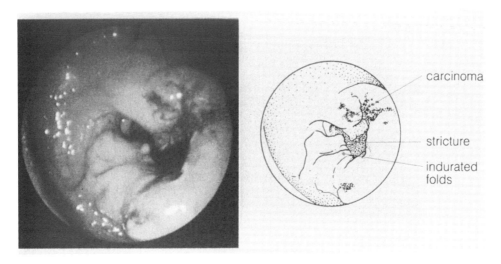

Figure 4.5. View of a stenosing sigmoid carcinoma with submucosal spread of tumor. The folds at the entrance of the stricture were firm and indurated. The laser had been used at an earlier time to open the stenosis. (Reprinted with permission from Silverstein FE, Tytgat GN. Colon III: diverticular disease, vascular malformations, and other colonic abnormalities. In: Atlas of gastrointestinal endoscopy. J. B. Lippincott, Philadelphia, 1991:12.5) [Ref. 34].

Transabdominal Ultrasonography

There have been only a limited number of studies performed regarding the use of transabdominal ultrasonography (USG) in the diagnosis of acute diverticulitis (19–22). In theory, ultrasound should be helpful because it provides information about the bowel wall and surrounding structures. However, it is highly operator-dependent and some clinicians have found it to be unreliable (20). Proponents report that high-resolution real-time sonography permits identification of thickened bowel wall, inflamed surrounding omentum or pericolic fat, associated intramesenteric and adjacent collections, often the diverticula themselves, and luminal narrowing. To perform the examination, the transducer is compressed against the anterior abdominal wall, which will elicit tenderness in an inflamed area. Schwerk et al included the presence of local tenderness to gradual compression as one of the necessary criteria for the diagnosis of acute diverticulitis in their study (21). The diagnosis, therefore, relies on both USG and clinical findings. The sensitivity and specificity of USG in detecting acute diverticulitis in Schwerk's study using these criteria were 98%. Less spectacular results were reported in a similar study by Verbanck et al, in which the sensitivity was 84.6% and the specificity was 80.3% (22). These results are encouraging, but clearly additional studies will be needed to determine the future role of USG in the acute setting.

Although it is possible to make a case for the use of USG in diagnosing simple diverticulitis (23,24), there is no evidence to support the notion that USG can differentiate between complicated diverticulitis and perforated cancer. One of the two false-positive patients in the study by Schwerk et al, in fact, had a perforated sigmoid cancer. As is the case with CT, several of the USG findings are not caused by the cancer or diverticulitis but are due to inflammation or infection resulting from a perforation.

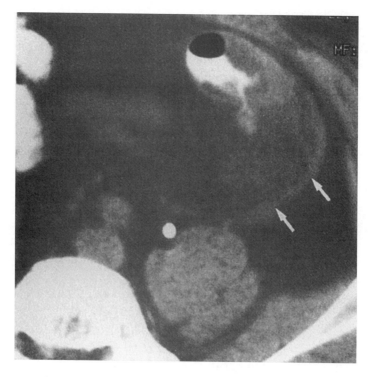

Figure 4.6. Contrast-enhanced CT view shows linear collection of fluid (arrows) at the base of the sigmoid mesentery in a case of diverticulitis. (Reprinted with permission from Padidar AM, Jeffrey RB, Mindelzun RE, et al. Differentiating sigmoid diverticulitis from carcinoma on CT scans: mesenteric inflammation suggests diverticulitis. Am J Roentgenol 1994;163:81–83.)

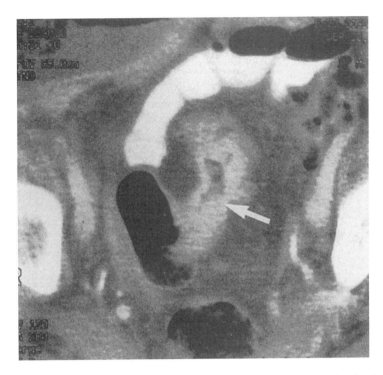

Figure 4.7. This CT scan shows a sigmoid carcinoma (arrow) that was not perforated at the time of operation. There is no fluid at the root of the mesentery, and there is a lack of vascular engorgement. (Reprinted with permission from Padidar AM, Jeffrey RB, Mindelzun RE, et al. Differentiating sigmoid diverticulitis from carcinoma on CT scans: mesenteric inflammation suggests diverticulitis. Am J Roentgenol 1994;163:81–83.)

Endoluminal Ultrasonography

Rigid transrectal and flexible endoluminal USG is being used for patients with rectal tumors to determine the depth of tumor invasion and the presence of lymph node metastases. Colonic tumors also can be evaluated using either a special scope with a transducer at its tip or via a small transducer that is passed through the working channel of a flexible endoscope. The precise role of endoluminal USG in the evaluation of colonic tumors is not currently clear, although the technique is promising. The use of these techniques for patients with suspected complicated diverticular disease will, most likely, be quite limited for the same reasons that colonoscopy is avoided in this setting (i.e., the risk of perforation and inability to examine the entire segment).

Other Diagnostic Tests

By using air to distend the bowel, it is possible to detect intestinal wall thickening as well as fistulas via MRI (25). In the future, MRI may play a role in the diagnosis of both simple and complex diverticulitis. Currently, however, MRI is not commonly used for this purpose. A literature search revealed not a single study concerning the use of MRI for diverticular disease.

Radionuclide scans can be used to identify abdominal infections and areas of inflammation. At this time, radiolabeled leukocytes are most commonly used for this purpose. Technetium-99 (^{99}Tc) labeled leukocytes are used for the diagnosis of acute infection, whereas indium-111 (^{111}In) is used for the evaluation of suspected chronic infection and inflammation (26). The imaging scan is performed within 2 hours after injection with Technetium-99 Hexamethylpropylene amine oxime labeled leukocytes; this is an attractive feature when evaluating acutely ill patients. Radionuclide scans, although sensitive, cannot differentiate between infection and inflammation. Furthermore, they provide no information about the bowel wall. Therefore, it is not likely that nuclear medicine techniques would be very useful when trying to differentiate between perforated diverticulitis and perforated colonic tumors. Presently, radionuclide scans are not frequently used in the setting of diverticular disease.

ARE COLON CANCERS MORE COMMON IN PATIENTS WITH DIVERTICULAR DISEASE?

There is no doubt that adenocarcinomas can arise in a diverticular segment of colon. Rarely, a tumor may actually develop within a diverticulum (27). Boulos et al reported that the incidence of neoplastic lesions in patients with diverticular disease is 34%: adenomas in 27.6% and carcinomas in 6.6% (8). The peak incidence was 40% and was noted in the patients between 60 and 79 years of age. Interestingly, rectal bleeding was a presenting complaint in 38% of patients without a neoplasm and 61% of patients with neoplasms ($P < .05$). The incidence of abdominal pain or a change in bowel habits in the two groups was not significantly different. The authors conclude that *if bleeding occurs in patients with known diverticular disease, then it should be investigated with either sigmoidoscopy or colonoscopy* (8). Hunt reported that in patients with diverticular disease who reported persistent rectal bleeding, there was an 11% incidence of carcinoma and a 14% incidence of adenomas (28).

Other investigators have found that the incidence of colon cancer in patients with complex diverticular disease ranges from 11 to 22% (11,29–32). The incidence of adenomas in the same population ranged from 16 to 21% (29,31). Stefansson et al, in a large retrospective study of more than 7000 patients with diverticular disease, found approximately a twofold increase in the incidence of left-sided colon cancer (33).

CONCLUSIONS

It is very difficult to distinguish between diverticular disease and perforated left- sided colon cancer. However, for the reasons outlined above, it is important to try to make this distinction. Patients with left lower quadrant tenderness and an associated mass are initially best evaluated by CT. Careful transrectal insufflation of contrast and/or air should be mandatory when CT is performed in the setting of suspected diverticular disease. Patients suspected of having diverticulitis who are without a left lower quadrant mass can be well evaluated by either CT or limited contrast enema. Endoscopy should be avoided in the acute setting. Patients who are successfully treated medically should undergo a thorough elective colon evaluation 4–8 weeks after the resolution of their acute process. Either colonoscopy or air-contrast barium enema plus flexible sigmoidoscopy can be used for this evaluation of the large bowel.

It is important to remember that it is possible for a patient to have both diverticular disease and cancer. In fact, there may be an increased incidence of colon cancer in patients with diverticular disease. Therefore, it is necessary to periodically screen all patients with diverticular disease.

EDITORIAL COMMENTS

Colon cancer and diverticular disease are both common; they frequently occur together, and it may be difficult to detect both with diagnostic evaluation. This is of particular importance, because an obscure carcinoma must not be overlooked. In a comprehensive discussion, in the era before CT and flexible endoscopy, the eminent radiologist Richard Schatzki said: "...there are still cases in which diverticulitis lends to such deformities as to make its differentiation from neoplastic disease extremely hard. In such a case one often asks oneself whether it would not be much better to transfer the responsibility to the surgeon and have him solve the problem..."(35). Establishing a diagnosis can be difficult, even in the operating room, and resection may be the only answer. In a recent procedure of ours involving a firm mass attached to the bladder, intraoperative endoscopy revealed diverticulitis and spared a partial cystectomy.

An extremely important issue raised is the importance of communication between the radiologist and surgeon when diverticulitis or perforated cancer may exist. An unsuspecting radiologist who fills the colon with barium may create barium peritonitis, a basis for malpractice suits and potential fatal outcomes from barium peritonitis. We favor *limited* examinations with gastrografin only in this setting, if significant perforation is suspected.

We favor CT as the initial examination, preferably with rectal contrast. At the same time, we realize its limitations and do not consider it definitive in differentiating carcinoma and diverticular disease. If possible, we avoid contrast enemas in the acute setting (unlike a number of European centers), preferring a later study with barium, when the risk of iatrogenic perforation is smaller. Contrast studies may define areas of stricture that are not possible to enter with the endoscope.

REFERENCES

1. Donaldson GA. The management of perforative carcinoma of the colon. N Engl J Med 1958;258:201–207. *A classic review of 182 cases. Describes the pathogenesis and clinical implications of fistulas, local abscesses, and free perforation.*
2. Glenn F, McSherry CK. Obstruction and perforation in colorectal cancer. Ann Surg 1971;173:983–992. *In a study of 1815 patients with colorectal carcinoma, 5.5% had perforation and 1.7% combined obstruction and perforation. The 5-year survival rate was only 6.7% with combined obstruction and perforation, partly attributable to a 31% operative mortality.*
3. Schnyder P, Moss AA, Thoeni RF, et al. A double-blind study of radiologic accuracy in diverticulitis, diverticulosis, and carcinoma of the sigmoid colon. J Clin Gastroenterol 1979;1:55–66. *Review of barium enema studies in 73 patients with diverticular disease of the colon with and without associated neoplasm. The neoplasm was recognized correctly in approximately one-half of the cases.*
4. Hulnick DH, Megibow AJ, Balthazar EJ, et al. Perforated colorectal neoplasms: correlation of clinical, contrast enema, and CT examinations. Radiology 1987;164:611–615. *CT is recommended in case of suspected or proven colorectal tumors or when contrast studies are indeterminate or suggestive of perforated neoplasm.*
5. Hiltunen KM, Kohlemainen H, Vuorinen T, et al. Early water-soluble contrast enema in the diagnosis of acute colonic diverticulitis. Int J Colorectal Dis 1991;6:190–192. *No complications were seen with the use of early water-soluble contrast enemas of the left colon. If no diverticulitis is seen, further investigations can be done without delay.*
6. Steffanson T, Bergman A, Ekbom A, et al. Accuracy of double contrast enema and sigmoidoscopy in the detection of polyps in patients with diverticulosis. Acta Radiol 1994;35:442–446. *Neither double contrast barium enema or sigmoidoscopy alone detected all sigmoid lesions in patients with sigmoid diverticulitis.*
7. Baker SR, Alterman DD. False-negative barium enema in patients with sigmoid cancer and coexistent diverticula. Gastrointest Radiol 1985;10:171–173. *Extensive diverticulosis limits the sensitivity of barium enema examinations. Twenty percent of tumors were missed in patients with more than 15 diverticula.*
8. Boulos PB, Cowin AP, Karamanolis DG, et al. Diverticula, neoplasia, or both? Early detection of carcinoma in sigmoid diverticular disease. Ann Surg 1985;202:607–609. *In a study of 105 patients with symptomatic diverticular disease, endoscopy is recommended, especially for patients older than 60 years of age with rectal bleeding.*
9. Dean ACB, Newell JP. Colonoscopy in the differential diagnosis of carcinoma from diverticulitis of the sigmoid colon. Br J Surg 1973;60:633–635. *Thirty-six patients had barium enemas suggesting the possibility of carcinoma in a segment of diverticular disease. Colonoscopy failed to visualize the diseased segment in 17 cases.*
10. Brewster NT, Grieve DC, Saunders JH. Double-contrast barium enema and flexible sigmoidoscopy for routine colonic investigation. Br J Surg 1994;81:445–447. *Double contrast enema and fiberoptic sigmoidoscopy were complementary in the diagnosis of diverticular disease, although the barium enema was more sensitive.*
11. Glerum J, Agenant D, Tytgat GN. Value of colonoscopy in the detection of sigmoid malignancy in patients with diverticular disease. Endoscopy 1977;9:228–230. *Colonoscopy is a valuable adjunct for detecting cancer in patients with diverticular disease.*
12. Doringer E. Computerized tomography of colonic diverticulitis. Crit Rev Diagn Imaging 1992;33:421–435. *A review. CT is preferable to contrast enema for showing pericolic inflammation.*

13. Hulnick DH, Megibow AJ, Balthazar EJ, et al. Computed tomography in the evaluation of diverticulitis. Radiology 1984;152:491–495. *A study of 43 cases of colonic diverticulitis. CT should be the initial procedure, particularly if contrast enema is contraindicated.*

14. Doringer E, Ferner R. CT of colonic diverticulitis. Rofo Fortschr Geb Rontgenstr Neven Bildgeb Verfahr 1990;152:76–79.

15. Johnson CD, Baker ME, Rice RP, et al. Diagnosis of acute colonic diverticulitis: comparison of barium enema and CT. Am J Roentgenol 1987;148:541–546. *A retrospective study of 102 patients with the clinical diagnosis of colonic diverticulitis or of surgically confirmed diverticulitis. The contrast enema is the recommended initial examination and CT is reserved for patients who have inadequate contrast enemas, a suspected abscess, or a lack of response to medical treatment or who are candidates for possible percutaneous drainage.*

16. Cho KC, Morehouse HT, Alterman DD, et al. Sigmoid diverticulitis: diagnostic role of CT-comparison with barium enema studies. Radiology 1990;176:111–115. *A prospective study of 56 patients with presumed acute sigmoid diverticulitis. CT was recommended over contrast enema for the initial study because of its sensitivity and specificity and its ability to detect extracolonic abnormalities such as small bowel obstruction.*

17. Neff CC, vanSonnenberg E. CT of diverticulitis. Diagnosis and treatment. Radiol Clin North Am 1989; 27:743–752. *Provides numerous illustrations of complicated diverticulitis and discusses the use of percutaneous drainage.*

18. Padidar AM, Jeffrey RB, Mindelzun RE, et al. Differentiating sigmoid diverticulitis from carcinoma on CT scans: mesenteric inflammation suggests diverticulitis. Am J Roentgenol 1994;163:81–83. *CT findings of fluid at the root of the mesentery and vascular engorgement are useful in differentiating sigmoid diverticulitis from carcinoma of the sigmoid.*

19. Parulekar SG. Sonography of acute diverticulitis. J Ultrasound Med 1985;4:659–666. *A description of the sonographic findings in 16 patients with diverticulitis of the colon.*

20. Feczo PJ, Nish AD, Craig BM, et al: Acute diverticulitis in patients under 40 years of age: radiologic diagnosis. Am J Roentgenol 1988;150:1311–1314. *In a study of eight young patients with proven colonic diverticulitis, barium enema was accurate diagnostically in six of seven cases.*

21. Schwerk WB, Schwarz S, Rothmund M. Sonography in acute colonic diverticulitis: a prospective study. Dis Colon Rectum 1992;35:1077–1084. *High-resolution sonography with graded compression was highly sensitive and specific for detecting diverticulitis and possible abscess formation.*

22. Verbanck J, Lambrecht S, Rutgeerts L, et al. Can sonography diagnose acute colonic diverticulitis in patients with acute intestinal inflammation? A prospective study. J Clin Ultrasound 1989;17:661–666. *A prospective study of 123 patients. Eight large abscesses were drained percutaneously with sonographic guidance.*

23. Worlicek H. Sonographic diagnosis of colon cancer. Ultraschall Med 1991;12:164–168. *Ultrasonographic studies of a large number of patients with colon cancer.*

24. Shiralama M, Koga T, Ishibashi H, et al. Sonographic features of colon carcinoma seen with high-frequency transabdominal ultrasound. J Clin Ultrasound 1994;22:359–365. *Discusses a group of sonographic criteria for the diagnosis of colon cancer.*

25. Chou CK, Chen LT, Sheu RS, et al. MRI manifestations of gastrointestinal wall thickening. Abdom Imaging 1994;19:389–394. *A study of the MRI appearance of the gastrointestinal tract after the bowel is distended by air.*

26. Lantto E. Investigation of suspected intra-abdominal sepsis: the contribution of nuclear medicine. Scand J Gastroenterol 1994;203(Suppl):11–14. *Discusses the role of nuclear scans in suspected abdominal sepsis.*

27. Cohn KH, Weimar JA, Fani K, et al. Adenocarcinoma arising within a colonic diverticulum: report of two cases and review of the literature. Surgery 1993;113.223–226. *Because colonic diverticula are thinned-walled, cancers may penetrate the serosa at an early stage.*

28. Hunt RH. Colonoscopy in unexplained rectal bleeding. In: Abstracts of the 4th annual meeting of the World Congress of Gastrointestinal Endoscopy, Madrid, 1978.

29. Hunt RH. The role of colonoscopy in complicated diverticular disease. Acta Chir Belg 1979;78:349–353. *The presence of rectal bleeding strongly suggests a concomitant lesion.*

30. Greene FL, Livstone EM, Troncale FJ. Fiberoptic endoscopy in the management of colonic disease. South Med J 1974;67:105–110. *An early report of the indications for and findings during colonoscopic examinations.*

31. Hunt RH, Teague RH, Swarbrick ET, Williams CB. Colonoscopy in the management of colonic strictures. BMJ 1975;3:360–361. *Colonoscopy may prove that a stricture does not exist and avoid unnecessary laparotomy.*

32. Sugarbaker PH, Vineyard GC, Lewicki AM, et al. Colonoscopy in the management of disease of the colon and rectum. Surg Gynecol Obstet 1974;139:341–349. *Another early report on a center's experiences with colonoscopy. Some patients were spared operation by colonoscopy when it was difficult to differentiate carcinomas from diverticulitis by other means.*

33. Stefansson T, Ekbom A, Sparen P, et al. Increased risk of left-sided colon cancer in patients with diverticular disease. Gut 1993;34:499–502. *In a retrospective cohort study in Sweden of patients with discharge diagnoses of diverticulosis or diverticulitis of the colon, an increased risk of left-sided cancer was detected.*

34. Silverstein FE, Tytgat GN. Colon III: diverticular disease, vascular malformations, and other colonic abnormalities. In: Atlas of gastrointestinal endoscopy. J. B. Lippincott, Philadelphia, 1991:12.5.

35. Shatzki R: The roentgenologic differential diagnosis between cancer and diverticulitis of the colon. Radiology 1940;34:651–662.

5 Differentiation of Inflammatory Bowel Disease from Diverticulitis

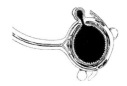

Carole S. Richard, MD
Tadaaki Hiruki, MD
Robin S. McLeod, MD

KEY POINTS

- Peak incidence at lower age with Crohn's disease
- Perianal disease suggestive of Crohn's
- Crohn's complicated by fistulas that are difficult to treat
- Extraintestinal manifestations more common with Crohn's
- Mucosa intact with diverticulitis (except at perforation)
- Endoscopy helpful but may be difficult
- Granulomas possible with diverticulitis

ILLUSTRATIVE CASE

A 50-year-old female presented with left lower quadrant pain, fever, and recurrent diarrhea. She had had several previous episodes, each responding to treatment with Cipro and Flagyl. On this admission, she had localized left lower quadrant tenderness and fullness. Rectal examination revealed a chronic fistula tract. Computed tomography (CT) scan showed pericolonic inflammation and streaking in the mesentery without abscess. She improved with intravenous therapy and was discharged. Before scheduling elective resection, the patient underwent flexible sigmoidoscopy showing granular friable mucosa and linear ulcerations. Biopsies were consistent with Crohn's colitis. Her symptoms improved with medical therapy.

Case Comments

This patient presented with abdominal symptoms suggestive of recurrent diverticulitis. Of note, however, she had perianal inflammatory disease (chronic fistula tract), which should have been a "red flag" for possible Crohn's colitis.

Endoscopy proved to be of considerable value because it provided the correct diagnosis of Crohn's colitis. Instead of an elective sigmoid resection for presumed diverticulitis, the surgeon initiated appropriate medical treatment for Crohn's disease.

INTRODUCTION

Although Crohn's disease and diverticulitis are both inflammatory diseases affecting the colon, they usually differ in their clinical presentation, radiologic and pathologic features, and surgical findings. In some situations, however, distinguishing Crohn's colitis from diverticulitis can be challenging. Schmidt et al (1), in 1968, were among the first to report cases in which Crohn's colitis had been confused with diverticulitis. Subsequent reports (2–4) have confirmed this difficulty and have emphasized that criteria differentiating the two entities can be subtle. Because medical and surgical treatment can differ considerably, misdiagnosis can be potentially harmful to the patient.

Ulcerative colitis also is an inflammatory disease of the colon. Typically, there is rectal involvement, and rectal bleeding and discharge are prominent symptoms. As a result, ulcerative colitis and diverticulitis generally are not confused. Rarely, in cases in which there is an acute onset of ulcerative colitis with colonic perforation, there might be difficulty in differentiating this from an acute episode of diverticulitis. However, minimal investigations such as proctoscopy usually will confirm the diagnosis. Therefore, this chapter focuses mainly on guidelines to help differentiate Crohn's colitis from diverticulitis.

CLINICAL MANIFESTATIONS

The peak incidence of diverticulitis is in the late 60s, whereas Crohn's disease appears most frequently during the second decade of life. Age of onset would thus seem to be an important distinguishing feature. However, in the reported cases in which the two entities have been confused, age was not helpful (1–4). There is a second peak incidence of Crohn's disease during the sixth decade of life (5). Moreover, when Crohn's disease does appear at a later age, there is a higher tendency for colonic involvement (3). Therefore, Crohn's colitis is not uncommon in the older population. Diverticulitis is known to increase in frequency with age, but approximately 5–7% of patients with diverticulitis are reported to be younger than 40 years of age. In large series, 85% of these younger patients are in their third decade of life (6–8).

Both diseases are equally distributed between the sexes. However, when diverticulitis occurs at a younger age, there is a significantly higher proportion of males and they often are overweight (8). Therefore, the presence of symptoms compatible with either acute diverticulitis or Crohn's disease in a young obese male is more suggestive of diverticulitis.

The classical findings of diverticulitis are left lower quadrant pain, fever, and leukocytosis. Crohn's colitis can manifest similarly. Schmidt et al (1), from the St. Mark's Hospital, compared the characteristics of patients admitted with diverticulitis only with those who had diverticular disease and were subsequently diagnosed as having Crohn's disease. Abdominal pain was a less prominent complaint in patients with Crohn's disease than in patients with diverticulitis. A significantly higher proportion of patients with Crohn's disease had rectal bleeding compared with those with diverticulitis (77% versus 36%). The type and quantity of bleeding were not specified. There was no significant difference in the proportion of patients with a history of diarrhea, constipation, mucous discharge, and weight loss. Berman et al (2) also found that approximately half of their series of 25 patients who initially presented with diverticulitis, but in whom Crohn's disease was diagnosed subsequently, had rectal bleeding. Thus, *a history of rectal bleeding or an acute episode of diverticulitis associated with rectal bleeding should raise the possibility of Crohn's colitis.*

The presence or a history of perianal disease may be of importance in differentiating Crohn's disease from diverticulitis (1,3,4). Between 40 and 85% of reported patients in whom diverticulitis was diagnosed initially but who subsequently had Crohn's disease had experienced past or present perianal problems (1,3,4). In Berman et al's series (2), 19 of 21 patients had perianal abnormalities on physical examination, including fissures, fistulas, or anal ulcerations. In a series of 26 patients reported by Schmidt et al (1), 85% had anal lesions, including two patients who were found to have a rectovaginal fistula. Anal abnormalities must be sought in patients presenting with symptoms of diverticulitis. Any anal abnormalities found should be recorded and taken as a possible sign of Crohn's disease.

On abdominal examination, there are no pathognomonic findings of diverticulitis or Crohn's disease. Patients with either entity can have peritoneal signs, a palpable mass, or localized tenderness in the left or right lower quadrant. Signs and symptoms of any type of fistula, including the colovesical or colocutaneous varieties, can be associated with both entities. However, the presence of a colocutaneous fistula without prior surgery, one in an unusual location, and/or a complex presentation of a fistula are associated more frequently with Crohn's disease. This was substantiated by the Cleveland group (9), who reported on 93 patients with colocutaneous fistulas secondary to diverticular disease. Eighty-eight patients had developed the fistula after a colonic surgical procedure and only five patients had spontaneous occurrence of the fistula before undergoing a surgical procedure involving the colon. Of the 93 patients, 10 were found subsequently to have Crohn's disease. All of these 10 patients had colocutaneous fistulas that were more complex and difficult to treat than the fistulas associated with diverticulitis.

Endoscopy probably is the most useful diagnostic modality for differentiating Crohn's disease from diverticular disease. The problem, however, is that *in many of these patients with a complicated presentation, colonoscopy may be difficult or impossible to perform* because of a presence of a mass or stricture in the sigmoid colon. Characteristic endoscopic findings in Crohn's disease are ulcerations, deep fissuring, and serpiginous or rake ulcers. There typically is an uneven involvement of the mucosa. In differentiating Crohn's disease from diverticulitis, colonoscopy has been reported to be useful, because abnormalities are found in up to 88 to 96% of patients (1,2). Proctoscopy is of less benefit because only 20 to 50% of patients with Crohn's disease have rectal involvement (4,10). However, if abnormal rectal findings are seen on sigmoidoscopy, it increases the likelihood of Crohn's disease or even ulcerative colitis, and diverticulitis alone can be excluded.

Finally, the presence of any extraintestinal manifestations such as oral lesions, erythema nodosum, pyoderma gangrenosum, arthritis, and spondylitis must be sought and, when present, make the diagnosis of Crohn's disease more likely.

RADIOLOGIC FEATURES

Marshak et al (4), in the early 1970s, were among the first to describe the radiologic differences between diverticulitis and Crohn's colitis during barium enema examinations. These same criteria apply today (Table 5.1). Although they believed that fistula tracts tended to be short in diverticular disease, subsequent reports have, however, shown that the length of the tract is not a distinguishing feature. Long tracts have been found in association with both Crohn's colitis and diverticulitis.

CT currently is among the most useful diagnostic tests for the investigation of patients with acute diverticulitis. It aids in confirming the diagnosis and quantifying the severity of the episode (11). A study by Hulnick et al (12) found that contrast enemas underestimated the severity of diverticulitis compared with CT scan. Cho et al (13) compared CT scans and barium enemas for evaluation of diverticulitis in 25 different hospitals. They found CT scans to be more sensitive than contrast enemas (93% versus 80%) for the diagnosis of diverticulitis, and moreover, the diagnostic specificity of CT scans for

Table 5.1.   Radiologic Features of Diverticulitis and Granulomatous Colitis of the Descending and Sigmoid Colon

Diverticulitis	Crohn's Disease
Short process, 3–6 cm in length	Long, usually 10 cm or more
Diverticula sharply defined and frequently contain fecaliths but may, on occasion, simulate abscesses	Abscesses frequently have a triangular configuration but may be undistinguishable from the co-existent diverticula
When a diverticulum perforates, the abscess creates an extramural defect or an arcuate configuration of folds that stretch over the abscess	This is an ulcerating mucosal process; folds are straightened, perpendicular, picket-fence-like, and associated with a thick wall and secretions
No transverse fissures; folds may be straightened but more commonly have an arcuate configuration	Transverse fissures with marked edema of mucosa produce a stepladder configuration
A short paracolic tract may be seen occasionally (usually associated with an extramural defect); on rare occasions, a perforation may run parallel to the bowel wall	If a tract is seen, it is long, linear, and located in the submucosa or muscular layers

Adapted from: Marshak RH, Janowitz HD, Present DH. Granulomatous colitis in association with diverticula. N Engl J Med 1970;283:1080–1084.

diverticulitis was 100%. The radiologic features of diverticulitis on CT scan are inflammation of the pericolic fat, which is characterized by increased soft-tissue density within the mesenteric fat adjacent to and surrounding the involved segment of diseased colon (11). The severity of the episode may correlate with the severity of the pericolic inflammation, the presence of an abscess or phlegmon, and the quantity of free fluid within the peritoneal cavity (14). Complications such as extraluminal sinus tracts, fistulas, or even obstruction often will be visualized on the CT scan if contrast has been used.

Unfortunately, the CT scan findings with diverticulitis can resemble those of segmental Crohn's colitis. *However, in most circumstances, an experienced radiologist will be capable of differentiating the two entities.* Crohn's disease tends to involve a longer segment of bowel and the mucosal changes are more prominent and diffuse. There also can be skip areas. In diverticulitis, most of the inflammation is localized extramucosally in the surrounding pericolic fat; mucosal changes usually are quite localized, and the length of the diseased colon is more limited. Another benefit of CT scanning is its usefulness in percutaneous drainage when indicated.

OPERATIVE FINDINGS

In most patients with either diverticulitis or Crohn's disease, surgery is performed electively or semielectively after the correct diagnosis has been established clearly. However, in emergency situations in which the patient has generalized peritonitis or is in septic shock, an urgent laparotomy is required. At laparotomy, it may be difficult to differentiate between perforated segmental Crohn's colitis and perforated diverticulitis. In both situations, there may be a large inflammatory mass in the area of the diseased colon with a thickened mesentery. There may be surrounding inflammation of the adjacent large and small bowel. An abscess also can occur in both diseases. *If more than the sigmoid colon is involved, Crohn's disease is more likely.* Although differentiating the two entities may be difficult at emergency surgery, in reality, decision-making usually is unchanged. The extent of the resection will depend on the length of the involved colon irrespective of the responsible entity. After the resection has been performed, the state of the patient, the local abdominal conditions, and the status of the rectum will be the determining factors in deciding whether a primary anastomosis or an end stoma is performed. The etiology of the disease is of much lesser importance.

For cases in which it is impossible to differentiate between Crohn's colitis and diverticulitis at the time of surgery, one should remove the diseased segment and perform a Hartmann procedure. Additional investigation or treatment can then be guided by the pathologic diagnosis.

Berman et al (2) retrospectively reviewed the operative reports of 25 patients with presumed diverticulitis who were found subsequently to have Crohn's colitis. It was noted either that the procedure had been unusually difficult or that confusing intraoperative findings were present in all patients. Although some specimens were opened at the time of surgery, there was still difficulty in differentiating segmental Crohn's colitis from diverticulitis. In general, the findings of granularity or ulcerations on the mucosa of the opened specimen were suggestive of Crohn's disease.

The postoperative course of patients with Crohn's disease may potentially differ from that of patients with diverticulitis. One of the findings in Berman et al's series (2) was the high postoperative complication rate related to the distal segment. In their report, 16 patients were treated initially by diversion alone, whereas nine patients had resection with (2) or without (7) a proximal protecting stoma. In the latter group, seven patients required additional surgery for problems associated with the segment distal to the resection site and only two remained well. They concluded that late complications from the distal segment in patients operated on for presumed diverticulitis, such as intermittent or continued bleeding, late onset of sepsis, or fistula, or even signs of recurrent diverticulitis, should be regarded as probable signs of Crohn's disease. Schmidt et al (1) also concluded that if complications occur after a resection for diverticulitis, Crohn's disease should be considered. These patients may require investigation with CT scanning to exclude postoperative septic complications as well as colonoscopy and small bowel enema to search for Crohn's disease elsewhere.

PATHOLOGY

On gross examination of the resected specimen, *the mucosa in diverticulitis usually appears normal, except for the immediate area where the perforation has occurred.* The responsible diverticulum often can be found by probing the area of inflammation. Mucosal redundancy around the site of the inflammation caused by the muscular shortening may be a sign of diverticulitis (1). In cases of Crohn's disease, the usual macroscopic findings are mucosal inflammation with granularity, mucosal thickening, and patches of full thickness ulcerations. On the cut surface of the diseased bowel, the inflammatory component in diverticulitis is mainly pericolic and extramural with minimal changes on the mucosa, whereas in Crohn's colitis, there are macroscopic abnormalities on the mucosa in association with mesenteric thickening.

On microscopy, the pathognomonic finding of Crohn's disease is the presence of granulomas in the bowel wall. Transmural inflammation with fibrosis and deeply penetrating fissures or ulcers also are characteristic. Granulomas can be found in diverticulitis, but they are caused by foreign body giant cells secondary to pericolic abscesses, and they are not found in the bowel wall or in the nodes (1). *Therefore, if granulomas are seen on frozen section, the possibility of diverticulitis cannot be excluded.* In diverticulitis, the inflammatory reaction is concentrated in the surrounding extramural tissue, especially in the mesentery. Foci of lymphoid tissue may be found around the site of perforation, but they do not involve the submucosal and muscular part of the bowel as in Crohn's disease.

If there is uncertainty about the diagnosis preoperatively, biopsies may be helpful in differentiating between diverticulitis and segmental Crohn's colitis. In both entities, there may be nonspecific infiltration of the mucosa with inflammatory cells. However, in up to 30% of endoscopic biopsies in patients with Crohn's disease, there will be typical granulomas with the presence of Langhans giant cells (10).

In certain rare cases, diverticulitis and Crohn's disease do coexist. Meyers et al (3) have postulated several mechanisms for the pathogenesis of diverticulitis complicating granulomatous colitis. One of them is the development of a Crohn's ulcer in an isolated diverticulum. Because the bowel wall is very thin at the site of a diverticulum, the Crohn's disease ulcer can easily perforate and cause typical symptoms of diverticulitis in that segment of colon with Crohn's disease. Another proposed mechanism is that a segment of the colon contained a deep Crohn's ulcer adjacent to a diverticulum, and subsequently, the Crohn's disease fistulized in the diverticulum and caused diverticulitis.

CONCLUSION

Crohn's disease and diverticulitis are common inflammatory diseases that affect the colon. Fortunately, in most cases, the correct diagnosis can be made based on clinical presentation and endoscopic findings. Laparotomy and pathologic analysis of the diseased colon is rarely required for confirmation of the diagnosis.

In a small proportion of difficult cases, mainly those presenting acutely, differentiating these entities may be difficult. A high degree of suspicion must be maintained in such unusual cases. The presence of rectal bleeding, anal abnormalities, unusual fistulas, technical difficulties, and postoperative complications are all signs that Crohn's disease might be the responsible entity. In emergency situations, when time does not permit additional investigation, the safest approach is to resect the involved segment and defer reestablishment of intestinal continuity until final pathologic analysis is available.

EDITORIAL COMMENTS

This chapter deals with a difficult group of patients, both from standpoints of diagnosis and therapy. The authors have made a detailed but succinct summary of the features, such as the history, physical examination and radiologic studies (15), that help differentiate Crohn's colitis from diverticulitis (Table 5.2).

The two diseases overlap significantly in the clinical signs and laboratory tests, and therefore, the preoperative diagnosis is, at times, inaccurate (16), especially for elderly patients (17). Clouding the picture, the diseases may coexist in older patients (16–18) (Figs. 5.1 and 5.2), and there even may be a relationship to "malignant" diverticulitis described in Chapter 13 (19,20). Nevertheless, it is useful to emphasize a number of differential points that the authors have touched on.

Certainly diverticulitis is encountered much more frequently than Crohn's colitis. However, the surgeon should be alert to several points for patients who are presumed to have only diverticulitis: the young patient, perianal involvement (fistulas, suppuration, etc.), the presence of unusual fistulas,

Table 5.2.   Differential Diagnosis of Crohn's Colitis and Diverticulitis: History and Physical Findings

	Crohn's Disease	Diverticulitis
Age of onset:	Any age	Age older than 40 years
History:		
Pain	Frequent	Localized
Diarrhea	Frequent	Occurs
Bleeding	Variable	Unusual
Anal lesions	Common	None
Physical findings:		
Clubbing	Common	None
Mass	Common	Occurs
Anal lesions	Common	None
Rectovaginal fistula	Occurs	None

Adapted from: Lennard-Jones JE. Differentiation between Crohn's disease, ulcerative colitis and diverticulitis. Clin Gastroenterol 1972;1:367–375.

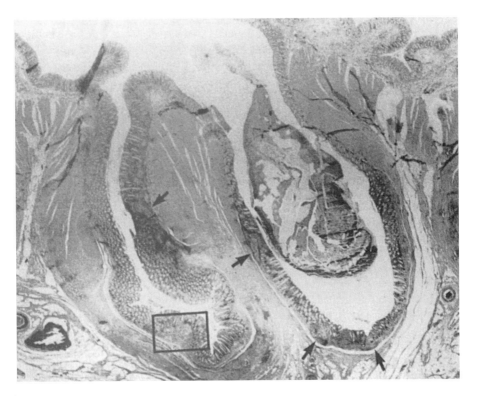

Figure 5.1. Noncaseating granulomas (arrows), typical of Crohn's disease, involving the mucosa of two sigmoid diverticula (×8). (Reprinted with permission from Meyers MA, Alonso DR, Morson BC, et al. Pathogenesis of diverticulitis complicating granulomatous colitis. Gastroenterology 1978;74:24–31.)

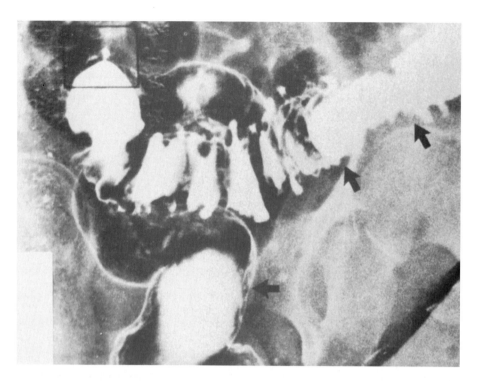

Figure 5.2.   Contrast study in patient with diverticulitis. Signs of Crohn's disease include the indentation and ulceration of the left side of the rectum and the gross changes in the proximal sigmoid colon (arrows). There also are multiple diverticula present. (Reprinted with permission from Meyers MA, Alonso DR, Morson BC, et al. Pathogenesis of diverticulitis complicating granulomatous colitis. Gastroenterology 1978;74:24–31.)

and especially recurrent disease following an appropriate resection suggest the possibility of Crohn's colitis. As part of the evaluation, the pathologic specimen from the first operation should be reviewed carefully, looking for mucosal involvement and taking additional sections if necessary. Endoscopy is useful because a rectal or colonic biopsy may be diagnostic of Crohn's disease (15); contrast studies may add information as well (long fistulous tracts may complicate both diseases, but short tracts usually are caused by diverticulitis) (21). Despite the development of complications, the mucosa remains intact in diverticular disease (22). Involvement of other portions of the colon and rectum and rectal bleeding should increase the suspicion of Crohn's disease (23). Very rarely, fistulas after an attack of diverticulitis are related to development of an infectious process such as actinomycosis (24).

Clearly, the medical and surgical treatment may vary depending on which diagnosis is made: steroids are useful for exacerbations of Crohn's colitis, but they are not indicated for attacks of diverticulitis. If Crohn's disease goes unrecognized in patients with presumed diverticulitis, significant morbidity could result. There also is evidence of significant morbidity following surgery for the combined diseases (22), even after proximal diversion and resection (2).

REFERENCES

1. Schmidt GT, Lennard-Jones JE, Morson BC, et al. Crohn's disease of the colon and its distinction from diverticulitis. Gut 1968;9:7–16. *A review of 26 patients with Crohn's disease in a segment of bowel containing diverticula. Most patients had an anal lesion or rectovaginal fistula, an abnormal sigmoidoscopy, and noncaseating granulomas on biopsies.*

2. Berman IR, Corman ML, Coller JA, et al. Late onset Crohn's disease in patients with colonic diverticulitis. Dis Colon Rectum 1979;22:524–529. *A discussion of 25 patients with presumed diverticulitis who turned out to have combined diverticulitis and Crohn's colitis. A classic description of the complex clinical course of this group of patients.*

3. Meyers MA, Alonso DR, Morson BC, et al. Pathogenesis of diverticulitis complicating granulomatous colitis. Gastroenterology 1978;74:24–31. *Discusses the radiologic signs of peridiverticulitis complicating granulomatous colitis. Involvement of the diverticula by the granulomatous colitis may predispose to peridiverticulitis and/or abscess formation.*

4. Marshak RH, Janowitz HD, Present DH. Granulomatous colitis in association with diverticula. N Engl J Med 1970;283:1080–1084. *In a study of 10 patients with combined diverticular disease and Crohn's colitis, the authors found that radiographic findings were among the most sensitive in making the correct diagnosis. Four patients had a past history of perirectal disease.*

5. Kirsner JB, Shorter RG. Recent developments in "non-specific" inflammatory bowel disease, Part 1. N Engl J Med 1982;306:775–785. *A comprehensive clinical review with 194 references.*

6. Rodkey GV, Welch CE. Colonic diverticular disease with surgical treatment. A study of 338 cases. Surg Clin North Am 1974;54:655–674. *One report of a series from the Massachusetts General Hospital.*

7. Rodkey GV, Welch CE. Changing patterns in the surgical treatment of diverticular disease. Ann Surg 1985;200:466–478. *Compares different surgical populations and operative procedures in two successive decades.*

8. Milsom JW, Singh G. Diverticulitis in young patients. Semin Colon Rectal Surg 1990;1:103–108. *Young patients have a lower surgical mortality than the "usual" patient.*

9. Fazio VW, Church JM, Jagelman DG, et al. Colocutaneous fistulas complicating diverticulitis. Dis Col Rectum 1987;30:89–94. *Reviews 93 patients who developed colocutaneous fistulas associated with diverticular disease. Eighty-eight fistulas occurred in the postoperative period. The 10 patients identified with Crohn's disease had complicated fistulas and recurrent fistulas.*

10. Strong SA, Fazio VW. Crohn's disease of the colon, rectum and anus. Surg Clin North Am 1993;73:934–963. *A review with 99 references.*

11. Hachigian MP, Honickman S, Eisenstate TE, et al. Computed tomography in the initial management of acute left sided diverticulitis. Dis Colon Rectum 1992;35:1123–1129. *CT stratifies patients according to disease severity and provides anatomic information useful for surgical planning. Early CT-guided percutaneous drainage downstages cases of complicated diverticulitis, avoids emergent operation, and permits elective one-stage resection and anastomosis.*

12. Hulnick DH, Megibow AJ, Balthazar EJ, et al. Computed tomography in the evaluation of diverticulitis. Radiology 1984;152:491–495. *Compares CT (43 cases) with contrast enemas (37 patients) and discusses the differential diagnosis of the CT findings.*

13. Cho KC, Morehouse DT, Alterman DD, et al. Sigmoid diverticulitis: diagnostic role of CT -comparison with barium enema studies. Radiology 1990;176:111–115. *A prospective study. CT should be the initial study in acutely ill patients, especially if the clinical features are atypical of diverticulitis.*

14. Birnbaum BA, Balthazar EJ. CT of appendicitis and diverticulitis. Radiol Clin North Am 1994;32:885–898. *CT is less invasive and has a greater diagnostic sensitivity and specificity than contrast enemas. The major benefit of CT is the identification of patients with pericolic abscesses. Includes 39 references.*

15. Lennard-Jones JE. Differentiation between Crohn's disease, ulcerative colitis and diverticulitis. Clin Gastroenterol 1972;1:367–375. *A summary including a detailed table of the differential diagnosis.*

16. Petros JG, Happ RA. Crohn's colitis in patients with diverticular disease. Am J Gastroenterol 1991;86:247–248. *The authors point out that it may be very difficult to establish the diagnosis of Crohn's disease before operation.*

17. Shapiro PA, Peppercorn MA, Antonioli DA, et al. Crohn's disease in the elderly. Am J Gastroenterol 1981;76:132–137. *A study of 33 patients older than 60 years of age with Crohn's disease. Differentiation from diverticulitis and ischemic bowel disease was difficult.*

18. Naouri A, Maroun J, Tissot E. diverticulose et maladie de Crohn sigmoidienne. Ann Chir 1992;46:67–70. *Discusses three cases of combined disease associated with high postoperative morbidity.*

19. Stephen Lock. Editorial: is malignant diverticulitis a true bill? BMJ 1980;280:1156. *Questions whether malignant diverticulitis may in some cases represent combined inflammatory bowel disease with diverticulosis.*

20. McLaren CA. A case of "malignant" diverticulitis associated with tuberculous colitis. Scott Med J 1989;29:112–113. *A patient having many operations for diverticulitis was eventually found to have associated tuberculous colitis.*

21. Marshak RH, Lidner AE, Maklansky D. Paracolic fistulous tracts in diverticulitis and granulomatous colitis. JAMA 1980;243:1943–1946. *A well illustrated review that goes into fine differential points between the two disorders.*

22. Tudor RG. The interface of inflammatory bowel disease and diverticular disease. In: Allan RN, Keighley MR, Alexander-Williams J, et al, eds. Inflammatory bowel disease. 2nd ed. Edinburgh: Churchill Livingstone, 1990:559–562. *An excellent summary of the topic.*

23. Small WP, Smith AN. Fistula and conditions associated with diverticular disease of the colon. Clin Gastroenterol 1975;4:171–199. *An interesting comprehensive discussion of the topic.*

24. Gingold BS, Fazio VW. Abdominal actinomycosis: a complication of colonic perforation. Dis Colon Rectum 1978;21:374–376. *Report of a patient with recurrent enterocutaneous fistulas assumed to be complications of perforated diverticulitis. The left colectomy specimen contained clumps of "sulfur granules" caused by actinomycosis, and the patient responded to intravenous penicillin therapy.*

6 Diverticular Hemorrhage

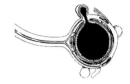

William Pennoyer, MD
Jeffrey Cohen, MD

> ## KEY POINTS
> - Bleeding ceases spontaneously in 80–90%
> - Right-sided diverticula account for 50% of the bleeding
> - Avoid barium studies during acute bleeding
> - Angiography and colonoscopy are studies of choice for localizing a source
> - Rebleeding occurs in as many as 50% after using vasopressin
> - Bleeding should be localized if possible before surgery to allow segmental resection
> - Nonlocalized bleeding treated surgically is managed with subtotal colectomy

ILLUSTRATIVE CASE

A 66-year-old man with a history of hypertension and exertional angina controlled with medication presented to the emergency room with a history of intermittent bright red rectal bleeding over the past 6 hours. He had been passing clots of blood, initially mixed with stool, but most recently only frank blood. He estimated at least four episodes during this time period. The patient had a history of similar bleeding 2 years earlier that required admission to the hospital and blood transfusions. At that time, colonoscopy had demonstrated extensive sigmoid diverticulosis.

Case Comments

This patient had a history of prior diverticular bleeding and presented with bleeding from either the same or a new source. Evaluation and resuscitation should proceed according to the algorithm and steps outlined in this chapter. Because of this patient's excessive bleeding, as manifest by numerous and ongoing bloody bowel movements, angiography might give the most useful and rapid results, avoiding the delay of a screening nuclear medicine scan. If there was any suspicion that the patient's bleeding had stopped or slowed to a level undetectable by angiography, screening with a nuclear scan might be more appropriate. If bleeding was localized by the scan alone, even within the first 2 hours of study, other localization procedures should be used before operative resection. If the patient's bleeding seemed to have stopped entirely, a mechanical bowel preparation and colonoscopy should be pursued.

If the source of bleeding can be localized by angiogram, one should proceed with segmental resection or superselective embolization. Embolization would be less invasive in this patient with angina pectoris. Transcatheter infusion of vasopressin would be inadvisable because of his

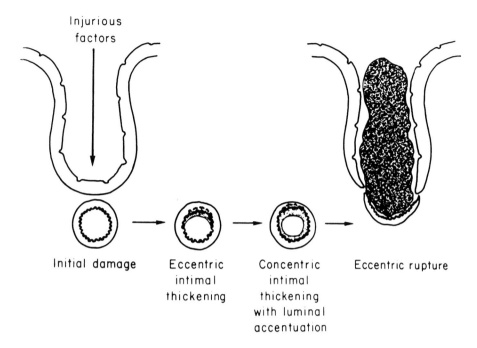

Figure 6.1.   Proposed pathogenesis of bleeding colonic diverticulosis. (Reprinted with permission from Meyers MA, Alonso DR, Gray GF, et al. Pathogenesis of bleeding colonic diverticulosis. Gastroenterology 1976;71: 577–583.)

cardiovascular history. If the angiogram proved negative, a skilled endoscopist might immediately prepare the patient and perform an emergent colonoscopy. With a negative initial angiogram, one might also consider the use of the experimental "pharmacoangiography" to improve the diagnostic yield in this patient with a second significant bleed.

INTRODUCTION

Hematochezia is a common and dangerous medical problem because severe bleeding in the acute setting has a mortality as high as 10–15% (1). In Western society, as many as 65% of the population will have diverticula by 85 years of age (2). Some estimate that as many as 20% of patients with diverticulosis coli will present with bleeding in their lifetime and 5% of patients will have severe hemorrhage (3). Although most diverticula are situated in the left colon, *right-sided diverticula account for approximately 50% of bleeding diverticulosis* (4). Bleeding will spontaneously cease in 80–90% of cases, and 25% of patients rebleed at some point in the future (3,5).

The pathogenesis of diverticular bleeding was elucidated by Meyer et al's histologic analysis of bleeding diverticula. The characteristic changes "include the asymmetric rupture of the vas rectum toward the lumen of the diverticulum precisely at its dome or the antimesenteric margin; conspicuous eccentric intimal thickening of the vas rectum, often with medial thinning and duplication of the internal elastic lamina at or near the bleeding point; and general absence of diverticulitis" (6) (Fig. 6.1).

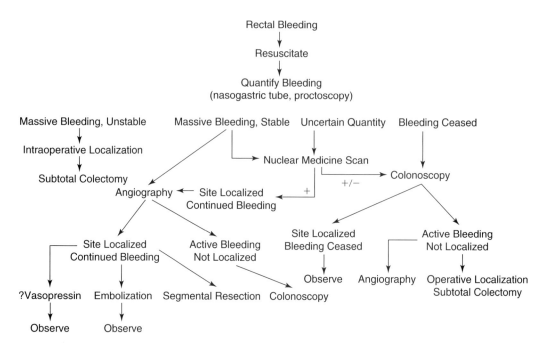

Figure 6.2. Algorithm with suggested approach to lower gastrointestinal hemorrhage.

The differential diagnosis of bright red blood per rectum is extensive; most cases occur because of diverticulosis and arteriovenous malformations. *Diverticulosis accounts for 30–50% of lower gastrointestinal bleeding* (7). An equal percentage originates from arteriovenous malformations. Other causes of bleeding distal to the ligament of Treitz include malignancy, polyps, inflammatory bowel disease, infectious complications, ischemia, and iatrogenic complications. Rectal and perianal lesions responsible for bleeding include hemorrhoids, fissures, ulcers, and trauma. It must be remembered that *as many as 10% of patients with hematochezia will have an upper gastrointestinal source for their bleeding and another 5% will have bleeding from the small intestine* (8).

The management of a patient with hematochezia is divided into phases of evaluation, resuscitation, localization/diagnosis and treatment; the assessment and resuscitation phases proceed simultaneously. The broad range of diagnostic procedures and possible therapeutic interventions reflects the large differential diagnosis and variable presentation of these patients. As a result, there is a lack of standardization in the treatment of lower gastrointestinal hemorrhage (Fig. 6.2).

EVALUATION/RESUSCITATION

The assessment of the bleeding can be divided into the history and physical examination. The history should include attempts to qualify and quantify the bleeding. Important characteristics include color, consistency, frequency, and duration of the bleeding and bowel movements. A history of bleeding can identify patients at risk for continued and recurrent bleeding. Symptoms of significant intravascular volume loss include weakness, fatigue, syncope, and palpitations. Comorbidities, particularly coronary artery disease, identify those at increased risk for complications of bleeding, resuscitation, and treatment.

Anticoagulant and nonsteroidal anti-inflammatory drugs (NSAIDs) affect the pathology of diverticular bleeding. Patients using NSAIDs tend to present with more severe forms of diverticular disease, being twice as likely to suffer a complication of diverticulosis than a similar control group with diverticula (9–11). The actual pathophysiology is uncertain.

Physical findings of tachycardia, hypotension, orthostasis, pallor, and mental status changes suggest a significant reduction of at least 10–20% of the circulating blood volume. A lack of these findings does not necessarily imply a minor bleed. A recent study at our institution showed that most patients (90%) with a positive angiogram for bleeding presented as normotensive or hypertensive. Only 30% of patients with positive angiograms were tachycardic and 56% were orthostatic. The digital rectal examination will allow an assessment of the amount and potential location of hemorrhage.

Intravenous access should be established and adequate fluid resuscitation should be initiated early in the evaluation. Laboratory studies of blood drawn on line placement should at least include a complete blood cell count, coagulation studies, type and cross match, and electrolytes. The inexpensive and quickly calculated blood urea nitrogen (BUN) and creatinine (Cr) ratio can be used at times to help distinguish upper from lower gastrointestinal bleeding. In one series, no patient with a BUN/Cr ratio higher than 36 had bleeding from a lower source. Snook et al described a 90% accuracy for defining an upper source with a similar ratio (12,13).

Resuscitation must proceed while the patient is being evaluated. Blood loss and volume status should be estimated and replaced with appropriate isotonic crystalloid and blood products. Coagulopathies should be corrected. Attempts should be made to keep the patient normothermic with a warm room environment, fluid warmers, and warming blankets. With normal renal function, Foley catheter placement should allow for assessment of the ongoing fluid replacements. Patients with massive hemorrhage, significant cardiac disease, or comorbidities would benefit from intensive monitoring, including systemic arterial, pulmonary arterial, electrocardiographic, and oximetric monitors. Patients with active bleeding require continuous care and frequent reassessments.

A nasogastric tube should be placed early in the evaluation. An upper gastrointestinal source for bleeding usually can be excluded if clear bile is seen in the tube when placed on suction following gastric lavage. Without the presence of bile, a duodenal source still must be considered. Even if clear bile is noted on gastric lavage, upper gastrointestinal bleeding may be seen in as many as 16% of patients (14). The nasogastric tube also may be used as access for a mechanical bowel prep with polyethylene glycol for early colonoscopy (15).

Rigid sigmoidoscopy can give a preliminary assessment of the quantity and possible source of bleeding. The findings of red blood, clots, melena, or even brown stool can help determine whether bleeding is ongoing. It is imperative to rule out an anorectal source for bleeding, such as a hemorrhoid, fissure, posttraumatic lesion, ulcer, or mass because "blind" subtotal colectomies will not cure rectal bleeding. Local control of perianal bleeding can be performed through an anoscope or sigmoidoscope. The appearance of the mucosa also can suggest a possible source of bleeding such as infectious, inflammatory, or ischemic colitis.

DIAGNOSIS

The diagnostic phase includes attempts at localization of the bleeding. Radiologic tests and endoscopy help in localization, diagnosis, and treatment. For the small percentage of lower gastrointestinal bleeding that does not stop spontaneously, it is imperative to identify the site to determine the appropriate treatment.

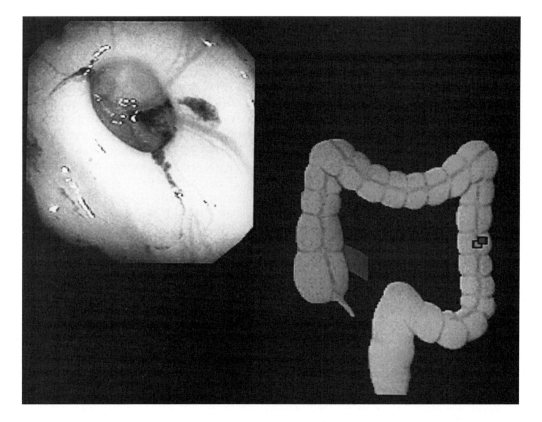

Figure 6.3.   Colonoscopic visualization of colonic diverticulum with visible, nonbleeding vessel.

Endoscopy

Endoscopic options include the use of anoscopy, rigid sigmoidoscopy, flexible sigmoidoscopy, and colonoscopy. With proper equipment, colonoscopy can be performed in the acute setting after adequate bowel preparation. Authors have described the use of a volume of saline, sulfate, or ethylene glycol ranging from 4 to 15 liters via mouth or flush through the nasogastric tube for adequate cleansing to permit diagnosis (1). The cathartic effect of blood in the gastrointestinal tract may aid in the preparation, thereby obviating the need for formal mechanical bowel preparation (1). The colonoscope must be advanced cautiously with adequate visualization of the lumen at all times. Frequent "jet" saline irrigation through the instrument port may be necessary. Changing the position of the patient will allow pooling of blood or fluid at sides of the bowel to more readily visualize the lumen. Emergent colonoscopy should be attempted only by skilled and experienced endoscopists (3). With or without the proper cleansing, the procedure may be performed at the bedside, in an endoscopy suite, or in the operating room.

The diagnostic accuracy varies widely between studies but can be as high as 94% when panendoscopy is performed (15). One report stresses the importance of having either multiple or large (> 3.7-mm diameter) suction channels to allow for irrigation and suction of stool and clot during the colonoscopy. Potential complications include fluid overload secondary to purge and perforation secondary to instrumentation. Although visibility may be decreased because of active bleeding, reported complication rates have been low (4%) (15).

Forde and Treat described their early experience with one perforation in 40 emergent colonoscopies (3). Irvine et al noted a 17% rate of failure to advance the colonoscope to the cecum (16). Findings at colonoscopy that help to localize the site are active visualized bleeding, fresh blood in an area, and adherent clot (1) (Fig. 6.3). Most authors support the practice of "turnaround exam (retroversion)" of the endoscope in the rectum to recognize any rectal pathology missed on the usually difficult rigid sigmoidoscopy (15).

Colonoscopy is helpful for patients who have stopped bleeding as well as in those who continue to hemorrhage. Most sources of colonic hemorrhage can be evaluated with a high percentage of accuracy using the colonoscope. Rossini and colleagues reported an accuracy of 76% in the acute setting (17) (Table 6.1). Polyps, cancers, arteriovenous malformations, colitis, ulcers, and diverticula all can be identified readily. The presence of any of the above does not confirm the actual source of hemorrhage unless the previously stated stigmata of active bleeding are noted. In one series, Jensen and Machicado stated that 73% of patients with diverticula had another cause for lower gastrointestinal hemorrhage found at colonoscopy (15). They also stressed the capability of the colonoscope to define the actual anatomic site or segmental area of bleeding to help guide any additional interventions (15). Tedesco et al noted the usefulness of colonoscopy in self-limited rectal bleeding, arguing that it is the examination of choice for those who have stopped bleeding (18). If one is merely trying to identify the presence of diverticula and does not intend to pursue mesenteric angiography, barium enema may have a higher sensitivity than the colonoscope (51% versus 34%) (19). Barium enema also may be used to compliment an inadequate colonoscopy or sigmoidoscopy.

Nuclear Medicine

Nuclear medicine offers two radionuclide scintigraphic techniques for localization of bleeding points: intravenous infusion of technetium-99 sulfur colloid (Tc-SC) and transfusion with technetium-labeled red blood cells (Tc-rbc). In the acute setting, Tc-SC is injected intravenously and serial studies are then performed to identify extravasation. Tc-SC can reveal blood loss at a rate as low as 0.1 mL/minute (20). The Tc-SC is cleared actively from the circulation by the reticuloendothelial system and thus requires that the patient be actively bleeding at the time of injection for the scan to be diagnostically valuable. Concentration of technetium in the liver and spleen may obscure bleeding located in the upper abdominal portions of the colon (21).

Tc-rbc scans are reported to be sensitive to bleeding at rates as low as 0.05–0.1 mL/minute (22) (Fig. 6.4). The tagged red blood cells have an extended half-life, and repeated imaging may be used to detect intermittent or recurrent bleeding for as long as 36 hours after initial injection of the erythrocytes (23). The scans are safe and cause no known morbidity. Early sensitivities of the studies were reported to be higher than 90%; however, more recent literature suggests that true sensitivities may be less than 50% (21,24). Older studies may not have included patients with negative scans or confirmed

Table 6.1.   Efficiency of Diagnostic Colonoscopy

Study	Diagnostic Efficiency
Rossini et al (17)	76%
Forde and Treat (3)	85%
Jensen and Machicado (15)	70%

localization by other diagnostic means. In a recent review of 72 Tc-rbc scans performed at our institution, 44 (61%) showed active bleeding. Seventy-one percent of the positive scans accurately localized the site of bleeding as confirmed by surgery, angiography, or endoscopy. A review of most series show that localization accuracy varies among institutions; the overall average is 77% (253 localized/330 scans) (Table 6.2). It is probable that an operative procedure based on a bleeding scan alone has a high chance (25%) of inadequately identifying the source and thus leading to rebleeding (22). Some authors have suggested they can reliably (100% in 19 cases) localize a site of bleeding if the Tc-rbc is positive within the first 2 hours and an upper gastrointestinal source has been excluded (25). It is important to note that *a large percentage (35–60%) of patients with a positive bleeding scan will require operative intervention to control bleeding and should undergo additional localization workup* (Table 6.2).

The value of radionuclide scans as a screening tool before angiography is unclear (26). In our review, bleeding scans did not reduce the number of negative angiograms. Only 13 of the 44 patients (30%) with a positive bleeding scan went on to have bleeding demonstrated on angiography. Active bleeding was identified in 45 of 131 (34%) patients undergoing angiography without prior radionuclide scan. Other studies have failed to show any increase in the percentage of positive angiograms using the bleeding scan as a screening test (Table 6.3). The exact role of nuclide scans therefore has not been established. The scans still may prove useful, because early positive scans may be more accurate in localization. The examinations are minimally invasive, inexpensive, have low complication rates, and may alert the physician to patients who may require operative intervention. At this point, *it is not safe to limit a diagnostic workup to and to base treatment on a radionuclide scan alone. The scan should be used in conjunction with other diagnostic modalities.*

Angiography

Selective mesenteric angiography has been used consistently to both localize and treat lower gastrointestinal bleeding. Extravasation can be noted at bleeding rates of 0.5 mL/minute (20). Corman suggests that the actual rate must be higher in humans because

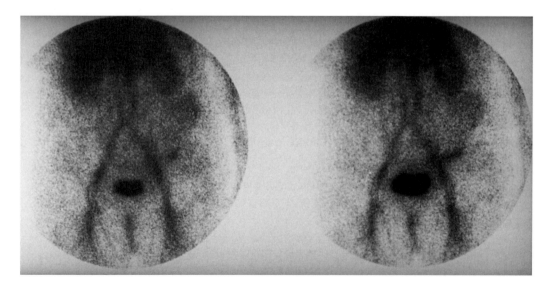

Figure 6.4.   Technetium-labeled red blood cell scan demonstrating bleeding in the left colon.

Table 6.2.   Nuclear Medicine Scanning in the Diagnosis of Lower Gastrointestinal Bleeding

Scanning Study	Total No. Scans	No. Positive Scans	No. Localized Scans (%)[a]	No. Positive to Surgery (%)
Alvai and Ring (60)	43	23	21/23 (91)	—
Nicholson et al (61)	43	31	29/31 (93)	15(48)
Ryan et al (24)	—	28	9/9(100)	10(35)
Bentley and Richardson (26)	162	98	24/46 (52)	—
McKusick et al (62)	80	51	39/47 (82)	25(49)
Szasz et al (63)	71	46	30/37 (81)	16(34)
Markisz et al (64)	39	17	10/11 (90)	6(35)
Orecchia et al (65)	76	26	15/16 (93)	16(61)
Hunter and Pezim (22)	203	52	9/22 (40)	19(36)
Dusold et al (25)	153	90	33/44 (75)	39(43)
Voeller et al (66)	103	85	—	18(21)
Present series	72	44	35/44 (80)	21(47)
Totals:			253/330 (79)	167/385(43)

[a]Localization confirmed by endoscopy, angiography, or surgery.

Table 6.3.   Nuclear Medicine Scan Screening Before Mesenteric Angiography

Study	Total No. of Positive NM Scans	Angiography Positive	Angiography Negative
McKusick et al (62)	38	25	13
Bentley and Richardson (26)	26	14	12
Voeller et al (66)	9	5	4
Present series	39	13	26
Totals:	112	57	55

NM, nuclear medicine.

of their larger size and bowel gas patterns than the animals studied (27). The pathognomonic finding of diverticular bleeding is pooling of contrast in the diverticulum (28). The limitation of the study is that the patient must be actively hemorrhaging at the time of injection (Fig. 6.5). Because of this, continuous monitoring of vital signs, cardiac rhythm, and oximetry in the radiology suite is imperative. Prompt and early angiography (after nasogastric tube, proctoscopy, and laboratory studies) has increased sensitivity to 72% (36 of 50 patients) in one larger series (29). Data from our institution over a 12-year period suggest a lower sensitivity of 34% (45 of 132 patients) with emergent and elective mesenteric angiograms for hemorrhage (Table 6.4). There are numerous reasons why hemorrhage may not be detected by angiography. The rate of bleeding may be below a certain threshold. Colonic bleeding often is intermittent in nature or may have stopped permanently. Technical difficulties and atherosclerotic anatomy may decrease the sensitivity of the study (30). Colonic bleeding may originate from small vessels (15). Angiograms are much more sensitive for arterial and capillary bleeding than for venous or variceal hemorrhage (21). In our series, 21 of 107 (19%) patients with negative

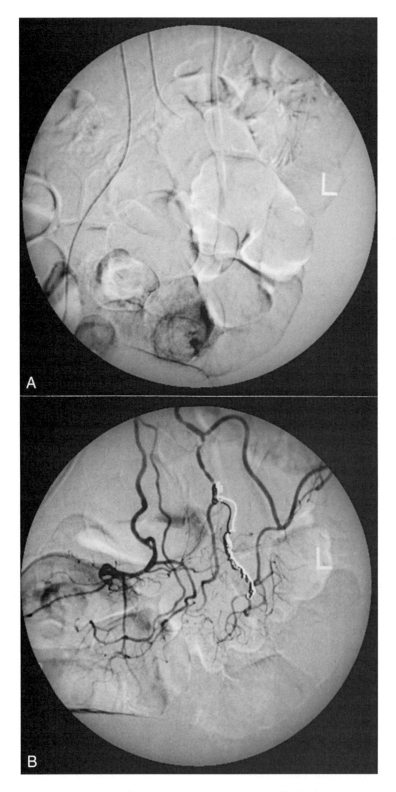

Figure 6.5.   **A.,** Mesenteric angiogram demonstrating extravasation. **B.,** No further extravasation is seen after superselective embolization with coils.

Table 6.4.   Review of Mesenteric Angiographies

Study	Total No. Angiographies	Positive Results	Percentage
Browder et al (29)	50	36	72
Welch et al (67)	59	22	37
Britt et al (68)	40	23	58
Wright et al (55)	14	12	86
Boley et al (69)	43	28	65
Casarella et al (70)	60	40	67
Uden et al (49)	28	16	57
Koval et al (32)	63	29	46
Leitman et al (7)	68	27	40
Moncure et al (4)	104	72	69
Parkes et al (56)	28	14	50
Wagner et al (50)	45	24	53
Farrands and Taylor (5)	9	5	55
Allison et al (71)	160	125	78
Whitaker and Gregson (72)	49	29	59
Present series	152	45	34
Totals:	972	547	56

angiograms required operative control of hemorrhage. Before resection, these patients required endoscopy, repeat angiography, or intraoperative localization procedures.

Complications of angiography include dissection, embolization, thrombosis, aneurysmal disease at the puncture site, bleeding, hematoma, allergic reaction to contrast material, and nephrotoxicity. Our data revealed four complications as a direct result of 132 (3%) mesenteric angiograms. Aggressive attempts have been made to increase the diagnostic sensitivity of angiography with the use of heparin, tolazoline vasodilatation, urokinase, and streptokinase (4,31). Koval et al improved the diagnostic efficiency from 32 to 65% with such "pharmacoangiography" (32). However, they noted some increase in transfusion requirements and complications with these techniques (32).

Angiography, when positive for bleeding, can reliably localize bleeding to an anatomic region of the bowel. Segmental bowel resections may be performed confidently on the basis of angiographic findings with little risk for rebleeding (29). *Angiography and colonoscopy remain the studies of choice in attempting to diagnose and localize lower gastrointestinal hemorrhage.* In patients with a negative angiogram, additional evaluation with colonoscopy or repeat angiography should be pursued because 25% of patients will require operative control of hemorrhage.

Barium Studies

Barium contrast studies should play little or no role in the diagnosis and localization of active diverticular bleeding. A barium enema will demonstrate the location of diverticula but will not identify any particular site of bleeding nor will barium enema diagnose colonic arteriovenous malformations, a major cause of hematochezia. On colonoscopy, Forde and Treat found pathology in 9 of 38 patients (24%) with a normal barium enema (3). Tedesco and colleagues noted that of 85 patients with diverticula noted on barium enema, 29 patients (34%) were found to have another source of bleeding at colonoscopy (18). Air-contrast barium enema (ACBE) should demonstrate tumors larger than 1 cm in diameter, ulcers, diverticula, and mucosal irregularities. Rex et al showed in a controlled study that ACBE with flexible sigmoidoscopy was better able to define the presence of diverticula than colonoscopy alone (51% versus 34%) (19). ACBE is more apt to be completed all the way to the cecum than colonoscopic examination (90% versus 74%) (21). It has been proposed that the increased intraluminal pressure may even provide hemostasis in colonic bleeding (33). *Barium enema performed for active bleeding may exclude the possibility of subsequent mesenteric angiography*, because the retained contrast material in the colon may obscure the arterial contrast agent. Barium enema should prove useful, however, for patients with subacute, chronic, slow, or intermittent bleeding. Barium enema should be complimented with flexible or rigid sigmoidoscopy to improve diagnostic accuracy in the region of the rectum and distal sigmoid colon.

THERAPEUTICS

Endoscopy

At the time that an emergent diagnostic colonoscopy is performed for hemorrhage, the physician may attempt to control an active bleeding site. Colonoscopic capabilities for therapeutics include the monopolar polypectomy snare, needle injection, bipolar electrode, heater probe, and argon laser. Although all of these modalities are effective for numerous potential causes of colonic bleeding, only cautery, probe, and local epinephrine injection can be used for diverticular bleeding (34–36). No large series were found addressing the safety of these particular interventions. Caution should be exercised when using monopolar electrocautery on the thin colonic wall.

Vasopressin

When angiography documents a bleeding diverticulum, transcatheter infusion of vasopressin may be initiated for treatment purposes. The recommended starting dose is 0.2-units/minute continuous infusion with repeat selective angiography performed 20 minutes later to document effectiveness of the infusion. The infusion may be increased to 0.4–0.6-units/minute maximum dose to achieve hemostasis. It is continued at the effective dose for 24–36 hours and then tapered. The catheter remains in place until the patient has stabilized and also is available for additional angiographic study if necessary (37). Studies of dogs demonstrate that superior mesenteric arterial infusion of vasopressin reduces blood flow by 65%, as compared with a 45% reduction with systemic infusion (38). There are less systemic effects with transcatheter infusion because of early metabolism by the liver (39). Fluid and electrolytes should be monitored because of the antidiuretic effect of the systemic vasopressin. Potential complications include all of those for mesenteric angiography and an extended indwelling arterial catheter, as well as catheter migration, and systemic complications from vasopressin infusion. Conn et al have reported complication rates as high as 43%, including arrhythmias, bradycardia, hypertension, cardiac arrest, and respiratory arrest (40).

Success rates with vasopressin infusion vary among studies. Athanasoulis et al's study of colonic diverticular bleeding demonstrated that hemorrhage was temporarily controlled by vasopressin in 91% of patients and remained controlled after completion of infusion in 70% (41). *Despite high response rates, rebleeding is common after cessation of vasopressin, reported as high as 50% (29).* In our series of 29 patients with positive angiograms who were treated with vasopressin, only 17 (58%) had successful treatment. Twelve patients (41%) had rebleeding, 22 patients (75%) required additional transfusions, and 9 patients (31%) had to be taken to the operating room emergently or semielectively. Complications in these patients included hematoma, electrocardiographic changes, hypertension, congestive heart failure, respiratory failure, and death. However, in a selected group of patients who are free of coronary artery disease, vasopressin remains a potential option to control ongoing diverticular bleeding.

Embolization

Transcatheter embolization is becoming a popular therapeutic option for the treatment of colonic hemorrhage. No large studies have been published that support the safety and efficacy of this treatment modality. More experience has been published regarding upper gastrointestinal embolization, with success rates as high as 88% (21/24) (42). Resistance to application of this procedure for colonic bleeding is most likely due to the lack of collateral blood supply in the colon. Numerous case reports exist describing ischemic complications secondary to embolization (43–46). Experience suggests that use of a coaxial catheter with a steerable guidewire may help decrease ischemic complications in subselective/superselective embolization. In addition to the usual mesenteric angiographic complications, other potential pitfalls include unintentional embolization of another vessel, increased intimal injury, and increased dye load. In follow-up, bleeding has been reported to recur either from the same or another site secondary to recanalization of the embolized branch or through collateral flow.

The rate of recanalization depends on the materials used for embolization. Autologous blood thrombus, Gelfoam pledgets, large polyvinyl alcohol particles, wire coils, detachable balloons, and collagen suspensions all have been used. Rosen and Sanchez suggest avoiding the use of collagen suspensions (Avitene) because of increased distal thrombosis (37). Gelfoam powder and absolute alcohol are more likely to cause mucosal injury (37). Coagulopathic patients tend to have a higher risk of rebleeding following embolization (47). With the proper materials and superselective angiography, recent embolization series show promising results and a decrease in the complication rate. Guy et al were able to control bleeding in nine patients with colonic hemorrhage (48). A recent 2-year follow-up review at our institution has shown that in eight cases of superselective embolization, two patients had recurrent bleeding; no ischemic complications occurred (Fig. 6.5). *Early data seem to suggest that superselective embolization has lower risks of rebleeding and fewer complications than vasopressin infusion.*

Embolization does not have a well-defined role at this point. Patients with diverticular bleeding who are poor operative candidates and who possess contraindications to vasopressin might benefit most from superselective embolization. Embolization also may be used as a means of controlling massive hemorrhage in preparation for a definitive operative procedure. At this point, there is no role for blind embolization for a patient in whom a point of bleeding can not be defined by angiography. Colonoscopy and close monitoring may be used to follow a patient's response to embolization as well as to identify any complications.

Surgery

Most patients with diverticular bleeding stop spontaneously and never require surgical intervention. Surgery is required for patients for whom other modalities have failed to control the bleeding as manifest by continued hemodynamic instability, transfusion requirements, or acute overt rebleeding. In Farrands and Taylor's series, patients requiring 4 or more units of blood during the first 24 hours of treatment had a 50% chance of requiring operative intervention (5). Patients who have had repeated episodes over longer periods also may require surgical resection. Even some patients with a negative

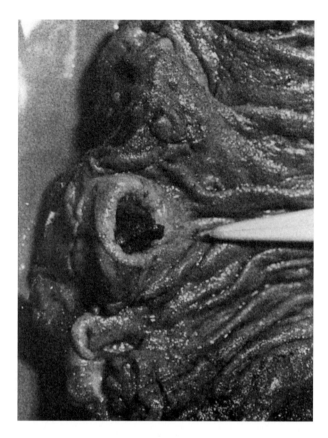

Figure 6.6. The diverticulum responsible for bleeding has been injected with resin in the right hemicolectomy specimen. (Reprinted with permission from Sabanathan S, Nag SB. Operative angiography in the management of massive rectal bleeding. J R Coll Surg Edinb 1984;29:96–99.)

angiographic and nuclear medicine evaluation may require operative intervention. Therefore, all patients with massive lower gastrointestinal bleeding should be evaluated and treated as though they may eventually require operative exploration and potential bowel resection.

There are no set criteria for when to operate. It is preferable to proceed with operative control after resuscitation, stabilization, and localization are complete. The instability of certain patients does not allow the usual diagnostic evaluation, and emergent surgery is sometimes required. If the patient's hemodynamic status allows, localization of bleeding preoperatively always should be attempted in an effort to decrease the overall morbidity and mortality. Browder and colleagues have shown that angiographic localization preoperatively has reduced morbidity from 37% to only 8.6% (29). Uden et al showed that attempts at angiographic localization reduced the mortality from 50% to 14% (49). If the stability of the patient allows, as many diagnostic modalities as necessary should be used to accurately localize bleeding, guide surgical treatment, and reduce morbidity and mortality.

If bleeding has not been localized, exploratory celiotomy is the final diagnostic modality. In the series reported by Wagner et al, the site of bleeding was localized operatively in seven of nine patients (78%) (50). In exploring for a site of bleeding, one may use transillumination, methylene blue staining, endoscopy, intraoperative angiography, and even colotomy to help localize the bleeding point (7,20,51–54). Because intraluminal bleeding may pass in both antegrade and retrograde directions and make direct visualization difficult, one may be forced to rely on any of these other modalities (20).

In the 1970s, subtotal colectomy was the treatment of choice for massive lower gastrointestinal hemorrhage. It had replaced blind segmental resections; this lowered the mortality rate to 10% (55). With the increased ability to localize bleeding preoperatively, segmental resections have become safer (Fig. 6.6). Most recent series support segmental resections for localized bleeding (7,56). Postoperative rebleeding rates with segmental resection range from 0 to 14 % (Table 6.5). The mortality rates for segmental resections are significantly lower than those for subtotal colectomies. *Total abdominal colectomy should be reserved for patients with a negative preoperative or intraoperative localization or for patients with multiple bleeding sites* (7,56). Even the recent mortality rates for these subtotal colectomies have improved, decreasing to lower than 10% (8). In the absence of a localized bleeding site, most authors support blind subtotal colectomy.

When operating for localized diverticular bleeding, one may find diverticula extending well beyond the segment of bleeding. There is no generalized consensus in the literature to support extended excision of the colon to include nonbleeding diverticula. Moncure and colleagues support subtotal colectomy for localized diverticular bleeding and for total colonic diverticula (4). Because of the lack of data and the low rebleeding rates following segmental resection, we support leaving nonbleeding diverticula behind.

The highest rate of complications occurred in patients who did not undergo angiography and received a segmental resection (56). Potential complications include death, sepsis, rebleeding after segmental resection, anastomotic leak, myocardial infarction, adult respiratory distress syndrome, pneumonia, and renal failure. Bender et al suggest considering the use of an ileostomy to avoid an anastomotic leak if more than 10 units of blood are transfused (57). Others have described the use of on-table lavage to prevent complications at an anastomosis (58,59). The decision to perform an anastomosis depends on the intraoperative conditions, as well as the patient's stability and comorbidities.

In conclusion, when a patient with massive lower gastrointestinal bleeding requires operative control, *every effort should be made to localize the source preoperatively*. If localized, a segmental resection may be performed safely, with low rates of rebleeding. Having excluded an upper gastrointestinal, small bowel, or a rectal source, severe, nonlocalized bleeding can be best treated with blind subtotal colectomy.

Table 6.5.   Segmental Colonic Resection Versus Subtotal Colectomy

Study Mortality	Segmental Resections	Postoperative Rebleeding (%)	Mortality (%)	Subtotal Colectomies	Postoperative Rebleeding	Mortality (%)
Britt et al (68)	8	1(13)	2(25)	9	0	2(22)
Browder et al (29)	17	0 (0)	0 (0)	18	—	—
Wright et al (55)	20	0	0 (0)	1	0	0 (0)
Welch et al (67)	11	0 (0)	0 (0)	3	0	1(33)
Leitman et al (7)	17	1 (6)	2(12)	7	0	3(43)
Parkes et al (56)	14	2(14)	1 (7)	10	0	3(30)
Bender et al (57)	—	—	—	49	—	13(27)
Boley et al (69)	7	—	0 (0)	4	—	2(50)
Cassarella et al (70)	—	—	—	39	0	2 (5)

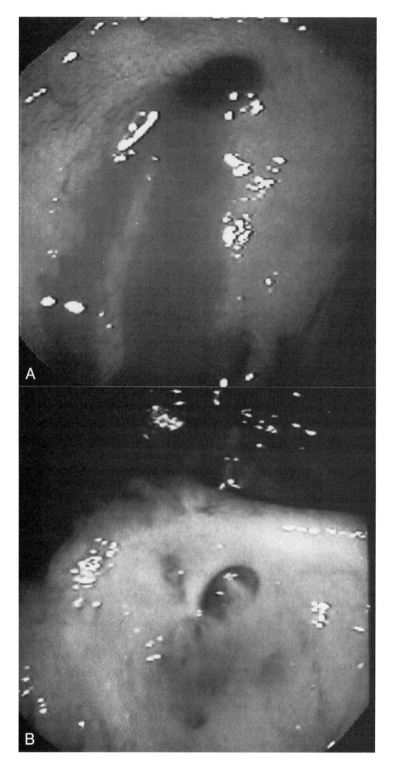

Figure 6.7.   A., This actively bleeding diverticulum was seen at colonoscopy. **B.,** The bleeding ceased after an epinephrine solution was injected into the region of the diverticulum. The patient did not require additional transfusions or emergency surgery.

EDITORIAL COMMENTS

Patients younger than 50 years of age rarely bleed from colonic diverticula (73,74). Conversely, elderly patients with colonic diverticular bleeding are hospitalized frequently. Virtually all of the episodes are self-limited and can be managed with resuscitation, monitoring, and endoscopy. Blood transfusions may be necessary, especially for patients with heart disease or anemia (75,76). A few authors aggressively prepare the bowel for endoscopy within 24 hours of admission (77); we tend to wait for 24–48 hours, when the bleeding tends to have ceased. Colonoscopy is useful at that time to search for diverticula, polyps, or malignancies (Fig. 6.7). The actual appearance of a diverticulum that has bled may have prognostic significance (78). We do not treat arteriovenous malformations of the right colon if they are not actively bleeding. If no abnormalities are found during colonoscopy, upper endoscopy and possible enteroclysis should be performed as well. A contrast study is not performed unless the bleeding has stopped and colonoscopy is not technically possible. In the rare incidence of massive bleeding from diverticulosis, we would monitor the patient carefully in an intensive care unit with Swan-Ganz monitoring if necessary. Attempts at localization should be made with arteriography, paying careful attention to the dye load, because of the risks to renal function. Results with vasopressin have been variable; based on our preliminary results, superselective embolization has been more effective and safe. The patient must be monitored continuously during angiography, and if the bleeding point can not be seen, pharmacoangiography can be used or the patient can be returned later to angiography for additional studies.

In the uncommon event that surgery becomes necessary, partial colectomy should be possible in most cases, based on accurate preoperative localization. Anastomosis should be avoided in the elderly patient who has been hypotensive preoperatively because of the risk of anastomotic leak (79).

SUGGESTED READINGS

1. Guy GE, Shetty PC, Sharma RP. Acute lower gastrointestinal hemorrhage: treatment by superselective embolization with polyvinyl alcohol particles. Am J Roentgenol 1992;152:521–526. *Largest published series in the literature to date for colonic embolization.*
2. Jensen DM, Machicado GA. Diagnosis and treatment of severe hematochezia. Gastroenterology 1988;95:1569–1574. *Describes the preparation and technique for emergent colonoscopy. Reports the experience with 80 patients having emergent colonoscopy for lower gastrointestinal bleeding.*
3. Meyers MA, Alonso DR, Gray GF, et al. Pathogenesis of bleeding colonic diverticulosis. Gastroenterology 1976;71:577–583. *A classic description of the pathology of diverticula and why they bleed.*
4. Rossini FP, Ferrari A, Spandre M, et al. Emergency colonoscopy. World J Surg 1989;13:190–192. *A review of the literature and personal experience with emergent colonoscopy for lower gastrointestinal bleeding.*
5. Shapiro MJ. Role of the radiologist in management of gastrointestinal bleeding. Gastroenterol Clin North Am 1994;23:123–181. *An excellent review article of nuclear medicine scans, angiography, and embolization of both upper and lower gastrointestinal bleeding.*
6. Schrock TR. Colonoscopic diagnosis and treatment of lower gastrointestinal bleeding. Surg Clin North Am 1989;69:1309–1325. *A detailed review of colonoscopy for diagnosis and treatment of both acute and chronic lower gastrointestinal bleeding.*

REFERENCES

1. Schrock TR. Colonoscopic diagnosis and treatment of lower gastrointestinal bleeding. Surg Clin North Am 1989;69:1309–1325. *A review of the role of colonoscopy in diagnosis and treatment of acute and chronic lower gastrointestinal bleeding.*
2. Painter NS, Burkitt DP. Diverticular disease of the colon: a deficiency of western civilization. BMJ 1971;2:450–454. *An important historical, geographic, and clinical review linking a low-residue diet and diverticular disease.*
3. Forde KA, Treat MR. Colonoscopy for lower gastrointestinal bleeding. In: Dent TL, Strudel WF, Turcotte JG, et al, eds. Surgical endoscopy. Chicago: Yearbook Medical Publishers, 1985:261–274.
4. Moncure AC, Tompkins RG, Athanasoulis CA, et al. Occult gastrointestinal bleeding: newer techniques of diagnosis and therapy. Adv Surg 1989;22:141–178. *A general survey with 55 references.*
5. Farrands PA, Taylor I. Management of acute lower gastrointestinal hemorrhage in a surgical unit over a four year period. J R Soc Med 1987;80:79–82. *A review of 107 patients with an algorithm for management of lower gastrointestinal bleeding.*
6. Meyers MA, Alonso DR, Gray GF, et al. Pathogenesis of bleeding colonic diverticulosis. Gastroenterology 1976;71:577–583. *Traumatic factors may induce asymmetric intimal proliferation and scarring of vasa recta, predisposing to rupture. There was a general absence of diverticulitis in this study of 10 colons with microangiographic techniques.*

7. Leitman IM, Paull DE, Shires DT III. Evaluation and management of massive lower gastrointestinal hemorrhage. Ann Surg 1989;209:175–180. *Forty percent of 68 patients had positive arteriograms.*

8. DeMarkles MP, Murphy JR. Acute lower intestinal bleeding. Med Clin North Am 1992;77:1085–1099. *A review with 64 references.*

9. Wilson RG, Smith AN, Macintyre IM. Complications of diverticular disease and non-steroidal anti-inflammatory drugs: a prospective study. Br J Surg 1990;77:1103–1104. *A prospective trial: patients admitted with complications of diverticular disease had a high incidence of intake of NSAIDs.*

10. Campbell K, Steale FJ. Non-steroidal inflammatory drugs and complicated diverticular disease: a case-control study. Br J Surg 1991;78:190–191. *This study suggested a strong association between the intake of NSAIDs and development of complications of diverticular disease.*

11. Langman MJ, Morgan L, Worrall A. Use of anti-inflammatory drugs by patients admitted with small or large bowel perforations and hemorrhage. BMJ 1985;290:347–349. *Patients with perforation or hemorrhage were more than two times as likely to take anti-inflammatory drugs.*

12. Richards RJ, Donica MB, Grayer D. Can the blood urea nitrogen/creatinine ratio distinguish upper from lower gastrointestinal bleeding. J Clin Gastroenterol 1990;12:500–504. *A BUN/Cr ratio of 36 suggests upper gastrointestinal bleeding, whereas a ratio lower than 36 does not help locate the source.*

13. Snook JA, Holdstock GE, Bamforth J. Value of a simple biochemical ratio in distinguishing upper and lower sites of gastrointestinal hemorrhage. Lancet 1986;1:1064–1065. *Eighty-seven percent of patients with upper gastrointestinal bleeding had a BUN/Cr ratio of 100; 95% of patients with lower gastrointestinal bleeding had a ratio lower than 100.*

14. Lichtenstein DR, Berman MD, Wolf MM. Approach to the patient with acute upper gastrointestinal hemorrhage. In: Taylor MB, Gollan JL, Peppercorn MA, et al, eds. Gastrointestinal emergencies. 1st ed. Baltimore: Williams & Wilkins, 1992:92.

15. Jensen DM, Machicado GA. Diagnosis and treatment of severe hematochezia. Gastroenterology 1988;95:1569–1574. *Urgent colonoscopy after an oral purge was effective, safe, and often diagnostic.*

16. Irvine EJ, O'Connor J, Frost RA, et al. Prospective comparison of double contrast barium enema plus flexible sigmoidoscopy v colonoscopy in rectal bleeding: barium enema v colonoscopy in rectal bleeding. Gut 1988;29:1188–1193. *Flexible sigmoidoscopy plus double contrast barium enema was superior to colonoscopy for detecting diverticular disease.*

17. Rossini FP, Ferrari A, Spandre M, et al. Emergency colonoscopy. World J Surg 1989;13:190–192. *A personal experience of 409 emergency colonoscopies; the test was a valuable diagnostic tool.*

18. Tedesco FJ, Waye JD, Raskin JB, et al. Colonoscopic evaluation of rectal bleeding; a study of 304 patients. Ann Intern Med 1978;89:907–909. *Significant lesions were found during colonoscopy in 41.5%.*

19. Rex DK, Weddle RA, Lehman GA, et al. Flexible sigmoidoscopy plus air-contrast barium enema versus colonoscopy for suspected lower gastrointestinal bleeding. Gastroenterology 1990;98:855–861. *A randomized controlled trial involving 380 patients. Colonoscopy is more cost effective in patients older than 55 years of age.*

20. Steer ML, Silen W. Diagnostic procedures in gastrointestinal hemorrhage. N Engl J Med 1983;309:646–649. *A discussion of current concepts.*

21. Shapiro MJ. Role of the radiologist in management of gastrointestinal bleeding. Gastroenterol Clin North Am 1994;23:123–181. *A comprehensive review article that discusses nuclear scans, angiography, and embolization of upper and lower gastrointestinal bleeding.*

22. Hunter JM, Pezim ME. Limited value of technetium 99m-labeled red cell scintigraphy in localization of lower gastrointestinal bleeding. Am J Surg 1990;159:504–506. *Performing an operation relying on localization by scan alone will lead to an undesirable result in at least 42% of patients.*

23. Owunwanne A, Abdel-Dayem HM. Radionuclide detection and localization of the site of gastrointestinal bleeding (letter). J Nucl Med 1988;29:130–131. *The authors point out that 99m DTPA detects gastrointestinal bleeding effectively in both the upper and lower abdomen.*

24. Ryan P, Styles CB, Chmiel R. Identification of the site of severe colonic bleeding by technetium-labeled red cell scan. Dis Colon Rectum 1992;35:219–222. *Scans correctly identified the site of bleeding in nine patients and avoided total colectomy in eight patients.*

25. Dusold R, Burke K, Carpentier W, et al. The accuracy of technetium-99m-labeled red cell scintigraphy in localizing gastrointestinal bleeding. Am J Gastroenterol 1994;89:345–348. *The scintigraphy was valuable if it was positive within 2 hours and a UGI source already had been excluded.*

26. Bentley DE, Richardson JD. The role of tagged red blood cell imaging in localization of gastrointestinal bleeding. Arch Surg 1991;126:821–824. *Tagged scans localized the site of bleeding in only 52% of patients.*

27. Corman ML. Vascular diseases. In: Corman ML, ed. Colon and rectal surgery. Philadelphia: JB Lippincott, 1993:860–900.

28. Athanasoulis CA. Angiography in the management of patients with gastrointestinal bleeding. Adv Surg 1983;16:1–23. *Embolization is not recommended in the mesenteric vascular bed (SMA and IMA).*

29. Browder W, Cerise EJ, Litwin MS. Impact of emergency angiography in massive lower intestinal bleeding. Ann Surg 1986;204:530–536. *Emergency angiography and vasopressin infusion may supplant emergency operation and permit segmental colectomy of the bleeding site.*

30. Sos TA, Lee JG, Wixson D, et al. Intermittent bleeding from minute to minute in acute massive gastrointestinal hemorrhage: arteriographic demonstration. Am J Roentgenol 1976;131:1015–1017. *Even acute massive gastrointestinal hemorrhage can vary greatly in intensity from minute to minute.*

31. Rosch J, Keller FS, Wawrukiewicz AS, et al. Pharmacoangiography in the diagnosis of recurrent massive lower gastrointestinal bleeding. Radiology 1982;145:615–619. *A good discussion of pharmacoangiography with case reports.*

32. Koval G, Brenner KG, Rosch J, et al. Aggressive angiographic diagnosis in acute lower gastrointestinal hemorrhage. Dig Dis Sci 1987;32:248–253. *Extravasation of contrast increased from 32 to 65% after introduction of pharmacologic techniques.*

33. Adams JT. The barium enema as treatment for massive diverticular bleeding. Dis Colon Rectum 1974;17:439–441. *Barium enema seems to arrest acute bleeding; if it does not, the author recommends resection of the portion of colon containing diverticula.*

34. Kim Y, Marcon NE. Injection therapy for colonic diverticular bleeding. J Clin Gastroenterol 1993;17:46–48. *A successful report of epinephrine injection in an elderly patient.*

35. Bertoni G, Conigliaro R, Ricci E, et al. Endoscopic injection hemostasis of colonic diverticular bleeding: a case report. Endoscopy 1990;22:154–155. *The neck of the diverticulum was injected with epinephrine solution, stopping the bleeding.*

36. Johnston J, Sones J. Endoscopic heater probe coagulation of bleeding colonic diverticulum (abstract). Gastrointest Endosc 1986;32:160. *The heater probe is a therapeutic alternative to treat a bleeding colonic diverticulum.*

37. Rosen RJ, Sanchez G. Angiographic diagnosis and management of gastrointestinal hemorrhage. Radiol Clin North Am 1994;32:951–967. *The risk of ischemia with embolization is significant only in the colon or if collaterals have been divided.*

38. Simmons JT, Baum S, Sheehan BA, et al. The effect of vasopressin on hepatic arterial blood flow. Radiology 1977;124:637–640. *Hepatic blood flow was inversely correlated with mesenteric blood flow.*

39. Baum S, Rosch J, Potter CT, et al. Selective mesenteric arterial infusion in the management of massive diverticular hemorrhage. N Engl J Med 1973;288:1269–1272. *Seven of 15 patients ceased bleeding after selective arterial infusion with a follow-up period of 6–30 months.*

40. Conn HO, Ramsby GR, Storer EH, et al. Intra-arterial vasopressin in the treatment of upper gastrointestinal hemorrhage: a prospective controlled clinical trial. Gastroenterology 1975;68:211–221. *Survival was not affected by vasopressin administration.*

41. Athanasoulis CA, Baum S, Rosch J, et al. Mesenteric arterial infusions of vasopressin for hemorrhage from colonic diverticulosis. Am J Surg 1975;129:212–216. *Nine of 24 patients studied had no recurrent bleeding within a 7- to 34-month follow-up period.*

42. Gomes AS, Lois JF, McCoy RD. Angiographic treatment of gastrointestinal hemorrhage: comparison of vasopressin infusion and embolization. Am J Roentgenol 1986;146:1031–1037. *The success rate was 88% with embolization and 52% with vasopressin infusion.*

43. Gerlock AJ, Muhletaler CA, Berger JL, et al. Infarction after embolization of the ileocolic artery. Cardiovasc Intervent Radiol 1981;4:202–205. *Occlusion of the cecal branches can devascularize the cecum and appendix, even if the colic and ileal branches are not occluded. Therefore, the ileocolic artery may not be a good candidate for therapeutic embolization.*

44. Uflacker R. Transcatheter embolization for treatment of acute lower gastrointestinal bleeding. Acta Radiol 1987;28:425–430. *Five patients with diverticular hemorrhage were embolized in the right or middle colic arteries with Gelfoam. A total of 13 patients with lower gastrointestinal bleeding of various etiologies are described; two patients developed large bowel infarction necessitating colectomy.*

45. Rosenkrantz H, Bookstein JJ, Rosen RJ, et al. Postembolic colonic infarction. Radiology 1982;142:47–51. *Embolization is recommended for patients in whom vasopressin treatment is contraindicated, when patients are refractory to vasopressin, or when rebleeding occurs after vasopressin infusion.*

46. Shiroy SS, Satchidanard S, West EH. Colonic ischemic necrosis following therapeutic embolization. Gastrointest Radiol 1981;6:235–237. *Ischemic necrosis of the transverse colon followed embolization of the middle colic artery.*

47. Encarnacion CE, Kadir S, Beam CA, et al. Gastrointestinal bleeding treatment with gastrointestinal arterial embolization. Radiology 1992;183:505–508. *Embolization is useful in patients with gastrointestinal bleeding together with coagulopathy.*

48. Guy GE, Shetty PC, Sharma RP. Acute lower gastrointestinal hemorrhage: treatment by superselective embolization with polyvinyl alcohol particles. Am J Roentgenol 1992;159:521–526. *Hemorrhage was controlled successfully in 9 of 10 patients with no cases of intestinal infarction.*

49. Uden P, Jiborn H, Jonsson K. Influence of selective mesenteric angiography on the outcome of emergency surgery for massive lower gastrointestinal hemorrhage. Dis Colon Rectum 1986;29:561–566. *Positive preoperative angiography allowed limited resection and decreased operative mortality.*

50. Wagner HE, Stain SC, Gilg M, et al. Systematic assessment of massive bleeding of the lower part of the gastrointestinal tract. Surg Gynecol Obstet 1992;175:445–449. *The source of bleeding was identified preoperatively in 74 of 83 patients.*

51. Flickinger EG, Stanforth AC, Sinar DR, et al. Intra-operative video panendoscopy for diagnosing sites of chronic intestinal bleeding. Am J Surg 1989;157:137. *Mucosal disease was found in 13 of 14 patients with intraoperative video panendoscopy.*

52. Bowden TA, Hooks VH, Mansberger AR. Intraoperative gastrointestinal endoscopy in the management of occult gastrointestinal bleeding. South Med J 1979;72:1532–1534. *A discussion of eight patients managed with intraoperative endoscopy; in six individuals, appropriate resection or local control of bleeding was accomplished.*

53. Sabanathan S, Nag SB. Operative angiography in the management of massive rectal bleeding. J R Coll Surg Edinb 1984;29:96–99. *A report of two patients on whom superior mesenteric angiography was performed through a catheter introduced into the ileocolic artery.*

54. Cohen JL, Forde KA. Intraoperative colonoscopy. Ann Surg 1988;207:231–233. *A study of 68 patients. Endoscopic evaluation influenced the outcome in 93%.*

55. Wright HK, Pellicia O, Higgins EF Jr, et al. Controlled semi-elective segmental resection for massive colonic hemorrhage. Am J Surg 1980;139:535–538. *A specific bleeding site permitting segmental colectomy was found in 92% of patients.*

56. Parkes BM, Obeid FN, Sorenson VJ, et al. Management of massive lower gastrointestinal bleeding. Am Surg 1993;59:676–678. *Subtotal colectomy should be reserved for massive bleeding with negative angiography.*

57. Bender JS, Wiencek RG, Bowman DL. Morbidity and mortality following total abdominal colectomy for massive lower gastrointestinal bleeding. Am Surg 1991;57:536–541. *Patients who have total abdominal colectomy and lose more than 10 units of blood should have ileostomy performed because of the risk of anastomotic leak.*

58. Scott HJ, Lane IF, Glynn MJ, et al. Colonic hemorrhage: a technique of rapid intra-operative bowel preparation and colonoscopy. Br J Surg 1986;73:390–391. *Describes a technique of operative orthograde colonic washout followed by colonoscopy in four patients.*

59. Radcliffe AG, Dudley HA. Intraoperative antegrade irrigation of the large intestine. Surg Gynecol Obstet 1983;156:721–723. *Describes a technique of lavage used in the treatment of 64 patients.*

60. Alvai A, Ring EJ. Localization of gastrointestinal bleeding: superiority of 99mTc sulfur colloid compared with angiography. Am J Roentgenol 1981;137:741–748. *The technique is considered simple and reliable.*

61. Nicholson ML, Neoptolemos JP, Sharp JS, et al. Localization of lower gastrointestinal bleeding using in vivo technetium-99m-labeled red blood cell scintigraphy. Br J Surg 1989;76:358–361. *The technique had a high predictive value.*

62. McKusick KA, Froelich J, Callahan RJ, et al. 99mTc red blood cells for detection of gastrointestinal bleeding: experience with 80 patients. Am J Roentgenol 1981;137:1113–1118. *This technique was useful in patients with melena as well as patients with passage of bright red blood per rectum.*

63. Szasz IJ, Morrison RT, Lyster DM. Technetium-99m-labeled red blood cell scanning to diagnose occult gastrointestinal bleeding. Can J Surg 1985;28:512–514. *The nuclear scan was preferable and more cost-effective than selective angiography as a first line diagnostic test.*

64. Markisz JA, Front D, Royal HD, et al. An evaluation of 99m Tc-labeled red blood cell scintigraphy for the detection and localization of gastrointestinal bleeding sites. Gastroenterology 1982;83:394–398. *Scintigraphy is a reliable test for screening patients before angiography.*

65. Orecchia PM, Hensley EK, McDonald PT, et al. Localization of lower gastrointestinal hemorrhage. Arch Surg 1985;120:621–624. *A study of 76 patients. Scans were accurate in localizing bleeding sites.*

66. Voeller GR, Bunch G, Britt LG. Use of technetium-labeled red blood cell scintigraphy in the detection and management of gastrointestinal hemorrhage. Surgery 1991;110:799–804. *Scintigraphy failed to localize hemorrhage in 85% of the patients.*

67. Welch CE, Athanasoulis CA, Galdabini JJ. Hemorrhage from the large bowel with special reference to angiodysplasia and diverticular disease. World J Surg 1978;2:73–83. *A series of 72 patients; in 85%, the bleeding originated in the right or transverse colon.*

68. Britt LG, Warren L, Moore OF. Selective management of lower gastrointestinal bleeding. Am Surg 1983;49:121–125. *Pitressin was more useful for control of diverticular bleeding than for bleeding from vascular ectasias.*

69. Boley SJ, DiBiase A, Brandt LJ, et al. Lower intestinal bleeding in the elderly. Am J Surg 1979;137:57–64. *Segmental colectomy was successful in patients with diverticular disease and positive angiography.*

70. Casarella WJ, Galloway SJ, Taxin RN, et al. "Lower" gastrointestinal tract hemorrhage: new concepts based on angiography. Am J Roentgen Radium Ther Nucl Med 1972;121:357–368. *Most bleeding colonic diverticula were proximal to the splenic flexure.*

71. Allison DJ, Hemingway AP, Cunningham DA. Angiography in gastrointestinal bleeding. Lancet 1982;2:30–33. *A study of 160 selective visceral angiograms and some embolizations.*

72. Whitaker SC, Gregson RH. The role of angiography in the investigation of acute or chronic gastrointestinal hemorrhage. Clin Radiol 1993;47:382–388. *Best results are achieved if angiography is done with minimal delay following negative endoscopy. This technique is also useful with continuing subacute blood loss when other studies are negative.*

73. Korkis AM, McDougall CJ. Rectal bleeding in patients less than 50 years of age. Dig Dis Sci 1995;40:1520–1523. *Five of the 102 patients had incidental diverticula not believed to be the bleeding source.*

74. Acosta JA, Fournier TK, Knutson CO, et al. Colonoscopic evaluation of rectal bleeding in young adults. Am Surg 1994;60:903–906. *Two percent of the patients had diverticular disease, which was considered to be an incidental finding.*

75. Bokhari M, Vernova AM, Ure T, et al. Diverticular hemorrhage in the elderly—is it well tolerated. Am Surg 1996;39:191–195. *The elderly tolerated nonoperative or operative treatment quite well, despite low initial hematocrits or substantial amounts of blood transfusions.*

76. Reinus JF, Brandt LJ. Vascular ectasias and diverticulosis. Common causes of lower intestinal bleeding. Gastroenterol Clin North Am 23:1-20, 1994. A *review with 56 references.*

77. Jensen DM. Current management of severe lower gastrointestinal bleeding (editorial). Gastrointest Endosc 1995;41:171–173. *Recommends colonic preparation and colonoscopy within 24 hours of severe hematochezia.*

78. Foutch PG. Diverticular bleeding: are nonsteroidal anti-inflammatory drugs risk factors for hemorrhage and can colonoscopy predict outcome for patients? Am J Gastroenterol 1995;90:1779–1784. *Combined exposure to NSAIDs and ASA may be worse than NSAIDs alone. Ulcerated diverticula led to less severe bleeding than diverticula with visible or adherent clot.*

79. McGuire HH Jr. Bleeding colonic diverticula. A reappraisal of natural history and management. Am Surg 1994;220:653–656. *Of 10 patients with "blind" colectomy and an emergency anastomosis to unprepared rectum, three leaked and three others had peritonitis or abscess.*

7 Recurrent Sigmoid Diverticulitis

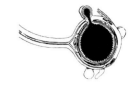

Charles W. Chappuis, MD
Isidore Cohn, Jr., MD

KEY POINTS

- Recurrent diverticulitis will occur in 33–45% of patients who have suffered one episode
- Flexible endoscopy and barium contrast studies are complementary tests: they delineate the extent of disease and rule out malignancy
- Elective resection best performed 8–10 weeks after acute attack
- Complete sigmoid resection to the rectosigmoid junction decreases recurrence rates
- The laparoscopic or open approach can be used

Although uncommon before 40 years of age, the incidence of colonic diverticular disease increases with advancing age, so that by the ninth decade, it is present in nearly two-thirds of the population. The incidence of diverticulitis also increases with advancing age. Studies by Horner found that the incidence of diverticulitis increased according to the length of time the patients were observed (1). The incidence of diverticulitis was approximately 10% after 5 years of observation and increased to higher than 35% at 20 years. Approximately 20% of patients diagnosed with diverticulitis will eventually require surgical intervention.

The sigmoid colon is involved in more than 90% of the cases of diverticulitis and is the only segment of bowel affected in roughly 50% of cases. Rodkey and Welch reviewed surgically treated cases of diverticular disease and found that 94.6% of all operative cases involved the sigmoid colon (2).

INDICATIONS FOR RESECTION

Episodes of diverticulitis complicated by obstruction, perforation, or urinary tract involvement frequently result in the need for operative intervention. In addition, the occasional inability to rule out a colonic malignancy may necessitate resection. In 1953, Welch and associates reported on 114 sigmoid resections with a mortality rate of 2.6%. They concluded that uncomplicated, recurrent acute diverticulitis must be considered an important reason for elective sigmoid resection (3). Also, it is estimated that 33–45% of patients who experience one attack of diverticulitis will subsequently have another. A review of 177 consecutive patients undergoing elective operation for sigmoid diverticular disease revealed that 70% had either two or more previous attacks or chronic symptoms (4). *Currently, the most common indication for elective sigmoid resection in diverticular disease is recurrent acute attacks of inflammation with chronic abdominal pain.*

CASE STUDY

The following case illustration describes a patient with recurrent diverticulitis. This case will be used to discuss diagnostic studies, preoperative preparation, intraoperative methods, and postoperative management.

A 60-year-old woman was seen with a history of recurrent attacks of lower abdominal pain associated with fever and an altered bowel pattern. These episodes of pain and fever had been treated with oral antibiotics in the past with prompt resolution of symptoms. At the time of evaluation, she complained only of occasional vague left lower abdominal discomfort. She had no fever, nausea, or diarrhea. Physical examination revealed mild left lower quadrant abdominal tenderness to palpation. No palpable abdominal mass was appreciated. Rectal examination was unrevealing and the stool was Hematest negative. Surgical history included appendectomy, hysterectomy, and tubal ligation. A diagnosis of recurrent diverticulitis was made and the following workup ensued.

Flexible sigmoidoscopy was performed to 20 cm showing a normal-appearing mucosa without evidence of diverticula. No other lesions were noted. Angulation of the bowel at 20 cm prevented further insertion of the endoscope. Air-contrast barium enema was performed and revealed numerous diverticula in the sigmoid colon without evidence of acute diverticulitis.

DIAGNOSTIC EVALUATION

Flexible endoscopy frequently is useful in evaluation of patients with diverticular disease. It is especially indicated when the presence of neoplasm cannot be ruled out on the basis of the contrast enema. Also, diverticular strictures are frequently overdiagnosed on the basis of contrast study alone. In this instance, flexible endoscopy often is useful in verifying the presence of a strictured segment of colon.

Because the sigmoid colon often is difficult to examine radiographically, some authors suggest the use of both endoscopy and contrast enema in the evaluation of patients with sigmoid diverticulitis. Boulos and associates performed colonoscopy on 105 patients with symptomatic sigmoid diverticular disease (5). Barium enema was found to be inaccurate in detecting adenoma and carcinoma in 43% of patients. Boulos and associates recommended endoscopic examination for patients with sigmoid diverticular disease, particularly those older than 60 years of age, and patients with rectal bleeding. The primary benefit of this diagnostic approach is early identification of occult sigmoid malignancy. We agree that these two studies complement one another. Flexible sigmoidoscopy followed by air-contrast barium enema can be performed on the same day to expedite the workup.

Most patients presenting with similar symptoms and a clinical diagnosis of diverticular disease should undergo an air-contrast barium enema. This study provides useful information regarding the number and distribution of diverticula. The most consistent finding in diverticular disease is secondary to the marked hypertrophy of the colonic muscle. The circular muscle layer becomes thickened, resulting in the serrated or saw-tooth appearance of the colon (Fig. 7.1).

We believe that rigid proctosigmoidoscopy has limited usefulness in evaluation of patients suspected of having sigmoid diverticular disease. The involved segment of bowel usually is above the 20- to 25-cm range visible with this instrument. In addition, sigmoid diverticular disease often is accompanied by significant angulation of the colon, which makes visibility difficult with a rigid instrument and also is frequently quite painful for the patient.

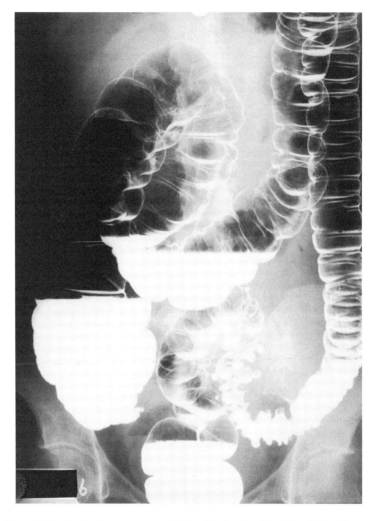

Figure 7.1. Sawtooth appearance of the colon involved by diverticular disease.

Although useful in the acute setting, we find little place for the use of ultrasonography, computed tomography (CT) scanning, or magnetic resonance imaging (MRI) in the diagnosis of uncomplicated, recurrent diverticular disease.

Intravenous pyelogram should be a routine part of the preoperative workup for all patients undergoing elective sigmoid resection for diverticulitis. It allows one to verify the function of both kidneys and to define the anatomic relationship of the ureter to the colon. Although unusual, the ureters occasionally may be involved in the inflammatory reaction adjacent to the involved segment of colon. In a review of 180 patients undergoing intravenous urography before colorectal surgery, Prager and associates found abnormalities in 43% of patients (6). Of these, 35% of the abnormalities were considered to be related to the primary colon disease. Preoperative intravenous pyelogram (IVP) allows the surgeon to anticipate and avoid injury to the urinary tract. Some authors advocate the placement of retrograde ureteral catheters before operation. We do not use this technique routinely but would rather reserve it for patients undergoing reoperative pelvic surgery or for those with significant ureteral abnormalities identified on the preoperative IVP.

Although expensive, a lighted ureteral stent can be especially useful for the obese patient with abnormalities identified on IVP. This also may be used when laparoscopic colectomy is to be performed.

SURGICAL MANAGEMENT

The timing of operation after an episode of sigmoid diverticulitis should depend both on the severity of the attack and on the response to medical management. *We believe elective resection should be performed 8–10 weeks after an acute attack.* This interval of time allows for resolution of the inflammatory reaction so that operation may be performed during a quiescent stage of the disease.

Preparation of the patient for elective colon resection should include both mechanical and antibiotic bowel preparation. The patient is placed on a clear liquid diet 24 hours before surgery. The two most commonly used techniques for mechanical bowel preparation use either cathartics, enemas, and a low-residue diet or whole gut lavage. We prefer the use of whole gut lavage using 4 liters of polyethylene glycol electrolyte solution administered over 3–4 hours starting at 9:00 AM on the morning before surgery. Mechanical cleaning of the bowel significantly reduces the total colonic content, and therefore the total microbial population, but does not reduce the number of microorganisms in any residual colonic content. Therefore, we use both oral and parenteral antibiotics along with the mechanical bowel preparation. Neomycin (1 g) and erythromycin base (1 g) are given at 1:00 PM, 2:00 PM, and 11:00 PM on the day before operation. In addition, we use parenteral broad-spectrum antibiotics given immediately before operation and one to two doses during the early postoperative period.

OPERATIVE PROCEDURE

An indwelling urinary catheter should be placed before initiation of the operation. This allows the bladder to remain decompressed during the course of the operation and is of particular importance when working in the pelvis with the patient in the Trendelenburg position. A nasogastric tube is also placed before beginning the operation. This allows decompression of the stomach and is especially important when a laparoscopic approach is desired.

Elective resection of the sigmoid colon should be performed in a controlled situation with adequate preoperative preparation and only after obtaining appropriate informed consent of the patient. Excellent results can be achieved with sigmoid resection for recurrent diverticular disease. In most cases, this resection should include the entire sigmoid colon. Equally acceptable results can be achieved with either an open resection or a laparoscopic colon resection.

If open resection is undertaken, we use either a stapled end-to-end anastomosis or a sutured end-to-end anastomosis using a single layer of 3–0 polyglycolic acid sutures. Either technique is very satisfactory. Use of the single-layer sutured technique allows one to tailor the anastomosis when there is a size discrepancy between the proximal and distal segments of bowel. When this discrepancy is marked, an antimesenteric (Cheatle) slit can be made on the smaller, usually proximal, side.

Our preference at this time is to use a laparoscopic approach with transanal, stapled, end-to-end anastomosis. Preoperative barium enema is useful in identifying the involved segment of bowel. *This is extremely important because of the loss of ability to palpate the bowel and identify the exact location of thickened hypertrophic bowel wall.* Because of this, our preference is to perform a resection of the involved sigmoid colon. The proximal line of resection is chosen based on both the barium enema findings and the appearance of the bowel during the course of inspection at the time of operation. The anastomosis should be performed in an area that is relatively free of diverticula.

Diverticulitis generally is confined to a short segment of the colon. The amount of bowel resected for sigmoid diverticular disease is debated frequently. Concern always exists about remaining diverticula proximal to the line of resection and the possibility of recurrent diverticulitis. We agree with Wolff and colleagues that it is not necessary to extend the proximal margin to include all of the diverticula-bearing portion of the colon (7). The distal margin of resection should be at the transition point from sigmoid colon to rectum, where there is loss of the taeniae coli (8) (see Chapter 25).

In all circumstances, the anastomosis must be fashioned with viable, well-vascularized proximal and distal margins in a tension-free manner. Resection of the involved segment of sigmoid colon and an anastomosis usually can be performed without the need for dissection of the splenic flexure. An extensive resection is not necessary, because the operation is being performed for benign disease.

The reader is referred to Chapter 8 for a detailed discussion of the techniques of laparoscopic resection.

POSTOPERATIVE MANAGEMENT

The indwelling urethral catheter and the nasogastric tube usually are removed on the morning after operation. A clear liquid diet frequently is started later the first postoperative day, if the patient does not experience nausea. This liquid diet is continued after discharge from the hospital until the patient has complete return of bowel function along with a desire for solid food. Early mobilization of the patient is advised, usually on the first postoperative day. Parenteral analgesics are used until the patients are able to tolerate an oral analgesic, which often occurs during the first postoperative day. Little postoperative pain is experienced with laparoscopic colectomy and, therefore, analgesic requirements are minimal. The patients are discharged from the hospital when they are able to tolerate a liquid diet without nausea and are able to ambulate without difficulty.

CONCLUSION

Recurrent sigmoid diverticulitis is the most common indication for elective resection of diverticular disease. Alleviation of symptoms occurs in most patients with a very low rate of recurrence. A laparoscopic approach to this disease is possible.

EDITORIAL COMMENTS

By nature of the symptoms that define recurrent diverticulitis, it may be difficult to distinguish this entity from other cases of recurrent abdominal pain. It is imperative to demonstrate objectively that the patient has diverticulitis, and it may be necessary to do this on more than one occasion. Most of the time, the diagnosis will be made by findings of perisigmoid inflammation on a CT scan.

If recurrent symptoms of abdominal pain develop in the absence of clinical findings, concern should arise that the underlying diagnosis may actually be irritable bowel syndrome. Even when operating for proven diverticulitis, the patient should be cautioned regarding the possibility that not all of the abdominal symptoms will resolve after performing a sigmoid resection (9). In one series, the best results after elective resection were correlated with several factors: male sex, preoperative bowel complaints of less than 1 year, left lower quadrant abdominal pain, and radiologic evidence of diverticulitis (10).

Regarding the question of when in the course of recurrent diverticulitis surgery is indicated, the answer is problematic. It is difficult to determine with certainty what the risk of additional attacks is in a particular individual. Studies of the natural history of diverticular disease are limited, and many were performed 20–30 years ago (11). According to one textbook of surgery, the risk of recurrence is 30% after one simple, uncomplicated episode of diverticulitis and increases to more than 50% after a second attack (12). Certainly, as noted in this chapter, recurrent attacks of mild to moderate severity represent an indication for operation.

However, considering the subjective grading of an individual attack, patients may come to surgery at different points in their course. It is safe to state that for most patients, a single attack is not an indication, considering the recurrence rate may not be more than 30%. As for surgery after a second attack, other factors may play a role, such as the patients' threshold for pain, their inherent fear of surgery, their work schedules and travel plans, or other issues that have little to do with the clinical situation. As a guideline, it is reasonable to suggest surgery for a patient with recurrent diverticulitis when the clinical course substantially interferes with the patient's daily living.

The editors would take issue with performing an IVP in the routine preoperative workup of a patient with diverticulitis. There is no evidence that obtaining an IVP will decrease the incidence of intraoperative injury to the ureters. Careful dissection through noninflamed planes before entering the diverticular inflammatory mass will best ensure the preservation of the ureters intraoperatively. In this era of cost-effective medicine, we would strongly discourage the use of routine preoperative IVP.

Another matter involves laparoscopic versus open colectomy. The authors clearly favor the laparoscopic operation. A satisfactory result can be achieved with each technique, if an adequate resection of the sigmoid colon is accomplished, but the ultimate approach taken will depend on the surgeon's preference and experience and on costs. On-table laparoscopic colonic irrigation has even been attempted in nonobstructed patients (13). There is some preliminary evidence that the length of stay and time to advances of diet are shorter in the laparoscopic group, but there is disagreement about overall costs in the literature (14,15). Presently, we are not using the laparoscopic approach frequently for elective resection and anastomosis of sigmoid diverticular disease.

REFERENCES

1. Horner JL. Natural history of diverticulitis of the colon. Am J Dig Dis 1958;3:343–350. *In this long-term study of a group of office patients, virtually none required surgery.*
2. Rodkey GV, Welch CE. Changing patterns in the surgical treatment of diverticular disease. Ann Surg 1984;200:466–478. *The indication for operation in 13% of this surgical series was chronic pain.*
3. Welch CE, Allen AW, Donaldson GA. An appraisal of resection of the colon for diverticulitis of the sigmoid. Ann Surg 1953;138:332–343. *A report of more than 100 colon resections during the era when elective procedures began to increase in numbers.*
4. Moreaux J, Vons C. Elective resection for diverticular disease of the sigmoid colon. Br J Surg 1990;77:1036–1038. *Of 177 patients having elective surgery for diverticular disease of the sigmoid, 52 had a history of two or more attacks of diverticulitis. Thirty-five percent of patients with chronic symptoms were found to have an unexpected abscess, and 18% of patients in this group had unsatisfactory results, perhaps related to irritable bowel syndrome associated with diverticulosis.*
5. Boulos PB, Cowin AP, Karamanolis DG, et al. Diverticula, neoplasia, or both? Early detection of carcinoma in sigmoid diverticular disease. Ann Surg 1985;202:607–609. *A study of 105 patients with symptomatic sigmoid diverticular disease that had colonoscopy. Endoscopy is recommended for patients with sigmoid diverticulosis, especially those older than 60 years of age and those with rectal bleeding.*
6. Prager E, Swinton NW, Corman ML. Intravenous pyelography in colorectal surgery. Dis Colon Rectum 1973;16:479–481. *Seventy-eight of 180 patients having IVP before colorectal surgery had abnormalities, including 41% of the patients with diverticulitis. The authors believe that injury is more likely to happen with distortions in normal anatomy and that preoperative knowledge is helpful in planning repair if an injury occurs.*
7. Wolff BG, Ready RL, MacCarty RL, et al. Influence of sigmoid resection on progression of diverticular disease of the colon. Dis Colon Rectum 1984;27:645–647. *If resection of the colon does not include the proximal rectum, the recurrence rate of diverticulitis is 11.4%.*

8. Benn PL, Wolff BG, Ilstrup DM. Level of anastomosis and recurrent colonic diverticulitis. Am J Surg 1986;151:269–271. *The authors recommend removal of the entire distal sigmoid colon when operating for diverticular disease with anastomosis to the proximal rectum.*
9. Charnock FM, Rennie JR, Wellwood JM, et al. Results of colectomy for diverticular disease of the colon. Br J Surg 1977;64:417–419. *Only 28% of patients were cured of their abdominal pain after colectomy.*
10. Breen RE, Corman ML, Robertson WG, et al. Are we really operating on diverticulitis? Dis Colon Rectum 1986;29:174–176. *Ninety-four percent of 77 patients followed after elective surgery for diverticulitis had satisfactory results. Patients with no inflammatory change apparent on histologic examination were less likely to have favorable results.*
11. Parks TG. Natural history of diverticular diseases of the colon. Clin Gastroenterol 1975;4:53–69. *A detailed, interesting account. The author reviewed several publications that suggested that the risk of recurrent attacks was 33–45%.*
12. Kodner IJ, Fry RD, Fleshman JW, et al. Colon, rectum and anus. In: Schwartz SI, Shires GT, Spencer FC, et al, eds. Principles of surgery. 6th ed. New York: McGraw-Hill, 1994:1191–1306.
13. Chung CC, Kwok SP, Kwong KH, et al. Technique of laparoscopically assisted on-table colonic irrigation. Br J Surg 1997;84:384. *Laparoscopic colonic irrigation was performed on two elderly men with sigmoid volvulus undergoing laparoscopically assisted colectomy.*
14. Bruce CJ, Coller JA, Murray JJ, et al. Laparoscopic resection for diverticular disease. Dis Colon Rectum 1996;39:S1–S6. *A retrospective comparison of laparoscopic (25 patients) and open (17 patients) resection of chronic diverticulitis. Diet was advanced more rapidly and hospital stay was shorter in the laparoscopic group (P < .001), but overall costs were higher with laparoscopic surgery because of significantly greater operating time.*
15. Liberman MA, Phillips EH, Carroll BJ, et al. Laparoscopic colectomy vs traditional colectomy for diverticulitis. Outcome and costs. Surg Endosc 1996;10:15–18. *The authors looked at 14 consecutive patients having laparoscopic sigmoid colectomy for diverticulitis and compared them with 14 matched patients having traditional open colectomy. Despite the greater operating charges for laparoscopic colectomy, the total hospital charges were less than those following open colectomy.*

8 Radiologic Evaluation of Diverticular Disease of the Small and Large Intestines

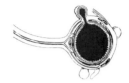

Stuart K. Markowitz, MD
Wanda Kirejczyk, MD

KEY POINTS

- CT scan diagnostic study of choice for acutely ill patients with suspected diverticulitis
- Contrast enema (*a*) provides complementary information, (*b*) can be initial diagnostic test for less acutely ill patients, (*c*) is secondary examination when CT results are equivocal
- Radiographic evaluation should be guided by the clinical presentation and specific examinations should be selected accordingly
- Diagnosis of unusual types of diverticulitis usually requires CT scan supplemented by contrast studies when needed
- Communication between clinician and radiologist to facilitate effective sequence of tests

ILLUSTRATIVE CASES

Case 1: A 65-year-old female presented to the emergency department with sepsis and 2 days of left lower quadrant pain and tenderness. On physical examination, a fullness was palpated in the left lower quadrant. Laboratory evaluation revealed marked leukocytosis. A diagnosis of diverticulitis was suspected and the patient underwent abdominal and pelvic computed tomography (CT) scan for additional evaluation (Fig. 8.1).

Case 2: A 68-year-old man with a known history of diverticulosis presented to the emergency department with a complaint of left lower quadrant pain, low-grade fever, and obstipation. On physical examination, the patient was in mild distress and slightly tender to palpation in the left lower quadrant. A contrast enema was ordered as the next diagnostic study (Fig. 8.2).

Case Comments

These two patients both seemed to have diverticulitis. The first patient had an abdominal mass and leukocytosis, suggesting a possible phlegmon or abscess. A CT scan was the procedure of choice, because it would define the degree of pericolonic inflammation, and if an abscess was seen, it might

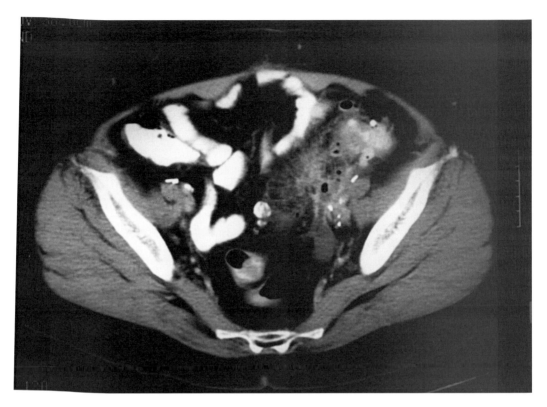

Figure 8.1.   Pelvic CT demonstrates extensive inflammation of the sigmoid colon and adjacent tissues with extraluminal gas confirming diagnosis of diverticulitis.

be amenable to percutaneous drainage. The second patient had symptoms and signs of a milder illness. An abscess or significant perforation was not suspected and he had no history of colon cancer. He would be evaluated most cost-effectively with a gentle contrast enema.

INTRODUCTION

Diverticular disease of the colon affects up to 65% of people older than 70 years of age in developed Western world countries (1). It is believed that these diverticula are an acquired abnormality resulting, at least in part, from a low-fiber diet. Complications of diverticulosis include bleeding, inflammation, and obstruction. Approximately 10–30% of patients will develop a complication as a result of their disease (2). The radiographic investigation of colonic diverticulitis traditionally has begun with the contrast enema; however, with the advent of CT and refinements in sonography, the diagnostic evaluation and therapeutic management may take many different courses.

Although it is a common entity, small bowel diverticulosis rarely is clinically significant. Small bowel diverticula may be found anywhere from the duodenum to the terminal ileum. In this chapter, we will present some of the radiographic signs of small bowel diverticular disease, including a discussion of their complications and several rare presentations.

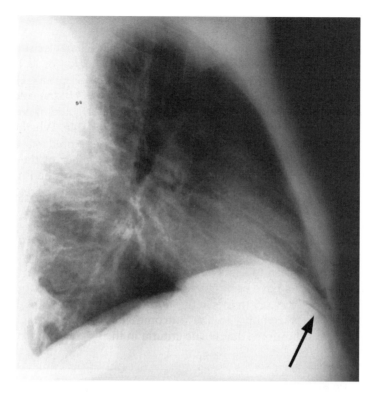

Figure 8.4. Small crescent of air is seen beneath the anterior portion of the right hemidiaphragm (arrow). The PA chest film was normal.

well as patient selection factors. Acutely ill patients imaged early in the course of their disease are more likely to have a positive study. Nevertheless, the contrast enema remains an excellent examination with low morbidity and cost.

This brings us to the question "When should a contrast enema be performed?" Any patient who is suspected of having diverticular disease is a potential candidate for this examination. *For patients who present atypically, a water-soluble enema can be performed initially and, if not diagnostic, a CT scan should be undertaken with minimal delay* because the contrast agent is absorbed rapidly or expelled and causes few artifacts during the CT study. The use of barium precludes immediate CT scanning because of artifacts created by the high-density barium agent. A contrast enema generally is contraindicated for patients with pneumoperitoneum who are hemodynamically unstable or who have undergone a deep colonic biopsy within the previous 7 days, because they are at high risk for complications from the procedure, particularly peritonitis.

The colon should not be prepared before the study. A water-soluble contrast material may be desirable, because extraluminal demonstration of contrast is the most reliable sign of diverticulitis. If spilled into the peritoneal cavity, water-soluble contrast is less irritating than barium, causes less reactive changes, and will be absorbed over time. Mucosal detail, however, is superior with barium. If peritoneal contamination occurs with barium, operative management of the patient becomes far more complex because barium is cleared less easily from the peritoneal cavity by the surgeon and it may incite a severe form of peritonitis. *The examination should be terminated after a diagnosis has been made.* Proximal disease may be coexistent, and a complete enema or colonoscopy can be performed at a later date (12,13).

Radiographic criteria of diverticulitis include a fistula (Fig. 8.7) or sinus tract (Fig. 8.8) extending from or involving the bowel wall, and/or a submucosal abscess as evidenced by the mass effect produced on the colonic lumen (Fig. 8.9). Extraluminal barium implies the perforation of a diverticulum (12,14) (Fig. 8.10). The characteristic tract may run perpendicularly to the bowel as a sinus tract or communicate with an adjacent abscess cavity or hollow viscus such as the small bowel, bladder, or vagina (Fig. 8.11). Cutaneous fistulas are rare (Fig. 8.12). The tracts may be single or multiple and may vary in contour from straight and smooth to markedly irregular and complex. The tract may course parallel to the bowel wall in the subserosal layer, most commonly in the sigmoid region. It may communicate with several diverticular sacs, which is called the "double tract sign" of diverticulitis (Fig. 8.13). The discovery of fistulous tracts and extraluminal collections occasionally may be confused with Crohn's disease, which also may present a similar double-tract appearance. However, in Crohn's colitis, the mucosa is involved and usually is edematous or irregular in appearance (15). Not uncommonly, filling of the abscess cavity or extravasation of contrast occurs after the patient evacuates due to a rise in intraluminal pressure generated during defecation. Therefore, the postevacuation film is mandatory when the initial films do not demonstrate a leak (12,13) (Fig. 8.14).

The most common radiographic finding seen in up to 65% of cases (14) is an extraluminal mass resulting from the intramural or adjacent abscess cavity. These appear as smooth,

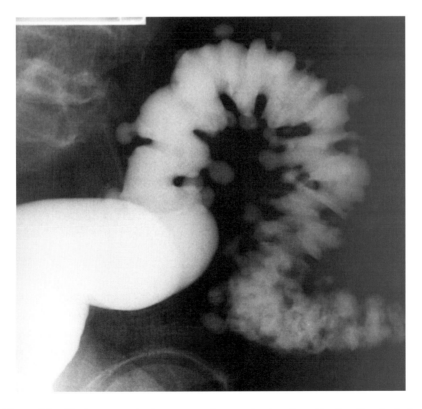

Figure 8.5.   Single contrast barium enema shows extensive sigmoid colon diverticulosis.

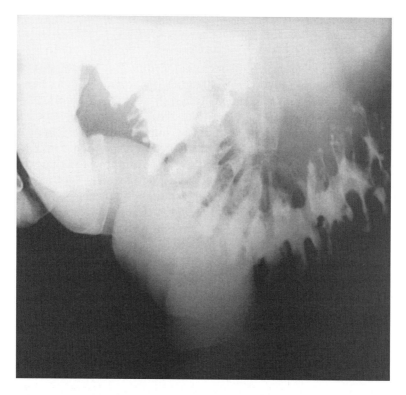

Figure 8.6. Marked muscle hypertrophy in this patient with long-standing diverticular disease creates a dramatic picket fence or sawtooth appearance on barium examination.

well-defined defects, most often with associated adjacent diverticula (Fig. 8.15). This appearance, however, may be created by a number of other entities, including carcinoma, metastases, and endometriosis (15). Ancillary findings that are suggestive of diverticulitis include diverticulosis, colonic spasm with tethering, and a "spiked" appearance of the mucosa, implying thickening (10). Retrograde obstruction also may be discovered, and this finding is difficult to distinguish from other etiologies of colonic obstruction, especially carcinoma. Radiographic findings that suggest diverticulitis rather than carcinoma include the involvement of a segment greater than 6 cm in length, as well as tapered rather than shouldered margins of the lesion and lack of mucosal destruction (15) (Fig. 8.16). In this particular situation, additional imaging with CT may be invaluable in suggesting the correct diagnosis.

The contrast enema remains the primary diagnostic imaging modality because of its widespread availability, ease of performance with no special preparation, high accuracy in diagnosis, low morbidity, and relatively low cost (16). *Its major limitation is its inability to fully evaluate the extent of the inflammatory process, particularly the extraluminal or extramural extent of disease.*

Computed Tomography

After the plain film examination, CT often is obtained in the evaluation of the patient with an acute abdomen. In the setting of diverticular disease, *CT has revolutionized both the diagnosis and management of patients with diverticulitis.* Many studies have looked at the sensitivity of CT as compared with the contrast enema. The results are somewhat varied. Smith et al (10) concluded that CT had a 90% sensitivity to abnormality as compared with 94% for the contrast enema. In a study reported by Cho et al (11), the sensitivity of CT was reported to be 93%, compared to 80% for the enema. Despite some of the variability in the findings, which may be influenced by scanning protocols and patient selection, it is clear that CT is an excellent imaging technique for the detection of diverticular disease. *The strength of CT is in the visualization of extraluminal disease and evaluation for nonoperative and operative management.*

Before scanning the patient, oral contrast should be administered to maximize bowel opacification. In addition to oral preparation, rectal contrast or retrograde air insufflation is suggested to enhance detection of bowel pathology. Scanning can be performed beginning at the abdomen or can begin at the level of the pubic rami and continue cephalad at no greater than 1-cm intervals. If a specific abnormality is seen, selected 5-mm cuts can be made through the area of concern for more precise delineation of extent of disease as well as to help detect subtle, early changes.

Diverticulitis is an inflammatory process of the bowel wall which is well seen with CT. The most frequent and sensitive indicator of diverticulitis is pericolic fat infiltration or phlegmon, which may be seen in as many as 98% of patients (17) (Fig. 8.17). In 1984, seven features of acute diverticulitis were described by Hulnick et al (17). These findings include sigmoid diverticula, pericolic inflammatory changes involving fat, colonic wall thickening

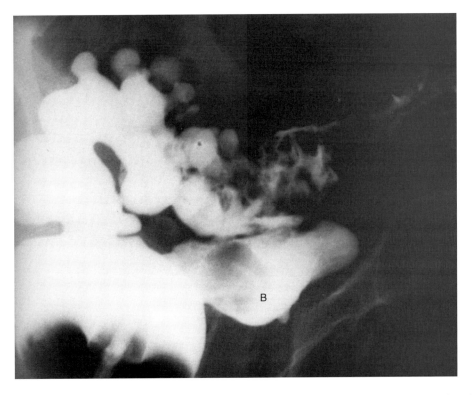

Figure 8.7. Barium enema shows extensive diverticulitis with long intramural fistulous tract extending along proximal sigmoid colon and fistula filling the bladder (B).

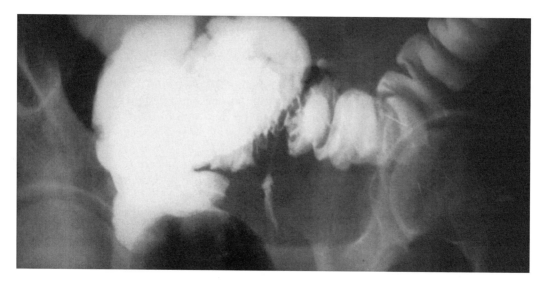

Figure 8.8. Long, thin sinus tract extends caudally from the sigmoid colon.

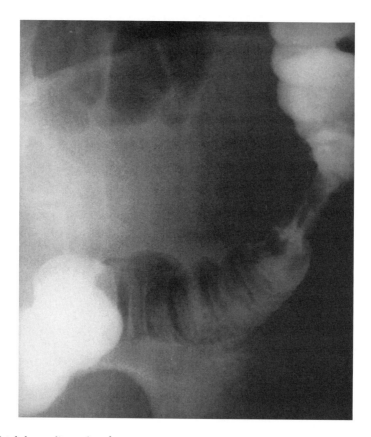

Figure 8.9. Distal descending colon shows concentric narrowing due to mass effect produced by intramural diverticular abscess.

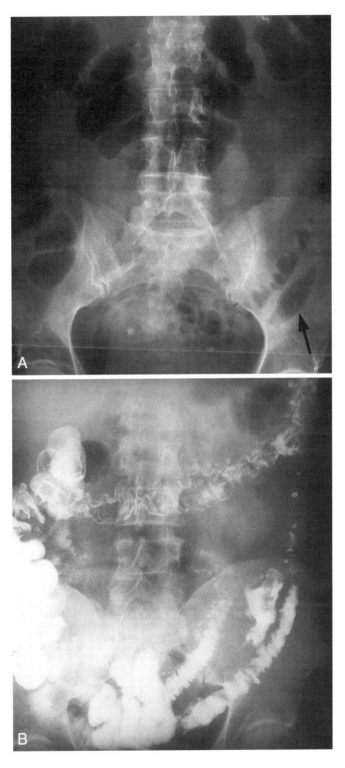

Figure 8.10.   **A.,** Preliminary film of the abdomen shows an ovoid gas collection paralleling the course of the descending colon (arrow). **B.,** Barium examination shows extravasation of contrast material into the diverticular abscess cavity.

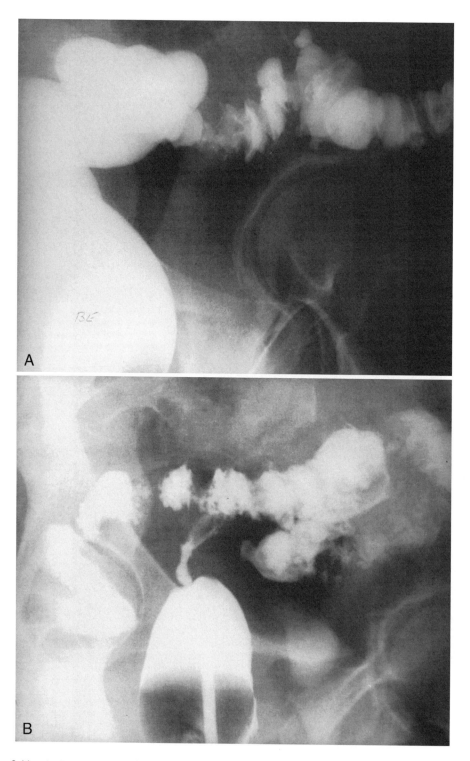

Figure 8.11.   A., Barium enema shows narrowed segment of sigmoid colon with adjacent diverticula but no extravasation or fistula. **B.,** Often, the colonic study will not demonstrate the fistula and the suspected organ involved must be evaluated. In this patient, contrast was injected into the vagina, subsequently demonstrating the fistulous communication to the colon.

greater than 4 mm (Fig. 8.18), fluid and/or contrast within the bowel wall indicating an intramural sinus tract, pericolonic abscess adjacent to an inflamed sigmoid colon (Fig. 8.19), extrapelvic abscess or peritonitis associated with an inflamed sigmoid colon, and fistula formation, especially sigmoidovesical fistula (18)(Fig. 8.20).

Abscesses identified on CT scan may appear fluid-filled or contain some air, creating a mottled appearance (Fig. 8.21). Although these collections are most commonly adjacent to the diseased segment of bowel, they may occur anywhere within the peritoneal cavity, retroperitoneum, or even extend into the groin and other remote sites.

Pitfalls in the use of CT include suboptimal detection of very early disease (19). Other factors limiting sensitivity include focal or concentric colonic wall thickening mimicking neoplasm (19). Most colonic carcinomas have marked thickening of the wall (greater than 2 cm); however, some will present with less than 1 cm of thickening (20). Useful signs to distinguish between carcinoma and diverticulitis were described by Padidar et al (21). Fluid at the root of the mesentery, which appears as a curvilinear band at the base of the reflection of the sigmoid mesentery, is suggestive of diverticulitis. Vascular engorgement also supports the diagnosis of diverticulitis. Lastly, microabscesses, intramural inflammatory exudate, and isodense-appearing infected intramural diverticula may escape detection with CT (19). A contrast enema is complimentary for these equivocal cases or for situations in which the clinical suspicion for diverticular disease remains high despite a negative study.

In summary, CT is advantageous because it can be performed in acutely ill patients and more readily allows the detection of extraluminal and extramural disease, even at sites

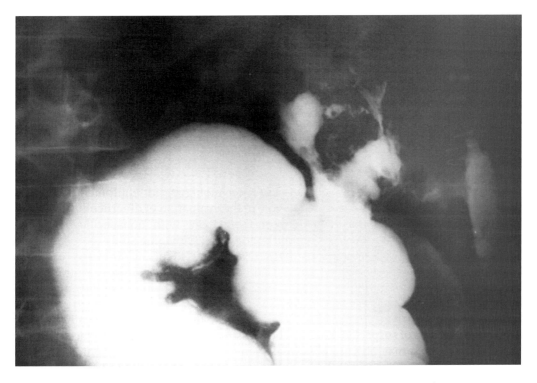

Figure 8.12. This patient had undergone a prior resection for diverticular disease. Left behind was a segment of involved sigmoid colon, which years later perforated and led to an enterocutaneous fistula to the anterior abdominal wall.

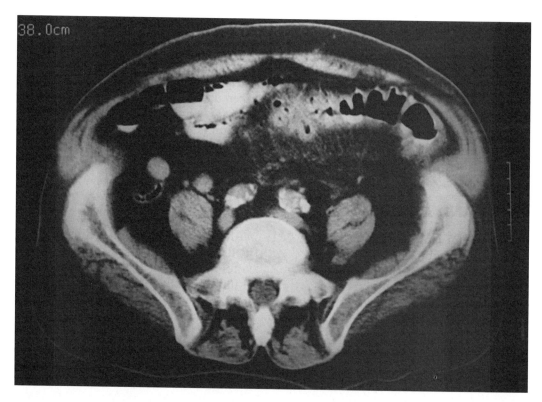

Figure 8.17.   As seen in Case 1 presented at the beginning of this chapter, the involved colon shows surrounding inflammatory changes or phlegmon with small bubbles of extraluminal air.

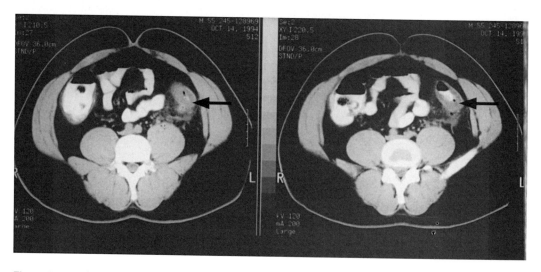

Figure 8.18.   The descending colon is thickened (arrow) to almost 10 mm with surrounding inflammation strongly suggesting perforation and therefore possible diverticulitis.

greater than 4 mm (Fig. 8.18), fluid and/or contrast within the bowel wall indicating an intramural sinus tract, pericolonic abscess adjacent to an inflamed sigmoid colon (Fig. 8.19), extrapelvic abscess or peritonitis associated with an inflamed sigmoid colon, and fistula formation, especially sigmoidovesical fistula (18)(Fig. 8.20).

Abscesses identified on CT scan may appear fluid-filled or contain some air, creating a mottled appearance (Fig. 8.21). Although these collections are most commonly adjacent to the diseased segment of bowel, they may occur anywhere within the peritoneal cavity, retroperitoneum, or even extend into the groin and other remote sites.

Pitfalls in the use of CT include suboptimal detection of very early disease (19). Other factors limiting sensitivity include focal or concentric colonic wall thickening mimicking neoplasm (19). Most colonic carcinomas have marked thickening of the wall (greater than 2 cm); however, some will present with less than 1 cm of thickening (20). Useful signs to distinguish between carcinoma and diverticulitis were described by Padidar et al (21). Fluid at the root of the mesentery, which appears as a curvilinear band at the base of the reflection of the sigmoid mesentery, is suggestive of diverticulitis. Vascular engorgement also supports the diagnosis of diverticulitis. Lastly, microabscesses, intramural inflammatory exudate, and isodense-appearing infected intramural diverticula may escape detection with CT (19). A contrast enema is complimentary for these equivocal cases or for situations in which the clinical suspicion for diverticular disease remains high despite a negative study.

In summary, CT is advantageous because it can be performed in acutely ill patients and more readily allows the detection of extraluminal and extramural disease, even at sites

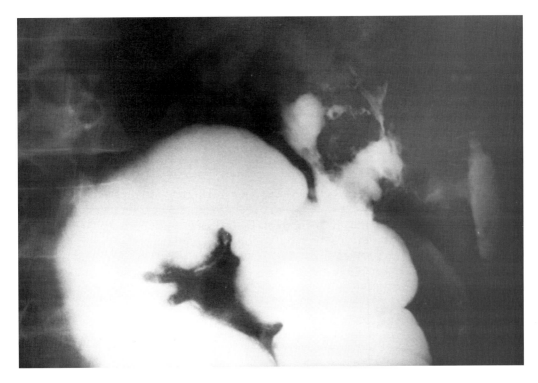

Figure 8.12.   This patient had undergone a prior resection for diverticular disease. Left behind was a segment of involved sigmoid colon, which years later perforated and led to an enterocutaneous fistula to the anterior abdominal wall.

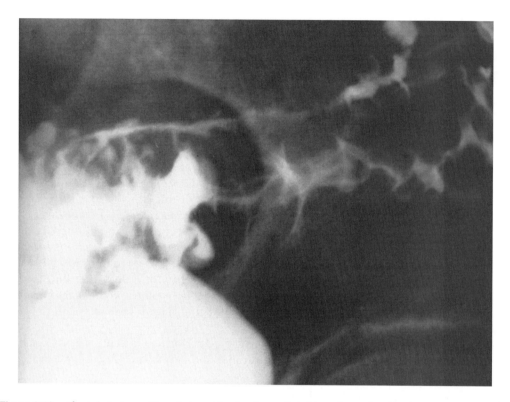

Figure 8.13. The inferiorly positioned sigmoid colon is paralleled by a long, thin fistulous tract creating the parallel tract or railroad tract sign of diverticulitis.

remote from the site of bowel abnormality (22). *Its use is limited currently by its relative nonavailability and higher cost compared to the contrast enema.* The full evaluation of fistulous communications is still best delineated with the contrast enema. Therefore, it is *likely that even with technologic improvements, these two examinations will remain complementary.*

Sonography

With the advent of improved transducer technology and equipment advances, sonography has dramatically expanded its role in the evaluation of diverticulitis, although its primary role remains the evaluation of the patient with nonspecific abdominal complaints. If an abscess is detected by this or some other imaging study, ultrasound can be helpful in guiding percutaneous biopsy and placement of drainage catheters. Ultrasonographic diagnosis can be followed immediately by percutaneous aspiration and drainage, thereby expediting the initiation of therapy (15). When a focal area of concern is raised or detected, a graded compression technique is used with a high-resolution transducer (5 or 7.5 MHz). The abdomen is scanned with the transducer gradually, pressing firmly over the area of suspected disease. The pressure of the transducer displaces air-filled bowel loops, which may obscure abnormal segments of bowel. Sonographic features of diverticulitis include hypoechoic thickening of the wall, greater than 4 mm, with a tubular pattern on longitudinal scans. The involved segment usually is 5 cm or longer. Thickened bowel has a target appearance on transverse scans due to muscular thickening and inflammatory changes in the wall (Fig. 8.22). This is the most common sonographic finding,

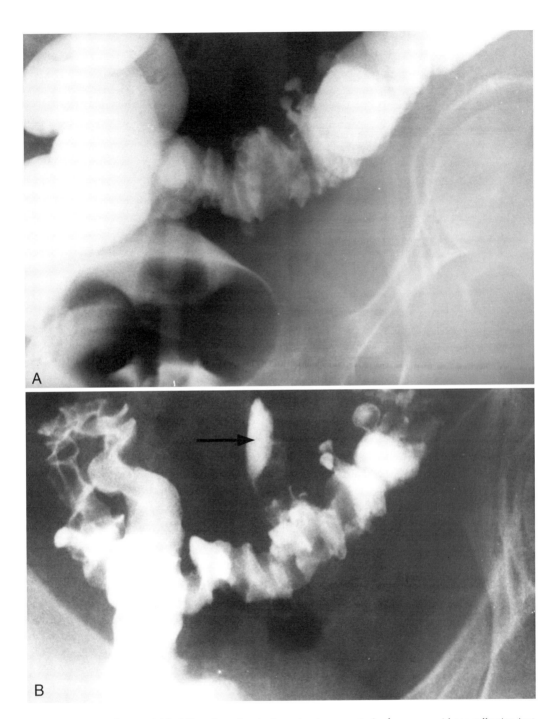

Figure 8.14.   A., The initial filled films from the single contrast enema study show an ovoid gas collection just above the midsigmoid colon adjacent to multiple small diverticula. **B.,** On evacuation, a follow-up film shows this cavity to fill with barium, diagnostic of a small communicating diverticular abscess (arrow).

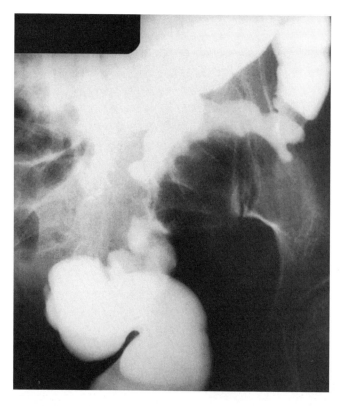

Figure 8.15.   The proximal descending colon is compressed by a large intramural or extrinsic mass, which was later proven to be a diverticular abscess.

occurring in up to 98% of cases (23). Tenderness and local pain must accompany the sonographic findings to make a diagnosis of acute diverticulitis. Diverticular disease without evidence of active inflammation may have a sonographically thickened bowel wall and may be confused with acute inflammation (23). Other signs of diverticulitis include hyperechoic diverticula and a hyperechoic halo representing peridiverticulitis. The inflamed mesenteric fat appears brightly echogenic. Pericolonic abscesses also may be evident as extraluminal hypoechoic collections with increased Doppler flow.

A potential pitfall in the use of sonography for evaluation of acute abdominal pain occurs when the findings of other disease processes such as Crohn's colitis, lymphoma, ischemic bowel, and ulcerative colitis mimic those of diverticulitis (23). Pericolonic abscesses and abnormalities in the mesentery also may be overlooked or obscured by overlying structures, especially air-filled bowel.

Magnetic Resonance Imaging

The use of magnetic resonance imaging (MRI) in the evaluation of bowel abnormalities currently is limited. Obstacles to accurate imaging include motion artifacts from peristalsis and respiratory excursion. In addition, metallic devices cause obscuring artifacts. The resolution of MRI is slightly inferior to that of CT and has not yet matched the sensitivity in detecting intestinal diseases seen with other imaging modalities (24).

Nuclear Imaging

The role of nuclear medicine in the imaging of diverticulitis is limited to the localization of a septic focus when a source is not evident clinically or by other imaging studies (25). [67]Gallium citrate or [111]Indium-labeled leukocytes can be used (Fig. 8.23). Both radiopharmaceuticals have limitations. [67]Gallium also is taken up by tumors and excretion into the bowel is normal. The large amount of bowel activity may limit its usefulness in detecting inflammatory conditions involving the gut. [111]Indium is expensive and requires special preparation. Neither agent can distinguish between an inflammatory mass and an abscess (25,26).

CECAL AND APPENDICEAL DIVERTICULAR DISEASE

The cecum is an uncommon site in the colon for the development of diverticula in patients living in the United States (Fig. 8.24). The diagnosis of cecal diverticulitis often is obscure and the clinical presentation is mistaken for appendicitis. Imaging of this entity often begins with either graded-compression ultrasound or CT looking for acute appendicitis. The diagnosis may then be apparent and appropriate treatment may be instituted. Often, however, the diagnosis is not made before the time of surgery (Fig. 8.25).

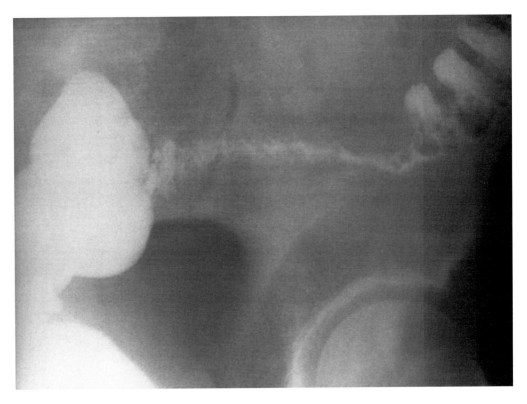

Figure 8.16. This patient presented with bowel obstruction. Barium enema demonstrated a long, narrowed segment of sigmoid colon. Note the tapered transition to the normal descending colon and the relative preservation of the mucosa in the involved segment. Surgery confirmed the diagnosis of diverticulitis.

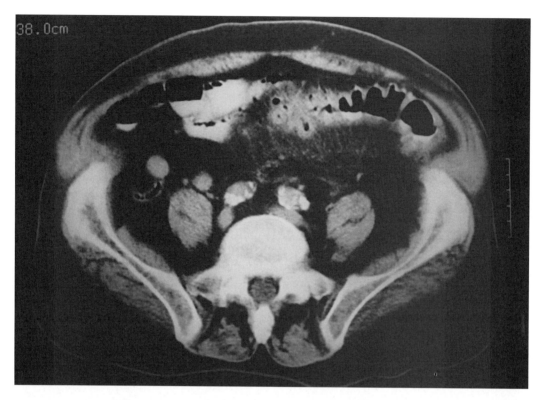

Figure 8.17.   As seen in Case 1 presented at the beginning of this chapter, the involved colon shows surrounding inflammatory changes or phlegmon with small bubbles of extraluminal air.

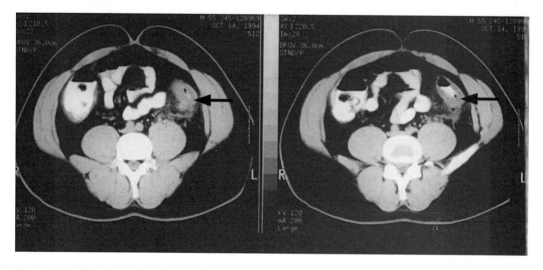

Figure 8.18.   The descending colon is thickened (arrow) to almost 10 mm with surrounding inflammation strongly suggesting perforation and therefore possible diverticulitis.

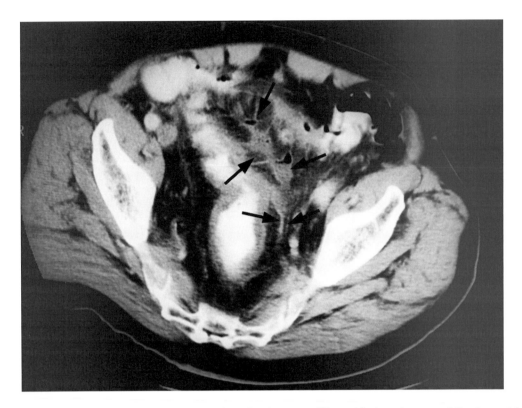

Figure 8.19. CT demonstrates a long, pericolonic fistulous tract filling with air and contrast following rectal contrast administration (arrows). There may be multiple sites of communication with the sigmoid colon.

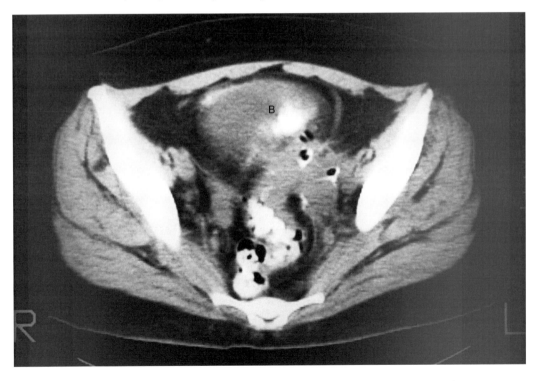

Figure 8.20. Rectal contrast administration just prior to beginning CT scanning is extremely helpful in better defining colonic anatomy and demonstrating associated pathology. In this patient, a sigmoidovesical fistula is diagnosed as contrast filling of the bladder is evident (B).

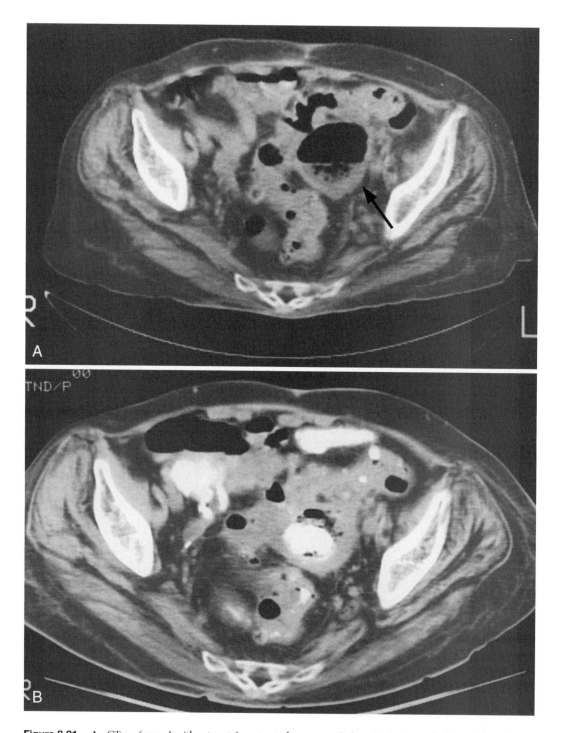

Figure 8.21.   **A.,** CT performed without rectal contrast shows rounded cavity filled with air, liquid, and stool that was difficult to distinguish from a flexure of the sigmoid colon. **B.,** Following contrast instillation, it was clear that this represented a large abscess cavity. Surrounding diverticula suggested diverticulitis as the likely diagnosis.

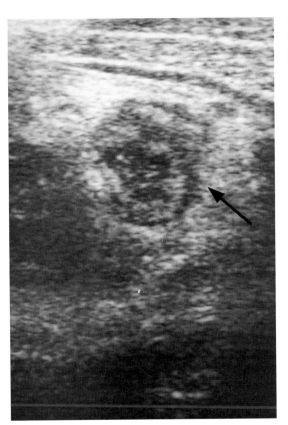

Figure 8.22. Transverse image of the thickened, inflamed descending colon shows the target appearance caused by edema and inflammation in the bowel wall (arrow).

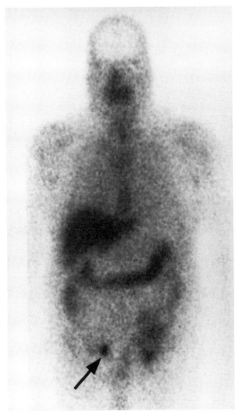

Figure 8.23. Twenty-four hours after intravenous injection of ^{67}Gallium citrate, imaging demonstrates a small focus of activity in the right lower quadrant adjacent to the sigmoid colon (arrow). The presumed diagnosis was appendiceal abscess, but surgery confirmed the presence of diverticulitis.

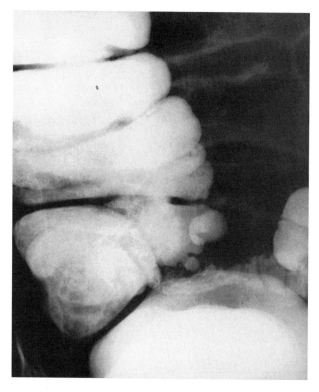

Figure 8.24.   Two small diverticula are seen arising from the medial aspect of the cecum just below the ileocecal valve.

Diverticulosis of the appendix is seen in approximately 1% of surgical specimens (Fig. 8.26). It frequently is reported in association with appendicitis and perforation. Although its exact significance is uncertain, it is suggested that patients in whom diverticula are seen involving the appendix should be followed closely, because they may be predisposed to developing acute appendicitis.

GIANT COLONIC DIVERTICULUM

Rarely, so-called giant diverticula may be found arising from the colon (Chapter 30. All but a few cases are reported as arising from the sigmoid colon. They may reach enormous size, in excess of 25 cm in diameter. They may present, merely due to their size, as a tympanic abdominal mass. Giant diverticula are vulnerable to all of the complications reported for typical colonic diverticula, and in addition, because of their large size, they are more likely to volvulize. They generally are believed to result from subserosal perforation of a diverticulum with formation of a pseudocyst, which slowly grows into a giant cavity. Others believe that a narrow-necked diverticulum undergoes a ball-valve effect and allows colonic air to enter but not exit. Over time, this typical diverticulum may enlarge to enormous proportions (27,28).

On plain film examination, giant colonic diverticula will appear as large gas-containing cystic structures typically overlying the pelvis and rising up into the midabdomen (Fig. 8.27). They may have air–fluid levels on upright films or may appear mottled on recumbent

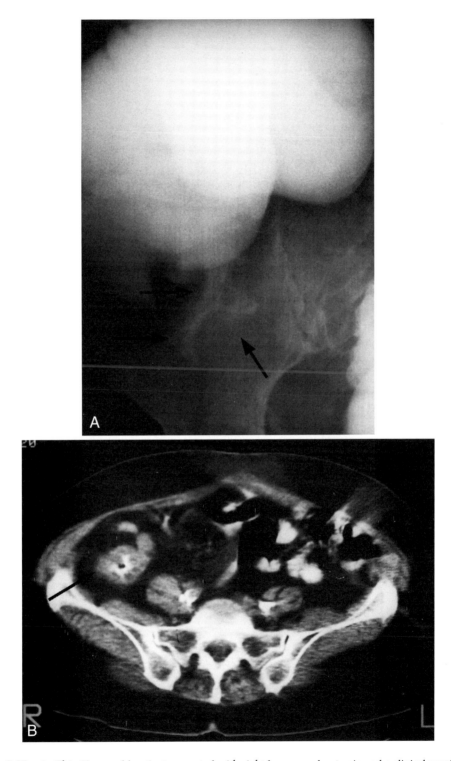

Figure 8.25.   A., This 65-year-old patient presented with right lower quadrant pain and a clinical suspicion of appendicitis. On barium enema, the cecum appeared contracted by an annular mass (arrows), raising strong suspicion of primary carcinoma. **B.,** CT was performed looking for a possible pericecal abscess, perhaps caused by a perforated carcinoma. The thickened cecum (arrow) again suggested neoplasm. At surgery, the final diagnosis of cecal diverticulitis was made.

studies. During contrast studies, barium will enter the diverticulum in approximately 60% of cases (27). The differential diagnosis of these collections must include colonic volvulus, giant abscess cavity, giant pancreatic pseudocyst, giant communicating intestinal duplication cyst, and other rare infected cystic abnormalities.

SMALL BOWEL DIVERTICULAR DISEASE

Duodenal Diverticular Disease

Most diverticular disease occurs in the colon. The second most common site is the duodenum (Fig. 8.28). It is estimated that 5–10% of patients have incidental duodenal diverticula (29,30). Although most of these patients remain asymptomatic, complications occur in approximately 5% (31), presenting a diagnostic challenge to the clinician. The lower incidence of complications as compared with colonic diverticula may be due to their larger size, more rapid flow of ingested materials and secretions through the duodenum, and the relatively sterile nature of duodenal contents. Duodenal diverticulitis does not have a "classic" clinical presentation, and the diagnosis often is elusive. Retrospective analysis of 56 cases reported before 1969 revealed that only 9% had been diagnosed correctly before surgery or postmortem examination (31).

The imaging findings also may be nonspecific. Plain film findings, if present at all, may demonstrate pneumoperitoneum or a mottled gas collection (31), suggesting an abscess. CT findings vary from identification of the diverticulum with thickened walls and

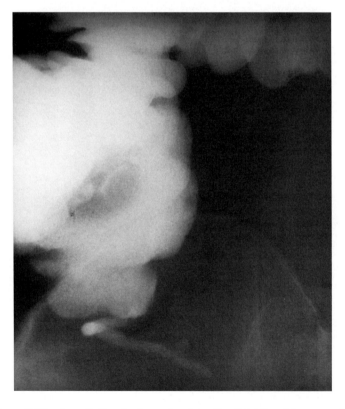

Figure 8.26.   A small diverticulum arises from the distal tip of the appendix.

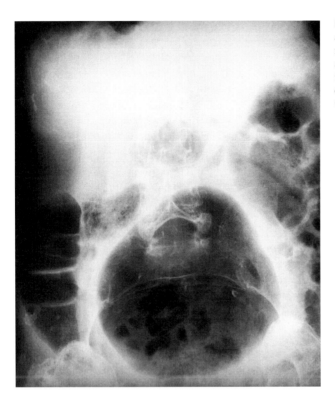

Figure 8.27. A huge ovoid gas collection arises from the pelvis and extends into the midabdomen. Although a large intra-abdominal abscess could be considered, this patient was asymptomatic and further evaluation revealed a giant sigmoid diverticulum.

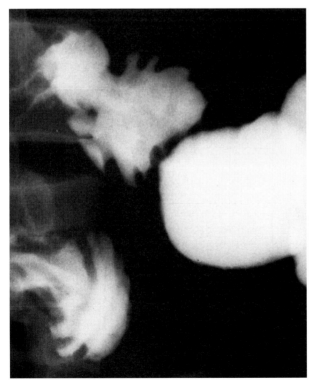

Figure 8.28. Multiple small diverticula are seen arising from the duodenal cap. They vary in size and shape. This clustering of diverticula in the first portion of the duodenum is uncommon.

surrounding inflammatory changes to that of a soft-tissue mass or extraluminal collection of contrast material and gas in the peripancreatic region (31). The upper gastrointestinal (GI) series may be the most suggestive test of the correct diagnosis, although perforation of the diverticulum rarely is demonstrated. The UGI may show a deformed diverticulum or more extensive deformity of the duodenum, suggesting ulcer disease as the diagnosis.

Several other pathologic processes mimic duodenal diverticulitis — pancreatitis, abscesses, penetrating duodenal or antral ulcers, necrotic pancreatic head neoplasms, adenopathy, Crohn's duodenitis, duodenal trauma with perforation, duodenal neoplasms, and infected duplication cysts. Therefore, arriving at the correct diagnosis is a clinical and diagnostic challenge (32–35).

It has been suggested for many years that noninflamed periampullary duodenal diverticula are significant, because they often are associated with anomalous insertion of the pancreatic and bile ducts and thereby predispose to formation of gallstones, cholangitis, and pancreatitis (36).

A rare variant of the duodenal diverticulum is the "giant" diverticulum, reaching sizes in excess of 20 cm. These may present as confusing air collections in the upper (Fig. 8.29) or even lower abdomen (Fig. 8.30) on plain films and, if not considered, may lead one to suggest an alternative diagnosis on cross-sectional imaging and other studies. The typical lateral position of these diverticula in the second or third portion of the duodenum may allow growth to a large size unrestricted by the medially positioned pancreas (37).

Jejunoileal Diverticular Disease

Diverticulosis of the small intestine is a poorly understood entity, the incidence of which is reported variably between 0.26 and 2.3% (38). The higher detected incidence is reported with enteroclysis examinations and is believed to be due to the greater distention achieved by this technique. These diverticula are more common in males, are larger in size, and are found more frequently in the jejunum than the ileum, generally on the mesenteric side of the bowel (Fig. 8.31). Pathologically, they are "pseudodiverticula," because they do not contain any muscular layers. Therefore, they are not seen to contract on contrast examinations and frequently remain distended with air on plain films and cross-sectional imaging studies. Although they may be seen in disorders involving the muscle or myenteric plexus such as scleroderma (Fig. 8.32), they generally are considered to be an acquired disease of unknown etiology. On contrast small bowel examinations, they usually are multiple and vary in size from 1 to 7 cm. The neck of the diverticulum by definition must be narrower than the outpouching, helping to distinguish it from sacculations of the intestines.

Most patients are asymptomatic. Vague abdominal complaints such as bloating have been reported but are difficult to attribute clearly to diverticulosis. The complications associated with this entity include malabsorption, diverticulitis, hemorrhage, pneumoperitoneum, volvulus, and pseudoobstruction (39). Malabsorption is related to stasis within diverticula and resultant bacterial overgrowth. Typically, B12 absorption is disturbed, causing a megaloblastic anemia. When extensive, a diffuse motor disorder known as "jejunal dyskinesia" may be recognized during fluoroscopic examination; this can create a form of intestinal pseudoobstruction (40).

Jejunoileal diverticulitis may result in perforation and development of an abscess or peritonitis. On contrast studies, extravasation may be demonstrated (Fig. 8.33). Mucosal edema, luminal narrowing, and an associated mass may be seen (41). CT may be helpful in suggesting the diagnosis by revealing an inflammatory mass or abscess within the mesentery (41).

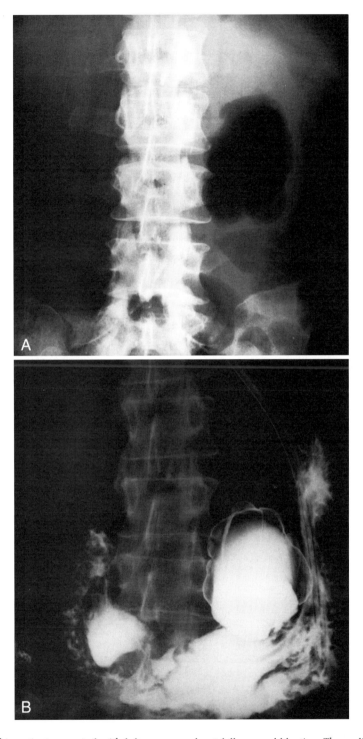

Figure 8.29. This patient presented with left upper quadrant fullness and bloating. The preliminary film **(A)** shows an unusual lobulated air collection in the left midabdomen. An upper GI series was performed **(B)**, clearly demonstrating this to be a large diverticulum arising from the fourth portion of the duodenum. Symptoms may have been related to intermittent distention of the diverticulum.

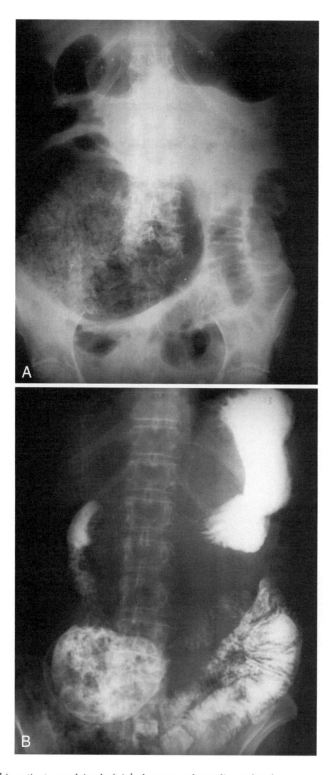

Figure 8.30.   A., This patient complained of right lower quadrant discomfort for many years. The plain film of the abdomen displayed a large collection of gas and particulate material filling the right lower abdomen. Perforation and abscess were considered, but the patient was afebrile and otherwise healthy. **B.,** An UGI series demonstrated a large diverticulum arising from the outer aspect of the third portion of the duodenum. Contrast is seen filling the diverticulum and outlining undigested food particles.

Meckel's Diverticulum

Meckel's diverticulum is the most common congenital anomaly of the GI tract. It results from failure of the intestinal end of the omphalomesenteric duct to close. It occurs in 1–3% of the general population. Although it has been demonstrated infrequently by conventional small bowel follow-through studies, enteroclysis has been shown to be the most reliable method for preoperative demonstration (42). Meckel's diverticulum is a "true" diverticulum arising on the antimesenteric side of the ileum, typically measuring 1–5 cm in size, most frequently encountered in the distal 2–3 feet of ileum, and occurring three times as frequently in males (Fig. 8.34).

Ectopic gastric mucosa may be found in 15–62% of cases (43), accounting for the most common clinical presentation — GI bleeding. Bleeding may be caused by peptic ulceration within the ectopic gastric mucosa or on the adjacent unprotected bowel wall (Fig. 8.35). The ectopic gastric mucosa causes a "hot spot" seen on technetium pertechnetate scans (Fig. 8.36). However, because of a high incidence of false-negative scans, particularly in adults, a negative scan should be followed by a small bowel enteroclysis study (44).

Plain films generally are unremarkable unless a rare enterolith is present (Fig. 8.37) or bowel obstruction has occurred. Small bowel contrast examination, preferably enteroclysis, may fill the blind antimesenteric sac and demonstrate the characteristic "triradiate" fold pattern (Fig. 8.38). With the ileum and diverticulum fully distended, a triangular area appears, which is void of mucosal folds. When the bowel and diverticulum collapse, the folds converge, creating the "triradiate" pattern. This appearance is pathognomonic of a

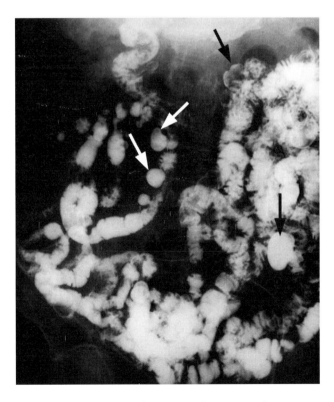

Figure 8.31.   Multiple diverticula are seen along the course of the jejunum. They vary in size from barely evident to several centimeters in this asymptomatic patient (arrows).

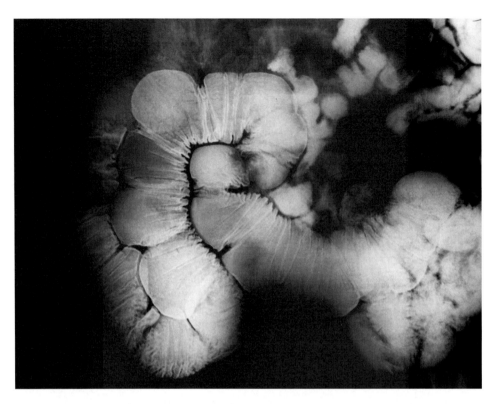

Figure 8.32.   Enteroclysis performed on this patient with scleroderma shows many clustered broad sacculations of the jejunum. The broad neck or wide-mouth appearance often is seen in scleroderma. In other patients, they must be distinguished from normal sacculations of the small intestines.

Meckel's diverticulum. The only other entity to be considered in the differential diagnosis is a communicating duplication cyst, which occurs on the mesenteric side of the bowel and whose long axis should parallel the bowel. These differential findings should help in making the proper diagnosis.

Meckel's diverticulitis often presents with abdominal pain, tenderness, fever, and leukocytosis. Clinically, it mimics acute appendicitis. If undiagnosed, it may perforate, producing an abscess or peritonitis. The diagnosis rarely is made preoperatively (Fig. 8.39).

Obstruction is another rare complication that may result from an inverted Meckel's diverticulum, serving as a leading point of intussusception or from volvulus of a loop of small intestine around the Meckel's diverticulum. Passage of the diverticulum into a hernial sac (Littre's hernia) also may produce obstruction and may be demonstrated on contrast small bowel or CT examination.

SUMMARY

Radiographic evaluation of the patient with suspected diverticular disease may take many different pathways. It must be guided strongly by the clinical presentation and usually begins with the plain film examination. *For the patient who is acutely ill and toxic, CT scanning is suggested as the best diagnostic procedure,* because it generally can be obtained quickly with minimal bowel preparation and can help differentiate patients who should be managed medically or by interventional radiology techniques from those in need of surgical exploration. *Patients who are less acutely ill and in whom diverticular disease of the colon is suspected may benefit from either contrast enema or CT evaluation*, and the decision should be guided by the acuteness and severity of the illness and the expected extent of the abnormality, i.e., abscess or localized inflammatory reaction or phlegmon.

Patients with possible small bowel diverticular disease, and especially those presenting with bleeding raising suspicion of a possible Meckel's diverticulum, are best evaluated with an enteroclysis study following radionuclide imaging. For rare cases in which small bowel diverticulitis may be suspected, CT should be ordered and followed with enteroclysis as needed.

The radiologic evaluation of these more unusual cases of diverticular disease of the GI tract require a strong suspicion on the part of the examining clinician and the diagnostic radiologist. Careful consultation before initiating the radiologic workup will produce the most cost-effective sequence of examinations and yield the highest success rate in preoperative diagnosis.

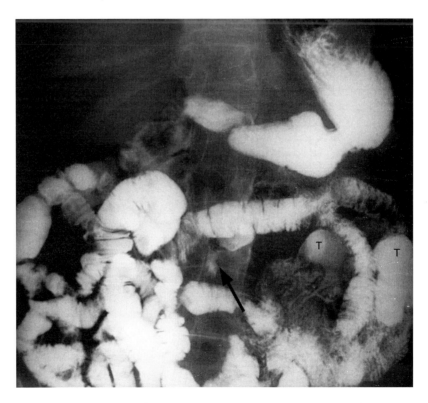

Figure 8.33.   This patient presented with nonspecific abdominal pain and fever. A small bowel series eventually was obtained that demonstrated extravasation from the tip of a jejunal diverticulum (arrow). Note other large jejunal diverticula in the left upper quadrant (T).

Figure 8.34. After several episodes of gastrointestinal bleeding, an enteroclysis was performed demonstrating this conical-shaped Meckel's diverticulum located approximately 2 feet from the cecum. At surgery, ulcerated gastric mucosa was evident.

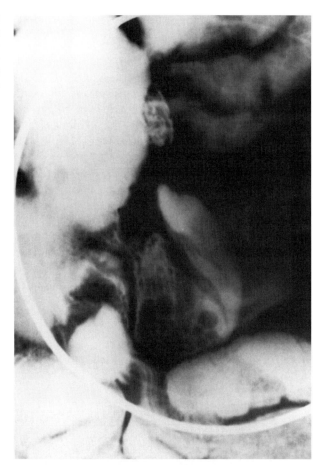

Figure 8.35. This 12-year-old boy presented with rectal bleeding. Colonoscopy and nuclear bleeding studies were negative. Enteroclysis demonstrated a contracted Meckel's diverticulum in the distal ileum located in the left lower abdomen. The mucosa appears edematous, and at surgery, an active ulcer was found in the ileum opposite the orifice of the diverticulum.

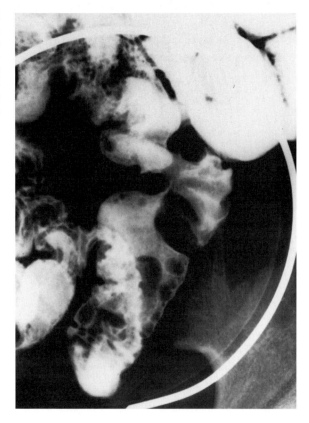

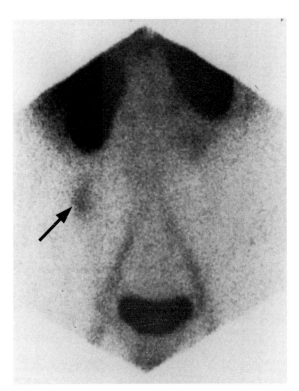

Figure 8.36. Technetium pertechnetate scan shows a focus of activity in the right midabdomen (arrow). At surgery, a bleeding Meckel's diverticulum was resected.

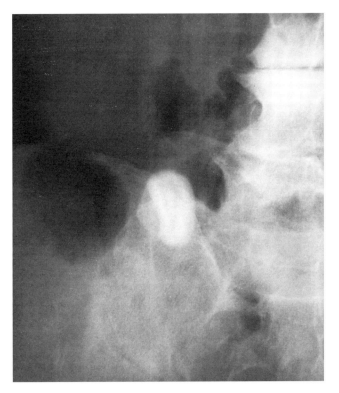

Figure 8.37. Laminated, calcified stone in the right lower quadrant initially was believed to be an appendicolith. Because of fever and pain, surgery was performed and an obstructed Meckel's diverticulum with a large enterolith was removed.

Figure 8.38. Enteroclysis small bowel examination readily demonstrates the triangular configuration of folds (arrows), caused by folds in the afferent and efferent portions of the ileum and at the base of the diverticulum.

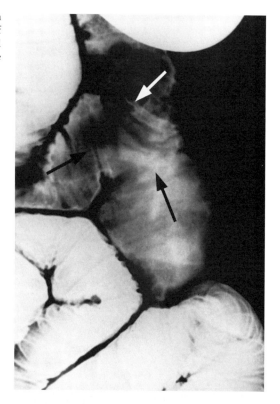

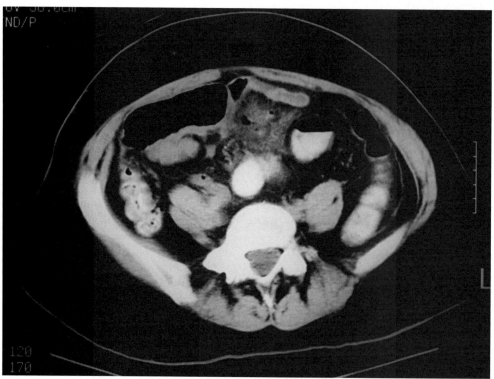

Figure 8.39. This young patient presented with a febrile illness and acute abdominal pain. CT shows an inflammatory process with extraluminal air in the small bowel mesentery. Many etiologies of this abscess were considered, including bowel perforation, but only at surgery was the diagnosis of perforated Meckel's diverticulum confirmed.

EDITORIAL COMMENTS

Working at the same institution with the authors, we concur with their diagnostic approach to diverticular disease of the colon. The importance of communication between the clinician and the radiologist cannot be overemphasized. A logical diagnostic approach should be guided by the severity of the patient's illness.

The CT scan is an extremely useful diagnostic test in the acutely ill patient with suspected diverticulitis because it is highly sensitive and provides useful additional information (i.e., associated phlegmon, abscess, or perforation), thus directing more appropriate treatment such as percutaneous drainage (45,46). The contrast enema should be considered as a complementary study providing information not readily available by CT scan.

Contrast enemas are most useful (a) for less acutely ill patients, (b) as a follow-up study to evaluate the intraluminal aspect of the bowel (for possible carcinoma or Crohn's disease), or (c) for cases of suspected diverticulitis in which the CT scan is negative.

Although these studies are used in most cases, patients with a clear-cut clinical presentation consistent with acute diverticulitis may be treated appropriately without the additional diagnostic costs.

The unusual types of diverticular disease mentioned by the authors that involve the colon and other parts of the GI tract are considered in much greater detail in other chapters.

SUGGESTED READINGS

1. Miller R, Nelson S. The roentgenologic demonstration of tiny amounts of free intraperitoneal gas. Am J Roentgenol 1971;112:574–585. *This is a landmark article from one of the great pioneer researchers in the field of diagnostic radiology. If not only for its historic significance, it is research science at its best. We have all learned how to evaluate the patient with suspected pneumoperitoneum, but few recognize that it was Dr. Miller, in this article, who first described the techniques that are so commonplace today.*
2. Balthazer EJ, ed. Imaging the acute abdomen. Radiol Clin North Am 1994;32:829–1049. *This volume is an excellent review of many relevant topics, including imaging, intervention, and management of the more common and pertinent abdominal conditions. Specifically, there are chapters on CT and sonography of appendicitis and diverticular disease.*
3. Gore R, Levine M, Laufer I. Textbook of gastrointestinal imaging. Philadelphia: WB Saunders, 1994. *This two-volume master text in gastrointestinal radiology includes 162 chapters and more than 2700 pages of text. It is, to date, the most comprehensive text in this field. Chapters are written by experts in the field from around the world. The chapters on diverticular disease include excellent drawings, pathologic specimen photographs, and radiograph reproductions. The book is strongly recommended as both a basic introduction to imaging diverticular disease and a reference to those studying or practicing advanced techniques.*

REFERENCES

1. Painter NS, Burkitt DP. Diverticular disease of the colon, a 20th century problem. Clin Gastroenterol 1975;4:3–22. *A summary of geographical distribution, autopsy findings, and etiology, with numerous references.*
2. Pohlman T. Diverticulitis. Gastroenterol Clin North Am 1988;17:357–385. *A general review with 166 references.*
3. Kourtesis GJ, Williams RA, Wilson SE. Surgical options in acute diverticulitis. Value of sigmoid resection in dealing with the septic focus. Aust N Z J Surg 1988;58:955–959. *Minimal morbidity and shorter hospitalization were accomplished when sigmoid resection was part of the initial procedure.*
4. Morris J, Stellato TA, Haaga JR, et al. The utility of computed tomography in colonic diverticulitis. Ann Surg 1986;204:128–132. *Evaluates CT in 41 patients with the clinical diagnosis of colonic diverticulitis. CT identified subtle and gross changes and extracolonic pathology.*
5. Hayward MW, Hayward C, Ennis WP, et al. A pilot evaluation of radiography of the acute abdomen. Clin Radiol 1984;35:289–291. *One hundred consecutive patients having chest x-rays and abdominal films were examined. A management change of 10% occurred based on radiologic findings. Patients with nonspecific abdominal pain had normal x-rays.*
6. Field S, Guy PJ, Upsdell SM, et al. The erect abdominal radiograph in the acute abdomen: should its routine use be abandoned? BMJ 1985;290:1934–1936. *Examines prospectively supine and erect abdominal films of 102 patients with acute abdominal symptoms. There was a small yield of positive information, a number of potentially misleading features, and a lack of effect on surgical management.*

7. Miller R, Nelson S. The roentgenologic demonstration of tiny amounts of free intraperitoneal gas. Am J Roentgenol 1971;112: 574–585. *Recommends a specific technique for demonstrating small amounts of pneumoperitoneum, based on clinical and experimental observations.*
8. Woodring J, Heiser M. Detection of pneumoperitoneum on chest radiographs: comparison of upright lateral and posteroanterior projections. Am J Roentgenol 1995;165:45–47. *The upright lateral chest film is more sensitive than the upright posteroanterior chest film in detecting small amounts of pneumoperitoneum.*
9. Johnson CD, Baker ME, Rice RP, et al. Diagnosis of acute colonic diverticulitis: comparison of barium enema and CT. Am J Roentgenol 1987;148:541–546. *The contrast enema is recommended as the initial and routine examination for patients with suspected diverticulitis.*
10. Smith TR, Cho KC, Morehouse TH, et al. Comparison of computed tomography and contrast enema evaluation of diverticulitis. Dis Colon Rectum 1990;33:1–6. *A study of 31 patients. Contrast enema is recommended as the primary mode of diagnosis.*
11. Cho KC, Morehouse HT, Alterman DD, et al. Sigmoid diverticulitis: diagnostic role of CT — comparison with barium enema studies. Radiology 1990;176:111–115. *Recommends CT as the initial study in acutely ill patients, especially if clinical features are atypical for sigmoid diverticulitis.*
12. Stein GN. Radiology of colonic diverticular diseases. Postgrad Med 1976;60(6):95–112. *Includes a series of barium enema views and promotes barium enema study to make the nonsurgical diagnosis of diverticulitis and most complications.*
13. Diner WC, Baznhard MJ. Acute diverticulitis. Semin Roentgenol 1973;8:415–431. *A general review of acute diverticulitis with 60 references.*
14. Nicholas GG, Miller WT, Fitts WT, et al. Diagnosis of diverticulitis of the colon: role of barium enema in defining pericolic inflammation. Ann Surg 1972;176:205–209. *Reviews 76 barium enemas performed preoperatively in patients with diverticulitis. In 4% of patients, there was no evidence of mass formation or peridiverticulitis.*
15. McKee RF, Deignan RW, Krukowski ZH. Radiological investigation in acute diverticulitis. Br J Surg 1993;80:560–565. *An assessment of the available radiologic techniques used in the management of acute diverticulitis, with 75 references.*
16. Doris PE, Strauss RW. The expanded role of the barium enema in the evaluation of patients presenting with acute abdominal pain. J Emerg Med 1985;3:93–110. *Recommends expanded use of barium enema examinations for evaluation of abdominal pain.*
17. Hulnick DH, Megibow AJ, Balthazar EJ, et al. Computed tomography in the evaluation of diverticulitis. Radiology 1984;152:491–495. *Compares CT in 43 patients with colonic diverticulitis with contrast enemas in 37 patients. CT is recommended as the initial procedure in patients with suspected diverticulitis, especially if the contrast enema is contraindicated.*
18. Neff CC, vanSonnenberg E. CT of diverticulitis. Diagnosis and treatment. Radiol Clin North Am 1989;27:743–752. *Discusses CT-guided percutaneous drainage and the use of CT for evaluation of extramucosal disease.*
19. Balthazar EJ, Megibow A, Schinella RA, et al. Limitations in the CT diagnosis of acute diverticulitis: comparison of CT, contrast enemas and pathologic findings in 16 patients. Am J Roentgenol 1990;154:281–285. *A minority of patients with diverticulitis have equivocal or misleading CT features; in most of these patients, contrast enema will make the correct diagnosis.*
20. Balthazar EJ, Megibow AJ, Hulnick D, et al. Carcinoma of the colon: detection and preoperative staging by CT. Am J Roentgenol 1988;150:301–306. *Negative CT findings do not help in staging a colonic tumor, whereas positive findings are highly indicative.*
21. Padidar AM, Jeffrey, RB Jr, Mindelzun RE, et al. Differentiating sigmoid diverticulitis from carcinoma on CT scans: mesenteric inflammation suggests diverticulitis. Am J Roentgenol 1994;163:81–83. *CT findings of fluid at the root of the mesentery and vascular engorgement are useful in distinguishing sigmoid diverticulitis from carcinoma of the sigmoid.*
22. Birnbaum BA, Balthazar EJ. CT of appendicitis and diverticulitis. Radiol Clin North Am 1994;32:885–912. *A well-illustrated review.*
23. Schwerk WB, Schwartz S, Rothmund M. Sonography of acute colonic diverticulitis: a prospective study. Dis Colon Rectum 1992;11:77–84. *High-resolution sonography with graded compression was highly sensitive and specific for the imaging diagnosis of acute colonic diverticulitis and abscess.*
24. Shaff MI, Tarr RW, Paetain CL, et al. Computed tomography and magnetic resonance imaging of the acute abdomen. Surg Clin North Am 1988;68:233–254. *Discusses benefits of CT in evaluation of the acute abdomen.*
25. Joseph AE. Imaging of intra-abdominal abscesses. BMJ 1985;291:1446–1447. *Recommends ultrasound as the first diagnostic choice, except when the site is better evaluated by CT (e.g., the retroperitoneum).*
26. McDougall IR. Diagnosis of abscesses by radionuclide scanning. Scott Med J 1979;24:263–265. *A brief discussion of different types of radionuclide scans.*
27. Kricun R, Stasik J, Reither R, et al. Giant colonic diverticulum. Am J Roentgenol 1980;135:507–512. *A clinical review of five patients with giant colonic diverticula.*
28. Rabinowitz J, Farman J, Dallemand S, et al. Giant sigmoid diverticulum. Am J Roentgenol 1974;121:338–343. *A discussion of five patients with giant colonic diverticula.*
29. Osnes M, Lotveit T, Larsen S, et al. Duodenal diverticula and their relationship to age, sex and biliary calculi. Scand J Gastroenterol 1981;16:103–107. *In all patients older than 40 years of age, the incidence of biliary calculi was higher with duodenal diverticula (86%) than without (38%).*
30. Stone EE, Brant WE, Smith GB. Computed tomography of duodenal diverticula. J Comput Assist Tomogr

1989;13:61–63. *CT visualized duodenal diverticula in 10 of 14 patients (71%) with diverticula visualized previously by upper GI series. CT may mistake duodenal diverticula for pancreatic pathology.*

31. Gore RM, Ghahremani GG, Kirsch MD, et al. Diverticulitis of the duodenum: clinical and radiological manifestations of 7 cases. Am J Gastroenterol 1991;86:981–985. *A study of seven patients. The abdominal CT was crucial in making the diagnosis in all patients.*

32. Hofer GA, Cohen AJ. CT signs of duodenal perforation secondary to blunt abdominal trauma. J Comput Assist Tomogr 1989;13:430–432. *Describes CT findings in two patients.*

33. Madrazo KL, Halpert RD, Sandler MA, et al. Computed tomographic findings in penetrating peptic ulcer. Radiology 1984;153:751–754. *Four patients with peptic ulcers penetrating the head of the pancreas were diagnosed by CT (that allowed the clinicians to make a confident diagnosis of this complication).*

34. Farah MC, Jafri SY, Schwab RE, et al. Duodenal neoplasms: role of CT. Radiology 1987;162:839–843. *CT allowed the accurate staging of 8 of 10 malignant lesions.*

35. Bar-Ziv J, Katz R, Nobel M, et al. Duodenal duplication cyst with enteroliths: computed tomography and ultrasound diagnosis. Gastrointest Radiol 1989;14:220–222. *The first description of enteroliths in a duodenal duplication cyst.*

36. Shemesh E, Friedman E, Czerniak A, et al. The association of biliary and pancreatic abnormalities with periampullary duodenal diverticula: correlation with clinical presentation. Arch Surg 1987;122:1055–1057. *Recommends ERCP for symptomatic patients with periampullary duodenal diverticula (especially with jaundice and pancreatitis) and a biliary drainage procedure in patients with periampullary duodenal diverticula and a dilated bile duct.*

37. Millard J, Ziter FM, Slover WP. Giant duodenal diverticula. Am J Roentgenol 1974;121:334–337. *Discusses the radiologic appearance in four cases.*

38. Maglinte DD, Chernish SM, DeWeese R, et al. Acquired jejunoileal diverticular disease: subject review. Radiology 1986;158:577–579. *A review of 12 patients with jejunoileal diverticula seen by enteroclysis. Discusses enteroclysis and the complications of the disease.*

39. Baskin RH, Mayo CW. Jejunal diverticulosis: a clinical study of 87 cases. Surg Clin North Am 1952;32:1185–1196. *Surgery was undertaken only for severe complications.*

40. Altemeier WA, Bryant LR, Wulsin JH. The surgical significance of jejunal diverticulosis. Arch Surg 1963;86:732–741. *Thirty-eight percent with multiple diverticula developed significant chronic symptoms or a serious complication treated surgically.*

41. Giustra PE, Killoran PJ, Root JA, et al. Jejunal diverticulitis. Radiology 1977;125:609–611. *Describes a number of radiologic manifestations in two patients with jejunal diverticulitis.*

42. Maglinte DD, Elmore MF, Isenberg M. Meckel's diverticulum: radiologic demonstration by enteroclysis. Am J Roentgenol 1980;134:925–932. *The diagnosis of Meckel's diverticulum was established preoperatively in 11 of 13 patients by enteroclysis.*

43. Rutherford RB, Akers DR. Meckel's diverticulum: a review of 148 pediatric patients with special reference to the pattern of bleeding and to mesodiverticular vascular bands. Surgery 1966;59:618–626. *Bleeding usually is painless and true suppurative diverticulitis is rare in children.*

44. Maglinte DD, Jordan LG, Van Hove ED, et al. Chronic gastrointestinal bleeding from Meckel's diverticulum: radiological considerations. J Clin Gastroenterol 1981;3:47–52. *The diagnosis of Meckel's diverticulum is still difficult, but nuclear imaging, enteroclysis, and angiography used appropriately can increase the preoperative diagnostic accuracy.*

45. Labs JD, Sarr MG, Fishman EK, et al. Complications of acute diverticulitis of the colon: improved early diagnosis with computerized tomography. Am J Surg 1988;155:331–335. *CT is especially useful in diagnosing suspected abscesses or fistulas complicating diverticulitis.*

46. Hachigian MP, Honickman S, Eisenstat TE, et al. Computed tomography in the initial management of acute left-sided diverticulitis. Dis Colon Rectum 1992;35:1123–1129. *Demonstrates the ability of CT scanning to recognize complications of diverticulitis and to stratify patients according to the severity of the disease.*

9 Small Bowel Obstruction Complicating Colonic Diverticular Disease

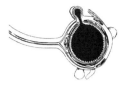

Richard L. Nelson, MD

KEY POINTS

- Operation should be prompt if ischemia is suspected
- Long or short tubes of comparable value for decompression
- Signs of small bowel obstruction obscured by diverticulitis
- Massively dilated small bowel must be decompressed
- Avoid blind colostomy that could be distal to obstruction

ILLUSTRATIVE CASES

Case 1: A 64-year-old male was admitted to the hospital complaining of weakness and a several-week history of crampy lower abdominal pain and diarrhea. The day of admission, the cramps became more pronounced in the periumbilical region and he vomited. He had undergone an appendectomy and cholecystectomy in the past.

His blood pressure was 140/90, pulse was 104, and temperature was 99.8°F. He appeared dehydrated with abdominal distention. The abdomen was tympanitic and minimally tender in the left lower quadrant with high-pitched, active bowel sounds. No masses were palpable. Rectal examination revealed a hemoccult negative stool.

The hematocrit was 40 percent, white blood cell count was 21,000 with a left shift, urinalysis was negative, blood urea nitrogen (BUN) was 34, creatinine was 1.5, potassium was 3.1, and the remaining electrolytes, glucose, and liver function tests normal. Abdominal radiographs revealed several dilated loops of small bowel and air–fluid levels on the erect view; there was minimal air in the colon.

He was given intravenous fluids and prepared for surgery. At operation, the small bowel was adherent to a site of localized perforation of the sigmoid colon. The small bowel appeared viable and was separated quite easily from the thickened colon (Fig. 9.1). A Hartmann procedure was performed. The specimen was opened in the operating room and appeared to be sigmoid diverticulitis with localized perforation; no mucosal lesions were appreciated. Postoperatively, he had moderate abdominal distention and hypoactive bowel sounds for 5 days.

Case 2: A 65-year-old male came to the emergency room with a history of 3 days of anorexia, progressive abdominal distention, nausea and vomiting, and a failure to pass either flatus or stool for 24 hours. He had experienced an attack of diverticulitis 1 year earlier that was treated medically. He had never undergone abdominal surgery. Upon examination, he was noted to be uncomfortable, nauseated, and somewhat dehydrated

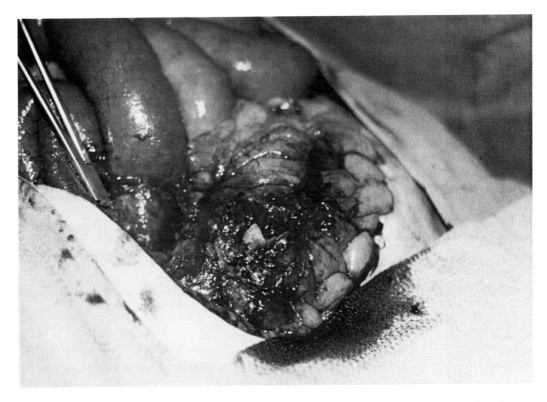

Figure 9.1. Small bowel obstruction caused by adherence of small bowel loops to a diverticular abscess. (Reprinted with permission from Welch JP. Operative techniques, decisions, and complications. In: Welch JP, ed. Bowel obstruction. Differential diagnosis and clinical management. Philadelphia: WB Saunders, 1990;423–448.)

with diminished skin turgor and dry mucous membranes. His pulse was 110 and thready, and his blood pressure was 120/65 with some orthostatic hypotension. The abdomen was distended with high-pitched bowel sounds but no localized tenderness was present. There were no hernias. Rectal examination revealed small amounts of stool, which was negative for occult blood. He took one medication for chronic essential hypertension.

A nasogastric tube was passed and infusion of intravenous fluids was begun. Initial radiographs demonstrated dilatation of the small intestine and no air in the colon. Upright films showed no free air under the diaphragm and noncollinear layering of the fluid menisci in the small intestine or inverted "J" loops (Fig. 9.2). Laboratory examination included a white blood cell count of 10,000 with a normal differential, hematocrit of 56%, normal blood gases, a potassium of 3, and a normal amylase, alkaline phosphatase, and creatine phosphokinase (CPK). A barium enema was performed because the patient had small bowel obstruction but no previous operations or hernias. It demonstrated numerous sigmoid diverticula, some sigmoid spasm, and muscular hypertrophy of the entire left colon, with free flow of barium to the cecum.

Case Comments

The patient in case 1 was suspected to have small bowel obstruction alone, rather than combined diverticulitis and small bowel obstruction. The symptoms of diarrhea and lower abdominal pain should have alerted the clinician to possible colonic disease and additional investigation preoperatively could have been of use (1). A gastrografin enema would have shown evidence of spasm and perhaps the localized site of perforation, whereas a computed tomography (CT) scan with contrast would have shown pericolic inflammation and possibly the site of perforation.

The patient in case 2 presented with a typical history of small bowel obstruction, although the cause was somewhat obscure. A colonic obstruction simulating a small bowel obstruction was ruled out with the contrast study. Adhesions that may have developed as the result of the previous diverticulitis could have been responsible. Other etiologies of small bowel obstruction were possible, including volvulus, internal hernia, and intussusception. Physical examination ruled out abdominal wall hernias, and auscultation of the lung ruled out a pneumonia that could cause ileus. The initial management of this patient was appropriate, including rehydration and nasogastric suction. Considering the high-grade small bowel obstruction, the surgeon should have a low threshold to operate, although it is conceivable that the small bowel would begin to decompress with antibiotic therapy and bowel rest.

DISCUSSION

Small bowel obstruction is a frequent cause of abdominal pain in patients coming to the emergency room. The diagnosis is made based on the characteristic symptoms of

Figure 9.2. Inverted "J" loops in small bowel obstruction.

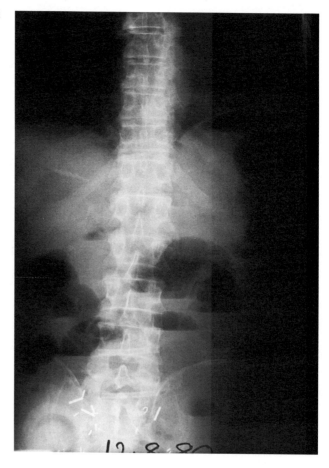

abdominal pain, vomiting, abdominal distention, and constipation. The actual complex of symptoms will depend on several factors, such as the degree (partial or complete), level (proximal or distal), and duration of the obstruction, and on the presence or absence of strangulation. This history, along with physical findings such as dehydration, low-grade fever, tachycardia, crampy abdominal pain, abdominal distention, and hyperactive or absent bowel sounds, is highly suggestive of the diagnosis. Abdominal radiographs typically show distended bowel loops and air–fluid levels on upright views.

Management of small bowel obstruction accompanying acute diverticulitis may be complex. First, if the clinician is aware that diverticulitis is present, the scenario is in some ways analogous to acute postoperative small bowel obstruction, in that *the usual signs upon which clinical decisions must be made are clouded by the additional entity.* Specifically, critical operative decisions are made in small bowel obstruction based on the estimate of risk that intestinal ischemia has occurred in a dehydrated patient with distended intestine (2). The signs that one uses to predict this likelihood are distention, elevation of the white blood cell count, localized tenderness, tachycardia, and a palpable abdominal mass. However, all of these are likely to be present in the patient with acute diverticulitis. In the case of acute postoperative adhesive small bowel obstruction, the danger of intestinal ischemia and the virtual impossibility of being able to detect it by the usual signs are frequently "put on the back burner" (because of incisional pain and distention) in favor of conservative therapy. It generally is believed that postoperative obstruction arises from soft adhesions that may well be reabsorbed. There are insufficient data in the literature to make such an assumption in the case of small bowel obstruction complicating acute diverticulitis; it also is likely that a significant proportion of such patients are treated operatively rather than conservatively.

Second, *the diagnosis of acute diverticulitis may not be apparent to the clinician until it is encountered in the operating room,* as in case 1. The symptoms of the superimposed small bowel obstruction or ileus may be dominant in the acute setting, and the symptoms of diverticular disease more chronic and less suspect. Any symptoms of changes in bowel habits suggestive of colonic disease, especially before the acute episode, should be considered during the workup and before the decision to operate precipitously.

The major early decision in the patient with suspected small bowel obstruction is between conservative management (intravenous hydration, nasogastric decompression, serial physical exams, white blood counts, and radiographs) and immediate operation. *An early operation is essential if intestinal ischemia is suspected (3), and most surgeons would operate if complete (rather than partial) small bowel obstruction was present.*

If medical management is chosen initially, additional diagnostic procedures and alterations in management might be undertaken. For patients with known diverticular disease, a contrast enema could be performed to rule out another episode; even more informative might be abdominal and pelvic CT or a technetium-99m-labeled white blood cell scan (Fig. 9.3). The author can obtain the latter examination on relatively short notice, with images becoming available within 4 to 5 hours. It is extremely sensitive in picking up inflammatory foci within the peritoneal cavity. It has been used both for the localization of intra-abdominal abscesses and in the diagnosis and management of patients with inflammatory bowel disease (4).

Regarding management, another controversy includes the type of intestinal decompression to be used. The choice is either nasogastric decompression or the passage of a "long" (nasointestinal) tube into the small intestine, with the intention of decompression as close as possible to the actual point of obstruction. Recently, long tubes have been avoided because retrospective descriptions stated that they were difficult to pass to the

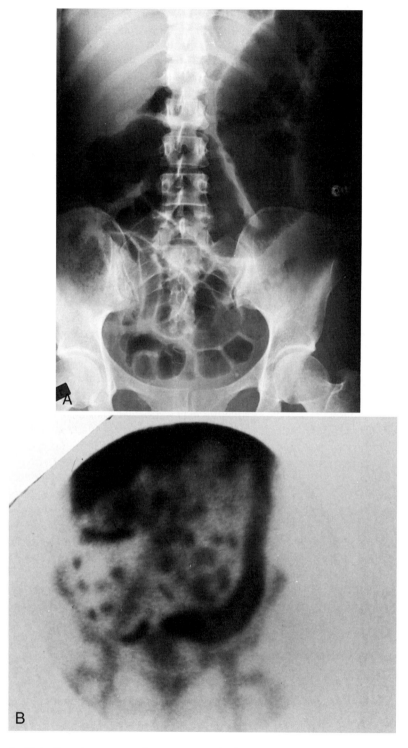

Figure 9.3.   **A.,** Plain film of a patient with toxic colitis who had obstructive symptoms. **B.,** Technetium-99m white cell scan showing colonic inflammation and diffuse small bowel ischemia. After resuscitation, the small bowel scanned negative and a workup for Crohn's disease was negative.

intended point of obstruction, and that surgery was delayed as a result of this difficulty (5). Morbidity and mortality from intestinal obstruction were increased, presumably because of this delay.

A recent study randomized patients with acute adhesive small bowel obstruction to either long tube or nasogastric decompression upon arrival in the emergency room. Patients who required operative intervention were defined as treatment failures. The variables assessed in the operative group included the interval between admission and operation, clinical indications for operation, operative findings, procedures performed, postoperative complications, and the length of postoperative ileus. There was very little difference in the outcomes of the two treatment groups, certainly much less difference than in previous retrospective studies. It also was noteworthy in this report to see that the authors were successful in passing a long tube into the small intestine in 89% of their patients (6).

Another issue is the risk of recurrence of adhesive obstruction. Does laparotomy, for example, create more adhesions and thus result in earlier or more frequent recurrence of obstruction than conservative therapy? There are no such data for patients with diverticulitis-induced adhesions, although it is likely that a major proportion of such adhesions resolve with antibiotic therapy. In a recent retrospective cohort study of 31 patients with adhesive small bowel obstruction managed operatively and 59 patients treated nonoperatively, the number of prior episodes was the strongest predictor of recurrence. Nonoperative management was recommended for stable patients having their first episode and operative therapy after the second episode; neither strategy had an acceptable outcome after the third or later episodes (7).

Are there any reliable methods of determining ischemia of the obstructed small bowel in patients with diverticulitis? *Even experienced clinicians have a limited ability to discriminate between simple and strangulation small bowel obstruction when examining patients* (8). If a diverticular abscess is drained completely with CT guidance, one would expect resolution of sepsis. If the septic process progresses, the possibility of small bowel ischemia would have to be considered: a CT scan, radionuclide-labeled white cell scan, or operation would help resolve this issue. *If an operation is performed because of florid sepsis, a blind-loop transverse colostomy in the right upper quadrant is to be condemned.* Failure to inspect the peritoneal contents would miss ischemic small bowel obstruction proximal to the colostomy and thus fail to resolve the patient's obstructive symptoms as well as the sepsis.

Whenever a laparotomy is performed for acute diverticulitis, in most instances, a resection of the sigmoid colon will be performed. If the patient had small bowel obstructive symptoms before the operation, the surgeon should run the small intestine to free adhesions. *If the small intestine is massively dilated, intraoperative decompression becomes a vital part of the procedure* (Fig. 9.4). The risk of ischemic infarction still exists in such patients unless intraluminal pressure can be decreased. There are several methods for accomplishing this. The most widely described and effective is the use of a long intestinal tube inserted in the operating room. This may be performed either by the nasogastric route, retrograde through a cecostomy, or best through a Stamm gastrostomy, with threading of the tube throughout the length of the small intestine and with aspiration during insertion (Fig. 9.5). The decrease in intraluminal pressure will immediately restore blood flow to the entire intestinal wall to normal and maintain it so postoperatively. Such a tube left in situ can be used for internal plication postoperatively so that as new adhesions form, they might be less likely to cause recurrent obstruction. This particular method of diminishing the likelihood of subsequent obstruction has been widely advocated, although the comparative studies needed to establish its efficacy have not been performed.

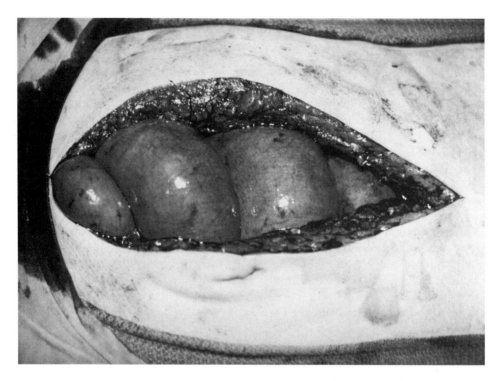

Figure 9.4.   Dilated small bowel requiring operative decompression. (Reprinted with permission from Welch JP. Operative techniques, decisions, and complications. In: Welch JP, ed. Bowel obstruction. Differential diagnosis and clinical management. Philadelphia: WB Saunders, 1990:423–448) [Ref. 10].

In a slightly different situation, when the patient's sepsis has been controlled by percutaneous abscess drainage but obstructive symptoms persist, essentially the same operative choices remain and blind colostomy is equally to be condemned. A definitive procedure may be performed to minimize the risk of subsequent diverticulitis, but concomitant with this should be exclusion of any obstructing mechanism in the small intestine, as well as decompression if indicated. Postoperative internal plication may minimize the risk of subsequent intestinal obstruction.

The placement of a long tube through a gastrotomy will ease the patient's postoperative course through the avoidance of a nasogastric tube, especially if the long tube used allows simultaneous gastric decompression. It takes approximately 14 days for fibrinous exudate to transform into fibrocollagenous scar and thus relatively permanent adhesion formation. It is therefore necessary to keep a plication tube in situ for this length of time to minimize the risk of subsequent adhesive obstruction (5).

CONCLUSIONS

1. Adhesive small bowel obstruction may occur because of a prior attack of acute diverticulitis. Operations should be performed when indicated for these individuals principally to prevent or treat suspected ischemia of the small intestine. Recurrent diverticulitis as the cause of the event should be considered and ruled out by diagnostic methods such as CT or radiolabeled white cell scan.

2. Small intestinal obstruction has been reported in patients with acute diverticulitis and should be considered in patients with obstructive symptoms in this setting (9).
3. A blind colostomy without exploratory laparotomy should never be performed on patients with acute diverticulitis and small bowel dilatation, because diversion may be performed distal to the point of obstruction.
4. Intraoperative decompression of the small intestine is a critical part of the operative management of patients with small bowel obstruction to improve blood flow to the intestinal wall.
5. The radiolabeled white cell scan is a sensitive method for detection of small intestinal ischemia and is useful for patients with diverticulitis in whom obstructive symptoms persist, especially beyond the initial resolution of sepsis related to diverticulitis (4).
6. Postoperative internal plication of the small intestine may diminish risk of the subsequent small bowel obstruction (5).

EDITORIAL COMMENTS

This chapter discusses a seldom-emphasized but important complication of acute diverticulitis—small bowel obstruction. The "obstruction" of the small bowel may be a form of adynamic ileus,

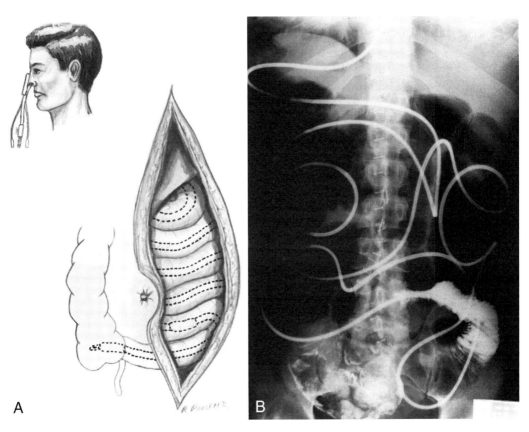

A

B

Figure 9.5. **A.,** Postoperative internal plication after nasogastric insertion of the long tube. **B.,** Postoperative radiograph of the plication tube.

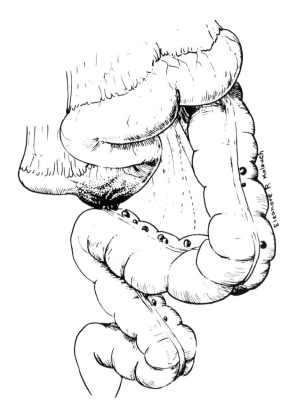

Figure 9.6.   Schematic view of small bowel obstruction induced by acute sigmoid diverticulitis with localized perforation. (Reprinted with permission from Welch JP. Inflammatory causes of small bowel obstruction. In: Welch JP, ed. Bowel obstruction. Differential diagnosis and clinical management. Philadelphia: WB Saunders, 1990:353–377) [Ref. 11].

or else a partial or high-grade mechanical process. The usual mechanism of obstruction is by adherence of the small bowel to the inflamed sigmoid colon (Fig. 9.6) (14). The adherence may be "filmy," as described above, or more tenacious, with adherence of the bowel and mesentery to the walls of a paracolic abscess (Fig. 9.7). In this setting, the involved intestinal loops should be freed carefully to avoid enterotomy. Fistula formation into the small bowel has been described (15), but is unusual, and should raise suspicion of Crohn's disease. The small bowel obstruction may persist, even with drainage of the abscess, and the dissection of the involved loops from the abscess cavity may be a wise idea (5, 14). Small bowel resection should be performed if the small bowel is injured during the operation.

We agree that the potential danger of the small bowel obstruction, intestinal ischemia leading to possible perforation or sepsis, can be overlooked and attributed to the acute diverticulitis. The failure to operate on such patients with direct treatment of the small bowel obstruction can have disastrous consequences. This requires exploratory laparotomy with inspection of the small bowel; the danger of a "limited look" with decompression of the colon by colostomy is deservedly emphasized as insufficient.

We do not have experience with the radiolabeled white blood cell scan and have relied more on serial physical examinations, abdominal radiographs, contrast studies (Figs. 9.8 and 9.9) (16), and CT scans (17). Just as with symptoms accompanying postoperative small bowel obstruction, the "danger signs" such as fever, tenderness, or leukocytosis may be attributed to the "other" factor, diverticulitis, rather than to the small bowel obstruction itself, thus diverting the surgeon from the appropriate treatment. General and colorectal surgeons are well aware of the dangers of small bowel

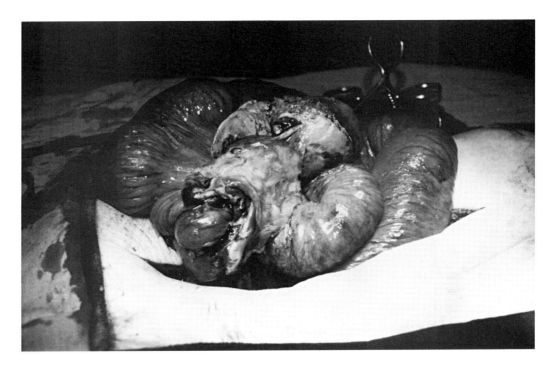

Figure 9.7. Thickening of mesentery of small bowel that was obstructed following adherence to an inflammatory focus of diverticulitis, with resultant kinking and small bowel obstruction. (Reprinted with permission from Welch JP. Adhesions. In: Welch JP, ed. Bowel obstruction. Differential diagnosis and clinical management. Philadelphia: WB Saunders, 1990:154–165) [Ref. 12].

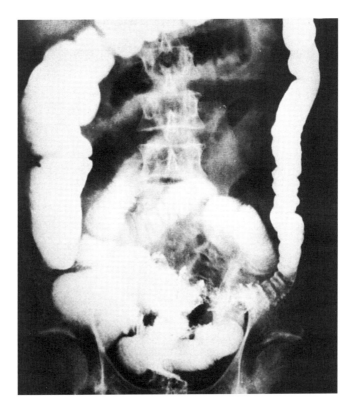

Figure 9.8. Barium enema view in a patient with small bowel obstruction related to entrapment in a sigmoid diverticular abscess. (Reprinted with permission from Welch JP, Warshaw AL. Isolated small bowel obstruction as the presenting feature of colonic disease. Arch Surg 1977;112:809–812.)

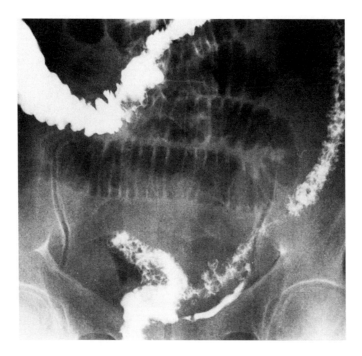

Figure 9.9.   Small bowel obstruction in a patient with sigmoid diverticulitis and a pelvic mass. There is extravasation of barium adjacent to the sigmoid.

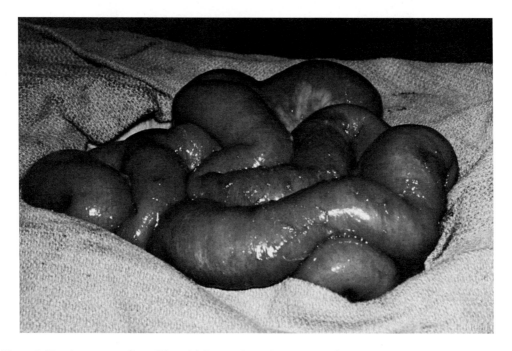

Figure 9.10.   Appearance of small bowel following lysis of numerous adhesions. An internal stent (Baker tube) was inserted into the small bowel during the operation to prevent additional episodes of small bowel obstruction. (Reprinted with permission from Welch JP. Intestinal intubation. In: Welch JP, ed. Bowel obstruction. Differential diagnosis and clinical management. Philadelphia: WB Saunders, 1990:122–153) [Ref. 13].

obstruction, especially if ischemia or high-grade obstruction are suspected. The role of early exploratory surgery following hydration should be kept in mind.

We have used long nasointestinal tubes for intraoperative decompression at times but less frequently as of late. The tube should be introduced through the stomach or cecum, not the jejunum (18). Usually, the small bowel contents can be milked back into the stomach by the surgeon and suctioned out; internal stenting is rarely used. Furthermore, stenting may be no more effective then enterolysis alone (19). We would reserve internal stenting with a Baker tube for patients with numerous adhesions or serosal injury (20) who are believed to be at high risk of developing postoperative obstruction (Fig. 9.10).

REFERENCES

1. Welch JP, Warshaw AL. Isolated small bowel obstruction as the presenting features of colonic disease. Arch Surg 1977;112:809–812. *Five patients with small bowel obstruction are described who had a variety of colonic disorders, including one case of sigmoid diverticulitis. Judicious use of contrast enemas will aid in evaluating possible colonic pathology.*
2. Kukora JS, Dent TL. Small intestinal obstruction. In: Nelson RL, Nyhus LM, eds. Surgery of the small intestine. Norwalk, CT: Appleton and Lang, 1987:267–282.
3. VerSteeg KR, Broders CW. Gangrene of the bowel. Surg Clin North Am 1979;59:869–876. *A study of 87 patients. The mortality was nearly three times higher following mesenteric vascular accidents than following strangulation. The length of gangrenous bowel correlated with mortality.*
4. Kipper SL. Radiolabeled leukocyte imaging of the abdomen. Nucl Med Ann 1995;__ :81–128. *A review discussing the use of this technique for evaluation of acute abdominal pain or abdominal sepsis, with 127 references.*
5. Nelson RL, Nyhus LM. Intubation of the small intestine and enteral feeding. In: Nelson RL, Nyhus LM, eds. Surgery of the small intestine. Norwalk, CT: Appleton and Lange, 1987:401–410.
6. Fleshner PR, Sigmand MG, Slater GI, et al. A prospective, randomized trial of short versus long tubes in adhesive bowel obstruction. Am J Surg 1995;170:366–370. *A prospective randomized trial comparing nasogastric tube and long tube decompression with respect to success of nonoperative treatment and morbidity of operation in 55 patients with acute adhesive small bowel obstruction. There was no advantage of one tube over the other.*
7. Barken H, Webster S, Ozaran S. Factors predicting the recurrence of adhesive small bowel obstruction. Am J Surg 1995;170:361–365. *A retrospective study of 31 patients with adhesive small bowel obstruction managed operatively and 59 managed nonoperatively. Nonoperative management was suitable for stable patients with a first episode; operation was best for those having a second episode. Neither method was satisfactory for the third or later episodes.*
8. Sarr MG, Bulkley GB, Zuidema GD. Preoperative recognition of intestinal strangulation obstruction. Prospective study of diagnostic capability. Am J Surg 1983;145:176–182. *This study included a prospective evaluation of the preoperative judgment of the senior attending surgeon for the determination of the presence or absence of intestinal strangulation. The surgeon detected strangulation in 10 of 21 patients with strangulation preoperatively (sensitivity, 48%).*
9. Ona FV, Salamone RP, Mehnart PJ. Giant sigmoid diverticulitis, a cause of partial small bowel obstruction. Gastroenterology 1980;73:350–352. *The wall of a giant diverticulum was adherent to a loop of terminal ileum, causing small bowel obstruction.*
10. Welch JP. Operative techniques, decisions, and complications. In: Welch JP, ed. Bowel obstruction. Differential diagnosis and clinical management. Philadelphia: WB Saunders, 1990:423–448.
11. Welch JP. Inflammatory causes of small bowel obstruction. In: Welch JP, ed. Bowel obstruction. Differential diagnosis and clinical management. Philadelphia: WB Saunders, 1990:353–377.
12. Welch JP. Adhesions. In: Welch JP, ed. Bowel obstruction. Differential diagnosis and clinical management. Philadelphia: WB Saunders, 1990:154–165.
13. Welch JP. Intestinal intubation. In: Welch JP, ed. Bowel obstruction. Differential diagnosis and clinical management. Philadelphia: WB Saunders, 1990:122–153.
14. Valerio D, Jones PF. Immediate resection in the treatment of large bowel emergencies. Br J Surg 1978;65:712–716. *Of 27 patients with diverticulitis requiring immediate resection for large bowel emergencies, three had small bowel freed from the colon at the time of colectomy.*
15. Marshak RH, Eliasoph J. Inflammatory lesions of the small bowel secondary to colonic diverticulitis. Am J Dig Dis 1961;6:423–428. *A well-illustrated report of three patients with small bowel involvement by adjacent diverticulitis. One patient developed a fistula into the jejunum.*
16. Greenall MJ, Levine AW, Nolan DJ. Complications of diverticular disease: a review of the barium enema findings. Gastrointest Radiol 1983;8:353–358. *A well-illustrated review including a case of diverticulitis associated with a mass that encased pelvic loops of ileum, causing small bowel obstruction.*
17. Frager D, Wolf EL, Frager JD, et al. Small intestinal complications of diverticulitis of the sigmoid colon. JAMA 1986;256:3258–3261. *A description of 10 patients, including three with small bowel obstruction. Diverticulitis should be considered in patients with no previous abdominal surgery or hernias, and diagnostic workup should be considered.*

18. Chilimindris CP, Stonesifer GL Jr. Complications associated with the Baker tube jejunostomy. Am Surg 1978;44:707–711. *Twenty-six of 39 patients having Baker tube jejunostomy had complications, including 10 reoperations. The authors recommend insertion of the tube through the stomach or cecum.*
19. Brightwell NL, McFee AS, Aust JB. Bowel obstruction and the long tube stent. Arch Surg 1977;112:505–511. *In a retrospective study of 58 cases, enterolysis alone was as effective or better than the long tube stent in treatment of adhesive small bowel obstruction.*
20. Weigelt JA, Snyder WH III, Norman JL. Complications and results of 160 Baker tube plications. Am J Surg 1980;140:810–815. *Baker tubes were inserted for widespread enteric serosal injury. The incidence of tube complications was 7% with 160 Baker tube plications, and the incidence of recurrent obstruction was 9%, with an average follow-up period of 3.9 years.*

10 Colovesical Fistulas

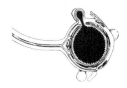

Albert Del Pino, MD
Herand Abcarian, MD

KEY POINTS

- Disease originates in bowel in virtually all cases and usually is diverticulitis
- Male predominance due to anatomic juxtaposition
- Patients have urologic symptoms such as recurrent urinary tract infection, pneumaturia, or fecaluria
- Usual symptoms of diverticulitis frequently are mild or absent
- CT scan is the most sensitive and cost-effective diagnostic study
- Barium enema or flexible endoscopy recommended to exclude malignancy

ILLUSTRATIVE CASES

Case 1: A 51-year-old Hispanic man with a medical history significant for pulmonary tuberculosis and ethanol abuse presented with severe lower abdominal pain of 2 weeks in duration. The patient also admitted to having feculent dark urine and occasional pneumaturia at the termination of voiding. Physical examination revealed a cachectic-appearing man, with left lower quadrant tenderness. No masses were palpated abdominally or per rectum, and the remainder of the examination was normal. The stool was positive for occult blood. Laboratory data demonstrated leukocytosis, and a clean-catch urinalysis showed more than 100 white blood cells (WBCs). Cultures grew more than 100,000 colonies of *Escherichia coli*. Examination of the sputum and urine were negative for acid-fast bacilli. A computed tomography (CT) scan of the abdomen and pelvis demonstrated a pelvic pericolic abscess with mesenteric thickening (Fig. 10.1). There was air in the urinary bladder, but no definite fistula was seen. A barium enema revealed diverticulosis and a colovesical fistula, with filling of the bladder with barium. The remainder of the colon, including the cecum, was normal (Fig. 10.2).

A CT-guided aspiration and drainage of the pericolic abscess was performed (Fig. 10.3). The following day, the patient's symptoms resolved. Cultures from the aspirate grew *Escherichia coli* and acid-fast bacilli. Intravenous antibiotics were continued for a course of 14 days and the patient was started on antituberculosis therapy comprising three drugs. He underwent colonoscopy 2 weeks later, revealing diverticular disease with edema and narrowing in the sigmoid colon. Biopsies of the narrowed segment were negative for acid-fast bacilli. Upon completion of a 3-month course of antituberculosis treatment, the patient was scheduled for surgery. Of note, he required treatment for a urinary tract infection on two occasions during the 3 months treatment for tuberculosis.

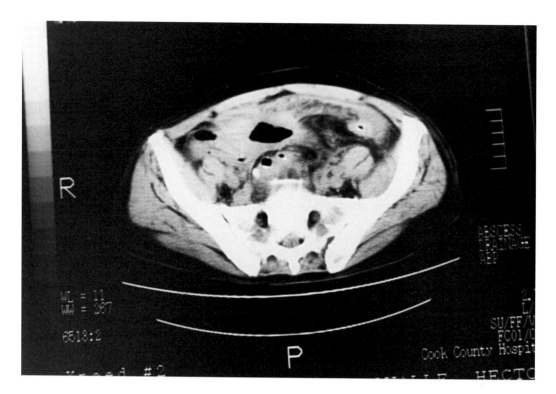

Figure 10.1. Pelvic pericolic abscess with mesenteric thickening.

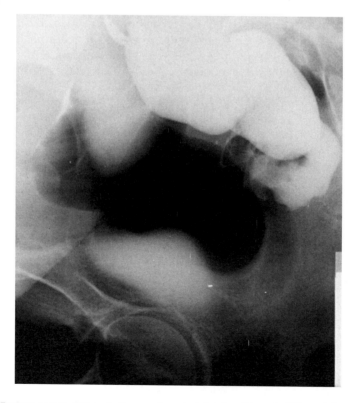

Figure 10.2. Barium enema demonstrating a colovesical fistula with early filling of the urinary bladder.

Stents were inserted intraoperatively. During the cystoscopy, the fistula was identified near the fundus of the bladder (Fig. 10.4). The patient underwent division of the colovesical fistula and left hemicolectomy with stapled colorectal anastomosis. The bladder side of the fistula was left alone and covered with omentum. He had an uneventful postoperative course and was discharged 10 days later after removal of the indwelling catheter.

Case 2: A 60-year-old woman presented with complaints of air expulsion during urination and recalled urinating corn kernels at one time. She was otherwise healthy, was taking no medications, and denied any previous hospitalizations, except for a hysterectomy 8 years earlier. She did not recall any episodes of severe abdominal pain, diarrhea, or fever, but had experienced occasional left lower quadrant abdominal cramps that she attributed to flatulence.

Physical examination revealed a well-healed infraumbilical midline incision and laboratory data were within normal limits.

A CT scan demonstrated air in the bladder, without signs of mesenteric inflammation (Fig. 10.5). Barium enema examination revealed a colovesical fistula with filling of the bladder with contrast (Fig. 10.6). Colonoscopic findings were consistent with chronic diverticulitis with sigmoid narrowing. A fistula could not be visualized.

She underwent cystoscopy, left ureteral stent placement, and a sigmoid colectomy with division of the colovesical fistula. The bladder defect was sutured closed and a primary colorectal anastomosis was performed without difficulty. Her postoperative course was uneventful.

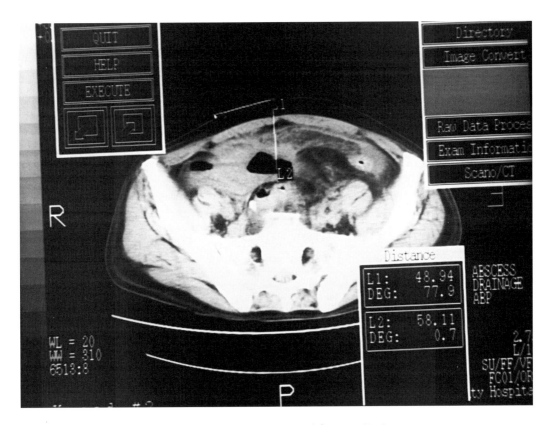

Figure 10.3. CT-guided drainage of the pericolic abscess.

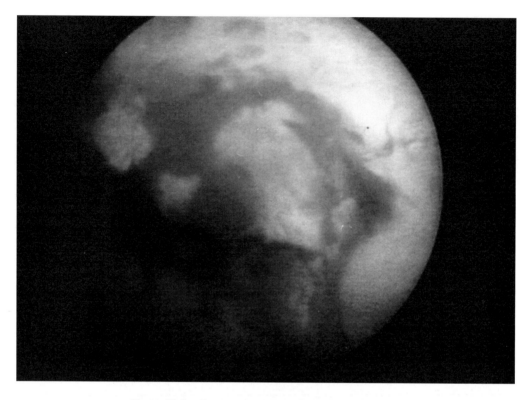

Figure 10.4.   Cystoscopic picture of a colovesical fistula.

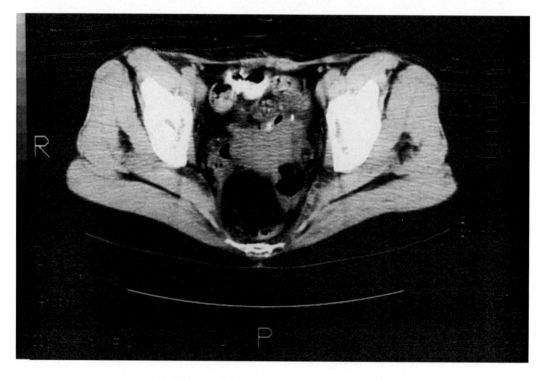

Figure 10.5.   CT scan of the pelvis demonstrating air in the bladder.

Case Comments

We agree with the early use of the CT scan in the evaluation of a suspected colovesical fistula. Air in the previously uninstrumented bladder is virtually diagnostic of an enterovesical fistula, although the remote possibility of emphysematous cystitis should be considered, especially in patients with diabetes. Juxtaposition of bowel (usually sigmoid colon) to the posterior aspect of the bladder in this situation also is highly suggestive of a fistula. In equivocal cases, we would recommend cystoscopy as the next diagnostic test.

Although barium enema or flexible endoscopy are necessary to assess the etiology of a colovesical fistula (i.e., diverticulitis, Crohn's disease, or carcinoma) and to rule out coexistent pathology, we have not found either test to be particularly helpful in actually demonstrating the fistulous tract. Because the surgical treatment of a malignant colovesical fistula may require an en bloc partial or total cystectomy, accurate diagnosis before resection is mandatory. Occasionally, we have used intraoperative endoscopy at the beginning of an operation on patients with equivocal barium enema findings.

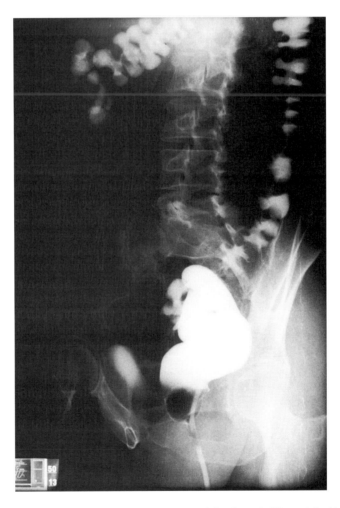

Figure 10.6.   Barium enema reveals a colovesical fistula with filling of the bladder.

Table 10.1.   Etiology of Colovesical Fistulas*

Diverticulitis	62%
Colon Cancer	18%
Crohn's Disease	7%
Genito-urinary Cancer	5%
Other	8%

*With permission from McConnell DB, Sasaki TM, Vetto RM. Experience with colovesical fistula. Am J Surg 1980; 140:80–84.

Table 10.2.   Symptoms Associated with Colovesical Fistulas*

Urologic symptoms:	
Cystitis	70–80%
Pneumaturia	60%
Fecaluria	40–70%
Hematuria	variable
Urine per Rectum	10%
Chronic epididymitis	rare
Suprapubic pain	30–90%
Clinical signs:	
Fever	20–50%

*With permission from Gray MR, Curtis JM, Elkington JS. Colovesical fistula after laparoscopic inguinal hernia repair. Br J Surg 1994;81: 1213–1214.

With respect to ureteral stents, our preference is to use them selectively. Indications for stent placement include reresection for recurrent diverticulitis, complex mass noted on physical examination or preoperative CT scan, low fistula in the region of the bladder trigone, or the presence of hydronephrosis. In addition, we strongly advocate intraoperative ureteral stent placement in the occasional case of an unanticipated difficult dissection in which anatomy and visibility of the ureters is unclear.

DISCUSSION

The first series describing colovesical fistulas was written by Cripps in 1888 (1). In 63 cases, the pathology originated in the bowel, usually as a result of diverticulitis. At that time, the procedure of choice was a colostomy. Uremia, secondary to urinary retention and recurrent urinary tract infections, was the most common cause of death.

Because of the rarity of this complication (2% of patients with diverticulitis) (2), there have been numerous retrospective reviews since 1888 (3–6). The etiology of colovesical fistulas has not changed remarkably (Table 10.1). In diverticulitis, authors speculate that colovesical fistulas originate from either of two processes: direct extension of a perforated diverticulum into the bladder or indirect spread through the erosion of an abscess into the bladder. *Intraperitoneal routes usually manifest near the dome and extraperitoneal lesions appear near the trigone of the bladder* (7). Crohn's disease is another major etiology of this complication. Other less common causes include pelvic irradiation for gynecologic cancers (8), iatrogenic injuries (9,10), and even prostatomegaly (11).

There is a male predominance because of direct contact between the sigmoid and the urinary bladder. In women, a hysterectomy precedes the complication in more than 50% of cases (12). The predominant age actually depends on the etiology: patients with diverticular or malignant disease usually are between 50 and 60 years of age. Although colovesical fistula is rare in Crohn's disease (2%) (13), it occurs in a younger population, usually younger than 30 years of age.

The symptoms are predominately urologic (Table 10.2). The patient typically gives a history of recurrent urinary tract infections (otherwise rare in men, <1%) and pneumaturia or fecaluria at the end of voiding. Urinary tract infections are even more prevalent if there is any degree of obstructive uropathy. Patients may have symptoms of chronic or subacute diverticulitis ranging from 2 weeks up to 8 years (median, 4 months). In fact, as many as half of the patients have no complaints (14). Colovesical fistulas usually do not complicate acute diverticulitis (as in case 1). Pneumaturia, one of the most common symptoms, is not pathognomonic of colovesical fistulas. It can be caused by cystitis due to gas-forming organisms (15) or by manipulation of the urinary system during catheterization.

Although it is not difficult to diagnose a colovesical fistula, demonstrating the etiology and location can be challenging. Excluding a recently instrumented patient, or one with cystitis from gas-producing organisms, pneumaturia is diagnostic, especially if food particles are expelled during urination. To identify the presence of a fistula, various dye studies using methylene blue or charcoal and the Bourne test have been described (16). More recently, radiologic and endoscopic studies have been found to be more useful in identifying the etiology and location of the fistula (Table 10.3).

Table 10.3.   Evaluation of a Patient Suspected of Having a Colovesical Fistula

Test	Advantages	Price	Identifies Fistula Presence/ Identifies Etiology
Abdominal radiograph	1. Air can be seen in the bladder in 22%.	$ 88	No information available
Infusion CT scan with rectal contrast	1. Excludes abscess. 2. Evaluates kidney function. 3. Locates ureters and their relationship to the lesion. 4. Allows drainage of abscess.	$722	>90%/>90%
Barium enema	1. May identify the fistula tract. 2. Very good in differentiating colon malignancy from diverticulitis.	$235	42% (5–90%)/>90%
Intravenous pyelogram	1. Evaluates kidney function.	$195	
Cystogram	1. Excludes bladder lesion as etiology.	$126	30%
Cystoscopy	1. Excludes bladder lesion.	$182	35% (suggestive in 80–100%)
Lower endoscopy	1. Excludes colon malignancy as etiology and identifies diverticulosis.	$700	<10%

A CT scan of the abdomen with narrow cuts of the pelvis together with intravenous and rectal contrast is undoubtedly the most sensitive and cost-effective study (17,18). Significant findings include a thickened bladder wall (90–100%), thickened bowel adjacent to the bladder (89%), gas in the bladder (90%), abscess or extraluminal mass (44–75%), opacified fistula (44%), and oral contrast medium in the bladder (22%). A barium enema or flexible sigmoidoscopy also is recommended to exclude malignancy (19). We have routinely performed cystoscopy before surgical intervention to evaluate the relationship of the fistula to the trigone and to allow ureteral stent placement if deemed necessary. Most fistulas are found in the fundus of the bladder.

Do all patients with colovesical fistulas require surgery? *It seems that, with few exceptions, surgery is indicated, irrespective of the primary disease process.* For instance, in diverticular disease, surgery is required not only because the fistula will not close spontaneously but to avoid the sequelae of recurrent urinary tract infection, specifically sepsis and renal failure (14). Surgery also is warranted if malignancy cannot be excluded. Anecdotal reports have appeared in the literature in which selected patients were treated nonsurgically and followed for many years without complications (20). These reports are rare and demonstrate a limited experience with clear-cut selection bias. Crohn's disease (13), malignant fistulas (13), and iatrogenic fistulas (9,10) also require operative intervention.

When is the optimal time for operative intervention and how should a patient be prepared? Unfortunately, there is a lack of good objective data to answer either question. In the past, most complications of diverticulitis were considered surgical emergencies, but more recently, the pendulum has swung to a more conservative approach. Bleeding is rare and usually self-limited. Pericolonic abscess can be treated by percutaneous drainage, and a colovesical fistula with cystitis can be managed with hydration and intravenous antibiotics. Aside from an unrelentless acute diverticulitis and cases with free perforation, *urgent surgery is rarely indicated.* Patients with complicated diverticular abscesses and colovesical fistulas can undergo surgery semielectively after proper preoperative evaluation.

For patients with acute diverticulitis and colovesical fistula, we believe that optimal time for surgical intervention follows subsidence of the acute inflammation. For patients with a chronic colovesical fistula and cystitis, a full course of antibiotic therapy for urinary tract infection is recommended before surgery.

Before surgery, a full bowel preparation, consisting of a mechanical cleansing agent together with oral antibiotics (aerobic and anaerobic coverage), is advised. Nutritional status should be assessed carefully and optimized by dietary counseling with appropriate supplementation if necessary. A stomal site should be marked on the skin before surgery. We have found that a properly located stoma significantly decreases the incidence of stomal complications (21).

Preoperative ureteral stents can be helpful. However, there is a lack of prospectively controlled data to evaluate the efficacy of prophylactic stents in preventing ureteral injury. One reason for the paucity of data is the rarity of ureteral injuries during colon operations (1–7%) (22). In the course of 198 colon resections (34 for diverticulitis), preoperative stent placement did not decrease the incidence of injuries but instead allowed early detection of an injury (23). Bothwell et al (24) published a 5-year retrospective chart review of 561 patients who underwent colonic surgery for various reasons (182 for diverticular disease). Ninety-two patients underwent placement of prophylactic ureteral stents. There were two surgical ureteral injuries in the control group (0.8%) and two in the stented group (2.2%). One injury in the stented group occurred during stent placement. They concluded that preoperative ureteral stenting should be used only in selected cases, because ureteral

Table 10.4. **Commonly Used Procedures in the Management of Colovesical Fistulas in Diverticulitis**

	Procedure	Indication
Three-stage	1. Drainage of abscess and diversion. 2. Division of fistula and anastomosis. 3. Colostomy closure.	Primarily of historic value. High-risk patients with an abscess, not amenable to percutaneous drainage or unsuccessfully drained.
Two-stage	1. Resection, including division of fistula, primary anastomosis, and diversion. 2. Colostomy closure.	Acutely ill patients with purulence in the pelvis or patients with a tenuous anastomosis.
	1. Resection and Hartmann procedure. 2. Colostomy closure with anastomosis.	Acutely ill patients considered unsafe to anastomose due to poor preparation or peritonitis, etc.
One-stage	Resection, including division of fistula and primary anastomosis.	Elective procedures.
	Intraoperative bowel preparation, primary resection with division of fistula, and primary anastomosis.	Elective procedure for patients who cannot be properly prepared.
Laparoscopic		Experimental at this time.

injuries are rare, and that stent placement may have complications. They also found that stent placement allowed early recognition of injuries. Unfortunately, both studies are plagued with the inherent biases of retrospective reviews and neither series had an adequate sample size (>2000 patients/group for $P<.05$) to show statistical difference in outcome. It has been our practice to perform preoperative cystoscopy and to use a left ureteral stent liberally in patients requiring surgery for complicated diverticulitis. Many of the complications from ureteral stent placement (reflux anuria and urinary tract infections) (24) seem to occur during prolonged stenting after surgery. We routinely remove the stents at the completion of an operation.

What are the surgical options? There has been a trend from colostomy without resection, commonly performed in the 1900s, to primary resection and anastomosis. A list of the common surgical options and indications are listed in Table 10.4.

The operative principles are as follows:

1. Early division of the proximal descending colon.
2. Early identification of the ureter.
3. Proximal to distal dissection of the diseased segment, remaining close to the colon (Fig. 10.7).
4. "Pinching off" the fistula between the colon and bladder (Fig. 10.8).
5. Resection of all distal diverticula with anastomosis to the rectum at the level of the sacral promontory (Fig. 10.9) (22).
6. Continuous bladder drainage for approximately 7 days (12).

Surgical Technique

The dissection is begun at the descending colon by dividing the colon at an area where it feels soft and free of inflammation. However, before dividing the colon, two factors must

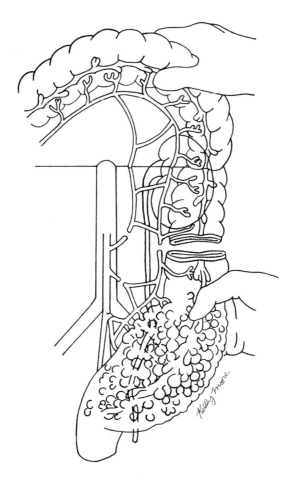

Figure 10.7.   Proximal-to-distal dissection of the diseased segment remaining close to the colon.

be considered. First, a proximal colostomy may be necessary and may require further mobilization of the splenic flexure. Second, it is necessary to ensure that there will be adequate blood supply to this segment.

The left ureter is identified early as it exits, just medial and deep to Gerota's fascia. The surgeon can then slide his hand between the colon and the kidney, staying superficial to the ureter, allowing for better exposure of the mesentery. The sigmoid vessels can be ligated proximally and the inferior mesenteric artery can be ligated distal to the left colic branch (22).

After complete mobilization of the diseased sigmoid colon, the colovesical fistula usually is encountered. At this point, the surgeon should place his hand horizontally in the pouch of Douglas and "pinch off" the colovesical fistula between his fingers. Occasionally, in a subacute colovesical fistula, one encounters a phlegmon (usually visualized on the preoperative CT scan) between the bladder and the anterior wall of the colon. Likewise, by placing a hand in the pouch of Douglas and pinching off the fistula, division can be accomplished (25).

If separation of the fistula is difficult, a malignant process should be suspected. Distending the bladder with saline often will facilitate fistula localization. Malignant fistulas have a poor prognosis; nevertheless, if an en bloc resection including the involved bladder wall is feasible, it should be performed (21).

A one-stage, hand-sewn or stapled colorectal anastomosis usually can be performed, even in the presence of an abscess or purulence. However, certain selection criteria must be met. The patient should have had an adequate preoperative bowel preparation or "on-table lavage," and the inflammatory focus must be completely removed (12). The literature clearly demonstrates that multiple-stage procedures are associated with increased morbidity and mortality, especially if the inflammatory process is not completely removed

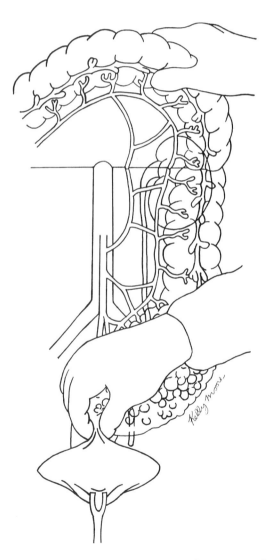

Figure 10.8. "Pinching off" the fistula between the colon and the bladder.

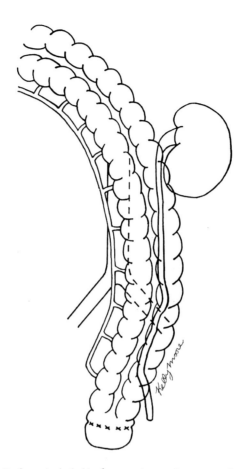

Figure 10.9.   All distal diverticula are included in the resection, and anastomosis to the rectum occurs at the level of the sacral promontory.

(26). The Hartmann procedure, for instance, can offer numerous advantages in certain situations involving the unprepared colon or free perforation or for the patient considered to have high risk for a primary anastomosis (25).

Management of colovesical fistulas in Crohn's disease does not vary a great deal from that of diverticular disease. Patients usually are younger, and the fistulas commonly originate from the small bowel (13). As in diverticulitis, the primary principle is to completely remove the diseased segment. It is not uncommon in Crohn's disease to find multiple fistulas and strictures during exploration. In this situation, only symptomatic problems should be approached surgically.

How should the defect in the bladder be managed? There are three options: primary closure, coverage with omentum, or neither. The only series that looked at this problem objectively came from the Cleveland Clinic (14), in which nothing was done in 58%, primary closure was performed in 20%, debridement and closure were performed in 22%, and omental interposition was performed in 27%. The outcomes were considered comparable between all groups (27). *Most authors believe that it does not matter how the bladder side of the fistula is treated, as long as continuous drainage is maintained for a minimum of 7 days* (12,14,27–29). However, in the literature, the most commonly used technique involves primary closure of the defect with omental interposition. If primary closure is attempted, the surgeon must be aware of the relationship between the bladder defect and the ureterovesical junction. Iatrogenic injury or ligation of the ureter is conceivable if large bites are taken too close to the defect near the trigone. Preoperative cystoscopy may help prevent this complication.

CONCLUSIONS

Colovesical fistulas are discovered most commonly during a subacute or chronic episode of diverticulitis. They rarely require urgent intervention. There usually is ample time for a thorough evaluation to identify the etiology and location of the fistula. CT scan and barium enema seem to be the most useful studies. Surgical intervention after adequate bowel preparation will, more often than not, permit division of the fistula and primary colorectal anastomosis with low morbidity. Preoperative ureteral stents may be helpful.

EDITORIAL COMMENTS

It has been estimated that 20% of patients with diverticulitis have genitourinary symptoms (30). A small number in this group have colovesical fistulas. Because most patients with colovesical fistulas present with urologic symptoms (31,32), they may have been evaluated by a urologist before referral to a surgeon. Often, cystoscopy has been performed, invasive bladder carcinoma has been ruled out, and the classic findings of bullous edema, erythema, granulation tissue, and less likely, the fistulous opening itself have been documented (Fig. 10.10). If cystoscopy is equivocal or has not

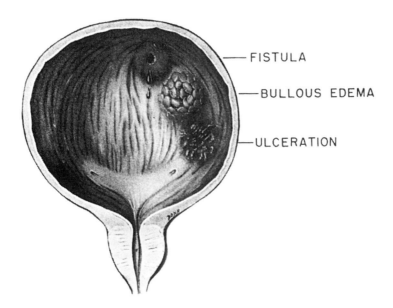

Figure 10.10. Depiction of some of the expected cystoscopic findings. There usually is bullous edema, granulating tissue, and an ulcerated area, rather than an actual fistular opening. (Reprinted with permission from Ward JN, Lavengood RW Jr, Nay HR, et al. Diagnosis and treatment of colovesical fistula. Surg Gynecol Obstet 1970;130:1082–1090.)

been performed, we find the CT scan to be extremely helpful and usually diagnostic (see Case Comments for further discussion of diagnostic evaluation).

If the clinical presentation is suspicious and the workup is equivocal, laparoscopy may be a useful diagnostic tool. If a colovesical fistula is confirmed, resection of the involved bowel, either laparoscopically (33) or open (depending on surgeon preference), can be performed. The possibility of Crohn's disease should be entertained in the younger patient (34).

We agree that most patients with symptomatic fistulas require surgery. A one-stage operation usually is possible because acute inflammation tends to have resolved in much of the operative field and bowel preparation is possible. Division of the fistula can be performed if cancer has been reliably ruled out. The pinching technique rather than sharp dissection minimizes the risk of bladder or ureteral injury. Every attempt should be made preoperatively and intraoperatively to rule out cancer, because a malignant fistula requires partial (or total) resection of the bladder en bloc (35,36) (see Case Comments). Preferably, the superior hemorrhoidal artery is preserved during the course of the dissection. The dome rather than the trigone will be involved in most cases (37). The current mortality rates are in the range of 0–3% (38).

A colovesical fistula is not an absolute indication for surgery: a nonoperative approach seems reasonable for patients with a high operative risk due to underlying medical problems, limited life expectancy (i.e., metastatic disease), or in asymptomatic patients when malignancy has been ruled out. Of interest, in one report, 11 patients with enterovesical fistulas secondary to Crohn's disease were followed medically for a mean period of 9 years; they had only intermittent symptoms without documented episodes of pyelonephritis or ascending infection. In addition, renal function was preserved (39). Similar series have been published (40). On the other hand, patients with urinary obstruction are more prone to develop ascending renal tract infections in this setting.

REFERENCES

1. Cripps WH. The passage of air and feces from urethra. London: JA Churchill Ltd., 1888.
2. Ward JN, Lavengood RW Jr, Nay HR, et al. Diagnosis and treatment of colovesical fistula. Surg Gynecol Obstet 1970;130:1082–1090. *A review of 18 patients. The authors obtained the best results with a three-stage surgical procedure.*
3. Couris GS, Block MA. Intesinovesical fistula. Surgery 1963;54:736–742. *In a series of 21 patients, diverticulitis was the underlying cause in 12 patients. At the time of this study, cystoscopy was the most reliable diagnostic test. Includes a literature review, with 42 references.*
4. Colcock BP, Stehmann FD. Fistulas complicating diverticular disease of the sigmoid colon. Ann Surg 1972;175:838–846. *A classic paper, reviewing 21 patients. Any pelvic structure may be involved. A significant number occurred as complications or failure of operations for diverticulitis. Includes 38 references.*
5. McConnell DB, Sasaki TM, Vetto RM. Experience with colovesical fistula. Am J Surg 1980;140:80–84. *Experience with 37 patients with adult colovesical fistula provides criteria for one-stage versus multi-stage surgical procedures.*
6. Mileski JW, Joehl RJ, Rege RV, et al. One-stage resection and anastomosis in the management of colovesical fistula. Am J Surg 1987;153:75–79. *Recommends cystoscopy as a diagnostic test and provides useful guidelines for one-stage resections.*
7. Small WP, Smith AN. Fistula and conditions associated with diverticular disease of the colon. Clin Gastroenterol 1975;4:171–199. *An excellent discussion of the clinical and anatomic aspects, with numerous references.*
8. Levenback C, Gershenson DM, McGehee R, et al. Enterovesical fistula following radiotherapy for gynecologic cancer. Gynecol Oncol 1994;52:296–300. *Retrospective review of rare radiation-induced enterovesical fistulae provides useful guidelines for clinical management.*
9. Nelson AM, Frank HD, Taubin HL. Colovesical fistula secondary to foreign-body perforation of the sigmoid colon. Dis Colon Rectum 1979;22:559–560. *First documented case of foreign-body-induced colovesical fistula presented.*
10. Gray MR, Curtis JM, Elkington JS. Colovesical fistula after laparoscopic inguinal hernia repair. Br J Surg 1994;81:1213–1214. *Case report of a colovesical fistula after laparoscopic inguinal hernia repair; discusses possible contributing factors.*
11. Abbas F, Memon A. Colovesical fistula: an unusual complication of prostatomegaly. J Urol 1994;152:479–481. *Case reports of an unusual form of colovesical fistula secondary to bladder outlet obstruction in the absence of intrinsic disease of the colon.*
12. Woods RJ, Lavery IC, Fazio VW, et al. Internal fistulas in diverticular disease. Dis Colon Rectum 1988;31:591–596. *Retrospective review of 84 patients with internal fistulas; most (65%) were colovesical followed by colovaginal (25%). Excellent discussion of criteria for one-stage resection presented.*
13. Greenstein AJ, Sachar DB, Tzakis A, et al. Course of enterovesical fistulas in Crohn's disease. Am J Surg 1984;147:788–792. *Experience with 38 patients with enterovesical fistulas in Crohn's disease; 95% of patients eventually required surgery. Location and pathogenesis discussed.*

14. Steele M, Deveney C, Burchell M. Diagnosis and management of colovesical fistulas. Dis Colon Rectum 1979;22:27–29. *Experience with 37 patients with colovesical fistulas presented; outlines role of diagnostic studies and surgical management.*

15. Ho KM, Sole GM. Pneumaturia due to gas-producing E. coli and urinary stasis. Br J Urol 1994;73:588–589. *Case report of pneumaturia secondary to E. coli cystitis emphasizes the importance of careful preoperative evaluation before surgery for a suspected colovesical fistula.*

16. Amendola MA, Agha FP, Dent TL, et al. Detection of occult colovesical fistula by the Bourne test. Am J Roentgenol 1984;142:715–718. *The Bourne test, consisting of radiography of centrifuged urine samples obtained immediately after a nondiagnostic barium enema, was positive in 9 of 10 patients.*

17. Labs JD, Sarr MG, Fishman EK, et al. Complications of acute diverticulitis of the colon: improved early diagnosis with computerized tomography. Am J Surg 1988;155:331–335. *CT scan recommended as the most sensitive and specific test for diagnosing complications of acute diverticulitis.*

18. Hachigian MP, Honickman S, Eisenstat TE, et al. Computed tomography in the initial management of acute left-sided diverticulitis. Dis Colon Rectum 1992;35:1123–1129. *Authors advocate early use of CT scan in diagnosis of acute left-sided diverticulitis, allowing stratification of patients according to severity of disease and, consequently, more appropriate clinical management.*

19. Jarrett TW, Darrocott VE Jr. Accuracy of computerized tomography in the diagnosis of colovesical fistula secondary to diverticular disease. J Urol 1995;153:44–46. *Retrospective data involving nine patients. Supports the use of CT scan as the diagnostic test of choice for the evaluation of suspected colovesical fistulas.*

20. Amin M, Nallinger R, Polk HC Jr. Conservative treatment of selected patients with colovesical fistula due to diverticulitis. Surg Gynecol Obstet 1984;159:442–444. *Although surgical resection of the diseased sigmoid colon is recommended by the authors, a nonsurgical approach was taken in a small select group of patients without complications of sepsis or renal failure.*

21. Bass EM, Del Pino A, Tan A, et al. Does preoperative stoma marking and education by the enterostomal therapist affect outcome? 1995, Dis Colon Rectum 1997;40;440–442.

22. Abcarian H: The difficult resection in diverticulitis. Semin Colon Rectal Surg 1990;1:97–98. *A brief technical description, discussing use of a left ureteral catheter and a proximal-to-distal dissection technique.*

23. Leff EI, Ciroff W, Rubin RJ, et al. Use of ureteral catheters in colonic and rectal surgery. Dis Colon Rectum 1982;25:457–460. *Authors present their extensive experience with routine use of ureteral catheters during colon and rectal surgery, confirming its minimal morbidity and ability to facilitate ureteral identification intraoperatively.*

24. Bothwell WN, Bleicher RJ, Dent TL. Prophylactic ureteral catheterization in colon surgery. A five-year review. Dis Colon Rectum 1994;37:330–334. *92 patients had ureteral catheterization; there was one ureteral injury as a direct result of ureteral catheterization.*

25. Kerner BA, Oliver GC, Eisenstat TE, et al. Use of the Hartmann procedure in the treatment of complicated acute diverticulitis. Semin Colon Rectal Surg 1990;1:87–92. *Summarizes the recent literature and confirms the advantages of the Hartmann procedure, including an acceptable morbidity and mortality.*

26. Bonello JC, Howerton R. Single-stage resection without colostomy in acute diverticulitis. Semin Colon Rectal Surg 1990;1:81–86. *Stresses the importance of patient selection and surgical judgment in deciding upon possible primary anastomosis. One of the most difficult settings involves rupture of an abscess with diffuse, nonfeculent peritonitis.*

27. Gordon PH. Diverticular disease of the colon. In Gordon PH, Nivatvongs S, ed. Principles and practice of surgery for the colon, rectum, and anus. St. Louis: Quality Medical Publishing, 1992:739–791.

28. Kirsh GN, Hempel N, Shuck JM, et al. Diagnosis and management of vesico-enteric fistulas. Surg Gynecol Obstet 1991;173:91–97. *Review of 56 patients with vesicoenteric fistulas identifies diverticulitis as the most common cause; outlines diagnostic workup and recommends single-stage surgical procedure.*

29. Mazier PW. Diverticulitis, in Mazier PW, Levien DH, Luchtefeld MA, ed: Surgery of the colon, rectum and anus. Philadelphia: WB Saunders, 1995:617–656.

30. Hafner CD, Ponka JL, Brush BE. Genitourinary manifestations of diverticulitis of the colon. A study of 500 cases. JAMA 1962;179:76–78. *Ten percent of the patients with genitourinary manifestations of diverticulitis had colovesical fistulas.*

31. Kovalcik PJ, Veidenheimer MC, Corman ML, et al. Colovesical fistula. Dis Colon Rectum 1975;19:425–427. *A study of 55 patients. Favorable factors for one-stage procedures were absence of pericolic abscess, little or no obstruction, and a well-prepared colon.*

32. King RM, Beart RW Jr, McIlrath DC. Colovesical and rectovesical fistulas. Arch Surg 1982;117:680–683. *Forty-three patients (39% of the entire series) had sigmoid diverticulitis as the cause of the fistulas. Cystoscopic examination had a 57% yield.*

33. Puente I, Sosa JL, Desai U, et al. Laparoscopic treatment of colovesical fistulas: technique and report of two cases. Surg Laparosc Endosc 1994;4:157–160. *Each operation took more than 5 hours, but the postoperative stays were short.*

34. Pontari MA, McMillen MA, Garvey RH, et al. Diagnosis and treatment of enterovesical fistulae. Am Surg 1992;58:258–263. *A study of 44 patients. An excellent description of the clinical characteristics of patients with Crohn's disease, carcinoma, and diverticulitis.*

35. Moss RL, Ryan JA Jr. Management of enterovesical fistulas. Am J Surg 1990;159:514–517. *A review of 51 patients with enterovesical fistulas; 41% of the fistulas were caused by diverticulitis. All multistage procedures were performed for fistulas complicated by abscess or bowel obstruction.*

36. Holmes SA, Christmas TJ, Kirby RS, et al. Management of colovesical fistulas associated with pelvic malignancy. Br J Surg 1992;79:432–434. *Thirteen patients are examined: seven had colonic carcinoma. Wide surgical excision is necessary, and in some cases, pelvic exenteration is also needed.*

37. Pollard SG, MacFarlane R, Greatorex R, et al. Colovesical fistula. Ann R Coll Surg Engl 1987;69:163–165. *Forty-seven of 66 fistulas studied (71%) were caused by diverticulitis.*
38. Kurtz DI, Mazier P. Diverticular fistulas. Semin Colon Rectal Surg 1994;1:93–96. *A succinct review of all types of diverticular fistulas. Colovesical fistulas account for 65%, and 55–75% of colovesical fistulas complicate diverticular disease.*
39. Gorcey S, Katzka I. Is operation necessary for enterovesical fistulas in Crohn's disease? J Clin Gastroenterol 1989;11:396–398. *Based on their evidence in 11 patients with enterovesical fistulas followed prospectively for up to 21 years, the authors believe that the presence of a fistula is not, in itself, an indication for surgical intervention.*
40. Margolin ML, Korelitz BI. Management of bladder fistulas in Crohn's disease. J Clin Gastroenterol 1989;11:399–402. *Six patients with enterovesical fistulas had no instances of pyelonephritis following medical therapy alone after a mean of 5.3 years.*

11 Colovaginal Fistulas

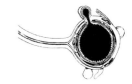

Bertram T. Chinn, MD
Theodore E. Eisenstat, MD

KEY POINTS

- Diverticular disease the most common cause
- Most patients have had hysterectomy
- Vaginal discharge frequent symptom
- 2–25% of all diverticular fistulas
- CT useful diagnostic test
- Vaginography is very helpful for identifying fistula
- Single-stage resection

CASE PRESENTATION

A 72-year-old female presented with a complaint of an increasing vaginal discharge. She had been treated for recurrent urinary tract infections over a 13-year period and her urine had begun to appear "more cloudy." Her history was remarkable only for bleeding fibroids resulting in a hysterectomy. Flexible sigmoidoscopy demonstrated extensive diverticulosis of the sigmoid colon but discomfort precluded examination beyond 40 cm. Vaginal examination revealed a malodorous discharge arising from the apex of the canal. A barium enema was performed and this confirmed extensive diverticulosis as well as a sigmoidovaginal fistula.

Case Comments

This scenario represents a common presentation of patients with colovaginal fistulas. When there is documentation of the fistula as well as the underlying etiology, it is reasonable to proceed with surgical intervention.

The patient underwent a mechanical and antibiotic bowel preparation. She was placed in stirrups before exploration. At operation, the inflammatory fistula was taken down primarily by blunt dissection. After this, a formal sigmoid resection with primary anastomosis to the proximal rectum was performed.

DISCUSSION

Formation of a fistula between the colon and vagina is uncommon. This process may be secondary to malignancy, radiation, iatrogenic or traumatic factors (including obstetric and foreign body), or from inflammatory conditions such as Crohn's disease and diverticulitis (1,2). The incidence of fistula formation associated with diverticulitis is reported to range from 5 to 40%; most reports suggest a frequency of 10–20% (3–5).

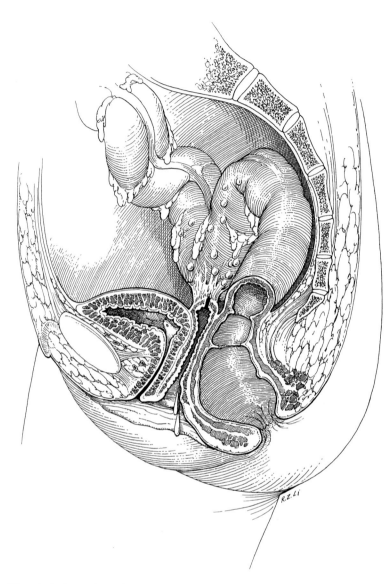

Figure 11.1.   Diverticulosis involving the redundant sigmoid colon. Prior inflammation resulted in fistulization at the vaginal cuff.

Although more than 50% of these fistulas involve the bladder, only 2–25% communicate with the vagina. Diverticular disease represents the most common cause of a colovaginal fistula (5–7).

The fistulization process is believed to involve the development of adhesions to adjacent viscera from the inflammatory reaction of diverticulitis. An abscess may develop with subsequent decompression back into the colon or into the adherent viscus (8,9). *In most cases of a colovaginal fistula, prior hysterectomy facilitated direct contact between a redundant and inflamed segment of colon and the vaginal cuff* (Fig. 11.1). However, colovaginal fistulas also have occurred in cases with the uterus in place (5,10). In this situation, the fistula develops through the thin peritoneum of the pouch of Douglas and penetrates directly into the posterior fornix of the vagina.

A 10-year review of our practice from January 1985 through December 1994 identified 12 women with colovaginal fistulas (Table 11.1). Nine were related to diverticular disease. The average age of these women was 66 years (range, 38–85 years). We found that many women experienced symptoms for several months to years before addressing this embarrassing problem with their physician and that each woman had undergone a hysterectomy. Virtually all patients complained of a foul vaginal discharge or the passage of feces through the vagina (Table 11.2). Abdominal and pelvic pain, alterations in bowel function, and symptoms consistent with diverticulitis also were described frequently, but there also are reports of colovaginal fistulas in individuals who have had no prior symptoms of diverticulitis (5). Less commonly encountered were complaints of the passage of air from the vagina, which also would be consistent with recurrent symptoms of a urinary tract infection, vaginitis, or other forms of sepsis.

Sigmoidoscopy should be performed on initial presentation, and we found that a flexible examination yielded more information than a rigid sigmoidoscopy. Although the actual fistulous opening is not seen commonly, identification of granulation tissue or inflammation in conjunction with an appropriate history suggests the presence of a fistula. Diverticulosis also can be confirmed and other pathology such as a malignancy can be excluded. Vaginal examination should be performed with a speculum or rigid sigmoido-scope in an attempt to identify granulation tissue or drainage. In our review, these findings were present in virtually all patients who had a colovaginal fistula, most frequently at the apex of the vaginal cuff or at the posterior fornix (Table 11.3).

Table 11.1.   Etiology of Colovaginal Fistulas

Etiology	N
Diverticular disease	9
Neoplasm	1
Crohn's disease	1
Anastomotic leak	1
Total:	12

Table 11.2.   Symptoms

Symptom	N	Percentage
Vaginal discharge	11	92
Abdominal pain	4	33
Pelvic pain	1	8
Pneumaturia	1	8
UTI/urinary frequency	1	8
Fever/sepsis	1	8

Table 11.3.   Clinical Examinations

Finding	RS	FS	VS
Fistula	0	1	1
Stool/drainage	n/a	n/a	7
Erythema/inflammation	0	1	1
Granulation	0	1	1
Neoplasm	0	1	1
Bowel fixation	2	2	n/a

RS, rigid sigmoidoscopy; FS, flexible sigmoidoscopy; VS, vaginoscopy; n/a, not applicable.

Radiographic studies may be useful diagnostically. A barium enema may identify the fistula on lateral and oblique views. The literature, however, reports that this study is only 30–50% accurate. *CT imaging not only provides the most information regarding the diseased bowel and adjacent viscera but may demonstrate the fistula with the use of contrast or may suggest it by the presence of vaginal air on multiple cuts* (11).

Although these studies together with the appropriate history generally have provided the necessary information to confirm the diagnosis of a colovaginal fistula, other methods also have been described. *Vaginography using a Foley catheter has been reported to be very sensitive in identifying a fistula* (3,12,13). Grissom and Snyder in their review noted a 90% accuracy of vaginography, compared with 19% for sigmoidoscopy and 49% for barium enema (3). With the patient in the supine position with her legs adducted, a 30-mL balloon is used to occlude the vaginal canal and a water-soluble contrast is instilled under the force of gravity. Typically, only 30 mL of contrast is necessary before the fistula is identified under fluoroscopy (Fig. 11.2).

Tandem colovaginoscopy also has been used to diagnose colovaginal fistulas (14). Simultaneously, a vaginoscopy is performed using a fiberoptic gastroscope to identify the distal fistula or granulation tissue near the vaginal cuff or posterior fornix and a colonoscopy is performed to identify the light from the gastroscope through the fistula. A chronic fistula tract may be cannulated with a soft catheter or flexible biopsy forceps. Charcoal ingestion has been used to identify colovesical and colouterine fistulas; we believe it may be helpful in confirming the diagnosis of a colovaginal fistula (15).

Although there are various approaches to the management of a rectovaginal fistula, such as fecal diversion or staged procedures, the only definitive approach for a colovaginal fistula secondary to diverticular disease is resection of the diseased bowel and division of the fistula. General surgical principles should be followed, including the use of a bowel preparation and perioperative antibiotics. The acute inflammatory phase of diverticulitis usually has resolved at the time of exploration, perhaps due to abscess decompression by the fistulous tract. Additionally, we believe that the placement of ureteral catheters is extremely helpful in identifying and protecting the ureters in the pelvis that had been operated on previously (16,17).

In our experience, *a colovaginal fistula can be managed safely with a one-stage procedure* and the length of hospitalization is shortened compared with staged procedures (3,5,13). Eleven of the 12 fistulas were managed by a sigmoid resection and primary anastomosis. There were no intra-abdominal complications such as anastomotic dehiscence or pelvic abscess; however, two patients developed wound infections that did not impede their overall recovery. One patient developed an adhesive partial small bowel obstruction requiring readmission (Table 11.4). The remaining case presented as an anastomotic leak with a pelvic abscess that could not be drained percutaneously, and a staged resection/repair was performed subsequently.

Division of the fistula often can be accomplished by attenuating the surrounding tissue and the tract between the thumb and index finger. Fibrosis may prevent a complete division using this blunt technique, and sharp dissection and division of the fistula may be required. Oversewing the vaginal ostium is not necessary because it will close by secondary intention (18). We also attempt to interpose a segment of omentum between the bowel and vagina to facilitate the closure of the distal fistulous opening (Fig. 11.3).

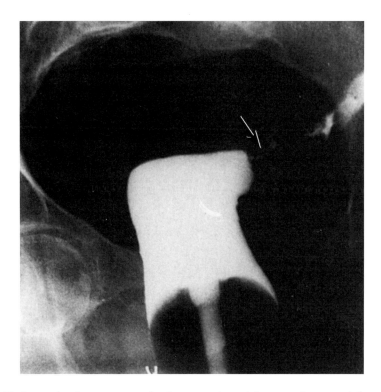

Figure 11.2.   Vaginography demonstrates a fistulous tract (arrow) between the apex of the vagina and the sigmoid colon. (Reprinted with permission from Reeves KO, Young RL, Gordon AN, et al. Sigmoidovaginal fistula secondary to diverticular disease. A report of three cases. J Reprod Med 1988;33:313–316.)

Table 11.4.   Complications After Primary Resection

Complication	N
Wound infection	2
DVT	1
Chronic obstructive pulmonary disease exacerbation	1
Partial small bowel obstruction (requiring readmission)	1
Anastomotic stricture	1

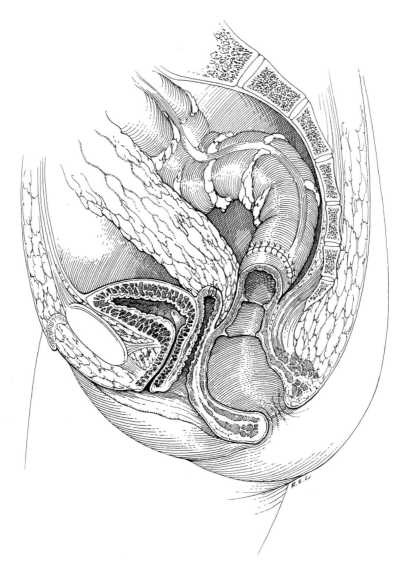

Figure 11.3.   Resection of diseased bowel and primary anastomosis. Interposition pedicle of omentum placed between the anastomosis and the vagina.

In summary, colovaginal fistulas are uncommon. They usually are caused by diverticular disease. Most women experience symptoms of a malodorous discharge, discomfort, or the passage of air from the vagina. Physical examination identifies stool or granulation tissue at the apex of the vagina. The uterus seems to provide an anatomic barrier against the formation of a colovaginal fistula, because most women in whom this fistula has developed have had a prior hysterectomy. One-stage repair of a colovaginal fistula should be safe for the appropriate patient, and an interposed pedicle of omentum may be useful in its repair and in preventing recurrence.

EDITORIAL COMMENTS

A colovaginal fistula should be suspected in any woman with vaginal discharge who has had a hysterectomy. Gynecologists must be particularly aware of this in the aging female population. Foul vaginal discharge, in itself, may be an adequate indication for operation on the patient with a clinical diagnosis of sigmoid diverticulitis. The authors and others have shown the lack of sensitivity of barium enema or of endoscopy in identifying the fistula itself; vaginography is quite accurate, however. We agree that primary resection and anastomosis usually are possible.

REFERENCES

1. Heyen F, Winslet MC, Andrews H, et al. Vaginal fistulas in Crohn's disease. Dis Colon Rectum 1989;32:379–383. *Describes 28 patients with vaginal fistulas. These fistulas do not close with conservative therapy or with a proximal defunctioning stoma alone.*
2. Stumpf PG. Stenosis and fistulae with neglected vaginal foreign bodies. A case report. J Reprod Med 1985;30:559–560. *Discusses a rectovaginal fistula due to a retained vaginal foreign body.*
3. Grissom R, Snyder TE. Colovaginal fistula secondary to diverticular disease. Dis Colon Rectum 1991;34: 1043–1049. *A comprehensive literature review. Most patients had a history of hysterectomy and had fistulas near the vaginal apex. The surgical trend is toward a one-stage resection and anastomosis.*
4. Wisniewski PM, Coonrod T, Thonet MA, et al. Early diagnosis of a diverticular colovaginal fistula with colposcopy. A case report. J Reprod Med 1988;33:705–708. *Multiple areas of purulent drainage were seen with colposcopy.*
5. Woods RJ, Lavery IC, Fazio VW, et al. Internal fistulas in diverticular disease. Dis Colon Rectum 1988;31:591–596. *A review of 84 patients with internal fistulas at the Cleveland Clinic from 1960 to 1986; 23 fistulas (25%) were colovaginal. There was a significant decrease in staged procedures in the latter half of the series.*
6. Carpenter WS, Allaben RD, Kamouris AA. Fistulas complicating diverticulitis of the colon. Surg Gynecol Obstet 1972;134:625–628. *A study of 19 patients followed up to 19 years. Three fistulas recurred because of inadequate resection.*
7. Cross SB, Copas PR. Colovaginal fistula secondary to diverticular disease. A report of two cases. J Reprod Med 1993;38:905–906. *The authors uncovered 87 cases in the English literature. Barium enema was diagnostic of a fistula in only 30–40% of cases; fistulous openings were seen with a speculum 60–68% of the time. Proctosigmoidoscopy was of limited value in demonstrating a fistula.*
8. Reeves KO, Young RL, Gordon AN, et al. Sigmoidovaginal fistula secondary to diverticular disease. A report of three cases. J Reprod Med 1988;33:313–316. *Reviews 49 literature cases. Proposes that these fistulas will be seen more frequently by gynecologists.*
9. Rothenbuehler JM, Oertli D, Harder F. Extraperitoneal manifestations of perforated diverticulitis. Dig Dis Sci 1993;38:1985–1988. *A clinical description of five patients with unusual extraperitoneal presentations of diverticulitis.*
10. Fleshner PR, Schoetz DJ Jr., Roberts PL, et al. Anastomotic vaginal fistula after colorectal surgery. Dis Colon Rectum 1992;35:938–943. *Discusses nine patients with colovaginal fistulas complicating colorectal surgery. Colorectal resection is advocated for high fistulas and transanal repair is recommended for low fistulas.*
11. Nokes SR, Martinez CR, Arrington JA, et al. Significance of vaginal air on computed tomography. J Comput Assist Tomogr 1986;10:997–999. *Two of three patients with enterovaginal fistulas had a distended, air-filled vagina on multiple successive CT images.*
12. Arnold MW, Aguilar PS, Stewart WR. Vaginography: an easy and safe technique for the diagnosis of colovaginal fistulas. Dis Colon Rectum 1990;33:334–335. *Discusses a simple, accurate diagnostic technique.*
13. Colonna JO Jr., Kang J, Giuliana AE, et al. One-stage repair of colovaginal fistula complicating acute diverticulitis. Am Surg 1990;56:788–791. *Compares different forms of staged procedures in 14 patients.*
14. Adams DB, Perry TG. Tandem colovaginoscopy in the diagnosis of colovaginal fistula. Dis Colon Rectum 1988;31:653–654. *A brief technical discussion of a safe useful diagnostic technique; a planned one-stage repair was favored.*
15. Huettner PC, Finkler NJ, Welch WR. Colouterine fistula complicating diverticulitis: charcoal challenge test aids in diagnosis. Obstet Gynecol 1992;80:550–552. *Activated charcoal given orally was seen coming from the cervical os during pelvic examination the following day. The authors state that 17 cases of colouterine fistulas due to diverticulitis have been reported.*
16. Kyzer S, Gordon PH. The prophylactic use of ureteral catheters during colorectal operations. Am Surg 1994;60:212–216. *Discusses 120 ureteral catheterizations; retrospectively, this was deemed necessary 28% of the time. One ureter was cut and one was tied but recognized by palpation.*
17. Sheikh FA, Khubchandani IT. Prophylactic ureteric catheters in colon surgery — how safe are they? Report of 3 cases. Dis Colon Rectum 1990;33:508–510. *Three of 59 patients developed reflux anuria after the use of prophylactic catheters.*
18. Colcock BP, Stahmann FD. Fistulas complicating diverticular disease of the sigmoid colon. Ann Surg 1972;175:838–846. *Reviews 64 fistulas complicating diverticulitis, including seven colovaginal fistulas. Vaginal discharge was characteristic.*

12 Management of Coincident Diverticular Disease

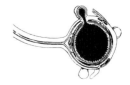

Thomas Stahl, MD

KEY POINTS

- Diverticular disease commonly found at laparotomy for other conditions
- The presence of diverticula is not an indication for resection
- Indications for resection unchanged when diverticula found unexpectedly at laparotomy

INTRODUCTION

Colonic diverticular disease is a common finding in patients older than 50 years of age, and hence, occasionally will be present in conjunction with other colonic or intra-abdominal pathologic processes requiring surgery. The purpose of this chapter is to discuss the potential significance of coincident diverticular disease, to identify those circumstances under which addressing this finding would be appropriate in conjunction with other intra-abdominal surgery, and to describe some of the technical considerations.

To deal with coexistent diverticular disease, it is important to understand the natural history of diverticular disease and the indications for elective resection.

ILLUSTRATIVE CASES

Case 1: A 68-year-old female was found to have a cecal cancer after colonoscopy performed for a heme-occult positive stool. Colonoscopy also revealed scattered diverticula throughout the sigmoid colon without inflammation or luminal narrowing. When questioned, the patient stated that she had been treated with an antibiotic for diverticulitis 6 years prior. She had been asymptomatic since that time.

Case 2: A 45-year-old female underwent elective laparoscopy for pelvic pain of presumed gynecologic origin. She was found to have an inflamed segment of sigmoid diverticulitis. There was no perforation, abscess, or obstruction. What should be done?

Case 3: An 81-year-old woman presented with several years of progressive rectal prolapse and difficulties with fecal incontinence. During her preoperative evaluation, she also was found to have significant diverticulosis of the left colon. She had experienced two episodes of diverticulitis during the last 3 years, requiring hospitalization and intravenous antibiotics. What would be the most appropriate operation for this patient?

Case 4: Mid-descending colon carcinoma was diagnosed in a 61-year-old man, who also was found to have diverticulosis involving the entire colon. He had no symptoms from his diverticular disease. How extensive an operation should this patient have?

Case Comments

In case 1, the patient's diverticular disease was limited to one mild episode several years previously and she had no symptoms or complications to justify sigmoid resection. Right colectomy without sigmoid resection should be performed in this case.

When faced with a situation such as that presented in case 2, the most logical question would be, if diverticulitis were suspected preoperatively, whether surgery would be required. The answer in this case would be no. The safest course would be to terminate the surgery and treat the patient for localized diverticulitis with intravenous antibiotics. If surgery is required subsequently, a planned one-stage procedure could then be undertaken.

For most surgeons, case 3 fulfills the criteria for elective sigmoid resection for diverticular disease. The alternatives for the patient's prolapse consist of an anterior resection, rectal fixation, or a perineal rectosigmoidectomy. Although the perineal approach might be least stressful for the patient, performing an anterior resection extending into the proximal rectum would obviously address both issues nicely, as long as the patient is otherwise fit to undergo an abdominal operation. The only precaution would be to accurately identify the proximal extent of the diverticular disease and either resect to that point or consider an open anastomosis if diverticula were in the vicinity.

In the setting of case 4, the options would be to perform a resection to take care of the colon cancer without regard to the diverticulosis, to perform a left colectomy to the rectosigmoid junction, and lastly, to perform a total abdominal colectomy with ileorectal anastomosis. Although the patient had no prior symptoms of diverticulitis or bleeding, he is comparatively young and has a modest chance of developing such problems over ensuing years. Because diverticulitis occurs almost exclusively in the sigmoid region, encompassing this within the resected specimen would seem reasonable. The only concern then would be anastomosing diverticula in the colon to the proximal rectum. Direct visualization of the anastomosis would help minimize the chance of including a diverticulum within the anastomotic suture line. Performing a total colectomy would seem to be excessive, and although completed with comparative safety in the elective setting, the consequences to bowel function are sufficiently unpredictable to warrant preservation of the proximal colon in this patient.

DISCUSSION

In the United States, diverticulosis is unusual in individuals younger than 40 years of age but becomes increasingly frequent in individuals older than 50 years of age. Although incidence figures vary somewhat among studies, approximately 30–40% of adults between the ages of 60 and 70 years will have some degree of diverticulosis, and by 80 years of age, this increases to 60% or greater (1,2). The gender differential is such that there is a slight female preponderance. Although there is a high incidence of diverticulosis in western societies, most of these patients remain asymptomatic. *The presence of diverticulosis alone is not an indication for resection.*

Indications for Elective Resection of Diverticular Disease

Regarding diverticulitis, there is little debate over the utility of semielective resection in complicated cases, which would include fistula, symptomatic stricture, or the inability to eliminate the possibility of carcinoma. *The advisability of elective resection for uncomplicated diverticulitis is where some uncertainty remains.* One must be cautious with the patient with chronic gastrointestinal symptoms in conjunction with diverticulosis when attributing these symptoms to the latter. When the symptoms are long-standing and not easily attributable to isolated inflammation of the sigmoid colon, the likelihood of a successful outcome after elective resection diminishes substantially.

What are the indications for elective resection with colonic bleeding attributable to diverticulosis? Some would argue that there is no such indication on an elective basis, whereas others would submit that because the likelihood of bleeding increases substantially after two episodes, elective resection would be reasonable. Obviously, this would be appropriate only if the bleeding site was identified clearly. Presently, clinical data do not give clear guidance in this situation.

DIVERTICULAR DISEASE IN CONJUNCTION WITH OTHER INTRA-ABDOMINAL SURGICAL CONDITIONS

In this section, consideration will be given to the handling of coincident diverticular disease encountered during surgery for an unrelated condition. The range of such an encounter would include elective versus emergency operation and primary colonic surgery versus noncolonic surgery.

Emergent Noncolonic Surgery

In the absence of unsuspected diverticular obstruction or abscess, it is never appropriate to perform colon surgery for coincident diverticular disease in the setting of a noncolonic emergency procedure. Therefore, during emergency surgery for appendicitis, cholecystitis, perforated gastric or duodenal ulcer, bowel obstruction (unrelated to diverticulitis), or traumatic injuries, attempting to address diverticular disease would be unwise. One would be working with unprepared bowel, the clinical significance of the diverticular disease would likely be unclear, and resecting the area would lengthen operative time and probably necessitate a colostomy. The added procedure would increase the risk of postoperative complications. In addition, the risks and benefits of elective surgery for diverticulitis should be discussed in detail with patients preoperatively.

Elective Noncolonic Surgery

As discussed above, it would be unwise to resect an area of possibly asymptomatic diverticular disease at the time of laparotomy for other pathology. Sigmoid resection, even under ideal circumstances, carries significant risks, including anastomotic leak, sepsis, and possible colostomy (3). In the event of unsuspected cancer, abscess, or obstruction, incidental sigmoid resection should not be performed without consent.

Emergency Colonic Surgery

In the event of urgent colonic surgery, the basic notion of addressing only that which is most pressing should prevail. Such settings could include perforated or obstructing colon cancer, toxic colitis from inflammatory bowel disease or infectious causes, irreducible colonic volvulus, uncontrollable hemorrhage, colonic trauma, and ischemia. In many of these circumstances, a colostomy will be a component of the operation, and the patient's diverticulosis can be quantified and the history (if any) of related problems can be ascertained before reversal of the colostomy. The latter operation would occur at a more appropriate time to address the diverticular disease. To perform a subtotal colectomy and either an ileostomy or ileorectal anastomosis to encompass diverticular disease coincident with the primary colonic pathology would, under most circumstances, be unjustifiable. The complications with emergent ileorectal anastomoses can sometimes be high, and subsequent bowel function is unpredictable (4,5). Furthermore, the indications for resecting coexisting diverticulosis may not be ascertainable in emergent circumstances; proceeding with a resection probably would be difficult to defend, particularly if doing so led to complications that otherwise might not have occurred or if the patient was left with substantially altered bowel function.

Elective Colon Surgery

During elective colon surgery, there is time to carefully evaluate the significance of coexisting diverticular disease and, if appropriate, include the symptomatic segment in the resection (Fig. 12.1). The mere presence of diverticulosis in the absence of symptoms or complications probably should be left alone. However, if the patient has had symptoms related to diverticular disease that independently would justify resection, then proceeding to do so at the time of the nondiverticular colonic surgery would be reasonable. Therefore, it is the patient with, for instance, an unlocalized prior lower gastrointestinal bleed or a mild single

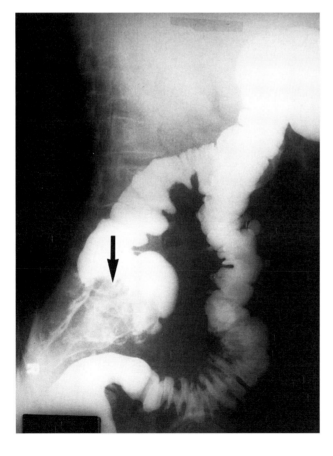

Figure 12.1. This oblique barium enema view shows a cecal carcinoma (arrow) as well as diverticular disease in the left colon.

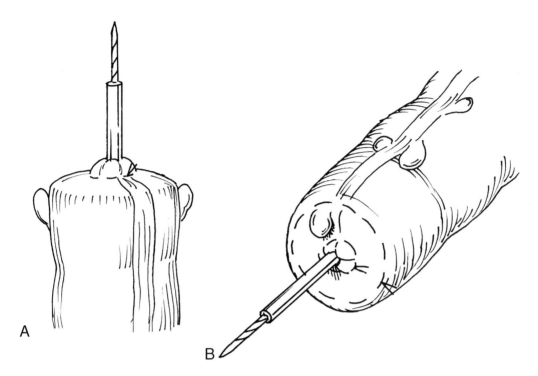

Figure 12.2.   Technical approach to circular stapled anastomosis when diverticula lie outside the anvil after the pursestring suture of 2–0 prolene is secured around the anvil **(A)**. A diverticulum is brought into the segment of bowel that is excised in the course of stapling using an inverting suture of 3–0 vicryl **(B)**.

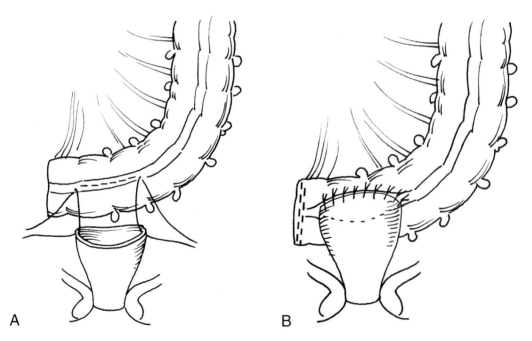

Figure 12.3.   Method of hand-sewn anastomosis involving a segment of colon containing multiple diverticula. This side-to-end coloproctostomy allows the suture line to lie on the antimesenteric border of the colon, which is rarely involved with diverticula. The anastomosis is constructed as depicted in **(A)** and is completed as shown in **(B)**.

previous episode of diverticulitis that presents the challenge. It is this circumstance in which common sense and good judgment are invaluable. In these equivocal cases, it would be reasonable to recommend coincident resection, because the likelihood of recurring episodes of bleeding or inflammation are low but real and could potentially be avoided by removing the segment of bowel in one encompassing operation. The argument to this would be predicated on whether one or two anastomoses would be involved, how much colon would be excised in total, and the patient's ability to tolerate an operation of potentially greater magnitude. Obviously, a left colectomy for a descending colon carcinoma and sigmoid diverticulitis represents a straightforward circumstance, whereas a cecal carcinoma coexisting with pandiverticulosis is an entirely different situation.

Occasionally, there will be a situation in which resection of a colonic lesion involves an anastomosis in the presence of diverticulosis. Extended resection of colon is not necessarily required, as long as normal full-thickness bowel wall is available for anastomosis. In this setting, an open anastomotic technique probably is best, because it allows identification of all diverticula and sutures can be placed outside the diverticula (Figs. 12.2 and 12.3). After diverticula are trimmed away from the proposed site of anastomosis, anastomotic sutures are placed through full-thickness bowel wall. Stapled or closed anastomoses introduce the risk of leak if a diverticulum is incorporated in the anastomosis.

SUMMARY

Despite the high incidence of diverticular disease, it is *rare* that unplanned sigmoid resection must be performed when operating for other indications. In the setting of careful preoperative evaluation and discussion with the patient, elective sigmoid resection may be combined with other procedures with low morbidity and a good outcome.

EDITORIAL COMMENTS

Diverticular disease is encountered very frequently when operating on abdominal conditions such as colon cancer (Fig. 12.1). In many cases, the diverticula have not been a source of symptoms, and we concur that no direct surgical intervention is needed at that time. On the other hand, if there is any suggestion of lower abdominal symptoms related to the gastrointestinal or urinary tracts, it would be wise to evaluate the colon involved with diverticular disease more fully using computed tomography (CT) or contrast studies. Frequently, a colonoscopy already will have been performed in evaluation of a colon cancer. For a patient with confirmed symptomatic diverticular disease or previous attack(s) requiring hospitalization, consideration should be given to subtotal colectomy. The issue of bowel function must be weighed for elderly patients, however, if subtotal colectomy (4,5) is considered; this is especially important if sphincter tone or continence are subnormal. As an option, two separate colonic resections and anastomoses can be performed, without significant increased risk over a single anastomosis, as long as care is taken to meet the criteria of safe anastomoses (6).

A well-known management problem involves patients with concurrent abdominal aortic aneurysm and colon carcinoma (7–9). The issue is not nearly as vital when diverticular disease is involved, because the disease is benign and the aneurysm is of greater import. In the case of complicated diverticular disease, an abscess would have to be drained before aortic aneurysmectomy could be considered (10), and large bowel obstruction conceivably could require urgent intervention. In some instances, a retroperitoneal approach to the vascular procedure is feasible to lessen the risk of prosthetic graft infection. The known risk of aneurysm rupture after laparotomy also must be considered when making a decision (11).

SUGGESTED READINGS

1. Parks TG. Natural history of diverticular disease of the colon. A review of 521 cases. BMJ 1969;4:639–642. *A widely quoted early study, one of many by the author.*
2. Veidenheimer MC, ed. Colonic diverticulitis. Semin Colon Rectal Surg 1990;1:63–115.
3. Goron PH, Nivatvongs S. Principles and practice of surgery for the colon, rectum and anus. St. Louis: Quality Medical Publishing, 1992:739–797.
4. Keighley MR, Williams NS. Surgery of the anus, rectum, and colon. London: WB Saunders Company, 1993:1128–1211.

REFERENCES

1. Keighley MR, Williams NS. Surgery of the anus, rectum and colon. London: WB Saunders, 1993:1132–1135.
2. Rodkey GV, Welch CE. Colonic diverticular disease with surgical treatment: a study of 338 Cases. Surg Clin North Am 1974;54:655–674. *A 1-decade summary of the surgical experience at Massachusetts General Hospital.*
3. Bokey EL, Chapuis PH, Pheils MT. Elective resection for diverticular disease and carcinoma: comparison of post-operative morbidity and mortality. Dis Colon Rectum 1981;24:181–183. *Patients having surgery for diverticular disease had a higher morbidity and mortality.*
4. Bender JS, Bouwman DL. Total abdominal colectomy: conditions defining outcome. Am Surg 1994;60:205–209. *Mortality was 10 times higher (56%) if the procedure was performed as an emergency or when perioperative transfusion requirements reached 10 liters.*
5. Ottinger LW. Frequency of bowel movements after abdominal colectomy with ileorectal anastomosis. Arch Surg 1978;113:1048–1049. *Sixteen percent of patients having ileorectal anastomosis had high and potentially disabling stool frequency. Patients with diverticulosis had more frequent bowel movements than those with neoplastic conditions.*
6. Whalen RL, Wong WD, Goldberg SM, et al. Synchronous bowel anastomoses. Dis Colon Rectum 1989;32:365–368. *It is safe to perform synchronous anastomoses without diversion if several criteria are met: a well-prepared bowel with minimal fecal soilage intraoperatively, a lack of tension, and an adequate, well-vascularized anastomosis.*
7. Robinson G, Hughes W, Lippey E. Abdominal aortic aneurysm and associated colorectal carcinoma: a management problem. Aust N Z J Surg 1994;64:475–478. *The authors recommend giving an aortic aneurysm greater than 6 cm preferential treatment or simultaneous resection, because of the high risk of rupture.*
8. Bickerstaff LK, Hollier LH, Van Peenen HJ, et al. Abdominal aortic aneurysm repair combined with a second surgical procedure — morbidity and mortality. Surgery 1984;95:487–491. *One hundred thirteen patients underwent one or more nonvascular procedures (no colectomies) together with aneurysmectomy. Because of the risk of additional complications, procedures in addition to aneurysmectomy should be performed with caution.*
9. Nora JD, Pairolero PC, Nivatvongs S, et al. Concomitant abdominal aortic aneurysm and colorectal carcinoma: priority of resection. J Vasc Surg 1989;9:630–636. *If the carcinoma is not symptomatic and localized, the aneurysm should be resected initially.*
10. Hugh TB, Masson J, Graham AR, et al. Combined gastrointestinal and abdominal aortic aneurysm operations. Aust N Z J Surg 1988;58:805–810. *No mention was made of diverticular disease in the operative notes; one patient developed diverticulitis during the postoperative period.*
11. Swanson RJ, Littooy FN, Hunt TK, et al. Laparotomy as a precipitating factor in the rupture of intra-abdominal aneurysms. Arch Surg 1980;115:299–304. *The authors reported 10 patients who had ruptured abdominal aneurysms (previously asymptomatic) within 36 days of laparotomy. Collagen lysis in the aneurysm wall is greatest during the first postoperative week.*

13 "Malignant" Diverticulitis

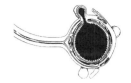

Leon Morgenstern, MD

> **KEY POINTS**
>
> - Incidence is less than 5% of all patients operated on for diverticular disease
> - Clinical similarities to granulomatous colitis
> - CT scan will demonstrate extensive pelvic phlegmonous changes
> - Plan for a staged resection
> - Attempt stenting of both ureters
> - If only diversion performed, allow 6–12 months before attempting resection
> - Diversion does not usually eliminate the inflammatory process, which may continue to "smolder"

"Malignant" diverticulitis (1) is a variant form of diverticular disease of the distal colon in which the basic features are extensive intramural inflammation, often extending below the peritoneal reflection; a great tendency to fistulize into adjacent structures or viscera; and the frequent association of obstruction, perforation, and abscess formation. The inflammation, chronic in nature, is phlegmonous, extensively involving the adjacent pelvic structures and obscuring normal anatomic relationships. *Attempted resection is fraught with great difficulty and complicated postoperatively by a tendency to anastomotic disruption, sepsis, and a potentially lethal outcome.* There is precedent for use of the term "malignant" for this disease, as exemplified in the commonly accepted terms of malignant hypertension, malignant hyperthermia, and malignant exophthalmos. All are benign conditions that have a complex, often adverse course to distinguish them from the more benign variants in the same disease spectrum (2,3).

ILLUSTRATIVE CASES

Case 1

These case studies are excerpted from actual recent cases at the author's hospital.

PREOPERATIVE PHASE

A 57-year-old woman had recurrent attacks of lower abdominal pain, chills, and fever over a 6-month period. Because of increasing constipation and increasing frequency of attacks of pain, fever, and chills, she was admitted to the hospital, where a gastrografin enema showed extensive sigmoid diverticulitis, pericolic abscess formation, and a suggestion of a sigmoidovesical fistula. A computed tomography (CT) scan showed an intrapelvic phlegmonous process. The patient was scheduled for sigmoid resection and primary anastomosis.

OPERATION

The left ureter could not be catheterized. The patient was explored through a long midline incision. The inflammatory process in the distal sigmoid and proximal rectum was considered very severe, with dense pericolonic adhesions and a phlegmonous inflammation involving the left lower quadrant and pelvis. Dissection in the vicinity of the bladder resulted in excessive bleeding, requiring use of a topical hemostatic agent. For identification of the left ureter, intravenous injection of indigo carmine was required. To free the diseased sigmoid for resection, it was necessary to open the peritoneal reflection in the cul-de-sac. The distal segment of involved sigmoid was freed with difficulty, and when transected, the lumen was almost nonexistent, with small intramural abscesses at the resection margin. On the proximal side, the splenic flexure was mobilized to allow a tension-free anastomosis. A stapled anastomosis was performed between the left transverse colon and the proximal rectum. Finally, a right transverse colostomy was performed.

POSTOPERATIVE COURSE

One week after operation, the patient developed spiking fevers and drainage of purulent material from the rectum. CT scan showed a large pelvic abscess. At reoperation, the abscess was drained and the anastomosis was found to be completely disrupted. The distal rectum was oversewn and the proximal sigmoid segment was stapled closed.

After the second operation, an ileal fistula, a vesical fistula, and a large ventral hernia developed, requiring months of parenteral alimentation and hospital care. An attempt to close the enteral fistula by a subsequent operation failed.

After 2 years of intermittent hospitalizations, multiple operative procedures for the fistulas, and parenteral alimentation, it was finally possible to resect the fistulas and reestablish colonic continuity. A large ventral hernia was repaired at a later date.

CASE COMMENTS

This is an example of the horrendous complications that can ensue when operating on patients with this form of diverticulitis.

When encountering such a situation, the surgeon should exercise judgment, restraint, and careful technique. Major decision-making involves the safety of both resection of the involved sigmoid and of primary anastomosis. Here, the surgeon should have given consideration to terminating the sigmoid dissection when widespread phlegmonous inflammation was encountered in the pelvis. Although diversion may not prevent a "smoldering" of the inflammatory process, it will avoid dissection through severely inflamed tissue planes. Even if the dissection is successful, it cannot be assumed that healing will occur without incident. Furthermore, possible difficulties with the anastomosis may have been predictable, considering the condition of the transected distal segment (narrowed lumen with intramural abscesses); if indeed the resection had been performed, consideration should have been given to a Hartmann procedure.

Of note, despite execution of a diverting colostomy, a complete anastomotic disruption developed, followed by multiple additional complications.

Case 2

PREOPERATIVE PHASE

An 81-year-old woman was known to have diverticular disease for at least 1 year, on the basis of contrast enemas performed for increasing constipation. Her presenting complaints just before admission to the hospital were fever, dysuria, a "whistling noise" on urination, and increasing constipation. Gastrografin enema revealed an abrupt narrowing of the sigmoid just above the rectosigmoid junction, with scant flow of contrast into the narrowed sigmoid with known diverticular disease. Contrast was also seen to enter the bladder. Cystoscopy showed a fistulous opening in the bladder wall just above the trigone. A CT scan was not performed. The patient was scheduled for sigmoid resection with possible transverse colostomy.

OPERATION

In this case, the left ureter was catheterized without incident. The vesical fistula was visualized during the cystoscopy. The abdomen was entered through a left paramedian incision. Exploration revealed an extensive phlegmonous inflammatory process involving the entire length of the sigmoid colon, extending deeply into the pelvis. Intimately involved in the phlegmon were the abdominal wall, uterus, left tube, and pelvic floor. With difficulty, the left ureteral catheter could be palpated deep to the inflammatory mass.

After a brief, futile attempt to delineate planes of dissection, the surgeon determined that the pelvic dissection and sigmoid resection was neither safe nor feasible. A right transverse colostomy was performed, and another attempt at resection was planned in 6 months.

POSTOPERATIVE COURSE

Although the second stage (sigmoid resection) was planned 6 months after the colostomy, the patient deferred operation for 18 months. Urinary infections ceased, and the patient's general condition was better than it had been for the first operation. At the second-stage operation, the phlegmonous inflammation had subsided sufficiently to allow mobilization of the distal sigmoid. A segment of small bowel contiguous with a fistulous tract in the diseased sigmoid was resected. The actual fistula into the bladder could no longer be demonstrated, but the area of adherence to the bladder was oversewn. A hand-sewn anastomosis was performed between the left transverse colon and the proximal rectum. The colostomy was left undisturbed. Recovery from this stage was uneventful.

Eight weeks after the second stage, closure of the colostomy was performed without incident. Now 83 years of age, the patient was able to resume her usual activities.

CASE COMMENTS

The surgeon took a much less aggressive approach in this classic example of malignant diverticulitis, and a potentially disastrous clinical course was avoided in this octogenarian.

The decision to perform diversion was made because the resection was "neither safe nor feasible." The degree of inflammation subsided significantly after fecal diversion and resulted in sharper dissection planes at the second operation. This can be contrasted with the possible ineffective role of fecal diversion in protecting against anastomotic disruption (case 1) or against the complications of sepsis in patients with perforated diverticulitis and pelvic sepsis.

CLINICAL FEATURES

Malignant diverticulitis characteristically occurs between the fifth and eighth decades of life. The estimated incidence is less than 5% of patients operated on for diverticular disease. It is not to be confused with the acute virulent diverticulitis that has been described in younger individuals (4).

The chronic symptoms consist of recurrent left lower quadrant pain over months or years, increasing constipation, and evidence of fistulization, as evidenced, for example, by pneumaturia. The acute complications that mandate elective, semiurgent, or emergency operation are colonic obstruction, perforation with abscess formation, complex fistulization, or pelvic sepsis.

IMAGING FINDINGS

Imaging studies that should suggest the possibility of malignant diverticulitis are the contrast enema and the CT scan. In the contrast enema, preferably performed with gastrografin, the suggestive findings are (1) a long segment of diverticular disease in the distal sigmoid, with characteristic spiculization and deformity of the normal colonic architecture (Fig. 13.1); (2) intramural sinus tract formation (Fig. 13.2); (3) perforation and abscess formation, particularly when juxtaposed to the proximal rectal segment in the cul-de-sac (Fig. 13.3); (4) sigmoidoenteric fistulas; and (5) marked narrowing of the distal sigmoid, obstructing retrograde flow of contrast (Fig. 13.4). The contracted distal sigmoid may show an abrupt transition to the rectosigmoid, raising the possibility of a constricting neoplastic lesion.

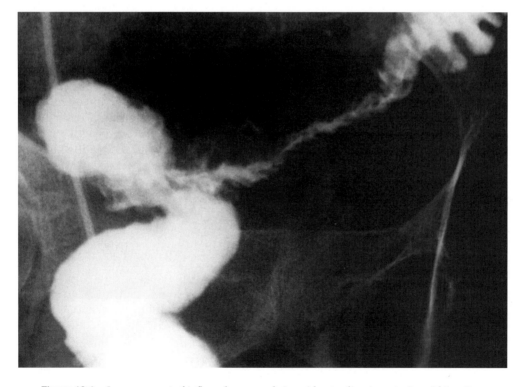

Figure 13.1.   Long segment of inflamed narrowed sigmoid extending to rectosigmoid junction.

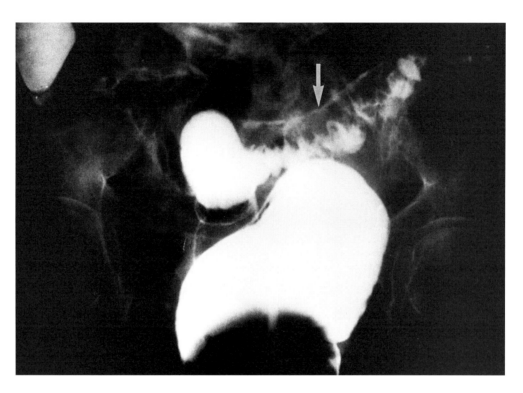

Figure 13.2.   Intramural sinus tract (arrow) in sigmoid diverticulitis.

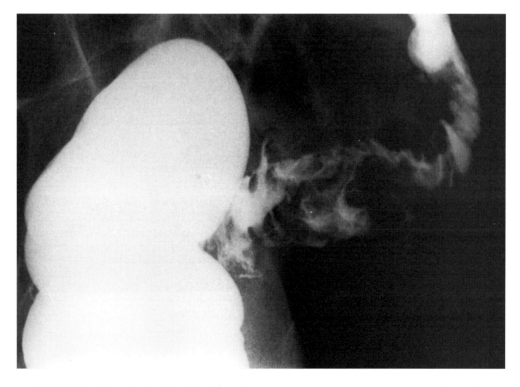

Figure 13.3.   Sigmoid diverticulitis with perforation; process impinging on rectosigmoid junction.

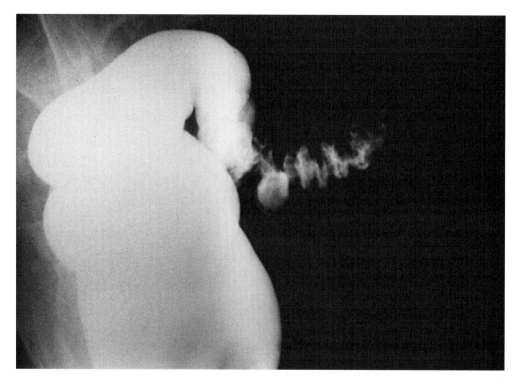

Figure 13.4. Obstruction of retrograde flow of barium in case of malignant diverticulitis (case 2).

CT scans of complicated diverticular disease delineate the extent of the disease process more accurately than the contrast enema (5,6). In malignant diverticulitis, *the pathognomonic finding is evidence of phlegmonous inflammation of the parasigmoidal and pararectal tissues with involvement of all pelvic structures in the inflammatory process* (Fig. 13.5). The CT scan also shows the status of the kidneys, ureters, and bladder.

PREOPERATIVE PREPARATION

Because patients with malignant diverticulitis who present for operation all have an acute inflammatory component to their diverticular disease, coverage with broad-spectrum antibiotics should precede operative intervention. Bowel preparation in nonemergent situations should include a liquid diet for at least 2 days before surgery, bowel cleansing with hyperosmolar oral fluids, and standard antibiotic bowel preparation. Informed consent should be worded to include the possibility of colostomy, whether the latter is performed as a part of a Hartmann procedure or as a diverting colostomy. Provision should be made for the catheterization of both ureters. In the event that ureteral catheterization is impossible or difficult, indigo carmine should be available for intravenous administration during the operative procedure.

OPERATIVE FINDINGS

Initial exploration of the sigmoid colon area reveals a more extensive inflammation than is usually anticipated. The phlegmonous inflammation not only involves the distal colonic segment but also adjacent pelvic structures, extending below the peritoneal reflection. Dense adhesions to adjacent small bowel, bladder, and even contiguous large bowel (sigmoid or transverse colon) may be sites of fistulous communication whether shown by prior imaging studies or not. Normal anatomic planes, usually easily delineated by blunt dissection, are obliterated, requiring sharp dissection to identify individual structures and organs.

CHOICE OF PROCEDURE

If the disease process falls into the category of malignant diverticulitis, there are two acceptable options. In the more severe cases, as in case 2 above, persistence in the dissection of the phlegmonous mass is unsafe and should be abandoned. *A diverting transverse colostomy is an expedient temporizing measure, allowing safer dissection and resection at a later date.* Depending on the response to diversion, resection may be attempted again in 6–12 months. Diversion does not eliminate the inflammatory process; the latter "smolders" but usually does not progress. Pericolonic abscesses usually may be drained under CT guidance, another measure that aids in choosing a more favorable time for resection.

A second choice, when safe dissection is possible, is the Hartmann procedure, if a normal distal segment below the disease can be identified (7). It is not safe to transect rectosigmoid or rectum through frank disease, a maneuver that invites postoperative pelvic sepsis. If a Hartmann procedure is performed, the inflammation usually subsides sufficiently to allow reanastomosis in 3 months. Earlier restoration is an invitation to possible anastomotic disruption.

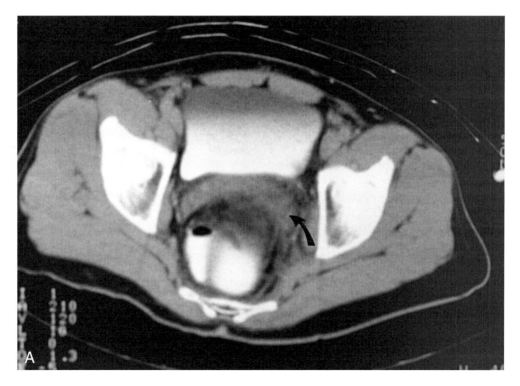

Figure 13.5. CT scans depicting three grades of severe diverticulitis in juxtaposition to rectosigmoid. **A.,** Pericolonic and pararectal inflammatory mass (arrow).

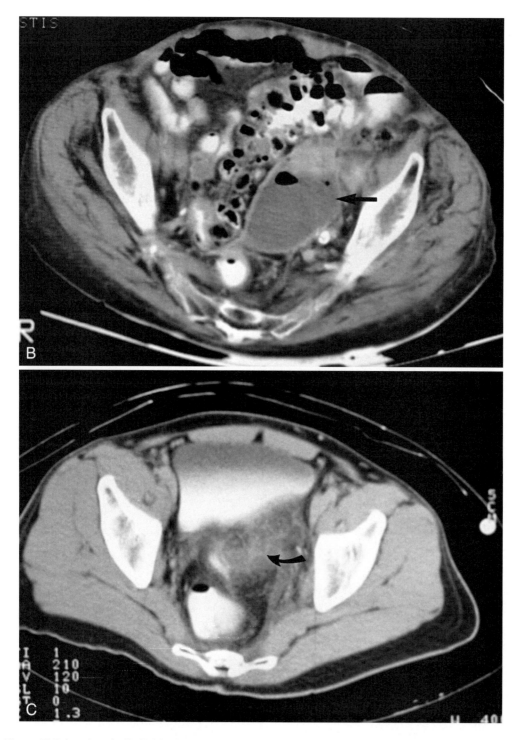

Figure 13.5. (*continued*)   **B.,** Pelvic abscess secondary to ruptured diverticulitis with surrounding zone of pelvic inflammation (arrow). **C.,** Pelvic phlegmon (arrow) adjacent to diverticulitis involving rectosigmoid.

Resection and primary anastomosis are not options for this condition, whether "protected" by a proximal colostomy or not. In the presence of the severe pericolonic inflammation, fecal diversion does not guarantee proper anastomotic healing.

PATHOLOGY

The pathologic findings in resected specimens of malignant diverticulitis reflect the severity of the disease. Grossly, there is marked thickening and edema of the colonic wall, extending into the adjacent mesocolon (Fig. 13.6), with a high incidence of perforation, abscesses, sinuses, and fistulas. Intramural tracking (sinuses) within the colonic wall is common (Fig. 13.7). Microscopically, acute and chronic inflammatory cells permeate all layers of the wall from the lamina propria to the serosa, including the adjacent mesocolon. Fibrosis, crypt abscesses, intramural microabscesses, and noncaseating granulomas with foreign body giant cells are common (Fig. 13.8). Occasionally, there is a striking histiocytic response.

Although several of the features (intramural sinus tracts, fistulas, and granulomas) bear some resemblance to the gross and microscopic findings in Crohn's disease, *there is no mucosal involvement in the nondiverticular mucosa of malignant diverticulitis*. The two diseases are not related.

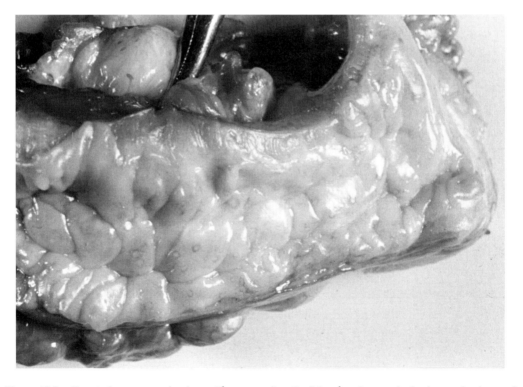

Figure 13.6. Resected segment of colon with severe diverticulitis, showing marked edema of colon and surrounding tissue. Note transection through edematous tissue.

Unrecognized acute and chronic inflammation or microabscesses at the resected margins (Fig. 13.9) may explain the high incidence of anastomotic failure with this condition. Inflamed colon is especially rich in collagenase (8), thus playing some role in failure of anastomotic healing (9).

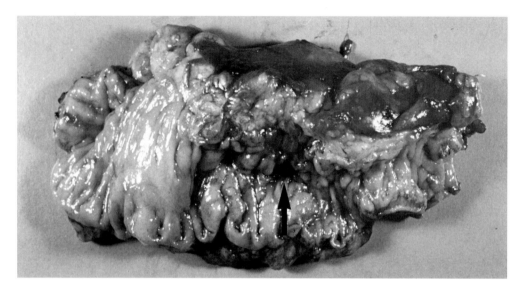

Figure 13.7.   Resected segment of colon with severe diverticulitis showing edema, distortion of normal architecture, and two central fistulous tract openings (arrow).

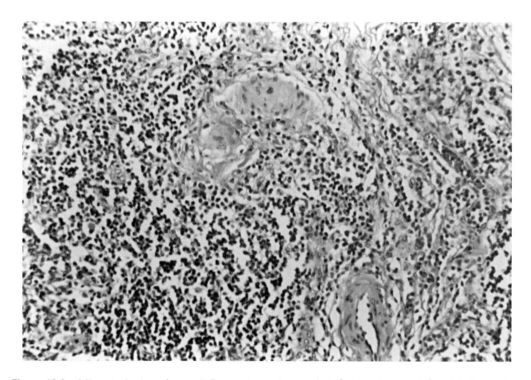

Figure 13.8.   Microscopic view of severe inflammation in diverticulitis showing acute and chronic inflammatory cells and noncaseating granuloma with giant cells.

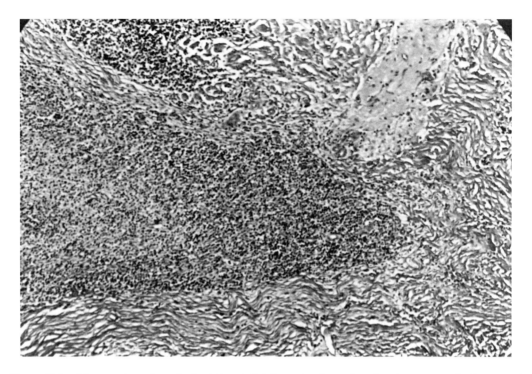

Figure 13.9. Microscopic section of colon taken at distal margin of resection, showing unrecognized acute and chronic inflammation.

CONCLUSIONS

Malignant diverticulitis is at the severest extreme of the diverticular disease spectrum. Although the incidence of this severe form of disease has decreased, it still occurs, demanding vigilance and good judgment on the part of the surgeon. *Errors in judgment can lead to catastrophic complications and, at worst, death.*

The following principles of management are offered as a guide to management:

1. Suspect malignant diverticulitis in elderly patients with chronic recurrent diverticular disease who present with obstruction and fistulization. Confirm by imaging findings, especially CT scan, seeking evidence of phlegmonous pelvic inflammation.
2. Plan for a staged resection if phlegmonous pelvic inflammation is present at operation.
3. Always catheterize both ureters. If the left ureter cannot be catheterized, use intravenous indigo carmine to aid in ureteral identification.
4. In the presence of severe phlegmonous inflammation of all pelvic structures, precluding safe dissection, limit the operation to transverse colostomy.
5. If safe dissection permits, limit the operation to a Hartmann procedure.
6. If a colostomy alone is performed, allow a 6- to 12-month waiting period before definitive resection is performed. Do not close the colostomy at the same time the anastomosis (second stage) is performed.
7. If a Hartmann procedure is performed, allow at least a 3-month waiting period before reanastomosis.

8. Do not perform a primary resection and anastomosis in this condition, with or without a complimentary colostomy.

Observance of these principles allows the safest course and most favorable outcome for patients with this most difficult variant in the spectrum of diverticular disease. Disregarding these principles for reasons other than patient safety and ultimate cure can be disastrous.

EDITORIAL COMMENTS

The present monograph expands on the wide spectrum of complications and disease severity that characterizes sigmoid diverticulitis. In this chapter, the author discusses the term "malignant" diverticulitis, coined in an earlier publication (1), as an extreme of this disease spectrum, characterized by extensive inflammation extending below the peritoneal reflection; the tendency toward obstruction, perforation, and fistula formation; and a relentless course. This process could just as well be termed "severe," "fulminating," or "phlegmonous" diverticulitis. The cause is unknown and perhaps could involve some infectious agent, just as the enigmatic "abdominal cocoon syndrome" that has been associated with encasing fibrosis and small bowel obstruction in different settings (10–12).

The resemblance to granulomatous colitis is striking, and indeed critics of the original publication point out that Crohn's disease may not have been entirely ruled out (13). These patients, for example, did not have endoscopy and biopsy before operation. On the other hand, Morgenstern points out that no mucosal involvement was seen in the final pathologic specimens to suggest inflammatory bowel disease (1,14).

We have seen patients with similar operative findings, but not often. Clearly, the interpretation of the findings might vary by individual surgeons: what may seem malignant to one surgeon may seem more routine in the opinion of another (perhaps more experienced) surgeon. Much more frequently, sigmoid diverticulitis tends to be relatively localized, and if fistulas are present, the process tends to be chronic rather than acute and phlegmonous. The findings described in this chapter are in stark contrast to those of free perforation, when tissue planes tend to be well defined, unless the patient has survived a sufficient period of time for extensive peritonitis to develop.

Is this process predictable? Perhaps the alert surgeon who notes inflammation extending into the pelvis on a CT scan will think of it. In other instances, the phlegmon will be extraordinary and unexpected, encountered either in the emergency or semielective setting, and the surgeon may run into operative difficulties or the "point of no return." If fistulas and/or an extensive phlegmon are suspected preoperatively, we favor the selective use of endoscopy, although this could prove very difficult considering the patient's clinical state and the narrowed, inflamed colon. In this way, the possibility of Crohn's colitis could be better investigated, perhaps obtaining histologic evidence, and further medical therapy could be initiated.

Above all, operative treatment of these patients requires judgment and a careful technical approach such as that recommended by Abcarian (15). The risks of both primary resection and anastomosis should be weighed carefully against lesser procedures such as fecal diversion alone. The significant risks of complications must be raised with the patient and family.

As a technical note, we have found that loop ileostomy is preferable to transverse colostomy as a mode of diversion. Although this may not be ideal for the elderly patients as described in the illustrative cases above, it has the benefit in younger patients of ease of closure and of lack of restriction of the mobility of the transverse colon for later anastomosis.

REFERENCES

1. Morgenstern L. "Malignant" diverticulitis: a clinical entity. Arch Surg 1979;114:1112–1116. *Discusses 17 patients meeting this definition; they represented 7% of patients operated on for diverticular disease during the same 14-year period.*

2. Rodkey GV, Welch CE. Changing patterns in the surgical treatment of diverticular disease. Ann Surg 1984;200:466–478. *A detailed review of the clinical course of 350 patients treated over a decade. The operative mortality was 6.3%, and 8.4% with sepsis died.*

3. Roberts PL, Veidenheimer MC. Current management of diverticulitis. Adv Surg 1994;27:189–208. *A concise review of the differential diagnosis and surgical treatment of diverticulitis, with 59 references.*

4. Schauer PR, Ramos R, Ghiatas AA, et al. Virulent diverticular disease in young obese men. Am J Surg 1992;164:443–448. *Sixty-one of 238 patients in this series were less than 40 years of age; young patients tended to be obese and the rate of perforation and fistula formation was higher than in older patients.*

5. Labs JD, Sarr MG, Fishman EK, et al. Complications of acute diverticulitis of the colon: improved early diagnosis with computerized tomography. Am J Surg 1988;155:331–335. *CT scans were sensitive in detecting intra-abdominal abscesses and colovesical fistulas.*

6. Hachigian MP, Honickman S, Eisenstat TE, et al. Computed tomography in the initial management of acute left-sided diverticulitis. Dis Colon Rectum 1992;35:1123–1129. *Fifty-four patients had early CT scans that allowed stratification of patients by disease, severity, and surgical planning based on extracolonic involvement and variations in anatomy.*

7. Rothenberger DA, Wiltz O. Surgery for complicated diverticulitis. Surg Clin North Am 1993;73:975–992. *This review recommends converting patients, if at all possible, from an emergency to an urgent or elective operative status with possible primary anastomosis.*

8. Yamakawa T, Patin CS, Sobel S, et al. Healing of colonic anastomoses following resection for experimental "diverticulitis." Arch Surg 1971;103:17–20. *Injection of a fecal suspension into the colonic wall in experimental animals was performed to simulate diverticulitis. After resection, collagen synthesis took 100% more time in the "diverticulitis" group.*

9. Morgenstern L, Yamakawa T, Ben-Shoshan, et al. Anastomotic leakage after low colonic anastomosis: clinical and experimental aspects. Am J Surg 1972;123:104–109. *The anastomotic leak rate was 20% after segmental colectomy, with a 3% operative mortality.*

10. Foo KT, Ng KC, Rauff A, et al. Unusual small intestinal obstruction in adolescent girls: the abdominal cocoon. Br J Surg 1978;65:427–430. *A review of ten cases of small bowel obstruction in adolescent girls involving a membrane encasing the small intestine like a cocoon. The authors postulated that a subclinical viral peritonitis secondary to retrograde menstruation was responsible.*

11. Cambria RP, Shamberger RC. Small bowel obstruction caused by the abdominal cocoon syndrome: possible association with the Leveen shunt. Surgery 1984;95:501–503. *A cirrhotic with a Leveen shunt developed intestinal obstruction in a fibrotic sac that encased the small bowel.*

12. Eltringham WK, Espiner HJ, Windsor CW, et al. Sclerosing peritonitis due to practolol: a report on 9 cases and their surgical management. Br J Surg 1977;64:229–235. *Reports on nine patients treated with the beta-adrenergic blocking agent practolol who developed a dense proliferation of the visceral peritoneum, causing formation of a dense white cocoon and small bowel obstruction.*

13. Editorial: Is malignant diverticulitis a true bill? Stephen Lock, ed. Br Med J 1980;1:1156. *Reviewing reference 1, the authors suggest that the diagnosis of Crohn's colitis has not been entirely ruled out. They suggest rectal biopsy as part of the initial evaluation and postulate that gram-negative anaerobes may have been responsible for the extensive inflammatory process.*

14. Morson BC. Pathology of diverticular disease of the colon. Clin Gastroenterol 1975;4:37–52. *The renowned pathologist in his detailed description of diverticular disease points out that the mucous membrane is normal apart from redundant mucosal folds. Granulomas can be part of a foreign body giant cell reaction to fecal material in the pericolic abscesses complicating diverticulitis as opposed to the granulomas of Crohn's disease.*

15. Abcarian H. The difficult resection in diverticulitis. Semin Colon Rectal Surg 1990;1:978–998. *If a sigmoid phlegmon is encountered, the author recommends use of a left ureteral catheter and a proximal-to-distal resection technique to avoid injury to the left ureter.*

14 Diverticular Stricture

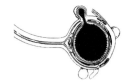

Andrew Feldman, MD
John P. Welch, MD

> ### KEY POINTS
>
> - Diverticular disease causes 10% of large bowel obstructions
> - Colonic obstruction may complicate acute or recurrent diverticulitis
> - Stricture formation usually follows recurrent attacks
> - Barium enema may fail to reveal cause of stricture
> - If cannot traverse stricture with flexible scope, consider operation because of cancer risk

ILLUSTRATIVE CASE

Case 1

A 58-year-old man presented with a 12-hour history of crampy left lower quadrant abdominal pain and mild nausea. He had experienced episodes of similar symptoms intermittently during the past several years, sometimes accompanied by fever. He also related a history of progressive, chronic constipation during the preceding 6 months. His medical history was otherwise unremarkable.

The patient was afebrile, and abdominal and rectal examinations were unremarkable. There was no leukocytosis, and plain radiographs of the abdomen were normal. Barium enema revealed a long, narrowed segment of sigmoid colon with spasm, as well as scattered diverticula. Carcinoma could not be ruled out. Attempted colonoscopy revealed diverticulosis with a stricture of the sigmoid colon, which could not be negotiated (Fig. 14.1). No mucosal abnormalities were evident. Random cytologic brushings were taken and were negative for malignancy.

Because of the chronic nature of the patient's symptoms and the inability to fully evaluate the stricture colonoscopically, sigmoid resection was undertaken in one stage, with a hand-sewn end-to-end anastomosis. Pathology revealed diverticulosis with fibrotic stricture, without evidence of cancer. The patient did well postoperatively and had no additional gastrointestinal symptoms.

CASE COMMENTS

This is not an uncommon scenario. Although diverticular disease is suspected to be the cause of the long stricture, the specter of carcinoma looms in the picture (Chapter 4). Thus, colon resection is indicated, not only to relieve the symptoms but also to treat the carcinoma that may be present.

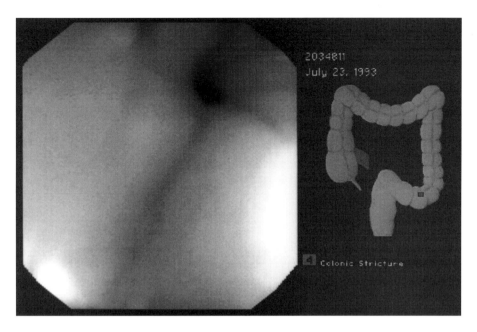

Figure 14.1. Colonoscopic view of a tight sigmoid stricture that could not be traversed despite the use of intravenous glucagon. Such patients have symptoms of partial large bowel obstruction and resection usually is necessary if cancer is to be ruled out reliably.

Case 2

A 74-year-old male with known diverticulosis presented with progressive constipation over 1 week, mild left lower quadrant pain, and abdominal distention. He denied vomiting, rectal bleeding, or weight loss. He had not undergone any previous abdominal operations. Plain films showed enlargement of the cecum to 8 cm in diameter; the descending colon was slightly dilated as well. The white blood cell count was 8000. A computed tomography (CT) scan suggested acute diverticulitis with phlegmon but no evidence of intra-abdominal abscess.

Treatment was started with intravenous antibiotics; a nasogastric tube was inserted, and the patient was to have nothing orally. Over 2 days, he began to pass flatus and his abdominal distention decreased. The nasogastric tube was removed. The white blood cell count decreased to 6000, and clear liquids were started. The patient became afebrile and was sent home on Flagyl® and Cipro®.

CASE COMMENTS

This picture is consistent with acute diverticulitis rather than chronic diverticulitis with stricture formation. The partial colonic obstruction was probably related to edema of the bowel wall; this was diminished after treatment for several days with intravenous antibiotics and bowel rest. Presumably, the edema of the bowel wall decreased rapidly and the patient did not require an emergent abdominal operation.

INTRODUCTION

Colonic stricture is seen most commonly in the sigmoid colon and may be due to diverticular disease, ischemia, inflammatory bowel disease, carcinoma, anastomotic stricture, or external compression. *Stricture due to diverticular disease occurs as a result of circumferential colonic and pericolic fibrosis, which follows recurrent attacks of diverticulitis, whether symptomatic or subclinical.* This frequently presents as partial colonic obstruction with chronic constipation, although high-grade obstruction sometimes ensues. Even complete obstruction may be seen, particularly with impaction of feces or a foreign body or with the inflammation of superimposed acute diverticulitis. Impaction of feces proximal to the point of narrowing may lead to stercoral perforation.

Diverticular disease is responsible for approximately 10% of cases of large bowel obstruction (other major causes are colonic carcinoma and volvulus). The major mechanisms are circumferential pericolic fibrosis and marked angulation of the pelvic colon when adherent to the pelvic sidewall (1). In a recent series of patients undergoing surgery for diverticular disease, 11% of operations were performed because of bowel obstruction (2). The median incidence of intestinal obstruction in the surgical literature between 1960 and 1984 was 12% (3). Many cases of obstruction seen with diverticular disease are a result of colonic strictures formed during the course of recurrent attacks of acute diverticulitis (see case 1). However, acute, high-grade colonic obstruction is an atypical clinical presentation in these patients.

The actual incidence of diverticular stricture is difficult to ascertain from the literature. Farmakis et al reported on 5-year follow-up of 120 patients who initially presented with complicated diverticulitis. Of these, eight patients returned with bowel obstruction, but it is unclear how many were ultimately found to have colonic strictures (4). In a retrospective study of 200 cases of diverticular disease in New Zealand (5), stricture was the most frequent reason for elective presentation (11 of 36 patients) and was the indication for 27% of 21 elective resections.

The critical elements in the management of patients with suspected diverticular stricture are the control of obstructive symptoms and the need to rule out carcinoma.

DIAGNOSIS

Typical gastrointestinal symptoms of diverticular stricture include constipation and narrowing of the stools, with or without other signs of intestinal obstruction such as nausea, vomiting, abdominal pain, and distention. *The diverticular origin of the obstruction may be suggested by known diverticulosis and particularly by a history of prior episodes consistent with diverticulitis.* Differentiation from carcinoma of the colon is particularly difficult, because presenting symptoms are similar, both diseases are common and occur in similar age groups, and almost 30% of colon cancers occur in the presence of colonic diverticula (Chapter 4).

Barium enema is an appropriate initial study to confirm the presence of an obstructing lesion of the sigmoid or left colon (Fig. 14.2). Historically, however, barium enema has been notoriously inaccurate at differentiating diverticular obstruction from that due to carcinoma. King et al reported on 11 patients who had barium enema before laparotomy for sigmoid stricture. In only two of these patients was barium enema accurate in distinguishing diverticular stricture from cancer (6). Forde and Treat reported 181 inconclusive studies in 184 consecutive patients undergoing barium enema for colonic stricture (7).

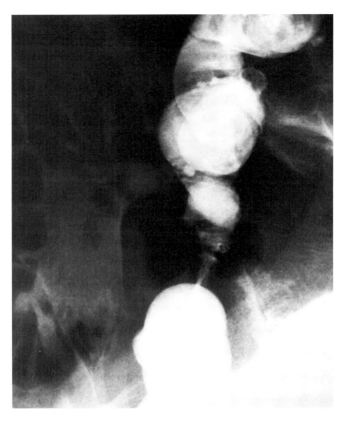

Figure 14.2. Barium enema view of a patient with a stricture caused by recurrent attacks of sigmoid diverticulitis. Attempts should be made to negotiate this with a narrow flexible scope. It also may be possible to define the stricture more accurately with contrast studies if the patient does not have clinical or radiographic evidence of antegrade colonic obstruction.

If barium enema findings are equivocal, colonoscopy may help distinguish diverticular stricture from cancer. Typical findings include the presence of diffuse spasm, the presence of diverticula, and no mucosal irregularities or ulceration. It has been suggested, however, that carcinoma of the colon can occur even in the presence of an intact mucosa.

Max and Knutson reported an 88% accuracy rate for distinguishing diverticular stricture from cancer in a series of 26 patients undergoing colonoscopy. The lesion could be traversed and visualized completely in 19 patients, and laparotomy was avoided in 16 patients. No false-negative studies were reported (8). Although diagnostic accuracy is up to 100% for patients in whom complete visualization of the colonic mucosa is reported, a long-term follow-up for patients avoiding laparotomy has not been fully reported.

Several authors have suggested that *the inability to negotiate a presumed stricture is an indication for resection,* because without direct visualization of the entire mucosa, exclusion of carcinoma is impossible (6). Along with the narrowing, poor bowel preparation, fixation, and sharp angulation interfere with traversal of the stricture (9,10). *Colonoscopy must be performed carefully and overinsufflation of air must be avoided; rigidity of the bowel and bowel fixation increase the risk of colonic perforation,* and at times, it is difficult to differentiate the lumen from diverticula when diverticulosis is pronounced (Fig. 14.3). When spasm significantly contributes to the inability to transverse a stricture, glucagon or Pro-Banthine®

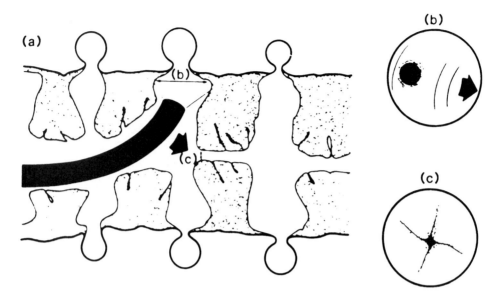

Figure 14.3.   There is some additional risk when inserting a colonoscope into a patient with a diverticular stricture **(A)**. Care must be taken to avoid pushing the scope deeply into a diverticulum **(B)**, which may turn out to have a wider lumen than the stricture. The stricture usually can be recognized by folds radiating into it **(C)**. (Reprinted with permission from Williams CB. Diverticular disease and strictures. In: Hunt RH, Waye JD, eds. Colonoscopy. Techniques, clinical practice and color atlas. London: Chapman and Hall, 1981:363–368) [Ref. 12].

have been used, with mixed results. Additionally, the use of a pediatric colonoscope has been helpful in negotiating these lesions (6).

King et al reported on 19 sigmoid strictures that could not be negotiated in a series of 1,039 consecutive colonoscopies. Of 15 patients who underwent laparotomy, six patients (32%) were found to have carcinoma (6). Forde and Treat reported a success rate in negotiating colonic strictures of 54% in a series of 181 colonoscopies for stricture (7).

Even when the mucosa is intact and all findings point to diverticular stricture, performing random biopsies to evaluate for the presence of cancer or severe dysplasia has been suggested (6). The utility of cytologic brushings as an additional diagnostic modality also has been emphasized (7). In 24 non-negotiable colonic strictures in which carcinoma was diagnosed, three cancers were diagnosed by positive cytology in the presence of negative biopsies. Notably, there also was one false-positive cytology. One advantage of cytology is the ability to obtain brushing from a region proximal to that which can be reached with colonoscopy.

TREATMENT

Operative treatment of diverticular stricture usually can be approached in an elective fashion. Symptoms typically have been present for more than 30 days, and in most cases, mechanical and antibiotic preparation are possible. For this reason, a one-stage resection can be performed in most cases, with a mortality of less than 3%. Mortality rises to 10–15% after emergent operation for diverticular obstruction, and mortality is higher than 50% in the presence of fecal peritonitis.

Giaccari et al reported success with medical therapy for postdiverticulitic stenoses in 79 patients with chronic low-grade obstructive symptoms (11). Patients were treated with alternating antibiotic treatment (oral rifaximin) and recolonization with lactobacilli; improvement in symptoms was reported in all cases without complications. The authors suggest that this success is due to the prevention of superimposed episodes of diverticular inflammation.

CONCLUSIONS

Colonic strictures account for most cases of large bowel obstruction complicating diverticular disease. It may be difficult to rule out carcinoma with diagnostic studies, and operation is necessary to make the final diagnosis. Usually, the bowel can be prepared before surgery, and resection and anastomosis are possible in one stage under elective conditions.

If the bowel cannot be prepared, on-table lavage can be used, or in the case of fecal loading and distended bowel, a Hartmann procedure is useful. There is little need for three-stage operations today in the management of these patients, with the exception of high-grade obstruction and marked bowel distention in high-risk patients.

EDITORIAL COMMENTS

Stricture formation is the usual mechanism of large bowel obstruction in diverticular disease. It represents a late pathologic stage of the disease, when fibrosis occurs based on previous episodes of inflammation (14) (Fig. 14.4). The major difficulty in these patients is ruling out carcinoma in the instances in which the stricture cannot be traversed with a flexible endoscope. This problem was evident to abdominal surgeons a number of years ago and continues to this day, despite modern

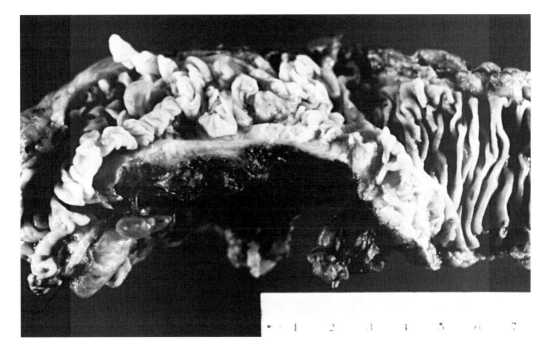

Figure 14.4.   Thickened sigmoid colon following resection. The appearance is typical of chronic diverticular disease, with thickening of the colonic wall and an intact mucosa. (Reprinted with permission from Welch JP. Diverticular disease. In: Welch JP, ed. Bowel obstruction. Differential diagnosis and clinical management. Philadelphia: WB Saunders, 1990:589–599.)

imaging methods such as spiral CT. At times, resection is the only way to rule out malignant disease. For a significant number of patients, surgery is required regardless by the time a stricture has become this narrow. We have no experience with the techniques mentioned in the report of Giaccari et al (11), although the concept is of interest for patients who have a rudimentary stricture.

Another common finding is a combination of ileus and inflammation that may give a clinical picture of large bowel obstruction (15). The bowel lumen is narrowed by a combination of edema and muscle spasm in an already shortened, irritable bowel with muscular hypertrophy. Usually, these types of symptoms abate with bowel rest and administration of antibiotics and surgery is not needed for relief of obstruction per se.

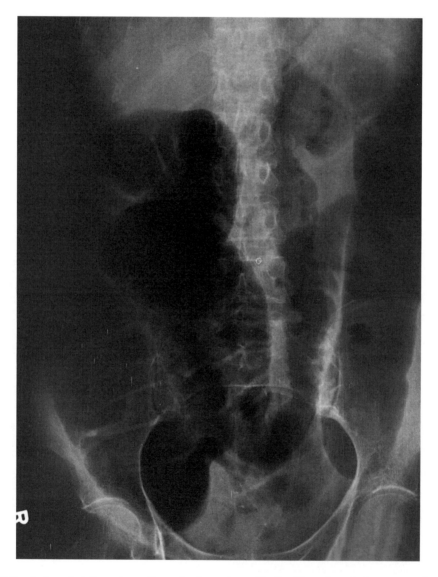

Figure 14.5.   A characteristic supine radiograph of a patient with distal large bowel obstruction. This finding is seen predominantly with colon carcinoma rather than with acute diverticulitis or diverticular stricture. (Reprinted with permission from Welch JP. Diverticular disease. In: Welch JP, ed. Bowel obstruction. Differential diagnosis and clinical management. Philadelphia: WB Saunders, 1990:589–599.)

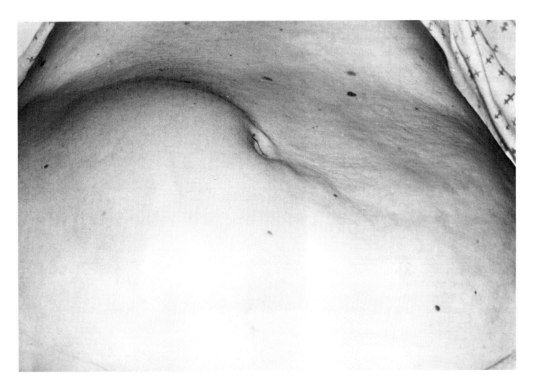

Figure 14.6. This patient had advanced dilatation of the cecum and a competent ileocecal valve. The bulge of the cecum is seen when visualizing the abdominal wall. (Reprinted with permission from Welch JP. Diverticular disease. In: Welch JP, ed. Bowel obstruction. Differential diagnosis and clinical management. Philadelphia: WB Saunders, 1990:589–599.)

Much less common is the appearance of high-grade obstruction, which must be treated like a high-grade obstruction caused by carcinoma. In one series of 205 patients with diverticulitis, only 3% had acute colonic obstruction (16) (Fig. 14.5). In these patients, abdominal distention is marked (Fig. 14.6), and there may be massive cecal dilatation (Fig. 14.7). These patients may be at risk of cecal perforation (17) (Figs. 14.8 and 14.9), and urgent surgery is indicated. If the patient is clinically stable and the cecum has not perforated, torn, or become ischemic, we might attempt on-table lavage/anastomosis/possible diverting ileostomy or the Hartmann procedure (Fig. 14.10). In advanced cases, the Hartmann operation is preferred; for the high-risk individual, decompression alone may be advised in the emergency setting (17).

During the last several decades, the surgical approach to diverticular obstruction has changed, even with high-grade obstruction: primary resections with or without anastomosis (18) are replacing three-stage operations (19,20,21). The technique of on-table lavage is facilitating this approach.

Of note, retrograde obstruction to contrast media can occur when the patient has no clinical signs of antegrade obstruction. In one study, 50% of patients with retrograde obstruction had no clinical evidence of obstruction (22). Later antegrade studies can be performed at times (23).

Interest in the use of self-expanding metallic stents has increased recently for treatment of patients with obstructing carcinoma of the rectum (24,25). It is conceivable that these stents could play some role in the management of a short diverticular stricture due to diverticulitis in a high-risk patient.

We would summarize the problem of colonic stricture with the statement that the surgeon should have a low threshold to operate (in all but high-risk patients) if the diagnosis is in any way unclear. The technique of on-table lavage facilitates this approach if there are clinical signs of significant large bowel obstruction.

15 Diverticular Abscess

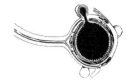

Steven H. Brown, MD
Paul V. Vignati, MD
Glenn W. Stambo, MD
Michael J. Hallisey, MD

KEY POINTS

- Most common complication of acute diverticulitis
- Can lead to significant morbidity and mortality from sepsis
- CT best diagnostic test if abscess is suspected
- Always resect involved colonic segment, unless the patient is unstable or the resection cannot be performed safely
- The ultimate goal, resection of involved colon with primary anastomosis, can be achieved in a high percentage, facilitated by percutaneous drainage or intraoperative lavage
- Decision to reanastomose colon must be addressed individually

ILLUSTRATIVE CASES

Case 1

A 47-year-old white female presented to the emergency room with a 3-day history of increasing bilateral lower quadrant abdominal pain. The pain was dull and nonradiating. She had noticed progressive constipation. She denied any hematochezia, melena, nausea, or vomiting. She had experienced chills on the evening before admission.

The patient's medical history was significant only for diverticulosis, with four episodes of pain in the previous year. She had not undergone prior abdominal surgery.

On examination, she was obese and clearly uncomfortable lying on the stretcher. Her blood pressure was 110/68, pulse was 130, temperature was 103°F. Examination revealed a soft, nondistended abdomen that was tender in both lower quadrants with concomitant suprapubic tenderness. There was involuntary guarding and no palpable mass. The rectal examination was normal and the stool heme-occult was negative. The white blood cell count was 17,200.

She was admitted and placed on intravenous metronidazole and ceftizoxime (a third-generation cephalosporin). After 48 hours of therapy, the patient continued to have temperatures as high as 102.4°F and a persistent leukocytosis of 18,400. A computed tomography (CT) scan of the abdomen and pelvis was obtained. This study revealed a large (7 cm) collection of fluid and air present in the pelvis. The patient's abscess was drained percutaneously without untoward sequelae. The catheter was removed on hospital day 5 because it had stopped draining; follow-up studies revealed complete resolution of the abscess. She was discharged on hospital day 9 on oral antibiotics.

Two weeks after drainage, she underwent a sigmoid resection with primary anastomosis. The perioperative course was uneventful, and she was discharged home on the fifth postoperative day.

CASE COMMENTS

This patient was suspected to have acute diverticulitis, based on the history of diverticulosis and recurrent episodes of abdominal pain. Appendicitis or small bowel obstruction were unlikely, considering the lack of vomiting or crampy midabdominal pain/distention, along with the x-ray findings.

It would have been preferable to perform the CT scan on the day of admission, considering the fever; the examination would have facilitated percutaneous drainage.

The patient was able to undergo a definitive elective resection early because of successful drainage that was documented by a repeat CT scan.

Case 2

A 52-year-old white female with an extensive medical history, most significant for steroid dependent interstitial lung disease, presented with a 72-hour history of chills, fever, anorexia, nausea, and lower abdominal pain. She had been discharged from the hospital 1 week previously on oral antibiotics (trimethoprim-sulfamethoxazole and metronidazole) after intravenous antibiotic therapy for barium enema-proven diverticulitis. On her prior admission, she had undergone abdominal ultrasound, which revealed no masses.

On physical examination, she was a cushingoid, obese female who appeared older than her stated age. She appeared in no apparent distress. Her vital signs included a temperature of 99.8°F, pulse of 80, respiratory rate of 20, and blood pressure of 132/90. On auscultation of her lung fields, diffuse rales with no audible wheezing were noted. Her abdomen was soft with normal-pitched bowel sounds. There was a questionable fullness in the infraumbilical region. Rectal examination was noncontributory. Her laboratory data revealed normal electrolytes and blood sugar, leukocytosis of 16,800, and 95% polymorphonuclear leukocytes.

She underwent CT of the abdomen and pelvis; the study was consistent with complicated acute diverticulitis. There was a large pelvic abscess (11 cm), posterior to the urinary bladder with cephalad extension. This collection was surrounded by colon and small bowel loops and was believed to be inaccessible to percutaneous drainage by ultrasonic or CT guidance.

She, therefore, was taken to the operating room, where she underwent a sigmoid colectomy, drainage of the abscess, and creation of a proximal end colostomy and a closed distal segment (Hartmann procedure). She recovered remarkably well after this operation and was discharged to an extended care facility on postoperative day 18.

CASE COMMENTS

It is not surprising that a pericolic and pelvic abscess developed in this immunosuppressed patient after a bout of acute diverticulitis. Her previous episode probably had never resolved.

This patient was not a candidate for percutaneous drainage because bowel loops were situated in the potential path of an aspirating needle. One could also argue that she was a poor candidate for definitive drainage, considering her steroid dependence.

Because the undrained pelvic abscess was large, it would have been risky to perform a pri-

mary anastomosis in the same region. The Hartmann procedure was the appropriate operation under these circumstances.

OVERVIEW

Complications associated with diverticular disease include bleeding, abscess, fistula formation, free perforation, and stricture formation. These complications are more often seen in patients younger than 50 years of age (1). Complications associated with acute diverticulitis rarely include bleeding, and stricture formation occurs late as a result of healing of the inflamed colon.

Diverticular abscess is the most common complication of acute diverticulitis and is seen in 10–68% of patients with complicated diverticular disease. There is a male : female preponderance (2:1) (2–6). Abscess formation occurs when the center of the inflammatory mass, or phlegmon, becomes necrotic (3). Clinically, an abscess usually manifests as an enlarging tender mass, in a patient with spiking fevers, chills, and leukocytosis. The mass often is palpable on abdominal, rectal, or vaginal examination (4).

A diverticular abscess can be pericolic or distant. An abscess usually originates in the sigmoid mesocolon, the sigmoid colon being the most prevalent site for diverticulitis (94%), but may track elsewhere and even manifest as extra-abdominal symptoms. Diverticular abscesses have been reported in the following sites: pericolic, retroperitoneal, retrorectal (3), psoas muscle, hip, buttock, flank, leg, inguinal region, or scrotum (7,8). An abscess can lead to hypovolemia, septicemia, ileus, or obstruction.

ROLE OF CT SCAN

For most patients, diverticulitis is a clinical diagnosis that can be ascertained from the patient's history and physical examination. Treatment is then instituted with bowel rest and broad-spectrum intravenous antibiotics. The diagnosis can be made with radiographs or ultrasonography, but *CT scanning has proved to be the best initial imaging study* for patients with suspected acute diverticulitis (4).

However, that does not suggest that all patients with suspected diverticulitis need a CT scan. In most patients, the CT scan will only serve to confirm the diagnosis. Most patients with uncomplicated diverticulitis will respond to treatment with intravenous antibiotics and bowel rest, manifest by a prompt decrease in abdominal tenderness, defervescence, and resolution of leukocytosis in the initial 48–72 hours.

A CT scan is most useful when *(a)* the initial diagnosis is unclear based on the history and physical examination; *(b)* complicated diverticulitis is suspected based on the patient's initial presentation (i.e., a mass is palpated) (5); and *(c)* the patient fails to improve or deteriorates clinically despite treatment with bowel rest and intravenous antibiotics, and a diverticular abscess is suspected (7).

The scan also provides the most complete information regarding acute colonic diverticulitis. This imaging technique can confirm the diagnosis, evaluate the severity of the inflammatory process, and detect complications such as abscess or fistula (9). Furthermore, the size and location of the abscess can be determined. In one study, abscess sizes ranged from 5 to 18 cm (mean size, 8.7 cm) and varied in location. They were identified in the pelvis (n = 9), pericolic (n = 8), retroperitoneum (n = 1), and multiple (n = 1) (pericolic, subphrenic, and right lower quadrant) (10). Despite this expanded technology, misdiagnoses occur. In one study, 24% of patients with a preoperative diagnosis of diverticulitis and abscess formation or fistula were found to have a perforated carcinoma upon abdominal exploration (7).

TREATMENT OPTIONS

Management of patients with diverticular abscess can be complex, requiring multispecialty coordinated input to incorporate drainage and facilitate resolution of the inflammatory focus. Treatment of patients with acute complicated diverticulitis begins with bowel rest and broad-spectrum intravenous antibiotics. Most patients with a peridiverticular microabscess will respond to antibiotics and bowel rest alone (10). In evaluating the microbiology of abscesses, Stabile et al found 100% (n = 19) to contain enteric bacteria. Seventeen of 19 culture isolates were polymicrobial with *Escherichia coli*, *Bacteroides*, and *Klebsiella* predominating. In one patient, only *Bacteroides fragilis* grew, and in another, *E. coli* was the only isolate. Ravo et al (8) found *E. coli*, *Enterococci*, and *Pseudomonas aeruginosa* to grow in the isolates from an abscess.

The surgical treatment options available for acute diverticulitis with abscess formation vary extensively, but have toward fewer operations per patient. The choice of a one-, two-, or three-stage procedure is multifactorial, based on the pathology involved (including size and location of the abscess and degree of induration), patient comorbidities, and surgeon's preference (11).

The single-stage procedure combines abscess drainage with resection of the diseased segment of colon and primary anastomosis. The two-stage operation involves resection of the diseased segment and drainage of the abscess with the creation of a proximal colostomy and closed distal segment (Hartmann procedure). Reanastomosis occurs at a second operation. The three-stage option provides diversion and drainage alone at the first operation. The second procedure provides removal of the offending diseased colon with anastomosis. Bowel continuity is restored during a third operation.

The three-stage procedure, touted in the 1940s, has been de-emphasized as a treatment option, because the diseased segment (septic focus) is not removed during the initial operation. Proximal diversion and drainage also fail to empty the left colon of stool and do not alter the pressure relationships, allowing for persistent sepsis (2,7,12). Drainage with proximal colostomy is associated with a 30–45% mortality rate versus 12% when resection is performed (13,14). Three-stage procedures in patients with abscesses are associated with a 26% mortality rate (12). Therefore, *only in extraordinary circumstances, such as intraoperative instability, should a three-stage procedure be performed* (7,15).

In evaluating patients with complicated diverticulitis, Hackford et al (12) compared cumulative mortality and morbidity in patients stratified to primary resection with anastomosis versus primary resection and anastomosis with a covering stoma versus two-stage operation without anastomosis versus three-stage procedure (Table 15.1).

Of note, therapy (closure of colostomy) was completed in 100% of patients with anastomosis and protecting stoma, but in only 71% of patients following Hartmann procedures, and in 76% of patients who started in the three-stage group.

Ideally, a one-stage procedure, including resection of diseased colon with associated abscess, together with primary anastomosis, is the goal of treating this disease. This approach usually eradicates sepsis and restores bowel continuity without the need for multiple operative interventions. There has been a historical trend that favors this therapeutic option, even in the face of pelvic peritonitis. Rodkey and Welch (16) reported performing a one-stage operation in 46.9% of patients in 1974–1983 compared with 10.6% in the previous decade. *The one-stage operation is most successful when the patient is not immunocompromised and is well nourished. Other factors that contribute to the success of a one-stage procedure include a colon that is free of edema and fecal matter and is well vascularized and has a localized abscess* (7,15,17).

Table 15.1.   Morbidity and Mortality of Various Procedures for Complicated Diverticulitis

	Cumulative Operative Morbidity	Cumulative Mortality
Primary resection and anastomosis	18%	1%
Primary resection and anastomosis with a covering stoma	22%	0%
Two-stage operation	23%	16%
Three-stage operation	24%	14%

Reprinted with permission from Hackford AW, Schoetz DJ, Coller JA, et al. Surgical management of complicated diverticulitis: the Lahey Clinic experience 1967 to 1982. Dis Colon Rectum 1985;28:317–321.

Under suboptimal conditions, some authors would advocate primary resection with anastomosis and a covering stoma (15) for protection. However, most of the current literature suggests, under these circumstances, performing a Hartmann procedure, especially in the presence of unprepared bowel or gross contamination (15).

Another option worth consideration, for a young, otherwise healthy individual with contained sepsis but an unprepared colon, is the use of on-table lavage. This can rid the colon of fecal matter to allow primary anastomosis. The intraoperative irrigation system, described by Dudley et al (18), as a modification of Muir's original description (19), has been supported by other reports for a variety of pathologic entities. The procedure that involves a proximal irrigation catheter and a distal tube for the siphoning of waste effluent is reported for colonic cleansing in colonic obstruction, stenosis, volvulus, hemorrhage, trauma, inadequacy of preoperative bowel preparation, and preparation for use of the colon as a conduit in replacement of the esophagus (Chapter 20) (20).

Some have suggested that this technique should be the standard of care in the treatment of emergencies involving the left colon (21). Others, although not suggesting this as the standard of care, have had good results with minimal morbidity and recommend this technique as the operation of choice for most patients with obstructive or inflammatory processes necessitating operation on the left colon without the benefit of a preoperative mechanical preparation (22,23). One, however, should *never perform an anastomosis in the presence of significant contamination*. With fecal spillage or purulence present, the proper management is resection and diversion in an otherwise stable patient in whom disease allows safe resection.

PERCUTANEOUS DRAINAGE

Percutaneous drainage of diverticular abscesses may allow the acute infection to resolve and the patient to recover. This facilitates preoperative bowel preparation as well as an operative field more conducive to primary anastomosis in patients who would otherwise have a multistage operative approach. Although percutaneous drainage began as a temporizing measure in elderly, debilitated patients deemed too septic and unstable for surgical intervention (24), the technique currently is used routinely for patients with diverticular disease.

Initially, percutaneous drainage catheters for diverticular abscesses were underused because of the concern of bacteremia. There was fear of secondarily formed enteric fistulas from blind instrumentation and of risky access routes to pelvic abscesses. These concepts have been remodeled due to development of CT-guided access routes, failure of fistula formation from precise instrumentation, and use of refined equipment. Colocutaneous fistulas are not a significant concern to the surgeon in operative management of these patients, because the fistulous tract can be excised as part of the operation.

Percutaneous drainage can be performed under either ultrasound or CT scan guidance. For patients who refuse surgery or who are poor surgical candidates, percutaneous drainage may actually be a curative modality as shown in three patients followed for 12–29 months (9). CT-scan-guided percutaneous drainage of adjacent and distant abscesses allows elective one-stage resection with decreased mortality when compared with staged resection in patients with complicated diverticulitis (2.2% versus 6.4%) (4).

Most patients are candidates for this intervention, with a few caveats. The abscess must be well defined and localized with a safe access route or "radiologic window" (9,15). In Figure 15.1, the abscess collection is inaccessible because of the bowel loops, bladder, and osseous makeup of the pelvis. Large abscesses not confined to the mesentery, extending into the pelvis, or contiguous with the uterus or urinary bladder may benefit from percutaneous drainage (9). Mueller et al (11) reported that 50% of patients with abscesses who underwent two-stage procedures may have benefited from percutaneous drainage, allowing for one-stage resection and re-anastomosis; this conclusion was reached after retrospective review of the operative findings in 13 patients based on location and size of abscesses.

Percutaneous drainage is not an appropriate option for patients with generalized peritonitis, pneumoperitoneum, or obstruction (10). Contraindications to percutaneous drainage include severe blood dyscrasias; extensive, poorly defined collections (9); lack of safe access route (15,25); or persistent symptoms after percutaneous drainage (7,15).

As Rodkey states, in the discussion of Stabile et al (10), *percutaneous drainage is not recommended for sicker, immunocompromised patients.* Other authors agree with this position, as the diagnosis and initiation of effective treatment may be unduly delayed in this population secondary to delayed, atypical presentation (15). This population, including transplant patients, patients with renal failure, patients with acquired immunodeficiency syndrome (AIDS) (15) or steroid dependence, cancer patients undergoing chemotherapy, patients with diabetes, and chronic alcoholics (2), are comparatively poorer surgical candidates and do not respond well to medical management of diverticulitis (7) and the complications of this disease (Chapter 22). Because of the unfavorable response to conservative, nonoperative treatment of complicated diverticulitis in the immunocompromised patient, a more aggressive approach should be taken with resection and creation of a Hartmann's pouch. This treatment results in fewer complications in this patient subgroup (13).

Small pericolic abscesses may resolve with bowel rest and intravenous antibiotic therapy alone (15). Patients with small (<5 cm) abscesses confined to the mesentery or pericolic region (bowel wall, epiploic appendages) are amenable to resection of the diseased segment en bloc with the abscess, thereby rendering percutaneous drainage unnecessary (9,11,14, 24–26).

APPROACH TO CT-SCAN-GUIDED DRAINAGE

As noted above, *the mere presence of a diverticular abscess is not an indication for percutaneous drainage.* Early CT scanning often will pick up small abscesses (i.e., smaller than 5 cm) that

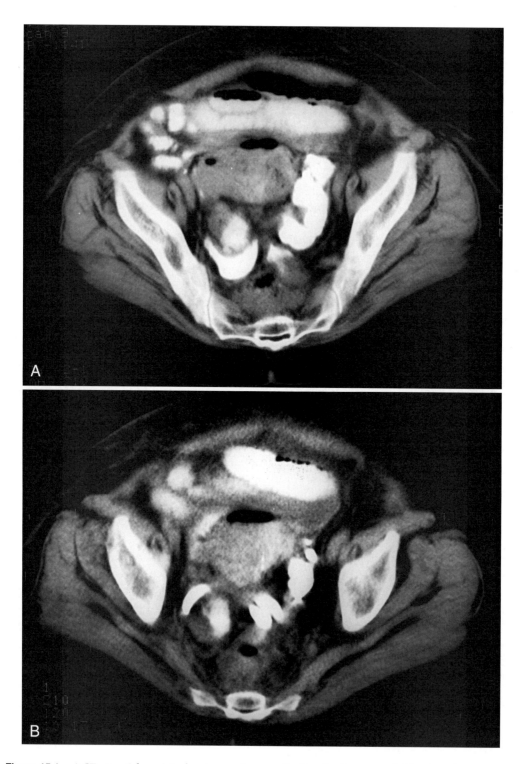

Figure 15.1. A CT scan of the pelvis showing an abscess collection that is surrounded by the pelvic sidewalls and is inaccessible to percutaneous drainage, as there is no "radiologic window," due to overlying small bowel, colon, and urinary bladder (A—C).   *(cont.)*

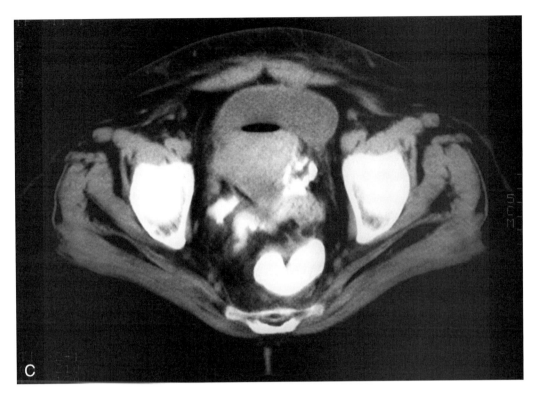

Figure 15.1. (*continued*)

may respond to standard treatment with intravenous antibiotics and bowel rest. Attempts at percutaneous drainage should be reserved for failure of conventional treatment.

Standard patient preparation includes intravenous sedation and analgesia and broad spectrum intravenous antibiotics. An 18-gauge sheathed needle is inserted, percutane-ously, into the collection according to premeasured depth and angulation (Fig. 15.2). CT is used to verify position. A small amount of fluid is aspirated for immediate gram stain and culture. A guidewire is passed through the sheath needle into the collection. The sheath needle is removed, and a series of dilators are used to dilate the tract. The appropriate catheter size, 7–14 French, is then advanced over the guidewire and coiled in the collection (Fig. 15.3). CT confirmation is then made. All catheter side holes should be coiled in the collection. Aspiration of the collection is performed until resistance to drainage is appreciated. The catheter is then irrigated with normal saline to dilute viscous material and break up loculations. High viscosity fluid, debris, and necrotic tissue are difficult to resolve, and routine saline flushes, with the possible addition of Mucomyst (27,28), increase the success rate of complete collection resolution.

Typically, a multiloculated fluid collection can be drained by one catheter due to the existing small communications between cavities. Manipulation using simple irrigation through a drainage catheter causes septations to be destroyed and permits free communication to occur, allowing drainage through a single tube.

If multiple distinct or multiseptated abscesses exist, then there is indication for two separate drainage catheters. If more than two drainage catheters are needed, surgical intervention should be considered seriously. *As a general rule, the number of drainage catheters is inversely proportional to the patient's recovery without surgery.*

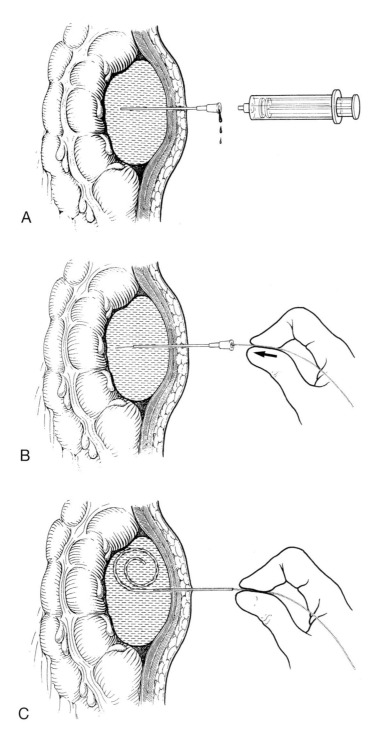

Figure 15.2.   Schematic view of percutaneous drainage of a paracolic abscess. **A.**, An aspirating needle is passed into the cavity. **B.**, A guidewire is passed through the needle. **C.**, A pigtail catheter (or, alternatively, a larger catheter following dilation of the tract) is passed over the wire into the cavity. (Reprinted with permission from Keighley MR, Williams NS. Surgery of the anus, rectum, and colon. Philadelphia: WB Saunders, 1993;2:1183–1184) [Ref. 34].

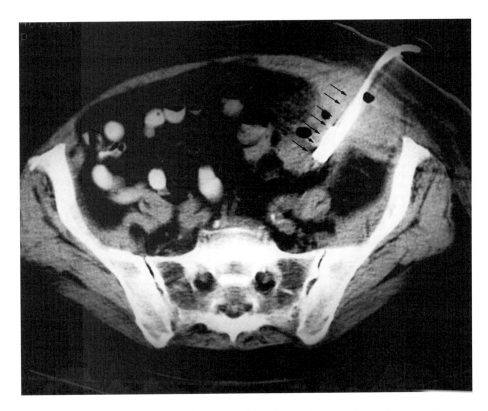

Figure 15.3.   CT scan illustrating successful catheter placement in an abscess cavity.

Access planning for draining fluid collections in the true pelvis remains difficult (29). Overlying bowel, uterus, bladder, and osseous structures often preclude anterior and lateral approach to these collections. The transgluteal approach (i.e., through the greater sciatic foramen) for abscess drainage requires precise anatomic knowledge of this route. The sacrospinous ligament serves as a marker for safe access to the pelvis because the major vascular and neural structures are located cephalad to this ligament as well as the piriformis muscle (29).

The access route of a pelvic fluid collection aspiration should be performed in a prone, prone-oblique, or lateral position. The puncture site should be as close to the sacrum as possible. A 20- or 22-gauge needle is inserted into the collection and fluid is aspirated. Fluid is sent as described earlier. Then, by the Seldinger technique, a catheter, 8.5–12 French, is inserted into the collection (Fig. 15.4). Contraindications to the transgluteal approach includes difficulty with placement of the catheter. The flexibility of the catheter makes transgressing through often-contracted gluteal muscles very difficult. Furthermore, local pain is directly attributable to impingement on branches of the sacral plexus and piriformis muscle (29).

Abscesses also can be drained internally, either transrectally (30) or transvaginally (9). In conjunction with the placement of an indwelling catheter, this can allow a convenient venue for control of sepsis. *We would avoid transrectal drainage if at all possible because this might necessitate a more extensive resection and lower anastomosis than would otherwise be required.*

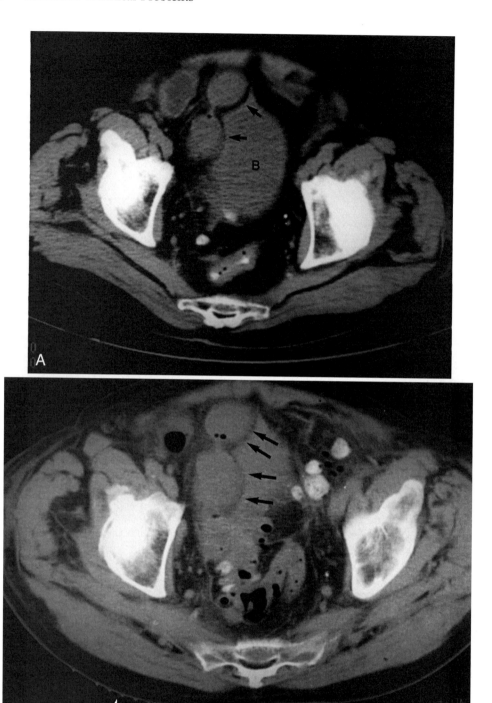

Figure 15.4. CT scan of the pelvis in a patient with an abscess accessible only by transgluteal approach. The patient is in the prone position. **A.**, Abscess cavity. **B.**, Planned approach marked (white arrows).   (*cont.*)

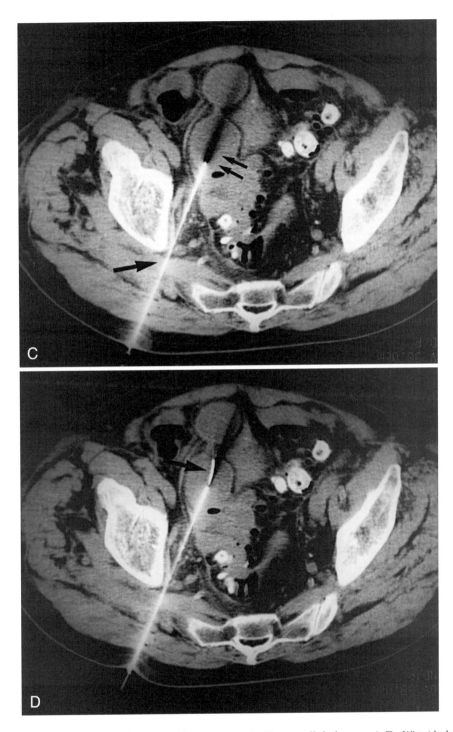

Figure 15.4.   **C.,** Needle (large dark arrow) in abscess cavity (two small dark arrows). **D.,** Wire (dark arrow) being advanced through needle.   (*cont.*)

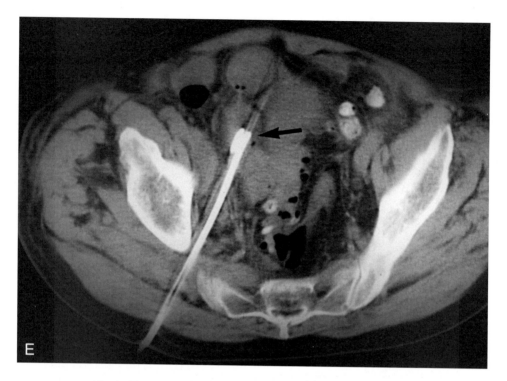

Figure 15.4. E., Catheter being advanced over wire into collection.

"Beaking" of the abscess cavity is an important clue to an occult fistula. The "beak" points directly toward the fistula and one can then reposition the catheter to obtain adequate drainage and definitively document a fistula (31). If catheter drainage exceeds 50 mL per day after the first 24 hours after insertion, suspicion of a fistula must be raised. *Fistula closure must be documented before catheter removal; otherwise, the catheter is removed at the definitive operation with excision of the fistulous tract.*

Resolution of the abscess cavity is determined by the patient's clinical condition. *High success rates have been reported with drainage of accessible abscesses.* Subsidence of sepsis manifest by decreased fevers, decreased abdominal pain, and resolution of ileus generally occurs by 72 hours after the procedure (9–11). In one report of 16 patients, 100% became afebrile 72 hours after percutaneous drainage (9). Others report success in 70–74% of patients (10,11).

Fifty-eight percent of ultrasound-visible abscess collections were treated successfully by ultrasound-guided percutaneous aspiration/catheter drainage in one study (32). With CT scan-guided drainage, higher success rates have been reported, up to 84–90% (10,25). High success rates, up to 82%, are associated with percutaneous drainage of simple abscesses (unilocular) with accompanying low complication rates around 5%. However, in complex fluid collections, success rates are considerably lower (at 45%) and are associated with a much higher complication rate of 21% (9).

After the patient has recovered and the drain output is minimal, the catheter may be removed. *Before catheter removal, a follow-up study documenting the collapse of the abscess cavity should be performed.* This may be either a CT scan or an "abscessogram" (Fig. 15.5), obtained by injecting water-soluble contrast into the catheter under fluoroscopic monitoring. If there is clinical or radiographic evidence of fistula formation, the catheter is left in place to be removed at the definitive operation.

At times, percutaneous drainage is not successful or the abscess is not accessible to the aspirating needle. As a general rule, patients who do not improve within 72 hours of drainage become candidates for resection.

Failure is related to multiplicity, multiloculation, or inadequacy of drainage and can sometimes be resolved by catheter manipulation (25). The higher complication rate is related to the multiplicity of catheters and catheter manipulation. Therefore, *the surgeon must dictate when catheter placement seems to be futile and surgical intervention is required.*

Complications encountered with percutaneous drainage can be subdivided into major and minor. Major complications include hemorrhage, ranging from hematoma to exsanguination, septicemia and sepsis, bowel laceration (9,33), and disseminated intravascular coagulopathy (33). Minor complications include transient bacteremia, incomplete abscess drainage, and infection at the catheter site (33).

What is the operative approach? Bowel preparation should be attempted if the patient's clinical condition permits. We favor a lavage-type preparation versus cathartic preparation in this situation. If the patient has significant ileus and bowel preparation cannot be completed, one can consider intraoperative colonic lavage when the conditions are suitable. We recommend placing the patients in Allen stirrups for this procedure. This allows performance of a transanal stapled anastomosis and will facilitate placement of ureteral stents if needed.

At laparotomy, one usually finds that the abscess is walled off either by the pelvic sidewall and colon or by other structures such as the bladder, uterus, or small intestine. Occasionally, the abscess is intramesenteric and can be resected with the sigmoid colon

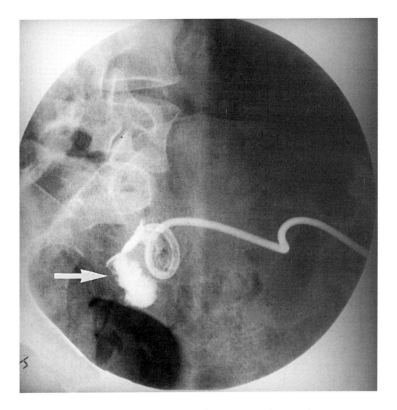

Figure 15.5.   Abscessogram; catheter study of drained cavity.

with no disruption of the abscess. This is less commonly the case. An attempt should be made to isolate this area before "breaking" into the cavity. All purulence should be aspirated after a culture is taken. The area should be irrigated and the involved colonic segment should be resected. Care should be taken to identify the left ureter, and ureteral stents may be helpful.

After the bowel has been resected, the decision to perform an anastomosis depends on the condition of the patient (i.e., well nourished, minimal cormorbidities, stable under anesthesia), condition of the proximal and distal bowel (i.e., well vascularized, well prepared with or without on-table lavage, and no tension), and the degree of contamination in the operative field. With significant fecal spillage and extensive purulence, one would favor the standard Hartmann procedure. One can consider anastomosis if contamination is limited. An often attractive alternative to the Hartmann procedure is anastomosis with proximal diversion (we favor a loop ileostomy as the diversion of choice). Although this does not eliminate the risk of anastomotic leak, it certainly decreases the clinical significance of a leak. Two months postoperatively, the ileostomy can be closed after contrast enema confirmation of a patent, leak-free anastomosis. The loop ileostomy can be closed through a small incision with a much shorter recuperation in the hospital than following a Hartmann closure.

The timing of surgery is quite variable. Reports have demonstrated successful outcomes with single-stage resection in 60–70% from 10 days to 6 weeks postdrainage (10,11). We have had success with both early and late operative intervention and base the decision on the patient's clinical condition, with a tendency to let the patient recuperate a bit longer after percutaneous drainage. Although this technique is highly successful, failure may be related to multiplicity or multiloculation of abscesses.

COST ANALYSIS

Analyses have shown considerable savings in both cost and disability with the reduction of operative interventions. However, few documented analyses of this cost benefit appear in the literature. Sparks et al (26) reported Medicare figures comparing two-stage resection with percutaneous drainage and one-stage resection with anastomosis. This revealed costs of $18,820 versus $11,428 for a savings of $7,392 (39.3%).

Rodkey and Welch (16) have shown that hospitalization and duration of disability is twice as long in patients treated with staged operations as in those treated with primary resection and anastomosis. In 1958, Colcock (1) reported hospital stays for one-stage resection of 9–24 days (average, 15 days) compared with patients undergoing three-stage resection with hospital stays of 37–84 days (average, 60 days). As indicated, length of disability should never influence the choice of operation if patient safety is a factor (16).

CONCLUSIONS

Diverticular abscess is the most common complication of diverticulitis. The goal of treatment in this complex condition involves control of the septic focus, removal of the diseased colonic segment, and restoration of intestinal continuity. With the advent of CT, percutaneous drainage techniques, and intraoperative colonic lavage, this goal can be accomplished with fewer operative stages, with lower morbidity and lower mortality.

The safety and efficiency in controlling the septic focus clearly takes precedence over the number of procedures and the cost of hospitalization. Therefore, sound clinical judgment is required in deciding which of the described approaches is best for each individual patient.

EDITORIAL COMMENTS

Abscess formation is the most frequent complication of diverticular disease. Most abscesses are small, contained within the colon wall or the mesentery; occasionally, large paracolic or pelvic abscesses occur (10,16). In part due to the frequency of diverticular abscesses, percutaneous drainage is a well-established modality for drainage of larger abscesses. Our radiologists have used this technique with a high degree of success, and we rarely encounter serious complications such as sepsis or major bleeding (34). However, the procedures do have their limits, and there are a few contraindications. In general, if an attempt at percutaneous drainage with one or more catheters fails to control sepsis (this happens in 20–30%), or if significant feculent drainage develops, we would proceed to surgery, barring prohibitive medical risks. Also, some immunocompromised patients are better treated with early resection as opposed to percutaneous drainage.

By avoiding some operative procedures and shortening the cumulative length of hospitalization, this drainage technique offers cost advantages without added morbidity that have gained particular importance in the managed-care era. Percutaneous drainage is another reason that three-stage procedures have become largely obsolete.

If percutaneous drainage cannot be performed, the type of operative procedure needed will be dependent on the operative findings. We would not attempt an anastomosis if the field contained a large abscess or contamination; poor-risk patients with diseases such as diabetes or advanced coronary disease can be treated effectively with the Hartmann procedure (35).

What is the appropriate interval between drainage and surgery? This is subjective and varies among patients and surgeons. A reasonable approach would be to assess the degree of inflammation seen by CT scan as well as the rapidity of the patient's response to the drainage procedure. In the case of a relatively small abscess and a rapid clinical response to drainage, operation could be performed during the same hospitalization. In the case of a large phlegmon, the most judicious approach would be a delay of at least 4–6 weeks, repeating the CT scan to visualize the degree of response. Because many of these patients are elderly with some nutritional deficits and associated medical illnesses, some delay to surgery seems warranted in most cases, to allow the patient to rebound before the additional stress of a major operation.

REFERENCES

1. Colcock BP. Surgical management of complicated diverticulitis. N Engl J Med 1958;259:570–573. *A retrospective review of 131 patients who were operated on for complicated diverticulitis.*
2. Roberts PL, Veidenheimer MC. Current management of diverticulitis. Adv Surg 1994;27:189–208. *Review article on diverticulitis and treatment guidelines.*
3. Veidenheimer MC, Roberts PL. Colonic diverticular disease. Boston: Blackwell Scientific, 1991. *Textbook with overview of all aspects of diverticular disease.*
4. Hachigian MP, Honickman S, Eisenstat TE, et al. Computed tomography in the initial management of acute left-sided diverticulitis. Dis Colon Rectum 1992;35:1123–1129. *Report on efficacy of CT scan as the initial study in 59 patients with the clinical diagnosis of acute sigmoid diverticulitis.*
5. Labs JD, Sarr MG, Fishman EK, et al. Complications of acute diverticulitis of the colon: improved early diagnosis with computerized tomography. Am J Surg 1988;155:331–336. *Review of CT scan in evaluating 68 patients with suspected complications of acute diverticulitis.*
6. Ambrosetti P, Robert J, Witzig JA, et al. Incidence, outcome, and proposed management of isolated abscesses complicating acute left-sided diverticulitis: a prospective study of 140 patients. Dis Colon Rectum 1992;35:1072–1076. *A prospective evaluation of 140 consecutive patients with acute left-sided CT scan diagnosed diverticulitis.*
7. Rothenberger DA. Surgery for complicated diverticulitis. Surg Clin North Am 1993;73:975–992. *A review of the complications associated with diverticulitis and management strategies.*
8. Ravo B, Khan SA, Ger R, et al. Unusual extraperitoneal presentations of diverticulitis. Am J Gastroenterol 1985;80:346–351. *Case report and review of the literature.*
9. Fabiszewski NL, Sumkin JH, Johns CM. Contemporary radiologic percutaneous abscess drainage in the pelvis. Clin Obstet Gynecol 1993;36:445–456. *Discussion of etiologies of pelvic abscesses and management issues.*
10. Stabile BE, Puccio E, vanSonnenberg E, et al. Preoperative percutaneous drainage of diverticular abscesses. Am J Surg 1990;159: 99–105. *Review of 19 patients followed after drainage of paracolic or pelvic abscesses.*
11. Mueller PR, Saini S, Wittenburg J, et al. Sigmoid diverticular abscess: percutaneous drainage as an adjunct to surgical resection in 24 cases. Radiology 1987;164:321–325. *Report of 24 patients with pelvic fluid collections, drained percutaneously.*

12. Hackford AW, Schoetz DJ, Coller JA, et al. Surgical management of complicated diverticulitis: the Lahey Clinic experience 1967 to 1982. Dis Colon Rectum 1985;28:317–321. *Retrospective review of 140 patients with complicated diverticular disease treated at one institution.*

13. Perkins JD, Shield CF III, Change FC, et al. Acute diverticulitis: comparison of treatment in immunocompromised and non-immunocompromised patients. Am J Surg 1984;148:745–748. *Retrospective review of 90 patients admitted to one institution with the diagnosis of acute diverticulitis.*

14. Smirniotis V, Tsoutsos D, Fotopoulos A, et al. Perforated diverticulitis: a surgical dilemma. Int Surg 1991;76:44–47. *Review of 38 patients operated on for perforated diverticulitis over 14 years.*

15. Roberts P, Abel M, Rosen L, et al. Practice parameters for sigmoid diverticulitis-supporting documentation. Dis Colon Rectum 1995;38:126–132. *Describes guidelines from The Standards Task Force of The American Society of Colon and Rectal Surgeons.*

16. Rodkey GV, Welch CE. Changing patterns in the surgical treatment of diverticular disease. Ann Surg 1984;200:466–478. *Comparison of two sequential decades of diverticulitis at a major teaching hospital, discussing 688 patients.*

17. Tudor RG, Farmakis N, Keighley MR. National audit of complicated diverticular disease: analysis of index cases. Br J Surg 1994;81:730–732. *Details of 300 patients with complicated diverticular disease from 30 hospitals.*

18. Dudley HAF, Radcliffe AG, McGeehan D. Intraoperative irrigation of the colon to permit primary anastomosis. Br J Surg 1980;67:80–81. *Description of a new technique.*

19. Muir EG. Safety in colonic resections. Proc R Soc Med 1968;61:401–408. *An early description of important techniques used during the course of on-table lavage.*

20. Danne PD. Intraoperative colonic lavage: safe single-stage, left colorectal resections. Aust N Z J Surg 1991;61:59–65. *Fifty consecutive cases of intraoperative colonic lavage during left-sided colorectal operations.*

21. Allen-Mersh TG. Should primary anastomosis and on-table colonic lavage be the standard treatment for left colon emergencies? Ann R Coll Surg Engl 1993;75:195–198. *An assessment of treatment of 60 patients with left colon obstruction or infection managed by one group during a 2.5-year period.*

22. Stewart J, Diament RH, Brennan TG. Management of obstructing lesions of the left colon by resection, on-table lavage, and primary anastomosis. Surgery 1993;114:502–505. *An analysis of seventy-three consecutive patients presenting with left colon obstruction during a 5-year period, evaluating perioperative complications and long-term survival.*

23. Murray JJ, Schoetz DJ, Coller JA, et al. Intraoperative colonic lavage and primary anastomosis in nonelective colon resection. Dis Colon Rectum 1991;34:527–531. *Review of 25 patients requiring urgent segmental left colon resection and intraoperative colonic lavage.*

24. Neff CC, vanSonnenberg E, Casola G, et al. Diverticular abscesses: percutaneous drainage. Radiology 1987;163:15–18. *Results of percutaneous catheter drainage performed in 16 patients.*

25. Saini S, Meuller PR, Wittenberg J, et al. Percutaneous drainage of diverticular abscess: an adjunct to surgical therapy. Arch Surg 1986;121:475–478. *Describes 17 patients with acute diverticulitis, with selective drainage and follow-up.*

26. Sparks FC, Strauss EB, Corey JM. Percutaneous drainage of a diverticular abscess can make colostomy unnecessary in selected cases. Conn Med 1990;54:305–307. *Case report and cost analysis.*

27. Dawson SL, Meuller PR, Ferrucci JT. Mucomyst for abscesses: a clinical comment. Radiology 1984;151:342. *Review of efficacy of Mucomyst in the treatment of abscesses.*

28. van Waes PF, Feldberg MA, Mali WP, et al. Management of loculated abscesses that are difficult to drain: a new approach. Radiology 1983;147:57–63. *Report of 14 patients who had percutaneous drainage with one or more contraindications to external drainage procedure.*

29. Butch RJ, Mueller PR, Ferrucci JT, et al. Drainage of pelvic abscesses through the greater sciatic foramen. Radiology 1986;158:487–491. *A report of CT scan guided transgluteal drainage in 21 patients.*

30. Chester JF, Turner WH, Lloyd-Williams K, et al. Permanent transrectal drainage of a diverticular-related abscess with a double ended pigtail catheter. Br J Surg 1988;75:562. *Case report of drainage 10 years after diversion for complicated diverticulitis.*

31. Jeffrey RB. Percutaneous drainage of enteric abscesses. Semin Intervent Radiol 1988;5:167–178. *A discussion of principles and management schema.*

32. Schwerk WB, Schwarz S, Rothmund M. Sonography in acute colonic diverticulitis: a prospective study. Dis Colon Rectum 1992;35:1077–1084. *Prospective study of 130 patients who underwent ultrasound to aid in the diagnosis of acute and complicated diverticulitis.*

33. van Sonnenberg E, Mueller PR, Ferrucci JT. Percutaneous drainage of 250 abdominal abscesses and fluid collections: Part I. Results, failures, and complications. Radiology 1984;151:337–341. *Results of 250 percutaneous abscess and fluid drainage procedures.*

34. Keighley MR, Williams NS. Surgery of the anus, rectum, and colon. London: WB Saunders, 1993;2:1183–1184.

35. Rodkey GV, Welch CE. Surgical management of colonic diverticulitis with free perforation or abscess formation. Am J Surg 1969;117:265–269. *Discusses 22 patients with diverticular abscesses. One of the earlier studies encouraging two-stage procedures because of safety and cost savings.*

16 The Proper Surgical Treatment of Perforated Sigmoid Diverticulitis with Generalized Peritonitis

Marilyn B. Sanford, MD
John A. Ryan, Jr., MD

> **KEY POINTS**
>
> - 1–2% of cases of acute diverticulitis
> - Hartmann procedure standard operation
> - Purulent peritonitis: consider primary anastomosis
> - Fecal peritonitis: anastomosis contraindicated
> - Mortality
>   purulent peritonitis: 13%
>   fecal peritonitis: 43%
>   overall: 20–30%

ILLUSTRATIVE CASE

The classic presentation of acute diverticulitis with free perforation occurs in an older patient with the sudden onset of left lower abdominal pain. The patient may have previously diagnosed diverticular disease. Depending on the time course, the vital signs would show evidence of early to overt sepsis, including fever, tachycardia, and hypotension. Physical examination elicits signs of generalized peritonitis, including a boardlike abdomen and rebound tenderness. Abdominal films are the key to the diagnosis by demonstrating free air.

CASE COMMENTS

Although acute diverticulitis with free perforation usually is a sudden and clinically obvious event, some patients with this complication present with abdominal pain and tenderness that are largely localized to the left lower quadrant. On examination, only mild tenderness is noted in other quadrants. In this setting, plain films often do not reveal free intraperitoneal air and further diagnostic studies are indicated (Fig. 16.1). This is especially true in the immunocompromised host, in whom physical findings tend to be understated.

We favor early use of computed tomography (CT) scanning in such patients, not only to confirm the clinical suspicion of diverticulitis but to rule out free perforation, which may not be apparent after the initial clinical and radiographic evaluations. CT scans are sensitive

223

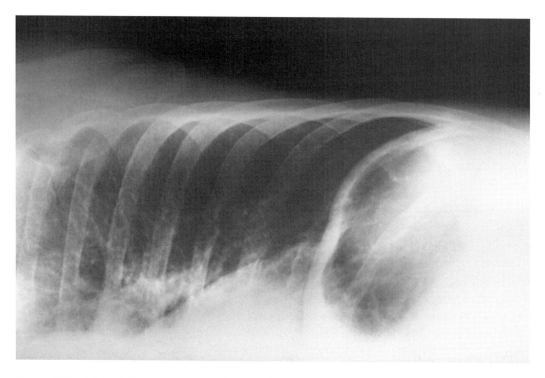

Figure 16.1.   A lateral decubitus view containing no free air of a patient who had freely perforated sigmoid diverticulitis.

for small foci of free air and limited amounts of free fluid suggestive of free perforation (Fig. 16.2). In the absence of free air or fluid by CT scan, most patients with acute diverticulitis do not require emergency laparotomy. They almost certainly will respond to medical therapy.

INTRODUCTION

Most episodes of acute diverticulitis do not require an emergency operation. Intravenous antibiotics, bowel rest, and supportive medical management will effectively treat most patients. When warranted, sigmoid colectomy can be pursued electively. However, *the entity of acute sigmoid diverticulitis with perforation and either generalized purulent or fecal peritonitis still demands immediate operation.* The challenge is not in making the diagnosis, nor is it in deciding who requires an operation, but is in selecting the appropriate procedure in the operating room. After an initial exploration, the surgeon must ascertain the feasibility of sigmoid resection. If the surgeon decides to resect the perforated colon, then either a descending end colostomy or a primary anastomosis must be performed. This decision remains controversial. This chapter reviews the issues surrounding the controversy and makes a recommendation.

HISTORIC BACKGROUND

The high concentration of gram-negative and anaerobic bacteria in the large bowel has posed a continuous and incompletely resolved difficulty for the surgeon. The current controversy is best understood when viewed within the context of the historical approach to emergency operations on the left colon.

The historic approach to perforated diverticulitis was the three-stage procedure, so named because three operations were necessary before the fecal stream regained continuity. The first operation controlled fecal contamination by forming a diverting colostomy proximal to the inflamed sigmoid colon and draining the actual perforation. During the second operation, the patient underwent sigmoid colectomy with primary anastomosis. The diverting colostomy remained to protect the new anastomosis. The third procedure was colostomy closure (1).

The three-stage approach has fallen into disfavor. First, the septic source, the fecal-laden perforated colon, remained in place and, thus the infection was not always controlled. Multiple operations with an elderly patient population resulted in high morbidity and mortality, excessive cumulative days of hospitalization, and frequent failure to complete all of the stages (2). Additionally, the possibility of recurrent diverticulitis or delay in diagnosis of a perforated colon cancer remained until after the colectomy was completed (3).

Surgical innovators realized that the three-stage procedure was unnecessarily cumbersome, with an unacceptably high morbidity and mortality, and several two-stage procedures evolved. Some two-stage procedures continued to limit the first operation to just a diverting colostomy without resection of the affected colon. These operations were associated with the same problems (ongoing sepsis and delayed diagnosis) as the three-stage procedure, prompting surgeons to try resecting the diseased segment at the initial operation with colostomy. Numerous reports in the late 1970s and early 1980s

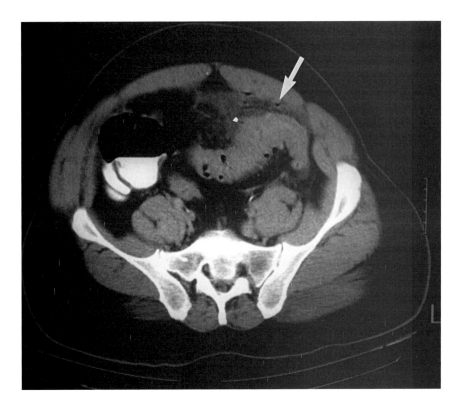

Figure 16.2.   CT scan of the patient described in Figure 16.1. Note the phlegmon involving the sigmoid colon and extracolonic gas indicated by the arrow.

demonstrated the feasibility and similar if not superior efficacy and safety of these approaches; the most common was the Hartmann procedure (2). The Hartmann procedure entails resection of the diseased sigmoid with an end colostomy and closure of the distal rectal pouch (4). The Hartmann procedure has gradually become the standard of care. However, it entails two operations on patients who tolerate surgery poorly, leading surgeons to question whether the benefits of a two-stage procedure outweighed the risks. Surgical innovators began to attempt resection with primary anastomosis on unprepped bowel in cases of trauma, obstruction, bleeding, and perforation. This chapter examines the proper surgical treatment of perforated sigmoid diverticulitis with generalized peritonitis.

ACUTE DIVERTICULITIS

Critical to the appropriate interpretation of the literature and understanding of the surgical issues is an understanding of the spectrum of disease labeled as acute diverticulitis. A growing body of evidence supports the theory that colonic diverticula form because of a motility disorder, which leads to spasm, mechanical obstruction, and thus the development of mucosal outpouchings. The diverticula form adjacent to the taenia libra and taenia omentalis, where perforating vessels cross the submucosa through the bowel wall out to appendiceal epiploica. During most acute attacks, the colon wall will be thickened and inflamed but not actually perforated. A second route to acute diverticulitis occurs when an individual diverticulum becomes plugged with inspissated fecal material leading to peridiverticular inflammation. The inflammatory process can coalesce to form a phlegmon, without an actual perforation. The above etiologies of acute diverticulitis respond best to conservative medical management (5).

Acute diverticulitis may also arise as a result of a colonic diverticular perforation. The perforation may present anywhere along a spectrum, from a limited perforation into the colonic mesentery to an abdominal catastrophe with fecal soiling of the peritoneal cavity. The management depends on the nature of the perforation. One useful system of codification divides acute perforated diverticulitis into four stages (5).

Stage I comprises mesenteric abscesses, specifically abscesses that result from inflammation of a diverticulum residing within the mesentery of the colon. The colonic mesentery functions as a barrier to contain the abscess.

Stage II contains walled-off abscesses. In these cases, a localized perforation in the peritoneum covering the abscess occurs. The leaking purulence causes inflammation of the surrounding organs (omentum, pelvic sidewall, uterus, bladder, and small bowel mesentery), which results in adhesions between the adjacent tissues. These adhesions enable the surrounding organs to "wall off" the escaping purulence, preventing spread throughout the rest of the abdomen.

In *Stage III*, the surrounding organs unsuccessfully control the perforated abscess, and purulent material thus spreads throughout the abdominal cavity with resulting generalized peritonitis. Fecal soiling does not occur because the inflammatory process has obliterated the neck of the diverticulum, effectively resealing the colon's lumen.

In *Stage IV* disease, the lumen is not effectively sealed off by the pericolonic inflammation, and there is spillage of stool into the peritoneal cavity, i.e., fecal peritonitis.

The host response differs according to the type of perforation, and consequently, so does the management. The management of contained perforations (stages I and II) differs significantly from that of free perforations (stages III and IV). We will limit our discussion to the controversy surrounding the intraoperative management of free perforations.

MAGNITUDE OF THE PROBLEM

Free perforation is a devastating complication of diverticulitis. Fortunately, it is relatively rare. *Free perforations comprise only 1–2% of all cases of acute diverticulitis.* The low incidence makes analysis of treatment options difficult. A large hospital might see only one or two cases each year. An individual surgeon may operate on patients with freely perforated diverticulitis only a handful of times throughout a busy career (6). A single surgeon or institution cannot accumulate enough patients to convincingly demonstrate an improved outcome with a new procedure. Therefore, surgeons must rely upon inferences within the literature and their own personal experience and judgment.

DATA FROM THE LITERATURE

A review of the literature on this topic is confusing because different surgeons reach nearly opposite conclusions from the same data. To minimize the confusion, we will first present the actual data in the literature. Subsequently, we will reconstruct the arguments for and against a primary anastomosis.

Patients do poorly when they undergo emergency operations for diverticulitis. The mortality of all approaches combined is approximately 20–30%. Older patients have a higher mortality rate, which reaches 50% for patients older than 70 years of age (7). Clinically significant anastomotic dehiscence (8) occurs approximately 20% of the time when surgeons operate on unprepped bowel (6). We do not know the incidence of anastomotic dehiscence for primary anastomosis performed in the setting of a free perforation. This information is not available because of the relative rarity of the condition and because authors neglected to stratify their patients with regard to contained perforations versus free perforations. Anastomotic leaks result in a mortality of approximately 30% with significant associated morbidity (9).

Many series have been published that attempt to correlate outcome with the type of surgical procedure chosen to manage the perforation. The earliest papers on this subject were intended to demonstrate feasibility of a primary anastomosis in unprepped bowel. In general, they had good results because of strict patient selection. Nearly all of these papers contain a disclaimer that this procedure should not be applied to patients with free perforation and generalized peritonitis. In 1978, Hinchey et al raised the issue that perhaps it would be reasonable to perform primary anastomosis in certain cases of acute diverticulitis but, to distinguish which patients might be appropriate candidates, surgeons needed to better classify the extent of the disease at operation (5). Table 16.1 is limited to papers that clearly separate free perforations from contained perforations and which have at least 10 patients with the former condition. Only retrospective reviews were found. The largest has only 51 patients with free perforation of the colon. For simplicity, the table omits patients who underwent a three-stage procedure.

The results from the above meta-analysis illustrate several facts. First, the numbers in each series are small, emphasizing that *acute perforated diverticulitis with peritonitis is a rare condition. Second, because of the small numbers, one cannot compare the two operations in any meaningful way. Third, patients with purulent peritonitis do much better than those with feculent peritonitis, with respective mortalities of 13% and 43%.*

Trauma provides another source of information. Primary closures are much more accepted in the trauma setting; however, trauma surgeons caution against a primary repair if the delay to operation has been greater than 6–12 hours. A large multicenter study concluded that gross fecal contamination is a contraindication to primary repair of the colon (14).

Table 16.1. Meta-analysis of the Mortality Associated with Two-Stage and One-Stage Procedures for Purulent and Feculent Diverticulitis

Study	Institution	Year	Duration of Review	Purulent No Anastomosis	Peritonitis Primary Anastomosis	Fecal No Anastomosis	Peritonitis Primary Anastomosis
Hinchey et al (5)	McGill University (Montreal, Canada)	1978	N/A	No. of patients: 6 Deaths: 0	0	2	0
Auguste and Borrero (10)	SUNY (Stony Brook, New York)	1985	1960–1983	No. of patients: 16 Deaths: 3	1	8	0
Krukowski et al (11)	University of Aberdeen (Aberdeen, UK)	1985	1977–1983	No. of patients: 5 Deaths: 1	0	3	2
Shepard and Keighley (12)	General Hospital (Birmingham, UK)	1986	1970–1983	No. of patients: 14 Deaths: 1	2	3	1
Sarin and Boulos (13)	University College (London, UK)	1991	1980–1987	No. of patients: 6 Deaths: 0	3	5	0
Totals:				No. of patients: 47 Deaths: 5 Mortality: 11%	6 0 0%	21 7 33%	1 1 3 2 66%

The Argument for a One-Stage Procedure

The basic premise of the argument for resection with primary anastomosis is that the mortality and morbidity from a second operation for colostomy takedown is greater than the risk of anastomotic dehiscence. Patients who do die succumb to cardiopulmonary disease, other preexisting conditions, or the underlying septic process. The additional operation carries a substantial risk in this generally elderly patient population. Studies clearly demonstrate that total mortality is equivalent if not better in patients who undergo a primary anastomosis, particularly for patients who have purulent peritonitis.

Death directly attributable to an anastomotic dehiscence is relatively rare in patients who undergo a primary anastomosis. Techniques for on-table colonic lavage aid the surgeon by allowing intraoperative colon preparation. Better antibiotics and the capabilities of interventional radiology reduce the impact of an anastomotic dehiscence. Some surgeons will make the argument that in a properly performed anastomosis, the bowel wall is inverted, preventing exposure of the suture line to the inflammatory intra-abdominal process. They believe that intra-abdominal infection and fecal loading have little affect on anastomotic healing (15).

Both the creation and the closure of the colostomy come with attendant risks and potential problems. The surgeon expects to encounter significant adhesions from the original inflammation. These adhesions obliterate the anatomic planes, placing the intra-abdominal organs at risk during the dissection. Many patients fail to come to colostomy takedown because of their age or general underlying infirmity. In most series, fewer than 50% of patients managed to regain gastrointestinal continuity. An emergent and therefore poorly placed stoma can be a constant source of difficulty for the patient. A long-standing Hartmann pouch may develop inflammatory changes (16).

The Argument Against a One-Stage Procedure

Fecal soiling is a contraindication to performing a primary anastomosis. As our meta-analysis demonstrates, the highest mortality occurred in patients with feculent peritonitis and a primary anastomosis. The literature lacks convincing evidence that patients benefit from a primary anastomosis, and the reported mortality is unacceptably high.

Trauma data confirm fecal soiling as a contraindication. After trauma, the surgeon is generally operating on an acutely injured but otherwise normal colon and the patients are generally young and healthy. One could argue that this would be the best circumstance in which to perform a primary anastomosis; however, the data show higher rates of infectious and intra-abdominal complications with primary closure in the presence of fecal soiling (14).

The data appear more muddled for patients with purulent peritonitis. It would seem that patients with a primary anastomosis do as well as, if not better than, those who undergo a Hartmann procedure. This is because of patient selection biases that are inherent to retrospective reviews. Retrospective series cannot eliminate the judgment of the surgeons when they selected which procedure to perform. Therefore, one should assume that resection with an unprotected primary anastomosis would only have been performed in the "best-risk" patients in those series, i.e., the patients with the least amount of contamination and who are in the best condition. Therefore, one would expect a group of select lower-risk patients to have a lower mortality and morbidity. Mortality often is similar after resection with primary anastomosis or the Hartmann procedure. Those opposed to a primary anastomosis will argue that this demonstrates that performing a primary anastomosis is inherently more risky: as a group, the patients that a surgeon would select for a primary anastomosis would certainly be those at lowest risk, and therefore, they should do better than patients undergoing the Hartmann procedure.

Inflammation and infection put the anastomosis at risk (17). Fecal soiling also negatively affects healing. Both poor bowel preparation at operation and fecal soiling are associated with dehiscence in 24% and 22% of cases, respectively (8). These factors will place a technically well performed anastomosis at risk of disruption. Furthermore, the associated generalized inflammation that occurs with a free perforation will make the added dissection that is necessary for a tension-free anastomosis more difficult and thus riskier. The added dissection further prolongs total operating time. Basic surgical teaching stresses that sick, septic patients tolerate operations poorly. The surgeon must limit the operation to give the patient the best chance of surviving the septic insult. It is an oversimplification to assert that the only difference between a Hartmann procedure and a primary anastomosis is the risk of anastomotic breakdown. The bigger operation with more dissection and more time in the operating room may result in more deaths and complications. Clearly, it is better to be alive with a colostomy than an operative mortality.

CONCLUSION

A two-stage procedure with resection of the perforated colon at the initial operation, such as the Hartmann procedure, is the standard of care for freely perforated sigmoid diverticulitis. It is the standard of care because the literature convincingly demonstrates improved mortality and morbidity with this approach when compared with the prior standard of care, the three-stage procedure (2,5,10). The literature demonstrates examples of surgeons performing single-stage operations for acute perforated sigmoid diverticulitis with generalized peritonitis. The literature, however, does not convincingly demonstrate superior efficacy of a one-stage procedure. *The literature fails to guide us for several reasons.* (a) *We cannot know the true affect that patient selection has on the outcome because of the retrospective nature of the literature.* (b) Perforated sigmoid diverticulitis with generalized peritonitis is a rare disease. *All of the published series have inadequate numbers of cases to allow for meaningful statistical analysis.* (c) *Current staging systems are not detailed enough to allow surgeons to identify subsets of patients with a free perforation who may benefit from a one-stage procedure.* Surgeons operating in the middle of the night on this rare condition should apply the standard of care and perform a sigmoid resection with colostomy.

EDITORIAL COMMENTS

The authors have analyzed a topic that is covered extensively in the literature, but in a confusing fashion. We, in essence, concur with their conclusions that are based on examination of reports that include at least 10 cases of free perforation.

As pointed out in the discussion of the illustrative case, the symptomatology and diagnostic examination can vary from localized abdominal tenderness with subtle changes on the CT scan to generalized abdominal rigidity with pneumoperitoneum (Fig. 16.3). Pus or feces can circulate within the abdomen (Fig. 16.4), setting the stage for sepsis and multiple system organ dysfunction. The abdomen may contain fibrinous debris and feculent material; if, by chance, barium is instilled through the perforation, it may be virtually impossible to lavage the abdomen clean. If possible, the perforation should be walled off early in the course of the operation and the abdomen should be irrigated profusely (Figs. 16.5 and 16.6).

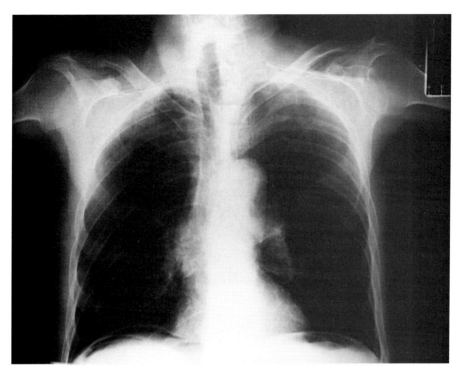

Figure 16.3.   Pneumoperitoneum (as seen under both hemidiaphragms in this upright chest radiograph) is a frequent manifestation of a free perforation of the colon.

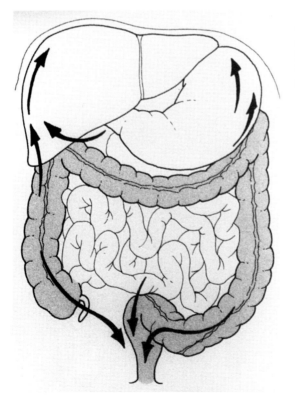

Figure 16.4.   This diagram shows the directions of spread that fluid and purulent material take after a perforation of sigmoid diverticulitis into the peritoneal cavity. (Reprinted with permission from Keighley MR, Williams NS. Surgery of the anus, rectum and colon. London: WB Saunders, 1993.)

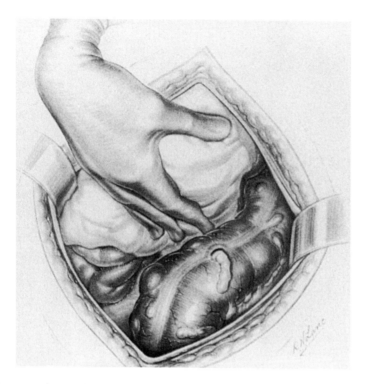

Figure 16.5. Exposure of a site of perforation in the sigmoid colon after the small bowel is packed away with laparotomy pads. (Reprinted with permission from Todd IP, Fielding LP, eds. Rob & Smith's Operative surgery. Alimentary tract and abdominal wall. 3. Colon, rectum and anus. 4th ed. London: Butterworths, 1983.)

Figure 16.6. Schematic representation of fibrinous debris between loops of small intestine in a case of purulent peritonitis. (Reprinted with permission from Todd IP, Fielding LP, eds. Rob & Smith's Operative surgery. Alimentary tract and abdominal wall. 3. Colon, rectum and anus. 4th ed. London: Butterworths, 1983.)

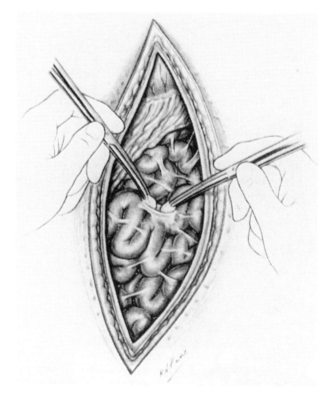

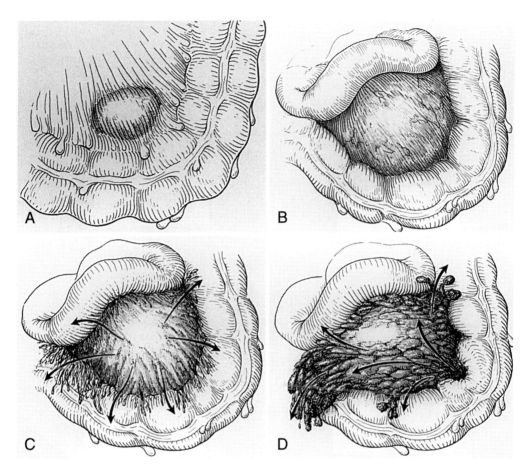

Figure 16.7.   The pathologic stages of perforated diverticulitis as devised by Hinchey and colleagues (5). In **(A)**, there is a localized pericolic abscess; in **(B)**, there is a large mesenteric abscess spreading into the pelvis; **(C)** depicts free perforation leading to purulent peritonitis; and **(D)** shows free perforation causing fecal peritonitis. (Reprinted with permission from Todd IP, Fielding LP, eds. Rob & Smith's Operative surgery. Alimentary tract and abdominal wall. 3. Colon, rectum and anus. 4th ed. London: Butterworths, 1983.)

The Hinchey classification is a useful system to compare patients with different forms of perforation (Figs. 16.7). Most of the controversy concerns patients with stage III and stage IV disease: in these patients, one could conclude that "it is better to be alive with a stoma than dead without." The Hartmann procedure is an excellent operation for the patient with freely perforated diverticulitis and feculent peritonitis (stage IV), because an anastomosis is unsafe in this setting (Figs. 16.8 through 16.10).

Choice of a procedure is more difficult in the setting of purulent peritonitis and limited sepsis (stage III). Judgment and experience are important when making the decision for or against a primary anastomosis. If in doubt, a staged procedure with resection and colostomy is an excellent initial operation; this is basically the gold standard. The use of on-table lavage and/or proximal diverting ileostomy or colostomy are useful adjuncts if anastomosis is to be considered (18,19). On-table lavage does have the disadvantage of increasing operative time, and perhaps risk, and it should be used judiciously for elderly patients. Although proximal fecal diversion does not prevent an anastomotic leak, it may ameliorate its septic effects.

Another tool in the setting of perforation, when anastomotic integrity is a concern, is the Coloshield (Fig. 16.11) (20,21). Although the principle of this device is intriguing, there has been little

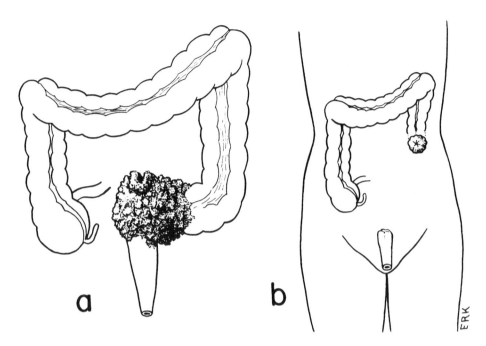

Figure 16.8.   Illustration of a locally perforated sigmoid diverticulitis **(a)** treated by a Hartmann procedure. The end colostomy and closed rectal segment are shown in **(b)**. (Reprinted with permission from Welch JP. Diverticular disease. In: Welch JP, ed. Bowel obstruction. Differential diagnosis and clinical management. Philadelphia: WB Saunders, 1990:589–599.)

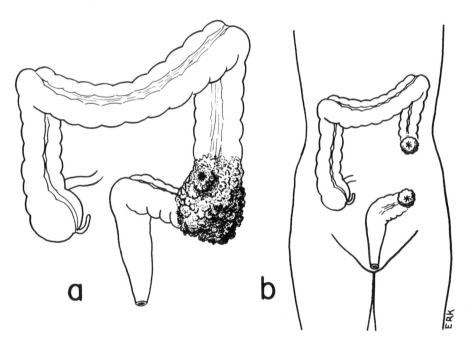

Figure 16.9.   Sometimes it is possible to construct an end colostomy and mucous fistula **(B)** after resection of perforated sigmoid diverticulitis (shown in **A**). This procedure is possible only with a suitably lengthy distal segment to construct the mucous fistula. Because the colon usually has a foreshortened mesentery when involved by diverticulitis, this procedure is performed infrequently. (Reprinted with permission from Welch JP. Diverticular disease. In: Welch JP, ed. Bowel obstruction. Differential diagnosis and clinical management. Philadelphia: WB Saunders, 1990:589–599.)

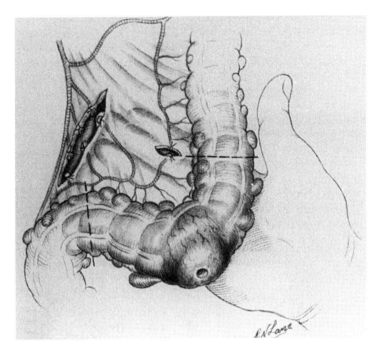

Figure 16.10. Commencing a sigmoid resection for perforated diverticulitis. Frequently, a Hartmann procedure is done in this setting. (Reprinted with permission from Todd IP, Fielding LP, eds. Rob & Smith's Operative surgery. Alimentary tract and abdominal wall. 3. Colon, rectum and anus. 4th ed. London: Butterworths, 1983.)

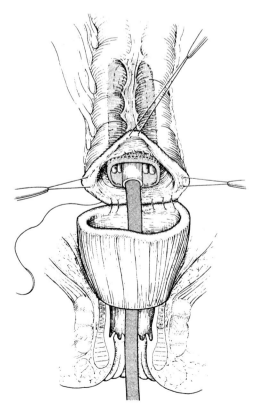

Figure 16.11. The Coloshield has been developed as a conduit for the bowel contents within the bowel when there is concern for anastomotic integrity. The shield eventually is passed spontaneously. (Reprinted with permission from Keighley MR, Williams NS. Surgery of the anus, rectum and colon. London: WB Saunders, 1993.)

mention of it in the recent surgical literature, and we have had no personal experience with it. There are many articles that the authors have not elaborated on, considering their criteria for inclusion in the meta-analysis (22–69). For the reader with further interest, some series published during the last three decades are listed in Table 16.2 (22–53). Most patients tabulated had generalized diffusing peritonitis, either purulent or fecal in type. Of interest, in this seriously ill population of patients (70), there has been little impact on median mortality. Of several papers that review this subject (23,25,32,71–75), a publication by Krukowski and Matheson is especially recommended (6). In the latter article, the authors conclude that the degree of localization of the peritoneal sepsis and the speed with which it develops probably are the most important determinants of outcome.

Individual cases will continue to be controversial, especially regarding the use of primary anastomosis; the Hartmann procedure generally is the most accepted operation (76). Prospective

Table 16.2.   Perforated Diverticulitis with Peritonitis: Other Selected Series

	Year	Number of Patients	Mortality (%)
1970s:			
Barabas (22)	1971	44	7
Byrne and Garick (23)	1971	15	26
Miller and Wichern (24)	1971	14	14
Watkins and Oliver (25)	1971	12	0
Whelan et al (26)	1971	25	28
Nahrwold (27)	1976	10	10
Nilsson (28)	1976	30	16
Taylor and Moore (29)	1976	60	18
Eng et al (30)	1977	8	0
Himal et al (31)	1977	26	
Howe et al (32)	1979	41	5
Median:			12
1980s:			
Theile (33)	1980	53	15
Edelmann (34)	1981	34	29
Sakai et al (35)	1981	32	28
Farkouh et al (36)	1982	15	7
Drumm and Clain (37)	1984	20	0
Underwood and Marks (38)	1984	12	8
Nagorney et al (39)	1985	121	12
Lambert et al (40)	1986	73	30
Finlay and Carter (41)	1987	37	27
Ravo et al (21)	1987	10	0
Alanis et al (42)	1989	12	
Berry et al (43)	1989	32	25
Median:			15
1990s:			
Hold et al (44)	1990	62	19
Peoples et al (45)	1990	50	22
Medina et al (46)	1991	6	10
Smirniotis et al (47)	1991	10	10
Nespoli et al (48)	1993	91	15
Kronborg (49)	1993	62	23
Saccomani et al (50)	1993	20	
Khan et al (51)	1995	60	21
Belmonte et al (52)	1996	11	0
Kumar et al (53)	1996	62	8
Median:			16

Table 16.3.   Acute Diverticulitis: Operative Pathologic Classification

Acute phlegmonous diverticulitis (no purulence)
Purulent diverticulitis
  1. Localized
       Localized peritonitis
       Abscess
  2. Diffuse
       Purulent
       Fecal

Modified after Krukowski ZH, Matheson NA. Emergency surgery for diverticular disease complicated by generalized fecal peritonitis: a review. Br J Surg 1984;71:921–927.

trials are very limited (49), individual experience is small, and the pathologic types of perforation are difficult to compare between studies. This, in part, reflects the great diversity of presentations that may complicate diverticulitis. More attention must be paid to stratifying these patients carefully by risk factors (48) and by stage of disease when comparing treatment methods; the reader is referred to excellent clinicopathologic analyses (77,78) and Krukowski and Matheson (6) for further information (Table 16.3).

REFERENCES

1. Smithwick RH. Experiences with surgical management of diverticulitis of the sigmoid. Ann Surg 1942;115:969–983. *A 15-year review of the Massachusetts General Hospital experience with the surgical treatment of diverticulitis. It specifically addresses the morbidity and mortality of the three-stage procedure.*
2. Graves HA, Franklin RM, Robbins LB, et al. Surgical management of perforated diverticulitis of the colon. Am Surg 1973;39:142–147. *A retrospective review comparing two-stage with three-stage procedures. They demonstrate improved mortality and morbidity with the two-stage procedure.*
3. Colcock BP. Surgical management of complicated diverticulitis. N Engl J Med 1958;259:570–573. *A review of the Lahey Clinic experience of complicated diverticulitis from 1947 to 1958. The conclusions emphasize the importance of early resection.*
4. Hartmann H. Nouveau procédé a'ablation des cancers de la partie terminal du colon pelvien. Cong Franç Chir 1923;30:411. *The original description of a two-stage procedure for management of emergency surgery on unprepped bowel. This procedure went on to become the standard of care and to carry the eponym of the author.*
5. Hinchey GC, Schaal GH, Richards MB. Treatment of perforated diverticulitis of the colon. Adv Surg 1978;12:85–105. *A retrospective review of patients with acute diverticulitis. Resection is recommended for most cases of acute diverticulitis. They propose a system of staging and then present their data using this system of codification. Contained perforations should be considered for primary anastomosis. Free perforations, however, should be managed with a Hartmann procedure.*
6. Krukowski ZH, Matheson NA. Emergency surgery for diverticular disease complicated by generalized fecal peritonitis: a review. Br J Surg 1984;71:921–927. *A meta-analysis of the numerous reviews comparing different surgical approaches to acute diverticulitis. They believe that the results support resection at the initial operation. Primary anastomosis may be considered in select cases with limited inflammation and soiling.*
7. Irvin GL, Horsley JS, Caruna JA. The morbidity and mortality of emergency operations for colorectal disease. Ann Surg 1984;199:598–603. *A detailed review from the VA Cooperative Studies Program, which demonstrates the high incidence of poor outcomes when surgeons operate on unprepped bowel.*
8. Irvin TT, Goligher JC. Aetiology and disruption of intestinal anastomosis. Br J Surg 1973;60:461–464. *This review concludes that patients with a poor bowel prep have a higher rate of anastomotic disruption.*
9. Schrock TR, Deveney CW, Dunphy EJ. Factors contributing to leakage of colonic anastomosis. Ann Surg 1973;177:513–518. *A thorough review of the cases of anastomotic dehiscence at UCSF. The paper specifically addresses the incidence and consequences of colonic suture line dehiscence. Additionally, it identifies risk factors for anastomotic disruption.*

10. Auguste L, Borrero E. Surgical management of perforated colonic diverticulitis. Arch Surg 1985;120:450–452. *A retrospective review of 116 patients with acute diverticulitis. They used the Hinchey classification and conclude that resection with primary anastomosis is a reasonable option. However, only one patient with free perforation received this treatment.*

11. Krukowski ZH, Koruth NM, Matheson NA. Evolving practice in acute diverticulitis. Br J Surg 1985;82:684–686. *A retrospective review from the University of Aberdeen that compares one- and two-stage procedures for acute diverticulitis.*

12. Shepard A, Keighley MR. Audit of complicated diverticular disease. Ann R Coll Surg Engl 1986;68:8–10. *A retrospective review looking at the mortality and morbidity of the different surgical approaches to acute diverticulitis.*

13. Sarin S, Boulos PB. Evaluation of current surgical management of acute inflammatory diverticular disease. Ann R Coll Surg Engl 1991;73:278–282. *A retrospective review of 31 patients who came to operation with acute diverticulitis. Fifteen of those patients had generalized peritonitis with a free perforation. They demonstrate the efficacy, the feasibility, and the improved mortality and morbidity of resection instead of diversion.*

14. Ross SE, Cobean RA, Hoyt DB, et al. Blunt colonic injury — a multicenter review. J Trauma 1992;33:379–384. *A multicenter review of blunt colon injuries. They conclude that gross fecal contamination is a strong contraindication to primary repair.*

15. Ryan P. The effect of surrounding infection upon leaking of colonic wound: experimental studies and clinical experience. Dis Colon Rectum 1970;13:124–126. *Dr. Ryan is a practitioner and proponent of primary anastomosis. This paper summarizes his clinical results and presents experimental data evaluating anastomotic healing in dogs with and without bacterial contamination surrounding the suture line.*

16. Haas PA, Haas GP. A critical evaluation of the Hartmann's procedure. Am Surg 1988;54:381–385. *The authors reviewed the clinical course of 150 patients who had undergone a Hartmann procedure. They report the rate of colostomy takedown and the incidence of complications related to the pouch.*

17. Hunt TK, Hawley PR. Surgical judgment and the colonic anastomosis. Dis Colon Rectum 1969;12:167–171. *A good discussion of the multiple factors that affect collagen synthesis and thus are implicated in anastomotic disruption.*

18. Koruth NO, Krukowski ZH, Youngson GG, et al. Intra-operative colonic irrigation in the management of left-sided large bowel emergencies. Br J Surg 1985;72:708–711. *In a consecutive series of 93 patients (including 36 with perforation and peritonitis), 61 had primary bowel resection with immediate anastomosis following intraoperative irrigation. Twelve patients with perforation and peritonitis had primary anastomosis, with one death.*

19. Murray J, Schoetz D, Coller J. Intraoperative colonic lavage and primary anastomosis in nonelective colon resection. Dis Colon Rectum 1991;34:527–531. *Of the 25 patients having urgent segmental left colectomy, 13 had diverticular disease that included five patients with obstruction, two patients with perforation, and four patients with abscess.*

20. Ravo B. Colorectal anastomotic healing and intracolonic bypass procedure. Surg Clin North Am 1988; 68:1267–1294. *A review of this technique with 131 references.*

21. Ravo B, Mishrick A, Addei K, et al. The treatment of perforated diverticulitis by one-stage intracolonic bypass procedures. Surgery 1987;102:771–775. *Twenty-eight patients with perforated diverticulitis, including 10 with peritonitis, underwent one-stage intracolonic bypass with no deaths or anastomotic leaks.*

22. Barabas AP. Peritonitis due to diverticular disease of the colon: a review of 44 cases. Proc R Soc Med 1971;64:253–254. *The author recommends that the surgeon use restraint in performing immediate resection, believing that antibiotic therapy without resection can be of great benefit.*

23. Byrne JJ, Garick EI. Surgical treatment of diverticulitis. Am J Surg 1971;121:379–384. *An informative review of the evolution of surgical procedures for treating complications of diverticular disease. The poor results with perforation and diffuse peritonitis are discussed; with 45 references.*

24. Miller DW Jr, Wichern WA Jr. Perforated sigmoid diverticulitis. Appraisal of primary versus delayed resection. Am J Surg 1971;121:536–540. *Of 200 patients having surgery for diverticular disease, 14 had free perforation and diffusing peritonitis. Immediate excision of the perforated segment is recommended; the dangers of immediate anastomosis are discussed.*

25. Watkins GL, Oliver GA. Surgical treatment of acute perforative sigmoid diverticulitis. Surgery 1971;69:215–219. *A review of 12 consecutive cases of acute diverticulitis with diffuse peritonitis treated successfully with exteriorization and later resection. The importance of eliminating the perforated segment from the peritoneal cavity at the initial operation is emphasized.*

26. Whelan CS, Furcinitti JF, Lavarreda C. Surgical management of perforated lesions of the colon with diffusing peritonitis. Am J Surg 1971;121:374–378. *A review of 25 patients. The perforated segment should be excised at the first operation.*

27. Nahrwold DL, Demuth WE. Diverticulitis with perforation into the peritoneal cavity. Ann Surg 1976; 185:80–83. *Ten consecutive patients were treated with sigmoid resection and temporary end colostomy, with one death.*

28. Nilsson LO. Surgical treatment of perforations of the sigmoid colon. Acta Chir Scand 1976;142:467–469. *The authors compare two groups of patients during different time periods; removal or exteriorization of the bowel was not associated with postoperative mortality, in contrast to drainage and colostomy (33% mortality).*

29. Taylor JD, Moore KA. Generalized peritonitis complicating diverticulitis of the sigmoid colon. J R Coll Surg Edinb 1976;21:348–352. *A retrospective study of 60 patients with generalized peritonitis. The prognosis was worse with fecal peritonitis (35% mortality) than with nonfecal peritonitis (12% mortality).*

30. Eng K, Ranson JH, Localio SA. Resection of the perforated segment. A significant advance in treatment of diverticulitis with free perforation or abscess. Am J Surg 1977;133:67–72. *None of the eight patients with generalized peritonitis died following primary resection.*

31. Himal HD, Ashby DB, Didnan JP, et al. Management of perforating diverticulitis of the colon. Surg Gynecol Obstet 1977;144:225–226. *A retrospective study including 26 patients with free perforation. The importance of removal of the septic focus is emphasized.*
32. Howe JH, Casali RE, Westbrook KC, et al. Acute perforations of the sigmoid colon secondary to diverticulitis. Am J Surg 1979;137:184–187. *Resection is the primary goal of therapy for these patients.*
33. Theile D. The management of perforated diverticulitis with diffuse peritonitis. Aust NZ J Surg 1980;50:47–49. *A review of 53 patients. Primary resection without anastomosis is advocated.*
34. Edelmann G. Surgical treatment of colonic diverticulitis: a report of 205 cases. Int Surg 1981;66:119–124. *Thirty-six patients had generalized peritonitis. All major types of complications are discussed as well in this series.*
35. Sakai L, Daake J, Kaminski D. Acute perforation of sigmoid diverticula. Am J Surg 1981;142:712–716. *This review includes 32 patients with free perforation (eight were on chronic steroid therapy). Control of the site of perforation and aggressive peritoneal irrigation are promoted.*
36. Farkouh E, Hellou G, Allard M, et al. Resection and primary anastomosis for diverticulitis with perforation and peritonitis. Can J Surg 1982;25:314–316. *In 15 patients, there was one anastomotic leak and one death from acute pulmonary edema.*
37. Drumm J, Clain A. The management of acute colonic diverticulitis with suppurative peritonitis. Ann R Coll Surg Engl 1984;66:90–91. *The authors propose a defunctioning transverse colostomy, drainage, and administration of antibiotics for perforated diverticulitis with purulent peritonitis.*
38. Underwood JW, Marks CG. The septic complications of sigmoid diverticular disease. Br J Surg 1984;71: 209–211. *A study of 41 patients with septic complications, including 12 with generalized peritonitis.*
39. Nagorney DM, Adson MA, Pemberton JH. Sigmoid diverticulitis with perforation and generalized peritonitis. Dis Colon Rectum 1985;28:71–75. *One hundred twenty-one consecutive patients with perforated sigmoid diverticulitis were examined: the mortality was 26% for patients treated by colostomy and drainage and 7% for those having colostomy and resection or exteriorization.*
40. Lambert ME, Knox RA, Schofield PF, et al. Management of the septic complications of diverticular disease. Br J Surg 1986;73:576–579. *A series of 105 patients, including 73 with communicating or noncommunicating purulent peritonitis.*
41. Finlay IG, Carter DC. A comparison of emergency resection and staged management in diverticular disease. Dis Colon Rectum 1987;30:929–933. *Emergency resection carried a lower morbidity than colostomy and drainage, but there was no statistically significant difference in mortality.*
42. Alanis A, Papanicolaou GK, Tadros RR, et al. Primary resection and anastomosis for treatment of acute diverticulitis. Dis Colon Rectum 1989;32:933–939. *Primary resection and anastomosis has satisfactory results in patients with stages I–III perforated diverticulitis.*
43. Berry AR, Turner WH, Mortensen NJ, et al. Emergency surgery for complicated diverticular disease: a five year experience. Dis Colon Rectum 1989;32:849–854. *This series included 32 patients with free perforations. Eight patients died after perforation and most had evidence of persistent sepsis. The possibility of rectal stump breakdown or inadequate resection during the Hartmann procedure is raised.*
44. Hold M, Denck H, Bull P. Surgical management of perforating diverticular disease in Austria. Int J Colorectal Dis 1990;5:195–199. *A countrywide study of 241 patients with a 9% operative mortality rate. The mortality was proportional to the extent of peritonitis.*
45. Peoples JB, Vilk DR, Maguire JP, et al. Reassessment of primary resection of the perforated segment for severe colonic diverticulitis. Am J Surg 1990;159:291–294. *In a retrospective review, colostomy and drainage were largely replaced by primary resection with colostomy, although the mortality increased from 14% to 19% in the same time interval.*
46. Medina VA, Papanicolaou GK, Tadros RR, et al. Acute perforated diverticulitis: primary resection and anastomosis. Conn Med 1991;55:258–261. *A study of six patients with fecal peritonitis complicating sigmoid diverticulitis. The authors believe that, depending on other factors, fecal peritonitis is no longer an absolute contraindication to immediate bowel reconstruction.*
47. Smirniotis V, Tsoutsos D, Fotopoulos A, et al. Perforated diverticulitis: a surgical dilemma. Int Surg 1991;76:44–47. *Resection of the perforated sigmoid with or without anastomosis is recommended.*
48. Nespoli A, Ravizzini C, Trivella M, et al. The choice of surgical procedure for peritonitis due to colonic perforation. Arch Surg 1993;128:814–818. *The mortality depended on the severity of peritonitis, not on the surgical procedure.*
49. Kronborg O. Treatment of perforated sigmoid diverticulitis: a prospective randomized trial. Br J Surg 1993;80:505–507. *Patients having transverse colostomy and suture of a perforation had a lower mortality than those having immediate resection in the presence of purulent peritonitis.*
50. Saccomani GE, Santi F, Gramegna A. Primary resection with and without anastomosis for perforation of acute diverticulitis. Acta Chir Belg 1993;93:169–172. *Twenty patients had generalized peritonitis. The importance of vigorous intraperitoneal lavage is stressed when performing resection and anastomosis.*
51. Khan AL, Ah-See AK, Crofts TJ. Surgical management of the septic complications of diverticular disease. Ann R Coll Surg Engl 1995;77:16–20. *Survival was worse in patients older than 70 years of age, in those with severe medical illness, in those with generalized peritonitis, and in patients with an APACHE II score higher than 11.*
52. Belmonte C, Klas JV, Perez JJ, et al. The Hartmann procedure. First choice or last resort in diverticular disease. Arch Surg 1996;131:612–617. *A study of the surgical course of 227 patients with diverticular disease, with a breakdown into pathologic stages. Eleven patients had purulent or feculent peritonitis.*
53. Kumar P, Sangwan YP, Horton A, et al. Distal mucus fistula following resection for perforated sigmoid

diverticular disease. J R Coll Surg Edinb 1996;41:316–318. *The authors believe that this operation may lead to higher reversal rates; it also reduces operating time and hospital stay without compromised outcome.*

54. Dandekar NV, McCann WJ. Primary resection and anastomosis in the management of perforation of diverticulitis of the sigmoid flexure and diffuse peritonitis. Dis Colon Rectum 1969;12:172–175. *The authors advocate primary resection and anastomosis after reviewing the hospital course of 26 patients with perforation and diffuse peritonitis.*

55. Large JM. Treatment of perforated diverticulitis. Lancet 1964;1:413–414. *All 18 patients had resection and immediate anastomosis; there were two postoperative deaths.*

56. Stelzner M, Vlahakos DV, Milford EL, et al. Colonic perforations after renal transplantation. J Am Coll Surg 1997;184:63–69. *This study spanning the period 1991–1995 includes 21 colonic perforations due to diverticulitis; 8 of the 26 patients with diverticulitis died.*

57. Dawson JL, Hanon I, Roxburgh RA. Diverticulitis complicated by diffuse peritonitis. Br J Surg 1965;52:354–358. *Seventy-nine patients in this series were operated upon: 68 had purulent peritonitis (19 died) and 11 had fecal peritonitis (6 died). In virtually all patients, diffuse peritonitis was the first significant manifestation of diverticulitis.*

58. Crile G. Dangers of conservative surgery in abdominal emergencies. Surgery 1954;35:122–123. *An editorial stressing the importance of removing the source of sepsis when the colon is perforated.*

59. Arnheim EE. Diverticulitis of the colon with special reference to the surgical complications. Ann Surg 1940;112:352–369. *A comprehensive examination of the different pathologic types of diverticulitis and a review of surgical treatment.*

60. Gregg RO. The place of emergency resection in the management of obstructing and perforating lesions of the colon. Surgery 1955;37:754–761. *The author outlines important principles of emergency surgery involving the colon. He emphasizes that resection of the perforated colon can be managed technically without undue difficulty.*

61. Arnheim EE. Diverticulitis of the colon with special reference to the surgical complications. Ann Surg 1940;112:352–369. *A detailed account of the pathologic forms of diverticulitis, including the history of medical and surgical treatment, with 31 references.*

62. Belding HH III. Acute perforated diverticulitis of the sigmoid colon with generalized peritonitis. Arch Surg 1957;74:511–515. *All four patients were treated with one-stage procedures.*

63. Lazarus JA. Perforated sigmoiditis with generalized peritonitis. Am J Surg 1933;22:284–289. *An early report of perforated diverticulitis in four patients. Inability to demonstrate the site of perforation does not rule out this condition.*

64. Smiley DF. Perforated sigmoid diverticulitis with spreading peritonitis. Am J Surg 1966;111:431–434. *Resection or exteriorization of the perforated colon is recommended; the mortality rate was 62% after proximal colostomy and drainage.*

65. Ryan P. Emergency resection and anastomosis for perforated sigmoid diverticulitis. Br J Surg 1958;45:611–616. *Immediate resection is recommended; an anastomosis is not advocated with extensive diffusing peritonitis.*

66. Large JM. Treatment of perforated diverticulitis. Lancet 1964;2:413–414. *Eighteen patients had peritonitis from free perforation or from rupture of a pericolic abscess; two patients died after operation. Aggressive resection of the diseased segment is recommended.*

67. Roxburgh RA, Dawson JL, Yeo R. Emergency resection in treatment of diverticular disease of colon complicated by peritonitis. Br Med J 1968;3:465–466. *A study of 25 consecutive patients; 24 had emergency resection. The 22 patients with purulent peritonitis survived, and the three patients with fecal peritonitis died.*

68. MacLaren IF. Perforated diverticulitis. A survey of 75 cases. J R Coll Surg Edinb 1957;3:129–144. *An in-depth analysis of the problem in this early study. Patients with feculent peritonitis frequently present in shock.*

69. Wara P, Sorensen K, Berg V, et al. The outcome of staged management of complicated diverticular disease of the colon. Acta Chir Scand 1981;147:209–214. *A study from the University of Aarhus that reviews many of the problems associated with a diverting colostomy.*

70. Bohnen J, Boulanger M, Meakins JL, et al. Prognosis in generalized peritonitis. Relation to cause and risk factors. Arch Surg 1983;118:285–290. *An analysis of 176 patients with generalized peritonitis, including six cases of perforated sigmoid diverticulitis with a 50% mortality rate.*

71. Greif JM, Fried G, McSherry CK. Surgical treatment of perforated diverticulitis of the sigmoid colon. Dis Colon Rectum 1980;23:483–487. *A retrospective literature review including 833 patients having emergency operation for perforated diverticulitis with diffuse peritonitis. The operative mortality decreased from 29% when the perforated segment was left in place to 12% when the perforated segment was exteriorized or resected.*

72. Scholefield JH, Wyman A, Rogers K. Management of generalized fecal peritonitis — can we do better? J R Soc Med 1991;89:664–666. *The authors promote the use of repeated abdominal lavage and debridement to reduce complications of generalized fecal peritonitis.*

73. Senapati A, Marks CG. Management of perforated diverticular disease. Ann R Coll Surg Engl 1995;77:161–162. *The authors recommend a multicenter trial to assess the optimal surgical management of perforated diverticulitis.*

74. Killingback M. Management of perforated diverticulitis. Surg Clin North Am 1983;63:97–115. *A well-illustrated discussion of the problem.*

75. Welch CE, Welch JP. Resection and anastomosis of the colon in the presence of peritonitis. In: Delaney JP, Varco RL, eds. Controversies in surgery II. Philadelphia: WB Saunders, 1983:341–349. *The authors believe it is more hazardous to attempt an anastomosis in the presence of peritonitis, because anastomotic healing is impaired. Includes 54 references.*

76. Pain J, Cahill J. Surgical options for left-sided large bowel emergencies. Ann R Coll Surg Engl 1991;73:394–397. *A survey of surgeons performing these types of procedures; the popularity of the Hartmann procedure for colonic perforation was confirmed.*

77. Hughes ES, Cuthbertson AM, Garden AB. The surgical management of acute diverticulitis. Med J Aust 1963;1:780–782. *An excellent early description of the various pathologic types of diverticulitis.*
78. Hughes LE. Complications of diverticular disease: inflammation, obstruction and bleeding. Clin Gastroenterol 1975;4:147–170. *Part of an excellent monograph on diverticular disease. The author presents the clinicopathologic aspects of various complications with much detail in a readable style.*
79. Keighley MR, Williams NS. Surgery of the anus, rectum and colon. London: WB Saunders, 1993 (Figs. 16.4, 16.11).
80. Todd IP, Fielding LP, eds. Rob & Smith's Operative surgery. Alimentary tract and abdominal wall. 3. Colon, rectum and anus. 4th ed. London: Butterworths, 1983 (Figs. 16.5, 16.6, 16.7, 16.10).
81. Welch JP. Diverticular disease. In: Welch JP, ed. Bowel obstruction. Differential diagnosis and clinical management. Philadelphia: WB Saunders, 1990:589–599 (Figs. 16.8, 16.9).

17 Subacute Diverticulitis

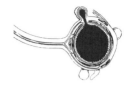

William V. Sardella, MD
James Pingpank, MD

> ### KEY POINTS
> - Characterized by "smoldering" lower abdominal pain, fever, altered bowel habits
> - Can present with localized perforation, abscess formation, or large bowel obstruction
> - Medical treatment may require hospitalization with bowel rest and broad-spectrum antibiotics
> - Whenever possible, surgical therapy should be deferred until the inflammatory process has been treated
> - Generally a single-stage resection is possible

ILLUSTRATIVE CASE

A 57-year-old male with a history of diverticulitis 3 years previously presented with 6 weeks of recurrent left lower quadrant pain and low-grade fever initially responsive to oral antibiotics. Over a 3-day period, he noted increased abdominal discomfort associated with fever to 102°F, chills, nausea, and obstipation.

Vital signs at the time of presentation included a temperature of 101.6°F, pulse of 120, blood pressure of 110/70, and a normal respiratory rate. The patient appeared ill but not toxic. Abdominal examination revealed moderate distention, tympany, and localized left lower quadrant tenderness. Rectal examination was unremarkable.

Among laboratory studies were a white blood cell count of 18,600, hematocrit of 42, and a normal amylase and urinalysis. Abdominal films showed moderate small bowel distention with air throughout a nondilated colon, consistent with ileus or early partial small bowel obstruction.

Initial management consisted of nasogastric tube decompression, intravenous hydration, and broad-spectrum antibiotics. Computed tomography (CT) scan revealed numerous diverticula and a large inflammatory mass or phlegmon involving the sigmoid colon and adjacent paracolic fat. Moderate small bowel distention was also noted, but without evidence of free fluid or extraluminal air.

During the following 48 hours, abdominal distention lessened with return of bowel function. However, despite intravenous antibiotics, temperature spikes to 101°F continued, as well as persistent left lower quadrant tenderness. After 5 days of treatment with antibiotics, in the absence of significant improvement, a repeat CT scan was performed, which revealed a persistent phlegmon involving the sigmoid colon with a discrete abscess visible within the adjacent mesentery. Numerous mildly dilated small bowel loops were noted adjacent to and overlying the phlegmon, precluding safe access for percutaneous drainage.

Because of failed medical treatment, the patient was taken to the operating room. A preoperative bowel preparation was well tolerated. Multiple dilated small bowel loops were found adherent to an inflammatory mass involving the sigmoid colon and its mesentery. Numerous inflammatory adhesions were divided, and an en bloc resection of the sigmoid colon and the adjacent mesenteric abscess was performed with a primary anastomosis. The patient experienced an uneventful recovery.

CASE COMMENTS

This case illustrates many of the challenging aspects of subacute diverticulitis, a form of "smoldering" inflammation despite antibiotic coverage that leads to ultimate failure of medical treatment and necessitates surgical intervention. Recurrent or persistent fever in such patients should prompt suspicion of an abscess, and a follow-up CT scan is indicated before surgical intervention. Whenever possible, discrete abscesses should be percutaneously drained preoperatively (see Chapter 15) to minimize intraoperative contamination and facilitate a one-stage resection.

In addition, a gentle or modified bowel preparation performed preoperatively is indicated and generally is well tolerated. At times, persistent ileus or associated small bowel obstruction will interfere with bowel preparation. In such cases, resection is performed and, in properly selected patients, on-table lavage can be used, followed by primary anastomosis (see Chapter 20).

Surgery for subacute diverticulitis can be quite challenging, and the technical aspects are detailed in this chapter. Certain aspects are worth reiterating. All patients should be placed in lithotomy position with both legs in stirrups for placement of ureteral stents when necessary or for use of intraluminal stapling devices. Dissection is begun in an area with limited inflammatory change, usually the proximal sigmoid or distal descending colon. The proximal ureter is identified early in the course of the procedure and followed distally as the inflammatory mass is mobilized. Difficulty in ureteral identification should prompt consideration of ureteral stents. The sigmoid colon should be mobilized completely before division of the mesentery. Significant induration of the paracolic mesentery or an intramesenteric abscess requires clamping of the mesenteric vessels near their origin below the level of inflammation. Upon completion of the resection, a one-stage procedure with primary anastomosis is possible in most cases (see Editorial Comments section).

CLINICAL PRESENTATION

Diverticulitis is a spectrum of illnesses and consequently may present with a variety of clinical manifestations. The classic constellation of fever, left lower quadrant pain, and leukocytosis, although usually present, may be conspicuously absent. Although free perforation usually is an acute, catastrophic, and clinically obvious event, chronic or subacute diverticulitis often is more subtle or less striking in its presentation and, at times, may even present with rather vague symptoms leading to confusion in diagnosis.

Subacute diverticulitis tends to be characterized by recurrent lower abdominal pain, low-grade fever, and alterations in bowel habits. Whereas most patients experience abdominal discomfort localized to the left lower quadrant, others may suffer from recurrent suprapubic, right lower quadrant, or more generalized abdominal complaints. Occasionally, patients experience a vague pelvic pressure rather than symptoms of true discomfort. *The varied clinical presentation can lead to diagnostic confusion and delayed or inappropriate treatment.*

Whereas most patients experience repeated flare-ups or attacks of similar symptoms with each episode, others may experience a more varied symptom complex, because recurrent inflammation leads to intramural fibrosis and chronic symptoms of partial colonic obstruction. *Subacute diverticulitis, therefore, includes a spectrum of illnesses from mild, intermittent attacks, perhaps punctuated with an occasional more severe episode, to a chronic, intractable variety with smoldering inflammation.*

DIAGNOSIS

Because of its varied clinical presentation, subacute diverticulitis must be distinguished from other intra-abdominal conditions that may require alternative treatment. The differential diagnosis includes carcinoma of the colon, inflammatory bowel disease, irritable bowel syndrome, intermittent volvulus, and partial intestinal and ureteral obstruction. In females, gynecologic causes of lower abdominal pain must be considered.

Initial evaluation of a patient with subacute diverticulitis is similar to that of patients with other intra-abdominal illnesses. A thorough history must be obtained, followed by an equally complete physical examination, focusing on the abdominal findings as well as information gleaned from rectal and pelvic examinations. Although a satisfactory diagnosis can be made from this information in most cases, additional information may be obtained from simple studies such as a complete blood count and urinalysis. Occasionally, a sedimentation rate and amylase or lipase level may be of additional diagnostic assistance.

Patients presenting with acute abdominal pain or signs of peritonitis warrant a more thorough evaluation, including radiographic studies. Plain abdominal films (two views) to evaluate for possible perforation or obstruction are a relatively simple and helpful next step. In some cases, additional radiographic studies such as a CT scan may be required, not only to help confirm the diagnosis of diverticulitis but to assess the degree and location of the inflammatory process, as well as the presence of complications such as localized perforation or abscess formation. Abdominal ultrasound, although traditionally helpful in diagnosing intra-abdominal abscesses, tends to be less informative than CT scan and, at times, less accurate due to technical limitations imposed by adjacent or overlying bowel gas. In milder cases of diverticulitis or after the acute inflammatory process resolves, a gentle or low-pressure barium enema examination may provide additional useful diagnostic information.

MEDICAL TREATMENT

Appropriate treatment of diverticulitis must be individualized and is based on the severity of the patient's clinical presentation, including the presence or absence of complications, as well as the underlying general medical condition. Mild cases of diverticulitis in healthy patients can be treated simply and effectively with oral antibiotics and a low-residue diet. More severe cases presenting with fever and significant but localized tenderness will likely require treatment with broad-spectrum intravenous antibiotics and bowel rest. Most cases of diverticulitis can be classified as mild to moderate in severity; these cases will resolve with medical management.

Clinically speaking, patients with *subacute* diverticulitis usually present with a history of prior multiple attacks of mild to moderate inflammation initially responsive to antibiotics, followed by a more substantial illness that does not readily respond to conventional medical therapy. The patient usually has fever, significant localized abdominal tenderness, and possibly abdominal distention or a palpable mass. Although, by definition, free intra-abdominal perforation has not occurred, a contained perforation with an associated paracolic phlegmon or abscess frequently is present. In addition, associated small or large bowel obstruction may further complicate the picture.

Medical treatment of such cases of subacute diverticulitis requires hospitalization, intravenous hydration, broad-spectrum antibiotics, and bowel rest. Bowel distention, whether secondary to illness or obstruction, may require decompression with a nasogastric tube. An indwelling urinary catheter will aid in assessment of the patient's fluid status.

Radiologic evaluation generally should include a CT scan (preferably with water-soluble oral and rectal contrast) to evaluate the location and degree of the inflammatory process as well as the presence of complications such as abscess or obstruction. Collections of pus, if localized and percutaneously accessible, should be drained whenever possible by a skilled, interventional radiologist (See Chapter 15). With aggressive medical management, most patients experience clinical improvement if not complete resolution of symptoms.

Occasionally, patients with subacute diverticulitis will fail to respond to the aforementioned medical treatment. These patients tend to have either severe localized inflammation in the form of a phlegmon alone or in conjunction with an undrained paracolic or mesenteric abscess. Clinical signs of ongoing inflammation, such as persistent fever, abdominal tenderness, and leukocytosis despite medical treatment warrant repeat radiologic evaluation to reassess for an abscess. In the absence of a drainable collection, a worsening clinical condition of the patient (increasing abdominal tenderness, distention, or overt signs of sepsis) warrant surgical intervention. *Fortunately, unless an undrained abscess is present, most patients with subacute diverticulitis either improve dramatically or resolve clinically with medical therapy, allowing a less urgent operative approach.*

SURGICAL TREATMENT

Indications

Surgical treatment of diverticulitis is reserved for recurrent attacks of mild to moderate severity or complications of acute or subacute inflammation such as free perforation, obstruction, or localized perforation with abscess formation. Whenever possible, in the absence of free perforation, surgery should be deferred until the inflammatory process can be assessed adequately and a trial of medical therapy can be initiated. Worsening clinical condition of the patient despite aggressive medical management warrants either additional imaging studies to reevaluate for delayed complications and/or surgical intervention. *Most patients with subacute diverticulitis present with either a history of smoldering inflammation or previous episodes of diverticulitis and should be considered for resection.*

Preoperative Preparation

Preoperative preparation includes a thorough knowledge of the extent and severity of the inflammatory process as well as associated medical illnesses. Patients should be hydrated well with attention to correction of electrolyte disturbances, anemia, and malnutrition. With the institution of medical therapy, the inflammatory process and associated ileus tends to resolve, allowing preoperative bowel cleansing. Whenever possible, a mechanical and antibiotic bowel preparation should be used. In the presence of recent diverticulitis, stimulant laxatives are best avoided and a lavage solution is preferred. Preoperative siting of potential stomal sites is recommended.

Usually the entire colon should be evaluated preoperatively by either barium enema or colonoscopy to confirm the diagnosis of diverticulitis and to rule out concurrent pathology. In the absence of a recent CT scan, an intravenous pyelogram (IVP) should be considered.

Technical Factors

Intraoperatively, the patient is placed in a supine position and general anesthesia is administered. Placement of the lower extremities in stirrups (lithotomy position) allows access to the perineum for placement of ureteral stents (if deemed necessary) or use of intraluminal stapling devices. Ureteral stents (although not necessary in most cases), allow ready identification of the ureters and are quite helpful in selected cases of severe acute or chronic inflammation with associated edema and/or fibrosis.

The peritoneal cavity usually is entered through a low midline incision. After a careful assessment of the disease process as well as examination of the remaining abdominal contents, the small bowel is packed away in the upper abdomen. A self-retaining retractor is quite helpful in providing and maintaining exposure of the operative field throughout the course of the procedure.

The dissection begins in an area of limited inflammation, usually the distal descending or proximal sigmoid colon. With this approach, normal tissue planes allow safe dissection along the lateral peritoneal reflection (line of Toldt) and mobilization of the sigmoid colon and its mesentery from underlying retroperitoneal strictures. The left ureter is identified proximally and followed distally as it enters the pelvis with careful surgical technique. With judicious use of ureteral stents in properly selected cases, most ureteral injuries can be avoided.

After the sigmoid colon has been well mobilized with its mesentery and the left ureter visualized clearly, the colon should be divided proximally through a soft and pliable area of the distal descending colon. This maneuver is facilitated by use of a linear stapling device but also can be accomplished quite satisfactorily with conventional bowel clamps.

Dividing the bowel proximally enhances access to the sigmoid mesentery, which is sequentially ligated and divided. *In the presence of subacute diverticulitis, the mesentery of the sigmoid colon is markedly thickened and indurated. In addition, the presence of chronic inflammation, fibrosis, or a mesenteric abscess may preclude safe dissection within the paracolic mesentery,* and a plane of dissection lower on the mesentery near its base may be necessary (Figure 17.1, p. 248). It is of paramount importance, therefore, to mobilize the sigmoid colon and its mesentery well so that injury to the left ureter and other retroperitoneal structures is avoided.

Uninflamed mesentery can be readily divided between clamps and ligated using standard techniques. Major branches of the inferior mesenteric vessels should be either doubly tied or suture ligated. *Whenever possible, when resecting the sigmoid colon for benign disease, both the left colic and superior hemorrhoidal branches of the inferior mesenteric vessels should be preserved,* because these vessels provide blood supply to both the proximal and distal ends of the bowel for subsequent anastomosis. A contained intramesenteric (paracolic) abscess can be resected safely, along with the sigmoid colon, and without risk of significant contamination. Rarely, an intramesenteric abscess may extend into or become adherent to retroperitoneal structures such as the left ureter or iliac vessels. In such a situation, mesenteric mobilization may be extremely dangerous and consideration should be given to drainage of the abscess and proximal fecal diversion.

The distal limit of dissection should be at the convergence of the teniae coli, usually near the level of the sacral promontory. The rectum at the distal margin of resection should be soft, pliable, and free of inflammatory changes. Division of the rectum may be accomplished with stapling devices or conventional bowel clamps based on the surgeon's preference and anticipated anastomotic technique. At the time of laparotomy, the surgical specimen should be examined to confirm the diagnosis.

Before anastomosis, the descending colon and its mesentery should be mobilized sufficiently along the lateral peritoneal reflection as well as posteriorly along the Gerota's fascia to enable a tension-free anastomosis. Occasionally, mobilization of the splenic flexure and/or rectum may be required.

A satisfactory anastomosis can be accomplished in a variety of ways using conventional hand-sewn or stapling techniques. However, it is imperative that the surgeon assess the bowel ends for adequacy of vascularity, completeness of bowel preparation, and absence of tension prior to performing the anastomosis. Lack of vascularity of either bowel end requires further resection to an area of well-perfused bowel. Inadequate bowel preparation should prompt consideration of a temporary colostomy (Hartmann procedure), anastomosis with proximal fecal diversion, or use of on-table lavage. Presence of anastomotic tension is unacceptable and further mobilization either proximally and/or distally is required.

SURGICAL OPTIONS — TO ANASTOMOSE OR NOT?

In the present era, the surgical treatment of diverticulitis should preferably involve resection of the diseased segment and anastomosis (one-stage) (1–9). Three-stage procedures are unduly morbid and are largely of historic interest. Occasionally, despite meticulous and appropriate management, the patient's condition will mandate that a two-stage procedure be performed. Specifically, *in the presence of significant inflammation, grossly distended or poorly prepared bowel, poor general medical condition, or an immunocompromised state, a one-stage procedure may be ill-advised and a Hartmann procedure should be performed.*

At times, under less than ideal circumstances, resection and anastomosis with proximal diversion are appropriate. Our preference is to use a loop ileostomy because of its ease of construction, excellent blood supply, "pouchability," and simplicity of closure. In our experience, transverse colostomy is harder to construct, more difficult to care for, a possible source of prolapse, and is, therefore, an inferior stoma. In most cases, the risk of disruption of a "protected" anastomosis is low, and the simplicity of the second-stage procedure (i.e., closure of the stoma) more than outweighs its limited risk. Although the immediate safety of a Hartmann procedure is apparent as a first-stage procedure, restoration of intestinal continuity requires a second major abdominal procedure, which can be technically challenging and is associated with considerable morbidity and occasional mortality (Chapter 19).

Acute diverticulitis with free perforation and feculent or diffusing peritonitis should be treated with a two-stage procedure, preferably resection of the perforated bowel with end colostomy and closure of the distal segment (10–12) (see Chapter 16). In the occasional patient with *severe* subacute diverticulitis or poor general medical condition, a Hartmann procedure may be required. Rarely, in the presence of hemodynamic instability or fixation

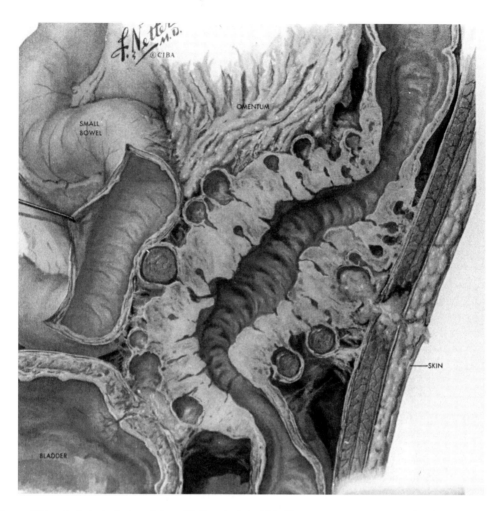

Figure 17.1. Artist's depiction of sigmoid diverticulitis. This illustration represents well the thickening in the pericolic area that characterizes a classic case of "smoldering" subacute diverticulitis. (Reprinted with permission from Oppenheimer E, ed. The CIBA collection of medical illustrations. Part II: Lower digestive tract. West Caldwell, N.J.: CIBA Pharmaceutical Co., 1962;3:131) [Ref. 14].

of the bowel or mesentery to retroperitoneal structures, a three-stage procedure with initial diversion and drainage is warranted.

CONCLUSIONS

Surgical treatment of subacute diverticulitis is challenging and requires considerable skill and judgment. In most cases, preoperative medical treatment with antibiotics and bowel rest allows the acute inflammatory component and associated ileus to resolve. Mechanical bowel preparation can thus be performed, followed by a one-stage surgical procedure if indicated. Whenever possible, intra-abdominal abscesses should be drained percutaneously to facilitate resolution of inflammation and/or sepsis prior to surgical intervention. With careful attention to detail both preoperatively and intraoperatively, most patients with subacute diverticulitis can undergo a one-stage procedure (resection and anastomosis) safely with expectation of a favorable outcome.

EDITORIAL COMMENTS

This chapter deals with a difficult variant of diverticulitis that can be described as persistent, relentless, progressive (13), smoldering, or ongoing. Management of these cases requires surgical timing and technical expertise to achieve a successful outcome. The pathologic changes are to be contrasted with those of free perforation with diffuse peritonitis or with recurrent diverticulitis (see Chapter 7), characterized by discrete attacks that usually resolve promptly with medical therapy. Persistent inflammation leads to increasing fibrosis and colonic thickening. The phlegmonous nature of inflammation is reminiscent of "malignant" diverticulitis, discussed in Chapter 13. Patients do not tend to fully recover from an attack and may continue to complain of abdominal pain, failure to thrive, and irregular bowel habits.

The goal of surgical treatment of subacute diverticulitis is to eradicate the diseased bowel while performing a safe, single-stage procedure. Careful attention to the details discussed within this chapter should allow this to occur in most cases.

Occasionally, as a result of associated medical problems or extensive inflammation, a modest increase in the risk of anastomotic complications is present and consideration should be given to performing a primary anastomosis and proximal diversion. In such cases, we prefer to use a loop ileostomy (see text). Actively septic or poor-risk patients should be treated with resection and colostomy (Hartmann procedure). Fortunately, for subacute diverticulitis, this is not commonly required. Furthermore, a three-stage procedure with initial proximal diversion and drainage is rarely indicated.

REFERENCES

1. Alanis A, Papanicolaou GK, Tadros RT, et al. Primary resection and anastomosis for treatment of acute diverticulitis. Dis Colon Rectum 1989;32:933–939. *Primary resection and anastomosis was satisfactory for most patients with Hinchey stages I–III perforated diverticulitis.*
2. Ambrosetti P, Robert J, Witzig JA, et al. Incidence, outcome, and proposed management of isolated abscesses complicating acute left-sided diverticulitis: a prospective study of 140 patients. Dis Colon Rectum 1992;35:1072–1076. *A prospective study of 140 consecutive patients. Mesocolic abscesses usually can be managed conservatively. Pelvic and intra-abdominal abscesses are more aggressive and require a two-stage surgical procedure if percutaneous drainage cannot be performed.*
3. Belmonte C, Klas JV, Perez JJ, et al. The Hartmann procedure: first choice or last resort in diverticular disease? Arch Surg 1996;131:612–617. *Primary anastomosis is safe with no abscesses and localized abscesses and should be performed selectively on patients with pelvic abscesses and peritonitis.*
4. Detry R, James J, Kartheuse A. Acute localized diverticulitis: optimum management requires accurate staging. Int J Colorectal Dis 1992;7:38–42. *An analysis of 120 patients with localized acute sigmoid diverticulitis. Most patients with acute phlegmonous diverticulitis did well with conservative treatment; high rates of recurrence and complications, however, were seen when pericolic abscesses were present.*
5. Hackford A, Schoetz D, Coller J, et al. Surgical management of complicated diverticulitis. Dis Colon Rectum 1985;28:317–321. *A study of 140 patients; 86 had resection and primary anastomosis with an 18% morbidity rate and 1% mortality rate. The average length of hospitalization for a one-stage procedure was 21 days.*
6. Levien D, Mazier P, Surrell J, et al. Safe resection for diverticular disease of the colon. Dis Colon Rectum 1989;32:30–32. *A retrospective study of 83 patients undergoing surgery for diverticular disease. The operative mortality was low. In complicated cases, primary anastomosis was performed in 43%.*
7. Moreux J, Vons C. Elective resection for diverticular disease of the sigmoid colon. Br J Surg 1990;77:1036–1038. *A series of 177 consecutive patients undergoing elective operation for diverticular disease. Most patients can have a safe one-stage procedure, even if an extracolic abscess is found.*
8. Murray J, Schoetz D, Coller J. Intraoperative colonic lavage and primary anastomosis in nonelective colon resection. Dis Colon Rectum 1991;34:527–531. *A review of 25 patients having intraoperative colonic lavage before emergency segmental left colectomy. Ten of the patients had an acute intra-abdominal inflammatory process. One pelvic abscess developed postoperatively, and there were three wound infections.*
9. Rodkey G, Welch C. Changing patterns in the surgical treatment of diverticular disease. Ann Surg 1984;200:466–478. *In this review of 350 surgical cases, 32% of the patients had perforation with local peritonitis or pelvic abscess.*
10. Grief J, Fried G, McSherry C. Surgical treatment of perforated diverticulitis of the sigmoid colon. Dis Colon Rectum 1980;23:483–494. *A retrospective review of 1353 surgical cases of perforated sigmoid diverticulitis. Operations in which the perforated segment was resected or exteriorized during the first operative procedure led to a lower mortality rate than procedures in which the perforated segment was not removed initially.*

Our first consideration is to avoid opening any unnecessary tissue planes. This minimizes potential spread of infection into uninvolved areas of the abdomen. More importantly, it avoids the difficulty of dissecting in areas that have been scarred down by previous unnecessary manipulation. *In particular, one should avoid the splenic flexure and the extraperitoneal rectum.*

Usually, the area of involvement with diverticulitis is in the sigmoid colon. This can be resected proximal to the thickened and inflamed site and a sigmoid or descending colon colostomy fashioned without mobilization of the splenic flexure. Dissection of the splenic flexure may carry bacteria into the subdiaphragmatic area. Subsequent mobilization of the descending and transverse colon also will be more difficult. It is not necessary to resect all diverticula at either operation. *At the initial operation, only the perforated or septic focus must be removed.* Ultimately, the proximal margin of resection should involve soft, pliable, well-vascularized bowel without significant muscular thickening and no diverticula in the immediate vicinity of the anastomosis.

Mobilization of the rectum from the sacral hollow at the initial operation also may allow spread of infection into the extraperitoneal space. More importantly, it may make the subsequent operation difficult if not impossible. Again, it is necessary initially to resect only the perforated or septic segment of the sigmoid. Diverticulitis almost never involves the rectum (18). The sigmoid can be divided a short distance below the area of involvement and closed with a linear stapler or sutures. *It is rarely possible to bring out the distal segment of bowel as a mucous fistula* due to the location of the area of involvement. When possible, however, this approach may make the second operation easier. In contrast to what is done for cancer, we suggest dividing the sigmoid mesentery relatively close to the bowel to be resected. This may avoid injury to the sympathetic nerves and also reduce the temptation to dissect behind the rectum.

Anchoring the rectal or sigmoid stump to the sacral promontory with one or two nonabsorbable heavy monofilament sutures may facilitate identification of the stump at the second operation. It also may prevent the rectum from collapsing on itself in an accordion fashion and producing shortening, which interferes with later insertion of an instrument from below.

Occasionally, the inflammatory segment of sigmoid will attach in the cul-de-sac and involve the anterior rectal wall with the inflammatory process. This is not an indication to resect that portion of the rectum. Instead, the sigmoid should be dissected free and the rectum should be left undisturbed. Over a period of a few months, the rectal wall inflammation will resolve, allowing reanastomosis to the full rectum.

In creation of the colostomy, we suggest avoiding sutures between the colon wall and the posterior peritoneum/rectus fascia because this may make subsequent mobilization of the stoma more difficult. We also do not attempt to close the lateral gutter or to tunnel the colon extraperitoneally. We have not found allowing direct egress of the colon to cause problems, and avoidance of these maneuvers may lessen the difficulty of mobilization of the stoma. Primary maturation of the stoma to the dermal edges should always be performed.

THE SECOND OPERATION

Timing of the Second Operation

Although many patients are eager to be rid of their stoma, we prefer to wait a minimum of 3 months before considering reoperation. This timing allows most patients sufficient time to recover from the first operation and to regain their strength. It also allows time for the inflammatory adhesions to mature sufficiently to facilitate dissection. Keck and associates suggested that a Hartmann's reversal should be delayed at least 15 weeks due to a reduction in density of adhesions (17). Occasionally, during the period of diversion, the patient will complain of drainage from the rectum. This may represent breakdown of the stump with drainage of a pelvic abscess or hematoma. The rectal mucosa also may appear inflamed and difficult to distinguish from inflammatory bowel disease. The usual cause of these mucosal changes is diversion colitis. The pathogenesis may be related to a nutritional deficiency of the colonic epithelium, specifically to an absence of short-chain fatty acids (SCFAs), predominantly N-butyric acid (19). This generally will resolve after reanastomosis, but if troublesome during diversion, may respond to an enema comprised of a solution of mixed SCFAs (mainly N-butyric, acetic, and propionic acids) (20).

Involvement of an enterostomal therapist will considerably lessen the psychologic and physiologic impact of having a colostomy. Modern appliances allow the patient to live an active life during the period of diversion. Irrigation of the stoma may permit the patient to have less concern for when the stoma will function. Some patients with irrigated stomas are able to wear only a stoma cap or gauze dressing.

Conduct of the Second Operation

Planning and attention to technical details may facilitate the reversal of the Hartmann procedure. After the patient has achieved optimal medical condition, the operation can be scheduled. A full mechanical and antibiotic bowel preparation is used. We favor neomycin and metronidazole orally and perioperative intravenous administration of a second-generation cephalosporin (cefotetan or cefoxitin). Intravenous fluids containing potassium are administered preoperatively. Only a tap water or Phospho-Soda enema is used for the rectal stump.

The patient is positioned in the modified dorsal lithotomy position. Our preference is to use Allen stirrups (Allen Medical Systems, Cleveland, OH). The sigmoidoscope is used to ensure adequate emptying of the rectal stump. Our preference for a midline incision has been mentioned previously but is repeated for emphasis. A figure-of-eight suture is used to close the colostomy and to allow traction for the mobilization of the stoma. After the abdomen is entered, adhesions are lysed and the rectal stump is exposed. (A one-sentence description of this step of the operation often does not do it justice!) *If there is difficulty identifying the distal bowel, a sigmoidoscope can be inserted from below to facilitate identification and dissection.* Often, if the suggestions made earlier about handling of the stump are followed, this is not necessary.

Generally, the rectum must be mobilized only enough to free the upper rectum and it is rarely necessary to go below the peritoneal reflection.

One of the important aspects of this operation is to ensure that the distal margin of resection is within the upper rectum, distal to the rectosigmoid sphincter of O'Beirne (21). The sphincter of O'Beirne, which lies approximately 1–2 inches above the superior rectal valve of Houston, is a high-pressure zone that may be responsible for anastomotic problems or recurrent diverticulitis. *The rectum may be identified by a variety of techniques.* These include going just below the sacral promontory, looking for the point at which the taenia spread out to cover the entire wall, and looking for disappearance of the sigmoid mesentery. The most reliable means of identifying the rectum, however, is to ensure that the diameter of the bowel enlarges to that of the rectum (usually at least 4 cm). We cannot emphasize enough the importance of making the distal limb of the anastomosis within the rectum. Almost always, when we are asked to see a patient who is having problems following resection for diverticulitis, we find that the anastomosis was created to the sigmoid colon.

When the distal bowel is suitable for anastomosis, the colostomy stoma can be mobilized. To allow a tension-free anastomosis, *the splenic flexure may need to be mobilized.* Guidelines for the proximal extent of the resection have already been described.

The anastomosis can be created either by hand or with staples. The authors' preference is a single-layer, hand-sewn anastomosis with continuous 4–0 monofilament absorbable suture (Maxon, Davis & Geck, Danbury, CT) (22). After dissection to the upper rectum, the bowel is divided either above a linear stapler or below a clamp. A pursestring suture of 0 polypropylene (Prolene, Ethicon, Somerville, NJ) is placed in the proximal bowel. The circular stapler, either the ECS 29-mm (Proximate ILS, Ethicon, Somerville, NJ) or CEEA 31-mm (Auto Suture, US Surgical Corporation, Norwalk, CT) model, is preferred because of the large anastomotic diameter. The anvil is placed into the proximal bowel and the pursestring suture is tied. Occasionally, additional proximal bowel must be resected to reach a segment of colon that is distensible enough to allow the anvil to be inserted. A pursestring suture also can be placed into the rectal stump to save the expense of another stapler. The stapler is then advanced through the rectum to the stump and the trocar is passed through the staple line or the pursestring is tied. After proper alignment of the bowel ends is ensured, the stapler is fired and withdrawn (Figs. 19.1 through 19.6). Our policy is to inspect the "doughnuts" and test the anastomosis with air instilled through the sigmoidoscope.

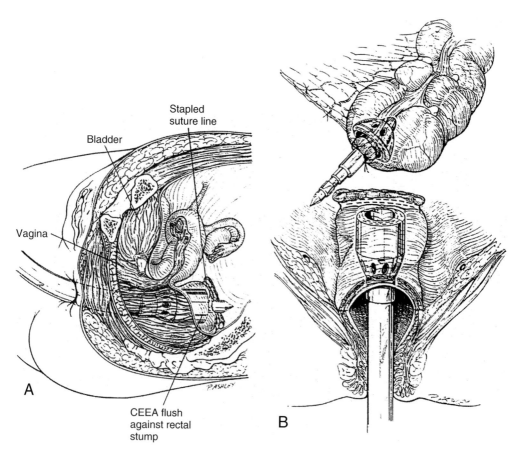

Figure 19.1.   Depiction of instruments used in stapled anastomosis (double-staple technique). **A.,** The circular stapler (CEEA) has been introduced through the anus, and with counterclockwise turning of the knob on the stapler, a spike pushes through the apex of the rectal stump. The spike is removed. **B.,** The anvil has been placed in the proximal bowel and the pursestring has been tied. (Reprinted with permission from Mazier WP, LeVien DH, Luchtefeld MP, et al. Surgery of the colon, rectum, and anus. Philadelphia: WB Saunders, 1995:637.)

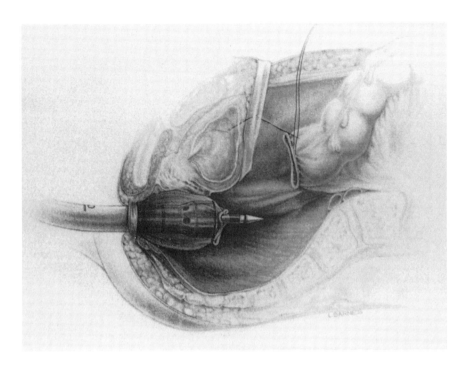

Figure 19.2.   Essential steps of double-staple technique. The stapler with trocar tip penetrates through the closed rectum at or adjacent to the linear stapler line. (Reprinted with permission from Corman ML. Colon and rectal surgery. 3rd ed. Philadelphia: JB Lippincott, 1993:663–669.)

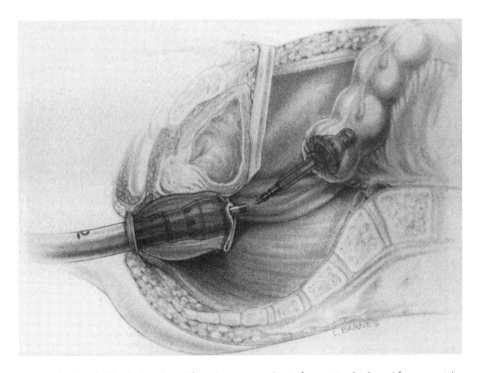

Figure 19.3.   The detachable shaft and anvil have been secured into the proximal colon with a pursestring suture of 2–0 Prolene. (Reprinted with permission from Corman ML. Colon and rectal surgery. 3rd ed. Philadelphia: JB Lippincott, 1993:663–669.)

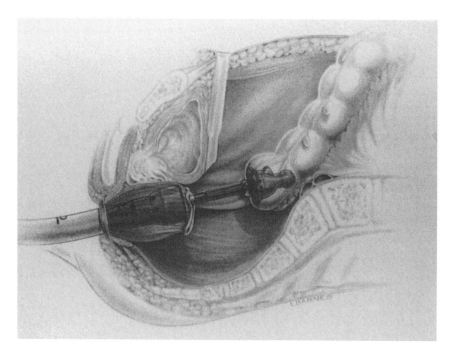

Figure 19.4.   The anvil shaft is reattached to the center rod. Care is made to avoid twisting of the sigmoid colon. (Reprinted with permission from Corman ML. Colon and rectal surgery. 3rd ed. Philadelphia: JB Lippincott, 1993:663–669.)

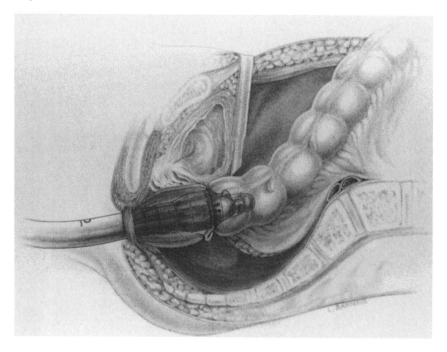

Figure 19.5.   The anastomosis is completed after the perineal operator brings the two ends of the colon and rectum together by rotating the knob of the stapler in a clockwise direction. Care is made to exclude pararectal tissue from the staple line. The integrity of the "doughnuts" of tissue in the stapler should be checked after the stapler is fired. (Reprinted with permission from Corman ML. Colon and rectal surgery. 3rd ed. Philadelphia: JB Lippincott, 1993:663–669.)

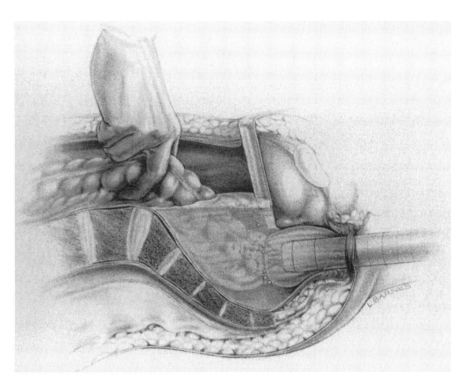

Figure 19.6.   Testing the integrity of the anastomosis with a rigid sigmoidoscope. As the proximal bowel is compressed with fingers or a noncrushing clamp, air is insufflated through the sigmoidoscope. A leak is demonstrated by bubbles leaking into saline in the pelvis. (Reprinted with permission from Corman ML: Colon and rectal surgery. 3rd ed. Philadelphia: JB Lippincott, 1993:663–669.)

SPECIFIC CONSIDERATIONS

Occasionally, the rectum is relatively nondistensible, making the passage of the stapler difficult if not impossible. The solutions to this problem involve either more extensive mobilization of the rectum or preferably creation of a hand-sewn anastomosis. The difficulty of inserting the anvil into the proximal bowel also may be managed by suturing. If the staple line was carried into the rectum during the first operation, the end of the stump may be too thick to allow a stapled anastomosis. In this circumstance, the upper portion of the rectum can be reresected, or the trocar can be passed through the anterior rectal wall just below the staple line. We have seen two instances in which the anastomosis was created to the anterior rectal wall, leaving a significant blind loop of sigmoid above. This may not create any functional problems but is certainly confusing to the endoscopist.

We generally do not drain the pelvis postoperatively unless it is necessary to mobilize the rectum from the sacral hollow. If needed, however, we prefer closed-suction drainage such as a 10-mm flat silicone Jackson-Pratt drain (Baxter Healthcare Corporation, Deerfield, IL). The skin at the colostomy site generally is closed loosely with two or three vertical mattress sutures, and the subcutaneous tissue is drained with Telfa gauze (Kendall Company, Mansfield, MA) cut into wicks that are removed after 4 days. We do not routinely use postoperative nasogastric decompression.

LAPAROSCOPIC CLOSURE

With the advent of laparoscopic colorectal surgery, there has been enthusiasm for reanastomosis following the Hartmann procedure by minimally invasive techniques (23) (Chapter 18). *If this is anticipated or considered, it becomes important that the bowel be resected into the upper rectum at the first operation.* This will avoid the need for a possibly difficult mobilization and additional resection performed laparoscopically. Likewise, the proximal resection should meet the guidelines we have listed for the ultimate point of resection. Enough mobility of the proximal bowel should exist to allow it to reach the rectum. Laparoscopic mobilization of the splenic flexure is not too difficult in experienced hands. *The pelvic and proximal dissections should be accomplished before mobilization of the colostomy, because this results in loss of pneumoperitoneum.* After the anvil is inserted into the proximal bowel, it can be replaced into the abdomen and the stoma site can be closed. It is difficult in our experience to get an air-tight closure of the peritoneum, but a high-flow insufflator usually will overcome this problem. The circular stapler is then advanced to the rectal stump, the trocar is advanced, and the anvil is mated with the stapler. The anastomosis is completed and tested. We have found this operation considerably more difficult than it sounds or appears in the edited videos.

CONCLUSIONS

Takedown following Hartmann operations remains a significant challenge due to both the frail nature of many patients and to technical difficulties that may be encountered. Preplanning the operations and attention to certain details may help minimize many of the technical problems that are encountered. This may ultimately reduce the number of patients forced to live with a permanent colostomy following resection for acute diverticulitis.

EDITORIAL COMMENTS

The authors have presented an excellent summary of the technical aspects of Hartmann closures. Other technical comments can be found in the literature for those interested, such as avoidance of rectal pouch mobilization (24,25) or maneuvers at the initial Hartmann procedure, including marking of the rectal pouch with long Prolene sutures (26) or suspending the rectal pouch (27). Hartmann closures, in particular, can be demanding, requiring an experienced operator with technical expertise. Over time, the mortality rate of the procedure has decreased to levels of 0–4% (9,28,29) and the morbidity rate has decreased to 10% (9).

A number of points should be emphasized.

1. At the initial resection, unnecessary opening of tissue planes should be avoided. However, if additional length is required to make a well-matured colostomy without tension, the splenic flexure should be mobilized. As the authors state, many of these stomas will be permanent.
2. Avoidance of the presacral space at initial operation makes the subsequent reanastomosis easier. We also recommend leaving the superior hemorrhoidal artery intact. This helps avoid entrance into the presacral space and may reduce shortening of the rectum, thus facilitating reanastomosis at the second procedure. In addition, preservation of this artery ensures a sufficient blood supply for a subsequent high rectal anastomosis (Fig. 19.7).
3. If the rectal segment is never closed, it should be surveyed occasionally with a proctoscope or sigmoidoscope for abnormalities such as polyps or carcinoma (30).

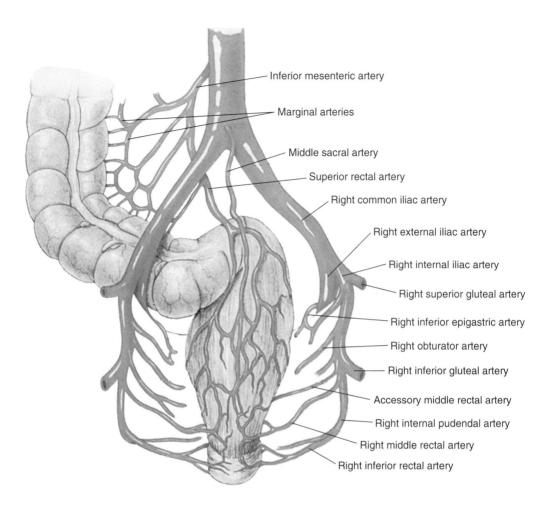

Inferior mesenteric artery

Marginal arteries

Middle sacral artery

Superior rectal artery

Right common iliac artery

Right external iliac artery

Right internal iliac artery

Right superior gluteal artery

Right inferior epigastric artery

Right obturator artery

Right inferior gluteal artery

Accessory middle rectal artery

Right internal pudendal artery

Right middle rectal artery

Right inferior rectal artery

Figure 19.7.   A posterior view of the rectum depicting the arterial blood supply. Note that the major supply to the upper rectum comes from the superior rectal (hemorrhoidal) artery; therefore, preservation of this vessel improves perfusion of the rectal segment for an anastomosis. (Reprinted with permission from Gordon PH, Nivatvongs S. Principles and practice of surgery for the colon, rectum, and anus. St. Louis: Quality Medical Publishing, 1992:21.)

4. We recommend colonoscopy or barium enema to rule out other colonic pathology before the elective Hartmann closure.

5. We also favor delayed closure after at least 3 months, especially if pelvic and/or abdominal peritonitis has occurred. Although most surgeons agree with the concept of delay (17,29,30,31), some disagree (3,32).

6. Any remaining sigmoid colon must be resected to minimize the risk of recurrent diverticulitis (Chapter 25) and to ensure a well-vascularized rectum for the anastomosis.

7. Identification of a low-lying rectal stump can be facilitated after insertion of a rectal tube, stapler sizer, or a lighted flexible sigmoidoscope (33,34).

8. Small circular stapler anvils should not be used because of the risk of an anastomotic stricture. If the anvil (33 or 29 mm) does not fit, the bowel should be mobilized to use the more capacious proximal colon. This may require mobilization of the splenic flexure, basing the blood supply in the middle colic artery. Alternatively, if the anvil will not fit, a hand-sewn anastomosis may be the best method of closure.

9. The success of laparoscopic Hartmann closure depends on the ability to free the small bowel off the rectal stump, allowing the necessary visualization. One cannot predict the extent of adhesions a particular patient may have, and it is reasonable for experienced laparoscopic surgeons to commence with the laparoscopic approach. If the pelvic adhesions are extensive, we favor early conversion to a laparotomy.

10. The anastomotic integrity is confirmed by inspection of the staple line with a proctoscope and by insufflation of air (Fig. 19.6).

REFERENCES

1. Rosenman LD. Hartmann's operation. Am J Surg 1994;168:283–284. *In Hartmann's original description, the rectum was closed at or below the peritoneal reflection. Complications seen today can occur with a long rectal stump with insufficient blood supply.*
2. Baaker FC, Holtsma HF, Den Otter G. The Hartmann procedure. Br J Surg 1982;60:580–582. *In 32% of the patients undergoing Hartmann procedures, intestinal continuity was restored later.*
3. Whiston JR, Armitage NC, Wilcox D, et al. Hartmann's procedure: an appraisal. J R Soc Med 1993;86:205–208. *Complicated diverticular disease was the most common benign disorder in this series; the most frequent complications were infectious and cardiovascular.*
4. Pain J, Cahill J. Surgical options for left-sided large bowel emergencies. Ann R Surg Engl 1991;73:394–397. *The popularity of the Hartmann procedure was evident in this questionnaire sent to 217 consultant general surgeons in the United Kingdom.*
5. Boyden AM. Two-stage (obstructive) resection of the sigmoid in selected cases of complicated diverticulitis. Ann Surg 1961;154(Suppl):210–214. *The author points out that two-stage resections were performed more frequently than three-stage ones at his institution in the previous decade.*
6. Rodkey GV, Welch CE. Surgical management of colonic diverticulitis with free perforation or abscess formation. Am J Surg 1969;117:265–269. *Promotes wider use of primary excision with proximal colostomy and distal closure or mucous fistula for complex cases; the operation combines the safety of staged operations with excision of the diseased bowel.*
7. Nunes GC, Robnett AH, Kremer RM, et al. The Hartmann procedure for complications of diverticulitis. Arch Surg 1979;114:425–429. *Recommends wider application of Hartmann procedure for complicated acute diverticulitis, based on removal of diseased bowel, no primary anastomotic risk, reduced hospitalization, and relatively low mortality.*
8. Liebert CW, DeWeese RM. Primary resection without anastomosis for perforation of acute diverticulitis. Surg Gynecol Obstet 1981;152:30–32. *The authors promote the Hartmann procedure for perforation with acute diverticulitis with or without abscess; transverse colostomy with drainage alone is associated with a high mortality under these conditions.*
9. Roe AM, Prabhu S, Ali A, et al. Reversal of Hartmann's procedure: timing and operative technique. Br J Surg 1991;78:1167–1170. *Discusses 69 patients having closures of Hartmann colostomies (48 had diverticular disease originally). There was no advantage (decreased complications) if closure was performed after 4 months; more stapled anastomoses after 4 months may have reflected shrinkage of the rectal stump.*
10. Eisenstat TE, Rubin RJ, Salvati EP. Surgical management of diverticulitis. The role of the Hartmann procedure. Dis Colon Rectum 1983;26:429–432. *The mortality rate was 4.5% in 44 patients undergoing Hartmann operations.*
11. Haas PA, Haas GP. A critical evaluation of the Hartmann's procedure. Am Surg 1988;54:380–385. *Reviews 150 Hartmann procedures. The operation is of low risk for diverticulitis; in general, it is a poor choice for inflammatory bowel disease.*
12. Bothwell WN, Bleicher RJ, Dent TL. Prophylactic ureteral catheterization in colon surgery. A five-year review. Dis Colon Rectum 1994;37:330–334. *Experienced surgeons requested these catheters in 16% of sigmoid or rectosigmoid colectomies. The risk of surgical ureteral injury with the catheter in place was 1%.*
13. Kyzer S, Gordon PH. The prophylactic use of ureteral catheters during colorectal operations. Am Surg 1994;60:212–216. *In a retrospective review, ureteral catheterization was considered necessary in 28% of cases.*
14. Sheikh FA, Khubchandani IT. Prophylactic ureteric catheters in colon surgery — how safe are they? Dis Colon Rectum 1990;33:508–510. *Three cases of reflux anuria developed in 59 patients with prophylactic ureteral catheters. Clinical factors differentiating anuria as a result of acute tabular necrosis or of this iatrogenic syndrome are discussed.*
15. Leff EI, Groff W, Rubin RJ, et al. Use of ureteral catheters in colonic and rectal surgery. Dis Colon Rectum 1982;25:457–460. *Recommends use of catheters in patients with previous pelvic or colonic surgery, complicated diverticulitis, and Hartmann closures.*
16. Zinman LM, Libertino JA, Roth RA. Management of operative ureteral injury. Urology 1978;12:290–303. *A review of the technical aspects of repair of ureteral injuries.*
17. Keck JO, Collopy BT, Ryan PJ, et al. Reversal of Hartmann's procedure: effect of timing and technique on ease and safety. Dis Colon Rectum 1994;37:243–248. *Patients having the reversal procedure within 15 weeks of the original operation had a longer hospital stay, a more difficult surgical dissection, and an increase in accidental enterotomies.*
18. Chiu TC, Bailey HR, Hernandez AJ. Diverticulitis of the mid-rectum. Dis Colon Rectum 1983;26:59–60. *An abscess involving a solitary diverticulum was drained through the diverticular opening with subsidence of rectal pain.*

19. Roediger WE. The starved colon-diminished mucosal nutrition, diminished absorption, and colitis. Dis Colon Rectum 1990;33:858–862. *A chronic lack of short-chain fatty acids or complete organ starvation together with other factors lead to mucosal hypoplasia with diminished absorption or diarrhea.*
20. Harig JM, Soergel KH, Komorowski RA, et al. Treatment of diversion colitis with short-chain-fatty acid irrigation. N Engl J Med 1989;320:23–28. *Diversion colitis may be treated effectively by local application of short-chain fatty acids.*
21. Ballantyne GH: Rectosigmoid sphincter of O'Beirne. Dis Colon Rectum 1986;29:525–531. *Anatomic and motility studies support the theory that a sphincter controls passage of stool from the sigmoid colon into the rectum.*
22. Max E, Sweeney WB, Bailey HR, et al. Results of 1,000 single-layer continuous polypropylene intestinal anastomoses. Am J Surg 1991;162:461–467. *The clinical suspected anastomotic leak rate was 1%; no deaths were due to anastomotic complications.*
23. Sosa JL, Sleeman D, Puente I, et al. Laparoscopic-assisted colostomy closure after Hartmann's procedure. Dis Colon Rectum 1994;37:149–152. *The laparoscopic procedure had comparable morbidity but was associated with a shorter hospital stay than the open operation.*
24. Caracciolo F, Castrucci G, Castiglioni GC. Anastomosis with EEA stapler following Hartmann procedure. Dis Colon Rectum 1986;29:67–68. *The authors test the anastomosis with instillation of saline into the rectum.*
25. Moesgaard F, Kirkegaard P, Nielsen ML, et al. A modified technique for stapled anastomosis after the Hartmann procedure. Acta Chir Scand 1984;150:693–694. *Describes stapling of anastomosis with mobilization of rectal stump.*
26. Madura JA, Fiore AC. Reanastomosis of a Hartmann rectal pouch. A simplified procedure. Am J Surg 1983;145:279–280. *Recommends use of polypropylene sutures to define rectal stump.*
27. Rushden RO, Kusminsky R. Closure of Hartmann's procedure. A technical note. Am Surg 1982;48:528. *Recommends suspension of closed rectal segment to the presacral fascia at original Hartmann operation to simplify the subsequent closure.*
28. Wigmore SJ, Duthie GS, Young IE, et al. Restoration of intestinal continuity following Hartmann's procedure: the Lothian experience 1987–1992. Br J Surg 1995;82:27–30. *No relation was found between timing and complications. Anastomotic stricture occurred more commonly in stapled anastomoses. The authors feel that operative expertise accounted for the low morbidity.*
29. Pearce NW, Scott SD, Karran SJ. Timing and method of reversal of Hartmann's procedure. Br J Surg 1992;79:839–941. *Six of 12 patients had clinical evidence of a leak when the interval between the Hartmann procedure and closure was less than 3 months: none of 40 patients died if the delay was more than 6 months.*
30. Haas PA, Fox TA Jr. The fate of the forgotten rectal pouch after Hartmann's procedure without reanastomosis. Am J Surg 1990;159:106–111. *Twenty-four patients with diverticulitis having Hartmann procedures were endoscoped at least 1 year later: 12 rectal pouches had proctitis and 2 had polyps.*
31. Khan AL, Ah-See AK, Crofts TJ, et al. Reversal of Hartmann's colostomy. J R Coll Surg Edinb 1994;39:239–242. *The morbidity was highest when colostomy closure was carried out within 3 months of colostomy creation.*
32. Geoghegan JG, Rosenberg IL. Experience with early anastomosis after the Hartmann procedure. Ann R Coll Surg Engl 1991;73:80–82. *In this series, early closure of the colostomy within 1 month did not increase patient risk.*
33. Criado FJ, Wilson TH Jr. Technique for re-establishing continuity after the Hartmann operation. Am Surg 1981;47:366–367. *Describes use of a rectal tube to help identify a rectal segment deep in the pelvis.*
34. Gervin AS, Fischer RP. Identification of the rectal pouch of Hartmann. Surg Gynecol Obstet 1987;164:176–178. *A fiberoptic sigmoidoscope in a darkened operative room facilitated identification of the rectal pouch.*

20 Intraoperative Colonic Lavage

An Option for Permitting Single-Stage Resection

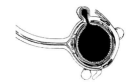

John J. Murray, MD
Edward C. Lee, MD

KEY POINTS

- Intraoperative lavage allows single-stage resection in selected cases of diverticulitis and other disorders
- Useful when primary indication for colostomy is lack of mechanical preparation of colon
- A safe, reproducible technique in trained hands

ILLUSTRATIVE CASE

A 59-year-old male presented to the emergency department with 5 hours of severe abdominal pain. The pain was initially localized to the left lower quadrant but had become diffuse. He was otherwise in good health. Evaluation revealed a temperature of 101°F and pulse of 110. Abdominal examination revealed diffuse peritonitis. Abdominal films confirmed the presence of free air. At laparotomy, the patient had a perforated sigmoid colon. There was minimal contamination. He underwent primary resection, on-table colonic lavage, and anastomosis. The hospital course was uncomplicated, and the patient was discharged on the seventh postoperative day.

CASE COMMENTS

Traditionally, patients with this history undergoing primary anastomosis have had proximal diversion at the time of the emergency procedure. Now there is sufficient evidence that on-table lavage is a safe and established technique, if performed by an experienced operator under the right conditions.

DISCUSSION

Approximately 20% of patients hospitalized for treatment of diverticulitis require urgent or emergency operation to relieve potentially life-threatening complications of the disease (1). The appropriate management of these individuals remains a controversial topic. *The relative merit and safety of resecting the diseased segment of large intestine at the initial operation and the optimal timing for restoration of intestinal tract continuity have been the central issues of debate.* Although segmental resection of the colon with primary anastomosis is the "standard" approach in the elective setting, resection of the involved colon with delayed anastomosis has become the most popular strategy for the emergency treatment of complicated diverticulitis.

Reliance on staged procedures in the acute setting reflects legitimate concerns of possible anastomotic dehiscence in the unprepped colon and in the presence of intra-abdominal sepsis. Critical evaluation of the success of staged procedures for acute diverticulitis must consider the *cumulative* morbidity and mortality that may accompany multiple operations, especially in elderly patients (2). In patients undergoing staged resection for complicated diverticular disease at the Lahey Clinic between 1967 and 1982, the cumulative mortality and cumulative morbidity were 11% and 23%, respectively. In addition, a significant proportion of patients embarking on a multistage approach fail to complete all phases of the procedure (3). Incomplete treatment usually reflects the consequences of postoperative complications and comorbid disease.

Availability of the circular, end-to-end anastomotic stapling instrument has made the Hartmann procedure the most commonly used technique for patients having emergency resection for complications of diverticular disease. Intestinal anastomosis following Hartmann resection can be technically challenging, however, and mobilization of the splenic flexure is frequently required to relieve tension on the anastomosis. Other alternatives for staged resection of the distal colon, including segmental colectomy with colostomy and mucous fistula and segmental colectomy with primary anastomosis and diverting loop colostomy, are less popular. *The prolonged cumulative hospitalization, the extended disability, and the cumulative morbidity that accompany staged operative procedures for diverticulitis justify a search for therapeutic alternatives* (4). Single-stage resection with primary anastomosis for the emergent treatment of complicated diverticulitis has a number of potential advantages. The incidence of anastomotic dehiscence in this setting has been reported to range from 0% to 33%, with an associated operative mortality of 0% to 20% (5–7). Eng and colleagues identified no difference in operative mortality when results with single-stage and two-stage procedures for treating perforated diverticulitis were compared (6).

Segmental resection and primary anastomosis are associated with the shortest period of hospitalization and the briefest term of postoperative disability. In general, however, the results reported with resection and primary anastomosis have involved small numbers of patients and may reflect a bias in patient selection. Postponing primary anastomosis of the colon following emergent intestinal resection avoids the septic complications that may accompany anastomotic dehiscence. *Fecal loading of the proximal colon may be the most significant factor jeopardizing anastomotic integrity.* Clinical and laboratory studies have confirmed an increased risk of anastomotic dehiscence after segmental resection of the left colon in patients with inadequate mechanical preparation (8,9).

The reason for the deleterious impact of fecal loading on anastomotic healing is uncertain. Mechanical disruption of the anastomosis may occur during passage of a fecal bolus in the early phase of anastomotic healing. Incomplete mechanical cleansing also may contribute to localized infection at the anastomosis that disrupts the usual pattern of collagen metabolism.

Objective evidence supporting the concept that intra-abdominal sepsis impairs healing of an intestinal anastomosis is less secure. Irvin and Goligher found no correlation between intraperitoneal sepsis and anastomotic complications in 204 patients undergoing segmental resection of the colon (9). It has been shown experimentally that defective anastomoses contain reduced amounts of collagen (10).

Studies suggesting an increased risk of anastomotic complications in the presence of intra-abdominal abscess or peritonitis often have failed to control for the quality of preoperative mechanical preparation of the intestine (11,12). *The technique for intraoperative antegrade lavage of the colon, first proposed by Edward Muir in 1968, eliminates the problem of fecal loading and facilitates primary anastomosis in patients who require urgent resection of the distal colon* (13).

The technique as modified by Radcliffe and Dudley involves mobilization of the segment of colon to be resected in standard fashion (14). The lumen of the bowel proximal to the diseased segment is occluded with a Dacron tape. The splenic flexure of the colon is mobilized routinely. Mobilization of the hepatic flexure also may be necessary to provide access to the proximal transverse colon during lavage. When mobilization of the colon is complete, the left colon is occluded and a colotomy is performed just proximal to the previously placed Dacron ligature. Sterile corrugated tubing is inserted through the colotomy and secured with a second Dacron tape (Fig. 20.1). The tubing is passed off the operating table to drain into disposable plastic containers (Fig. 20.2). The cecum is cannulated with a Foley catheter (20–24 French) passed through the base of the freshly amputated appendix (Fig. 20.3). If the patient has previously undergone appendectomy, the Foley catheter is introduced through an enterotomy in the terminal ileum and secured with a pursestring suture. Due to the risk for uncontrolled fecal spillage, the Foley catheter should not be introduced through a cecotomy. Saline solution that has been warmed to body temperature is infused through the Foley catheter to accomplish lavage (Fig. 20.4). Depending on the extent of fecal loading, 3–6 liters of solution usually are required (Fig. 20.5). Initially, it may be necessary to milk solid fecal material through the colon. This

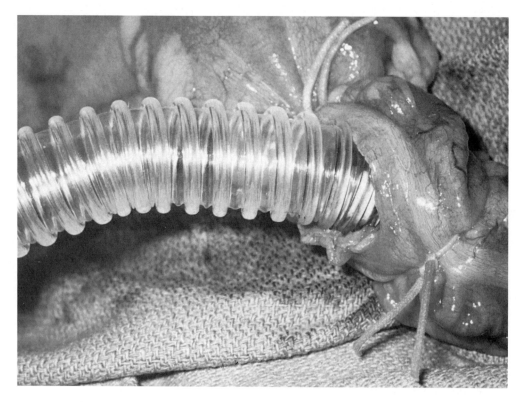

Figure 20.1.   The proximal sigmoid colon is occluded with a Dacron ligature. Sterile corrugated tubing, inserted through a colotomy proximal to the dacron ligature, is secured with a second dacron tape.

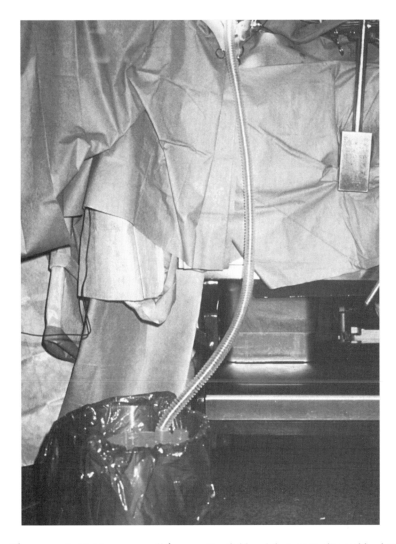

Figure 20.2.   The corrugated tubing passes off the operative field and drains into disposable plastic containers.

maneuver requires ready access to both flexures of the colon and explains the need for mobilization of the flexures before commencing lavage. When the lavage effluent is clear, 100 mL of a 10% povidone iodine solution is added to the last liter of irrigant as an antiseptic. In addition, all patients receive parenteral antibiotics effective against enteric pathogens during the perioperative period. When the lavage is completed, the Foley catheter is removed and the appendectomy is completed or the enterotomy is closed. The portion of large intestine containing the corrugated tubing is included in the operative specimen. In patients whose disease is complicated by large-bowel obstruction, the dilated lumen of the proximal colon usually is restored to normal caliber by the completion of lavage (3) (Fig. 20.6).

Depending on the technique selected for bowel anastomosis, the distal segment of colon is swabbed with a sponge soaked in povidone-iodine solution or is evacuated through a proctoscope. The latter method is used when anastomosis is performed with the circular end-to-end anastomotic stapling instrument. *The usual criteria for constructing a secure*

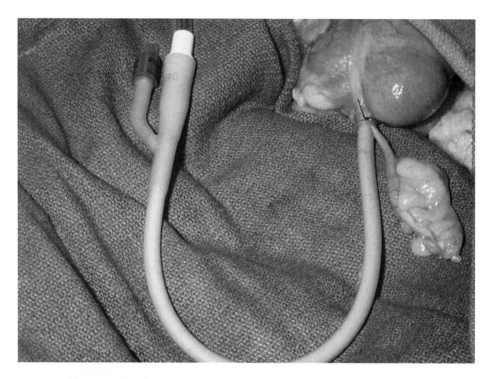

Figure 20.3.   The cecum is cannulated with a large-bore Foley catheter inserted through the base of the appendix or through an enterotomy in the terminal ileum.

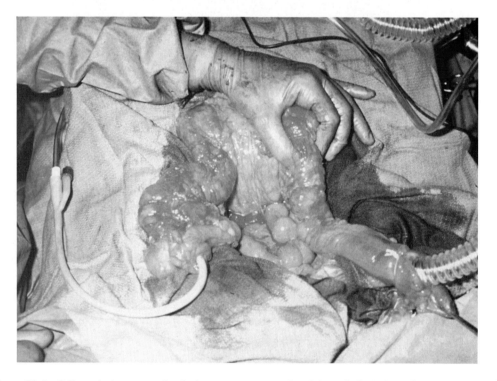

Figure 20.4.   Saline solution, warmed to body temperature, is infused through the Foley catheter to accomplish lavage.

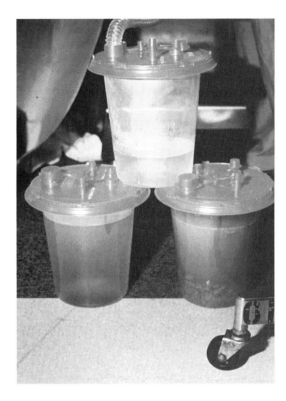

Figure 20.5.   Lavage effluent usually is clear after infusion of 3–6 liters of saline.

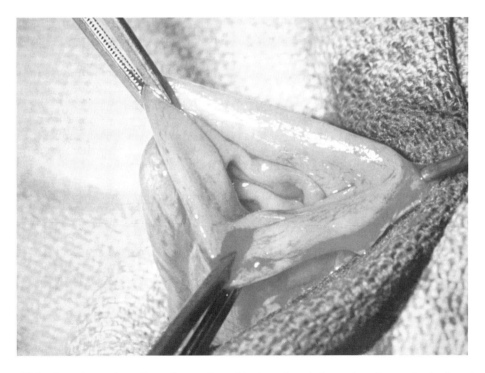

Figure 20.6.   In patients whose illness is complicated by large bowel obstruction, the proximal colon often is restored to normal caliber at the completion of the lavage.

intestinal anastomosis must be satisfied. The anastomosis must use intestinal segments that are well perfused, pliable, and uninflamed. The intestine should be approximated without tension.

Depending on the ease with which the flexures can be mobilized, intraoperative colonic lavage generally adds 25–50 minutes to the operating time.

Lahey Clinic Experience

Since 1987, 56 patients with complicated diverticular disease have required urgent operation at the Lahey Clinic (15). Thirty-two patients in this group have undergone segmental colectomy, intraoperative colonic lavage, and primary anastomosis (Table 20.1). The remaining 24 patients have been treated with Hartmann resection. The decision to perform a staged procedure has been based on the preference of the operating surgeon, the presence of generalized fecal or purulent peritonitis, or the identification of a large pelvic abscess. Large-bowel obstruction was the indication for urgent operation in 13 of the 32 patients (41%) treated with on-table lavage and primary anastomosis. An additional 13 patients required operation due to persistent, localized peritonitis despite treatment with antibiotics. In five patients (15%) treated by single-stage resection, a preoperative radiographic examination confirmed the presence of frank perforation of the sigmoid colon. One patient required emergency resection of the left colon to treat unrelenting diverticular hemorrhage.

We have classified our patients according to Hinchey's staging system for complicated diverticulitis (16) (Table 20.2). According to these criteria, 87% of our patients had stage I or stage II disease. Four patients (13%) had generalized purulent peritonitis (stage III). We have not used intraoperative lavage and single-stage resection for patients with feculent peritonitis.

Table 20.1.   Complications of Diverticulosis in 32 Patients

Indication for Operation	Patients
Obstruction	13 (41%)
Localized peritonitis/abscess	13 (41%)
Perforation	5 (15%)
Hemorrhage	1 (3%)

Table 20.2.   Clinical Staging of Diverticulitis

Stage	Patient
I: Pericolic abscess	18 (56%)
II: Pelvic abscess	10 (31%)
III: Purulent peritonitis	4 (13%)
IV: Feculent peritonitis	0 (0%)

Adapted from Hinchey EJ, Schaal PG, Richards GK. Treatment of perforated diverticular disease of the colon. Adv Surg 1978; 12:85–109.

Table 20.3.   Operative Procedures

Procedure	Number of Patients
Sigmoid colectomy	23 (72%)
Left colectomy	2 (6%)
Low anterior resection	2 (6%)
Hartmann resection	1 (3%)
Sigmoid colectomy, primary anastomosis[a]	4 (13%)

[a]1 diverting colostomy

Table 20.4.   Complications

Complications	Number of Patients
Intraoperative splenectomy	2
Ureteral laceration	1
Postoperative wound infection	6
Intra-abdominal abscess	2
Pulmonary	2
Phlebitis	1
Bacteremia	1
Urinary tract infection	1
Atrial fibrillation	1
Congestive heart failure	1
Dilantin toxicity	1
*Total:	13 (41%)

*Some patients had more than one complication

The procedures are listed in Table 20.3. Operation has included creation of a diverting colostomy in five instances (16%). Four of these patients have undergone primary anastomosis and diverting loop colostomy because the anastomosis rested within a large pelvic abscess cavity or because the rectal wall was thickened and indurated due to adjacent inflammation. In an additional patient, a persistent discrepancy in the caliber of the proximal and distal segments of intestine following intraoperative lavage was believed to preclude safe anastomosis. All five patients whose operation included creation of a colostomy were treated early in our experience with intraoperative antegrade colonic lavage.

There have been no postoperative deaths and no clinical or radiographic evidence of anastomotic complications in 31 patients having a primary colorectal anastomosis. Thirteen patients (41%) sustained one or more perioperative complications (Table 20.4), a figure comparable to the reported morbidity accompanying emergency intestinal resection in other large series. Three patients with intraoperative complications required corrective action. In two instances, this included splenectomy to control a splenic laceration sustained during mobilization of the colon. The third patient required ureteroureterostomy to repair a laceration identified after mobilization of a large pericolic phlegmon in the left paracolic

Table 20.5.   Applications of On-Table Lavage

Acute left colonic obstruction
   Carcinoma
   Diverticular stricture
   Volvulus
Left colonic trauma
Inadequate preparation left colon
Colonic interposition (esophageal cancer)
Diverticulitis
   Local abscess/peritonitis
Colonic hemorrhage

Modified after Danne PD. Intra-operative colonic lavage: safe single-stage, left colorectal resections. Aust N Z J Surg 1991;61:59–65.

gutter. *Wound infection was the most frequent postoperative complication.* Currently, we perform delayed primary closure of wounds that are judged to be excessively contaminated at laparotomy.

Despite the presence of an active inflammatory process at the time of laparotomy, postoperative intra-abdominal sepsis has been identified in only two cases. Percutaneous drainage of an abscess in the left subphrenic space was required in one individual whose initial operation had included splenectomy. A sinogram through the drainage catheter identified a gastric fistula that closed spontaneously after a period of gastric decompression and hyperalimentation. A 53-year-old woman required transvaginal drainage of a pelvic abscess after sigmoid colectomy for acute diverticulitis. A water-soluble contrast enema performed before drainage confirmed the integrity of the intestinal anastomosis.

The duration of hospitalization in this series has ranged from 8 to 24 days (mean = 13 days) after resection with intraoperative lavage and intestinal anastomosis.

SUMMARY

Our results suggest that intraoperative colonic lavage and primary anastomosis is a safe alternative for selected patients requiring urgent resection of the distal colon to manage complications of diverticular disease. In the absence of intraoperative lavage, all patients in our series would have required a multistage procedure. Candidates for primary anastomosis include individuals with acute diverticulitis complicated by localized peritonitis, intestinal obstruction, or a pericolic abscess that can be drained and largely excised during the course of segmental colectomy. Rather than representing an exception to the usual criteria for intestinal anastomosis, intraoperative lavage and primary anastomosis provide an alternative method for meeting those criteria, especially when the primary indication for colostomy is the lack of adequate mechanical preparation of the colon. *We would not recommend this approach for patients exhibiting the hemodynamic and pulmonary consequences of systemic sepsis. In addition, we would not pursue primary anastomosis in patients with feculent or fibrinous peritonitis or a large pelvic abscess.* For these individuals, the additional operating time required for intraoperative lavage and the potential consequences of anastomotic dehiscence pose too great a risk.

EDITORIAL COMMENTS

A decade ago, on-table lavage was rarely practiced or discussed; its origins can be traced back to techniques described by Muir in 1968 (13). Even today, the Hartmann procedure remains much more popular when emergency operations are performed for perforated diverticulitis, even in the United Kingdom (17), the source of most English language reports of on-table lavage at the present time (18–26).

The authors have presented one of the largest published series of the on-table lavage technique in the United States as part of an aggressive surgical approach to complicated diverticular disease. The major drawback to the procedure is added operative time, rather than technical complexity or a high morbidity and mortality rate. Despite the lack of controlled trials, the technique and modifications (26) are being disseminated gradually among colorectal surgeons in particular, and the number of applications is increasing (Table 20.5). As more surgeons become familiar with on-table lavage, its popularity will probably increase, and more patients will be spared colostomies.

This technique is another step in the evolution away from three-stage procedures for diverticulitis, with the potential for prolonged, cumulative lengths of hospitalization and numerous complications (27–29). On the other hand, on-table lavage should be used selectively; staged procedures such as the Hartmann operation are preferred when diffuse peritonitis, sepsis, or a large intra-abdominal abscess is present. A left colonic anastomosis can be extremely dangerous if performed under emergency conditions (30).

REFERENCES

1. Ambrosetti P, Robert JH, Witzig JA, et al. Acute left colonic diverticulitis: a prospective analysis of 226 consecutive cases. Surgery 1994;115:546–550. *Patients younger than 50 years of age were more prone to recurrences after conservative treatment; all of the patients required surgery more frequently during the first hospitalization.*
2. Rodkey GV, Welch CE. Changing patterns in surgical treatment of diverticular disease. Ann Surg 1984;200:466–478. *A study of 350 cases over a decade. Trends cited included increased disease severity in hospitalized patients, more immunocompromised patients, and an increased percentage of one-stage resections. The lowest mortality in patients with generalized peritonitis followed primary resection.*
3. Hackford AW, Schoetz DJ, Coller JA, et al. Surgical management of complicated diverticulitis. Dis Colon Rectum 1985;28:317–321. *A retrospective study of 140 patients comparing the results of one-stage and multiple-stage procedures.*
4. Auguste LJ, Wise L. Surgical management of perforated diverticulitis. Am J Surg 1981;141:122–127. *A retrospective review comparing groups having primary resection and staged procedures. The hospital stays and period of disability were longer in the staged group; the "cure" rate was lower in this group as well.*
5. Rodkey GV, Welch CE. Colonic diverticular disease with surgical treatment: a study of 338 cases. Surg Clin North Am 1974;54:655–674. *A review of the preceding decade. The authors noted more aggressive treatment of patients younger than 50 years of age, the importance of excising the source of sepsis, and the benefits of angiographic techniques for bleeding patients. High mortality rates following emergency procedures and significant morbidity rates represented persistent problems.*
6. Eng K, Ranson JH, Localio AS. Resection of the perforated segment. Am J Surg 1977;133:67–72. *The authors advocate primary resection of the involved colon with immediate or delayed anastomosis.*
7. Eisenstadt TE, Rubin RJ, Salvati EP. Surgical management of diverticulitis: the role of the Hartmann procedure. Dis Colon Rectum 1983;26:429–432. *For 44 patients undergoing the Hartmann procedure for complex diverticulitis, the mortality rate was 4.4%.*
8. Smith SR, Connolly JC, Gilmore OJ. The effect of fecal loading on colonic anastomotic healing. Br J Surg 1983;70:49–50. *In a prospective randomized control study in rats, anastomotic dehiscence appeared significantly more often with fecal loading than with an empty colon.*
9. Irvin TT, Goligher JC. Etiology of disruption of intestinal anastomoses. Br J Surg 1973;60:461–464. *In a series of 204 patients, 14% had clinical evidence of anastomotic dehiscence. A defunctioning colostomy did not decrease the risk of anastomotic complications; hypoalbuminemia and age older than 60 years were associated with increased risk.*
10. Irvin TT. Collagen metabolism in infected colonic anastomoses. Surg Gynecol Obstet 1976;143:220–224. *Rats with defective anastomoses had reduced amounts of collagen in the anastomoses compared with the control group.*
11. Schrock TR, Deveney CW, Dunphy JE. Factors contributing to leakage of colonic anastomoses. Ann Surg 1973;177:513–518. *The leakage rate was 0.6% after left colectomy for diverticular disease when no infection was present. Emergency left colonic anastomoses disrupted in more than 10%, regardless of whether infection was present. The dehiscence rate was 32% when massive hemorrhage was the indication for colectomy.*
12. Ravo B, Metwally N, Castera P, et al. The importance of intraluminal anastomotic fecal contact and peritonitis in colonic anastomotic leakages: an experimental study. Dis Colon Rectum 1988;31:868–871. *An experimental*

study in 64 dogs suggested that the intraluminal contact of fecal loading at the colonic anastomosis was a more important factor related to anastomotic dehiscence than peritonitis per se.

13. Muir EG. Safety in colonic resection. Proc R Soc Med 1968;1:401–408. *An excellent early discussion of the fundamentals of preoperative colon preparation and of on-table lavage techniques.*

14. Radcliffe AG, Dudley HA. Intraoperative antegrade irrigation of the large intestine. Surg Gynecol Obstet 1983;156:721–723. *A concise description of the technique of on-table lavage.*

15. Murray JJ, Schoetz DJ, Coller JA, et al. Intra-operative colonic lavage and primary anastomosis in nonelective colon resection. Dis Colon Rectum 1991;34:527–531. *Twenty-one of 25 patients having urgent left colonic resection had intraoperative colonic lavage with no deaths or clinically evident anastomotic leaks.*

16. Hinchey EJ, Schaal PG, Richards GK. Treatment of perforated diverticular disease of the colon. Adv Surg 1978;12:85–109. *An important review that classified perforated diverticulitis into four stages. Primary resection with or without anastomosis is advocated in most settings.*

17. Pain J, Cahill J. Surgical options for left-sided large bowel emergencies. Ann R Coll Surg Engl 1991;73:394–397. *The authors sent questionnaires to 218 consultant surgeons. The Hartmann procedure was the most popular operation for all conditions; on-table lavage was rarely used.*

18. Thomson W, Carter S. On-table lavage to achieve safe restorative rectal and emergency left colonic resection without covering colostomy. Br J Surg 1986;73:61–63. *A series of 122 consecutive single-stage resections, including 20 with acute obstruction, performed by 16 surgeons; the clinical anastomotic leak rate was 5%.*

19. Allen-Mersh TG. Should primary anastomosis and on-table colonic lavage be standard treatment for left colon emergencies? Ann R Coll Surg Engl 1993;75:195–198. *Fifteen consecutive patients treated by one surgeon with on-table lavage and primary anastomosis for left colonic emergencies (obstruction or peritonitis/pericolonic abscess) had a similar morbidity and mortality as a group of patients undergoing Hartmann procedures during the same time period. The importance of an experienced, suitably trained surgeon is emphasized.*

20. Koruth NM, Krukowski ZH, Youngson GG, et al. Intra-operative colonic irrigation in the management of left-sided large bowel emergencies. Br J Surg 1985;72:708–711. *One of the large early reports of on-table lavage, involving 61 patients having immediate anastomosis in the emergency setting for distal colonic lesions. Some patients with fecal peritonitis are included.*

21. Koruth NM, Hunter DC, Krukowski ZH, et al. Immediate resection in emergency large bowel surgery: a seven-year audit. Br J Surg 1985;72:703–707. *Discusses a 7-year experience involving emergency admissions for colonic complications under the care of one consultant surgeon. The safety of on-table lavage with primary anastomosis under appropriate conditions is emphasized.*

22. Donaldson DR, Hughes LE. Notes on "on table" lavage. Br J Surg 1987;74:465. *A modification of the lavage technique is described, using a long longitudinal colotomy to facilitate emptying of the colon more rapidly.*

23. Pollock AV, Playforth MJ, Evans M. Preoperative lavage of the obstructed left colon to allow safe primary anastomosis. Dis Colon Rectum 1987;30:171–173. *The lavage procedure took as much as 1 hour to perform.*

24. Stewart J, Diament RH, Brennan TG. Management of obstructing lesions of the left colon by resection, on-table lavage and primary anastomosis. Surgery 1993;114:502–505. *Seven of 73 consecutive patients with left colonic obstruction had diverticular disease as the cause.*

25. Gramegna A, Saccomani G. On-table colonic irrigation in the treatment of left-sided large-bowel emergencies. Dis Colon Rectum 1989;32:585–587. *Includes five patients with diffuse peritonitis and two patients with obstruction from diverticular disease. The only drawback to on-table lavage was a 40-minute increase in operative time.*

26. Danne PD. Intra-operative colonic lavage: safe single-stage, left colorectal resections. Aust N Z J Surg 1991;61:59–65. *Sixteen of 50 consecutive patients undergoing intraoperative colonic lavage had acute or subacute colonic obstructions. Candidates for this technique are discussed, as well as differing approaches for the nonobstructed colon versus the obstructed or trauma-disrupted colon.*

27. Wara P, Sorensen K, Berg V, et al. The outcome of staged management of complicated diverticular disease of the sigmoid colon. Acta Chir Scand 1981;147:209–214. *A retrospective study of 83 patients having staged procedures; the authors point out the permanence of many transverse colostomies and the serious anastomotic complications that occurred despite a proximal diverting colostomy.*

28. Mealy K, Salman A, Arthur G. Definitive one-stage emergency large bowel surgery. Br J Surg 1988;75:1216–1219. *Eighty-three of 126 procedures involving emergent large bowel conditions were treated with immediate resection and anastomosis. On-table lavage was not used; if fecal loading was present, the bowel was evacuated by manual compression into the bowel.*

29. Classen JN, Bonardi R, O'Mara CS. Surgical treatment of acute diverticulitis by staged procedures. Ann Surg 1976;184:582–586. *A report of 208 patients with acute diverticulitis treated at four urban hospitals; the overall mortality rate was 11%.*

30. Scott–Conner CE, Scher KS. Implications of emergency operations on the colon. Am J Surg 1987;153:535–540. *A retrospective study comparing patients having elective and emergency large bowel procedures. The mortality rates were 5% and 38%, respectively (P < .001). The mortality was 70% when a large bowel anastomosis was performed during an emergency operation.*

21 Complications of Surgery for Diverticulitis

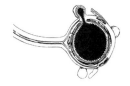

Jeffrey L. Cohen, MD
Glen Egrie, MD
William V. Sardella, MD
Paul V. Vignati, MD
John P. Welch, MD

KEY POINTS

- Morbidity and mortality higher with emergency procedures
- Control of hemorrhage and contamination important
- Carefully identify the ureters; stents if much inflammation
- Careful anastomotic technique to avoid leakage
- Usually manage intestinal obstruction conservatively
- Urgent management of suspected anastomotic leak
- Do CT scan if abscess suspected
- Numerous potential stomal problems exist
- Use of dilatation for anastomotic stricture

ILLUSTRATIVE CASES

Case 1

A 64-year-old male underwent an elective sigmoid resection because of recurrent hospitalizations for sigmoid diverticulitis. He had been on prednisone 5 mg p.o. daily because of chronic obstructive pulmonary disease. The postoperative course was smooth until the fourth postoperative day, when he developed abdominal distention, a low-grade fever, and lower abdominal pain.

CASE COMMENTS

This patient had worrisome clinical symptoms that should raise suspicion of an anastomotic leak. The study of choice in this situation would be a water-soluble enema with an agent such as gastrografin (Fig. 21.1). The films showed significant extravasation of contrast from the anastomosis. Such a complication, especially in the immunosuppressed patient taking steroids, warrants urgent laparotomy and, depending on the condition of the anastomosis, proximal diversion and drainage versus takedown of the anastomosis with diversion (see below). Early intervention lessens the risk of an additional cascade of symptoms and the possibility of multiple organ dysfunction, as discussed in Chapter 24.

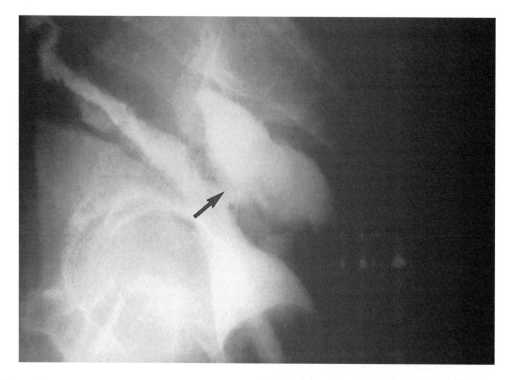

Figure 21.1.   Gastrografin enema study in a septic patient who had undergone sigmoid resection and anastomosis several days previously. Extravasation of contrast is evident at the arrow.

Case 2

A 70-year-old female underwent a Hartmann procedure. At operation, there was a phlegmon involving the midsigmoid colon and mesentery. Major bleeding at the base of the sigmoid mesentery was controlled with suture ligatures. The operation was otherwise uneventful.

On the fifth postoperative day, the patient complained of increasing lower abdominal pain. She had a low-grade fever; the white blood count was 17,000; electrolytes, liver function tests, blood urea nitrogen (BUN), and creatinine were normal. Because the pain was increasing, a computed tomography (CT) scan was performed, which showed a large fluid collection in the pelvis and lower abdomen that was homogeneous. Percutaneous drainage revealed serouslike fluid. No bacteria were identified in the fluid. A catheter was left in the collection and a later culture showed *Escherichia coli*. Because of continued output of fluid, the patient was given indigo carmine. There was colored fluid in the drainage catheter, and the creatinine level in the fluid was three times as high as the serum creatinine. She was returned to the operating room.

CASE COMMENTS

This patient had a ureteral injury that was not identified during the placement of suture ligatures in the inflamed pericolonic mesentery. The patient had no suggestive symptoms until the fifth postoperative day. Because the ureter was not ligated and obstructed, no flank pain developed and there were no signs of hydronephrosis on the CT scan. Operative management of this complication is difficult because of the delay in diagnosis. The ureter must be located within the urinoma and the inflammation before any type of repair can be attempted.

Case 3

A 76-year-old male underwent a one-stage resection of a colovesical fistula caused by diverticular disease. The bladder was drained with a Foley catheter. Of note, he had numerous intra-abdominal adhesions attributed to a perforated appendix many years earlier. On the fourth postoperative day, the lower part of the abdominal wound became erythematous. It was opened, and some purulence as well as a fecal odor were detected. During the next few hours, the dressing was soaked with enteric contents. A CT scan was performed with contrast: this showed no significant collection of fluid in the abdomen and no evidence of dilated bowel loops. No extravasation was seen from the anastomosis.

CASE COMMENTS

This patient seemed to have an enterocutaneous fistula, perhaps caused by an unrecognized small bowel injury that occurred during the enterolysis. A needle could have incorporated the wall of the small bowel during the abdominal closure, although the surgeon was confident that this was not the case. Because there did not seem to be an undrained fluid collection, the patient was not septic, and the anastomosis did not seem to be leaking, it was reasonable to treat him with bowel rest, intravenous alimentation, and wide-spectrum antibiotics. A fistulogram was performed that showed a connection with the midileum and no evidence of distal obstruction. The fistula output decreased from 150 to 10 mL/day within 1 week. He was subsequently started on a liquid diet and the hyperalimentation was tapered.

DISCUSSION

Numerous complications can occur both in the intraoperative and postoperative phases of surgery for diverticular disease (1–3). *These are especially likely to occur when operations are performed in the emergency setting (4), when sepsis may be established, preparation of the bowel has not occurred, and other organ systems are "stressed."* Also, with the introduction of laparoscopic procedures in colorectal surgery, there is evidence of a definite learning curve involving at least 50 cases (5). Beyond the phase of this discussion are problems such as atelectasis, pneumonia, pulmonary embolus, congestive heart failure, myocardial infarct, liver failure, renal failure, cerebrovascular accident, or coagulopathies. Some of these systemic illnesses are covered in Chapter 24.

During the operation, efforts should be made to control bleeding and contamination of the operative field by bowel contents. Postoperatively, the surgeon must be alert to wound, stomal, and abdominal complications involving the field of dissection, such as the mesentery, small bowel, spleen, and urinary system.

In a group of 78 patients undergoing sigmoid resection without anastomosis for perforated diverticulitis, intraoperative complications included hemorrhage requiring transfusions (37%), ureteral injury (1%), and small bowel injury (1%); postoperative complications consisted of wound infection (24%), intra-abdominal abscess (5%), wound dehiscence (4%), and stomal necrosis (1%) (6). In another series of 71 patients undergoing surgery for diverticulitis, the most frequent postoperative complications were wound infections, pneumonia, incisional hernia, and septic shock (7). Among a report of 338 patients, frequent postoperative problems consisted of wound abscess (4.4%), anastomotic leak (2.1%), abdominal/pelvic abscess (1.5%), cystitis (1.5%), pulmonary insufficiency (1.5%), and anastomotic stricture (1.5%) (8).

We have arbitrarily chosen a number of major complications that the surgeon must be on the lookout for during the patient's convalescence.

Ureteral Injuries

The best treatment of ureteral injury is prevention. Patients with an abdominal mass are more likely to have urologic abnormalities (9). Inflammation wrought by diverticulitis may distort the normal anatomy, where the ureter crosses over the bifurcation of the iliac vessels in the retroperitoneum. However, it is almost always possible to find the ureter proximally where there are normal tissue planes uninvolved by inflammation. The ureter can then be followed distally and separated from the sigmoid mesentery. We "pinch" the ureter gently with forceps, which leads to peristaltic contractions and ensures that the ureter is not confused with another structure such as a vessel. Although the ureter has a number of vessels supplying it, it should not be mobilized circumferentially to avoid possible devascularization (Fig. 21.2) (10).

If a difficult dissection is anticipated in the presence of a phlegmon, abscess, or in redo pelvic surgery, placement of ureteral stents can be very helpful in identifying the ureters. The stents are palpable, even in areas of thickening, and dissection in the inflamed tissue to look for the structures is not necessary. *Ureteral stents clearly save time in the operating room; however, they may not always prevent ureteral injury.*

If a ureteral injury is suspected, it can be confirmed by injecting indigo carmine or methylene blue intravenously; efflux will be seen through the injured ureter. After the injury has been identified, it is best repaired at the time of surgery. Urologic consultation should be sought if available. Small partial disruptions may be repaired primarily over a stent. Ureteral transections should be repaired primarily with a spatulated anastomosis over a stent.

The most common site of injury is at the level of the pelvic brim, involving the distal one-third of the ureter. If a substantial segment has been disrupted, then direct re-implantation into the bladder is the best option (ureteroneocystostomy) (Fig. 21.3) (10,11). If length is a problem, then a bladder-lengthening procedure may help. Generally, injuries within 4 cm of the ureterovesical junction are best managed by ureteroneocystostomy, and injuries more than 4 cm away are best managed by ureteroureterostomy (12). A crossover ureteroureterostomy should not be used, if possible, because complications could potentially jeopardize both kidneys.

Anastomotic Leak

Anastomotic leak is one of the most feared complications of surgery for diverticular disease. It can be devastating and potentially life-threatening, occurring clinically in 7–8% of cases (1,13). At the very least, it usually results in a return to the operating room for adequate drainage and fecal diversion. This prolongs the hospital course and leads to a series of operative procedures to achieve restoration of intestinal integrity.

One of the earliest signs of a potential anastomotic leak is a deviation from the previously steady postoperative course. *Although an anastomotic leak can present as an acute abdomen, more commonly, fever, tachycardia, and ileus herald the onset of trouble.* After this initial presentation, the patient usually will begin to complain of abdominal pain and distention, and examination will reveal increasing tenderness at the affected site.

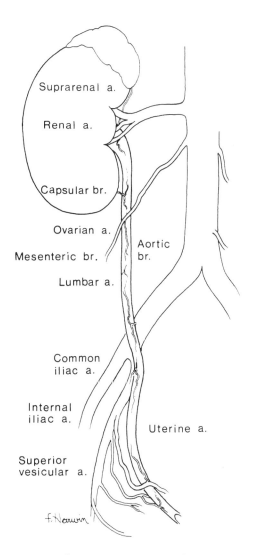

Figure 21.2.   Segmental blood supply of the ureter. (Reprinted with permission from Pearse HD, Barry JM, Fuchs EF. Intraoperative consultation for the ureter. Urol Clin North Am 1985;12:423–437.)

As a general guideline, the most likely time-frame for the development of a leak is between the fourth and sixth postoperative days. Predisposing factors include poor anastomotic technique involving excessive tension, compromised blood supply (14), or imperfect suturing. Although malfunctioning of a stapler has been implicated in many instances, it is far more common that the stapler has been used improperly or that the anastomosis has not been tested adequately. Other potential risk factors include poor bowel preparation, prolonged hypotension perioperatively, diabetes mellitus, immuno-suppression, medications such as steroids, obesity, and "low" rectal anastomoses. Although conclusive data are not available regarding many of these potential risk factors, it does seem that very low rectal or coloanal anastomoses are at significantly higher risk for anastomotic leak, and a diverting ileostomy should be considered at the time of surgery.

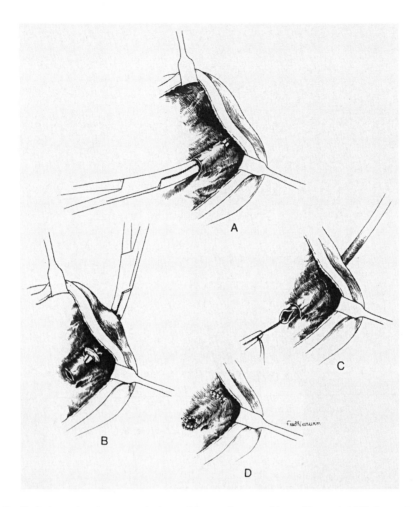

Figure 21.3.   Technique of ureteroneocystostomy. After a submucosal tunnel is created **(A)**, the ureter is brought through **(C)**, and the anastomosis is completed **(D)**. The proximal vesical hiatus is shown in **B.** (Reprinted with permission from Pearse HD, Barry JM, Fuchs EF. Intraoperative consultation for the ureter. Urol Clin North Am 1985;12:423–437.)

When there is clinical suspicion of an anastomotic leak, prompt evaluation must be performed. Although it has been reported that the radiologic leak rate is up to 10 times as high as the clinical leak rate, the use of either a CT scan with contrast (Fig. 21.4) or a gastrografin enema (Fig. 21.1) is the most accurate method of diagnosing a leak.

Radiologic confirmation mandates prompt intervention. *In most cases, fecal diversion is the treatment of choice.* Although it is optional regarding how diversion is accomplished, our own preference is a diverting loop ileostomy (15,16). It is relatively easy to create and usually is the easiest to reverse. Furthermore, creation of an ileostomy never jeopardizes the marginal circulation of the colon, which at times the anastomosis is dependent upon. As a general rule, it is unnecessary to take down the anastomosis; drainage of the site usually is sufficient. *Unless there is major disruption of the anastomosis or a long ischemic segment, it is likely that with proximal diversion and time, the anastomosis will heal and be functional.*

A few points from the literature deserve mention. A paucity of vessels in the midline of the rectum may explain, in part, the development of an anastomotic leak in some patients (17). The superior hemorrhoidal vessels should be preserved if at all possible during the original operation. If there is any bleeding tendency at the end of the original procedure, we sometimes insert a closed drain in the pelvis but remove it within approximately 48 hours because of the risk that the drain will disrupt the anastomosis if left in too long. Others have stated that accumulation of blood and serum in the pelvis may increase the anastomotic risk of a low anastomosis (18). In another series, there was a higher incidence of anastomotic leak after elective resection for diverticular disease when compared with resection of carcinoma (19). There are also data that patients converted from a laparoscopic-assisted colectomy to an open operation have an increased anastomotic leak rate, perhaps related, in part, to a lengthy procedure (20).

Perioperative Bleeding

Intraoperative and postoperative bleeding can occur in a number of locations, such as the bowel mesentery or the pelvic adnexal vessels in the region of the sigmoid colon. A potential cause of major intra-abdominal bleeding following colectomy is *splenic injury*, which occurs during mobilization of the splenic flexure to provide adequate length for a tension-free coloproctostomy. Splenic injury can also follow vigorous pulling on a retractor by an assistant. In one report involving mobilization of the splenic flexure in 260 patients, eight patients had splenic injuries (3.1%) (21). In a series of 185 incidental splenectomies, 9.7% were associated with left colectomy, 5.9% were associated with splenic flexure resection, 3.2% were associated with transverse colectomy, and 2.7% were associated with sigmoid resection (22). Splenic injury most commonly results from tension on the colon and greater omentum in attempts to mobilize the flexure (Fig. 21.5). Most injuries are minor. When operating for benign disease, we recommend mobilizing the colon from under the omentum. This involves lifting the omentum off the colon and dividing the flimsy

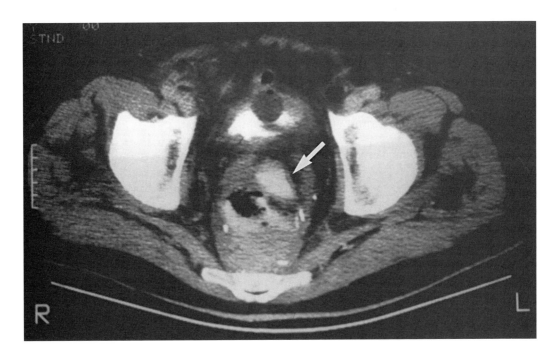

Figure 21.4.   A CT scan demonstrates extravasated contrast (arrow) from a recent colorectal anastomosis.

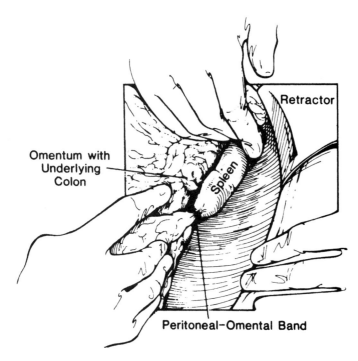

Figure 21.5. Example of a peritoneal–omental band attached to the inferior pole of the spleen. (Reprinted with permission from Langevin JM, Rothenberger DA, Goldberg SM. Accidental splenic injury during surgical treatment of the colon and rectum. Surg Gynecol Obstet 1984;159:139–144.)

attachments between the colon and omentum. The colon can then be safely rolled up off the retroperitoneum without a great deal of tension and essentially no tension on the spleen. Usually, there is a relatively bloodless plane immediately adjacent to the colon at the flexure (Fig. 21.6).

If possible, the spleen should be salvaged because of the dangers of postsplenectomy sepsis (23). Most avulsions or capsular injuries can be treated with topical Avitene, Surgicel, Gelfoam, or topical thrombin with good results. The argon beam coagulator can be of some help in controlling oozing from a large raw surface. Methods of suture repair also have been described (23). Significant bleeding, especially in an older, high-risk patient, warrants expeditious splenectomy. The risk of splenectomy is increased if the capsule is injured near the hilum (21).

In the pelvis, the *presacral venous plexus* can be difficult to control if disruption and bleeding occur. The superior hemorrhoidal artery is preserved, and only rarely does this plane need to be entered when resecting diverticular disease. If one has to open this plane, care should be taken to enter the presacral space above the presacral fascia—this is best performed under direct vision. Initial control of bleeding should involve packing. Because the blood loss may be considerable, attention should be paid to blood volume, temperature, and clotting parameters. Occasionally, suture ligation can be helpful. Placement of sterile titanium thumbtacks also has been described (24,25). If bleeding cannot be controlled, the pelvis should be packed and the patient should be transferred to an intensive care unit (ICU) for correction of the coagulopathy and warming. Rarely, there may be use for angiographic embolization or internal iliac artery ligation, although the bleeding tends to be of venous origin.

A rare source of postoperative bleeding is *the anastomosis* itself; this may occur in 1.8% of stapled colorectal anastomoses (26). Usually, this can be treated conservatively, with possible blood transfusions; endoscopic electrocoagulation also has been used successfully in a few cases (26).

Postoperative Small Bowel Obstruction

It is difficult to determine the actual incidence of early postoperative small bowel obstruction (occurring within 30 days of operation), although it has been estimated to be 0.7–0.8% (27,28). *The risk is particularly great following colonic and pelvic surgery* and, therefore, is of particular relevance to patients with sigmoid diverticulitis. Adhesions usually are at fault, the distal small bowel usually is involved, and strangulation is unusual.

A major diagnostic problem involves differentiating paralytic ileus from mechanical obstruction (Fig. 21.7) (29). There are a number of causes of paralytic ileus, such as pancreatitis, hypokalemia, pneumonia, or intra-abdominal abscess (Table 21.1) (30). Although small bowel activity returns within a few hours of an operation, gastric peristalsis is delayed for 24–48 hours and colonic motility is delayed for 48–72 hours. Crampy abdominal pain and peristaltic rushes suggest mechanical obstruction rather than ileus, and the development of such symptoms after the patient has established bowel movements a few days after surgery is particularly worrisome (28).

Another concern is the possibility that strangulation can occur, such as after volvulus of small bowel loops around an ileostomy stoma (Figs. 21.8 and 21.9). The difficulties of distinguishing strangulation obstruction from simple obstruction clinically have been

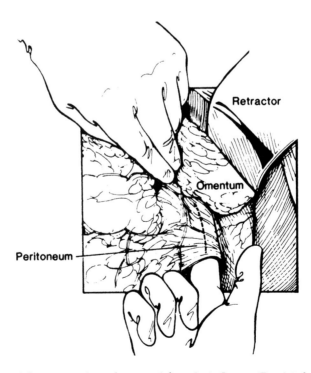

Figure 21.6. Exposure of the peritoneal attachments of the splenic flexure. (Reprinted with permission from Langevin JM, Rothenberger DA, Goldberg SM. Accidental splenic injury during surgical treatment of the colon and rectum. Surg Gynecol Obstet 1984;159:139–144.)

Figure 21.7. Plain radiograph (upright) shows air-fluid levels in dilated small bowel in patient with mechanical small bowel obstruction.

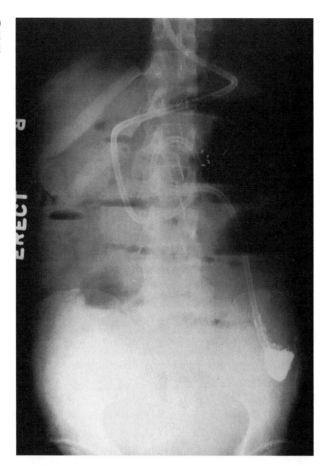

Table 21.1.   Causes of Postoperative Ileus

Drugs
    Anti-Parkinson agents
    Chronic laxatives
Hypokalemia
Pancreatitis
Pneumonia
Myocardial infarct
Pelvic/abdominal abscess
Anastomotic leak
Urinary tract infection

Modified after Nadrowski L. Paralytic ileus: recent advances in pathophysiology and treatment. Curr Surg 1983;40:260–273.

documented in a prospective study (31); complicating the problem is the fact that symptoms suggesting strangulation, such as persistent abdominal pain, tenderness, nausea, and constipation, are common findings during convalescence from abdominal surgery. Closed-loop small bowel obstruction may be found unexpectedly when operating for peritonitis.

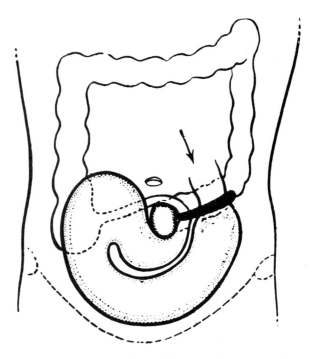

Figure 21.8. Schematic view of a paraileostomy hernia. This can lead to strangulation obstruction. (Reprinted with permission from Goligher JC. Surgery of the anus, rectum and colon. 5th ed. London: Bailliere Tindal, 1984:909) [Ref. 72].

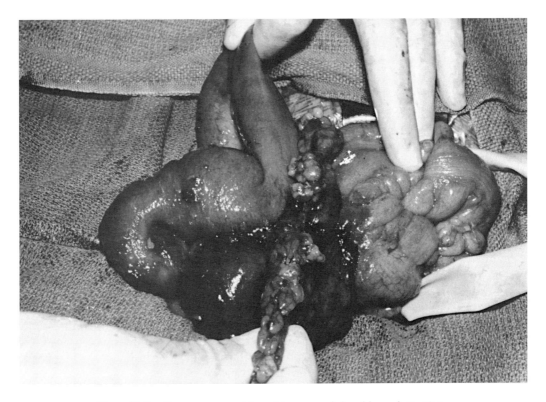

Figure 21.9. Gangrenous small bowel in a case of closed loop obstruction.

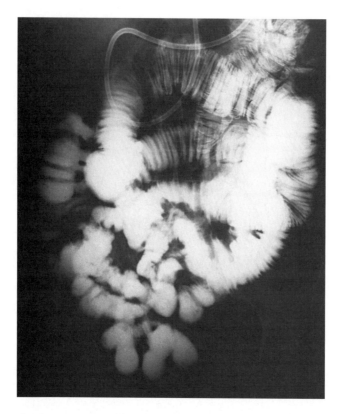

Figure 21.10.   Example of partial small bowel obstruction. Small bowel series shows dilated proximal small bowel and transition into collapsed small bowel.

Most cases of postoperative obstruction can be managed with intravenous fluids, tube decompression, and frequent physical examinations. As the situation improves, the tube can be clamped and clear liquids can be started. Contrast studies can be of some help in determining whether mechanical obstruction is present (Fig. 21.10) (32). If nasogastric outputs remain high or if the patient continues to have crampy pain (usually by the second postoperative week) with clamping of the tube, exploratory laparotomy should be considered (33). The abdomen must be entered carefully, with lysis of adhesions of bowel and omentum to the abdominal wall (Fig. 21.11). If gangrenous changes are found (Fig. 21.9), the Doppler probe (34) (Fig. 21.12) or fluorescein fluorescence (35) can help determine the margins of viable bowel if a substantial resection is entertained.

Postoperative Intra-Abdominal Abscess

One of the most serious complications of diverticular surgery is the development of an intra-abdominal abscess. Although the signs and symptoms are quite subtle at times, more frequently there is significant patient instability.

An abscess usually becomes apparent on the sixth to tenth postoperative days. Predictable signs and symptoms include fever, tachycardia, abdominal pain, distention, nausea, and inanition. If this constellation of symptoms develops or if a patient begins to deteriorate clinically during the appropriate time period, aggressive evaluation is warranted. *Clearly the most useful examination is a CT scan performed with oral and rectal*

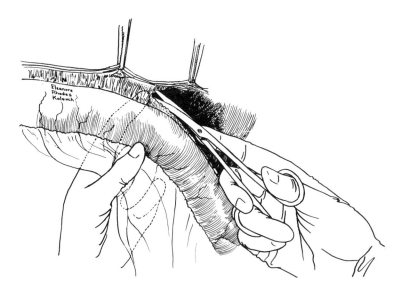

Figure 21.11. Lysing adhesions to the anterior abdominal wall must be done carefully when performing laparotomy in the postoperative period. (Reprinted with permission from Welch JP. Operative techniques, decisions, and complications. In: Welch JP, ed. Bowel obstruction. Differential diagnosis and clinical management. Philadelphia: WB Saunders, 1990:423–448) [Ref. 73].

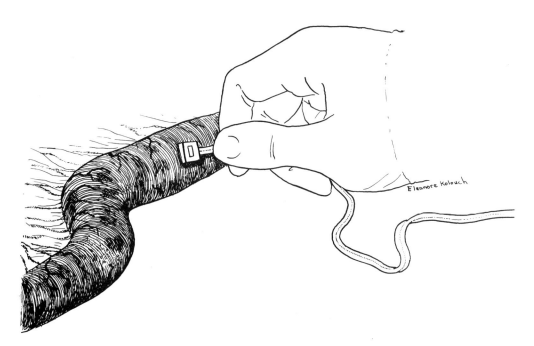

Figure 21.12. Use of the Doppler ultrasound in detecting ischemic small bowel. (Reprinted with permission from Welch JP. Operative techniques, decisions, and complications. In: Welch JP, ed. Bowel obstruction. Differential diagnosis and clinical management. Philadelphia: WB Saunders, 1990;423–448) [Ref. 73].

contrast. Not only will an intra-abdominal abscess be detected, but anastomotic leaks, which often lead to development of the abscess, also can be detected (Fig. 21.13).

After the abscess has been defined, *percutaneous drainage can usually be performed by the interventional radiologist to successfully treat the condition* (36). Transrectal drainage has also been performed successfully by the endoscopic route (37). In many cases, this obviates the difficult problem of reoperating in distorted, friable tissue planes. Interloop abscesses present a distinct problem for percutaneous drainage; usually, abdominal exploration is required for adequate drainage. Catheters placed for drainage should be left in place to ensure complete treatment of the abscess cavity. Furthermore, enteric drainage from the catheter may be the first indication of an underlying enterocutaneous fistula that can be studied further.

The APACHE II score has been correlated with survival of patients with intra-abdominal abscesses (38). Other studies have correlated certain factors with poor survival, such as the presence of subhepatic or lesser sac abscesses, advanced age, or organ dysfunction (39).

Wound Problems

Surgical incisions performed for the operative treatment of diverticulitis range from clean-contaminated (class II; see Table 21.2) to dirty (gross contamination, class IV) (40).

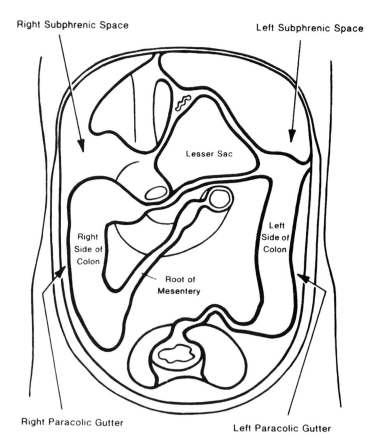

Figure 21.13. Potential spaces for collections of pus in the septic abdomen. The bowel mesentery is largely responsible for formation of these spaces. (Reprinted with permission from Ferrucci JT, van Sonnenberg E. Intra-abdominal abscess. Radiological diagnosis and treatment. JAMA 1991;246:2728–2733) [Ref. 74].

Table 21.2.   American College of Surgeons Wound Classification

Class	Wound Description	Examples
I	Clean	Uninfected wound Gastrointestinal tract not entered
II	Clean-contaminated	Gastrointestinal tract entered Minimal contamination
III	Contaminated	Wounds with major break in sterile technique Wounds contacting nonpurulent inflammation
IV	Infected	Wounds in contact with purulent infection

Modified from Coit DG. Care of the surgical wound. In: Wilmore DW, Brennan MF, Harken AH, et al., eds. American College of Surgeons, Care of the surgical patient. New York: Scientific American, Inc., 1992;VI:7:1–10.

The degree of contamination affects the surgical management of the wound as well as its subsequent risk of infection.

Elective procedures allow a conventional preoperative mechanical and antibiotic bowel preparation as well as prophylactic intravenous antibiotics given before the incision is made. These cases generally are classified as clean-contaminated and usually allow primary closure of the surgical wound with an acceptable risk of infection (less than 10%).

Emergency operations performed for bowel perforation or colonic obstruction usually are associated with significant contamination from either pus or stool, and primary closure of the wound carries an unacceptably high risk of infection. In the presence of gross contamination, wounds should be left open and packed with moist gauze. Dressings are changed several times daily, and most wounds can undergo delayed primary closure on the fifth postoperative day. If the wound is closed immediately adjacent to a stoma, it is easier to place a bag over the stoma. In some cases, wound management is complex (41,42).

In a group of patients undergoing Hartmann operations for perforated diverticulitis, the wound infection rate was 24% (6). It is not surprising that wound problems are frequent, because a septic focus is present in cases of acute diverticulitis (43).

Colostomy closure wounds should be considered contaminated and can be packed open initially, can undergo delayed primary closure as described, or can be closed loosely during the operative procedure over subcutaneous drains.

The primary risk factors for wound infection are the degree of contamination and the surgical management of the wound (i.e., primary closure versus open packing). Clearly, the goal is to obtain timely closure of the wound while minimizing the risk of infection (44). Other risk factors include an immunocompromised host due to diabetes mellitus or the intake of steroids. Obesity and the length of the surgical procedure affect the risk of infection as well.

Wound infections usually become apparent on the fifth to seventh postoperative days. Symptoms include increased incisional discomfort associated with fever, swelling, erythema, and sometimes drainage or separation of the wound edges. Wound cellulitis in the absence of purulent drainage or fluctuance can be treated initially with systemic antibiotics. The most common bacterial pathogens are enteric organisms such as *Escherichia coli*, *Klebsiella*, *Bacteroides*, and less commonly, *Staphylococcus aureus*.

When purulence is present, the wound must be opened and packed. Cultures of infected fluid should be obtained and antibiotics should be administered. A wound abscess requires opening of the wound and does not mandate antibiotics; when there is associated cellulitis, an antibiotic should be used. Most wound infections can be treated promptly with minimal adverse sequelae (45).

Wound Dehiscence

Fascial closure at the completion of an abdominal procedure can be accomplished well through a variety of techniques. *The goal of closure is to approximate margins of healthy fascia without significant tension* (Fig. 21.14). In most cases, the abdomen can be closed using fascial sutures of heavy nonabsorbable or long-term absorbable material placed in either an interrupted or running fashion. Some studies in the literature have promoted continuous closures because they are more economic and expeditious and are of similar strength as interrupted closures (46,47). Separate peritoneal closure is not necessary (48). Abdominal relaxation is paramount during this phase of the surgical procedure; whenever necessary, additional muscle relaxants should be given by the anesthesiologist to facilitate fascial reapproximation. Difficult closure secondary to visceral distention or poor fascial integrity should prompt consideration of placement of retention sutures. In such cases, our preference is to place multiple subfascial extraperitoneal "through-and-through" retention sutures of a heavy monofilament nonabsorbable suture. Wounds at high risk for dehiscence

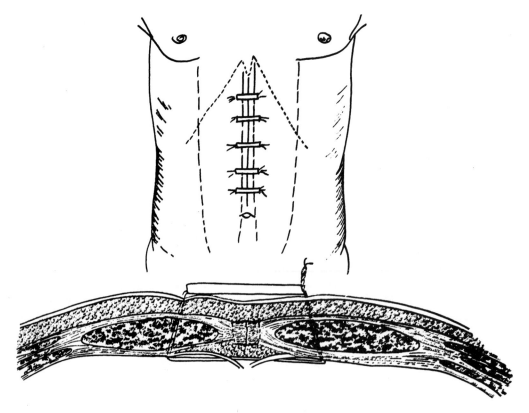

Figure 21.14. Method of closure of fascial dehiscence with all-layer retention sutures tied over bridges. (Reprinted with permission from Wilson SE, Kitts DG, Williams RA. Reoperation for abdominal wound dehiscence. In: McQuarrie DG, Humphrey EW, eds. Reoperative general surgery. St. Louis: Mosby Year Book, 1992:467–484.)

in elderly, obese, nutritionally depleted patients or individuals with severe pulmonary disease or liver disease with ascites should be closed in a similar fashion.

Although retention sutures do not eliminate the risk of fascial dehiscence, they do prevent evisceration when placed properly. Fascial dehiscence implies separation of the fascial edges and does not necessarily mandate reoperation. In contrast, *eviscerationor the passage of viscera outside of the peritoneal cavity requires immediate closure of the abdominal wound with placement of retention sutures.*

The management of fascial dehiscence requires considerable judgment. Usually, dehiscence of the fascial edges in the presence of retention sutures can be managed nonoperatively. In the absence of retention sutures, small localized areas of fascial separation can be observed closely without reoperation. Large areas of fascial separation, especially in the presence of ascites, malnutrition, pulmonary disease, increased intra-abdominal pressure, or obesity should be closed with retention sutures.

The diagnosis of evisceration is clinically quite obvious. Fascial dehiscence can be much more subtle. *Localized fascial separation with an intact skin closure can occur without obvious clinical symptoms or signs;* this, in part, explains the presence of incisional hernias recognized during office follow-up examinations weeks or months later. More extensive fascial dehiscence tends to be associated with a localized separation of the skin closure and serosanguinous drainage. *The presence of this form of drainage from the incision after the first 24 hours is virtually diagnostic of fascial dehiscence* (in some cases, it may be a spontaneously draining seroma). The fascial integrity is examined with a gloved finger or a surgical instrument (such as a Kelly clamp) using sterile technique.

The overall risk of wound dehiscence in abdominal surgery has been estimated to be 1–3% in one review (49), although this figure may now be approaching 1% (50).

Stomal Problems

Most colon resections for diverticulitis can be performed in one stage without a colostomy or ileostomy. However, if free perforation, sepsis, hemodynamic instability, or factors associated with poor wound healing are present, a two-stage operation with creation of a temporary ostomy (such as the Hartmann procedure) may be desirable. *A number of technical recommendations can be made in constructing a stoma in an attempt to reduce the number of possible complications.* Any anticipated stomal site should be marked by the operating surgeon or by an experienced enterostomal therapist before operation, if possible, to ensure the best positioning of the stoma away from belt lines, etc. After the resection is completed during the Hartmann procedure, the descending colon is mobilized along the lateral peritoneal segment, allowing sufficient length to reach several centimeters beyond the skin level at the stomal site without appreciable tension. Sometimes it is necessary to divide the inferior mesenteric artery or vein to gain sufficient length. It also is important to align and retract the skin and fascia toward the midline with clamps before the circular disc of skin is excised at the stomal site. The anterior rectus fascia is incised in a cruciate fashion and the ostomy opening is made into the abdomen. The aperture should be two to three finger-breadths in diameter and a larger opening may be needed to admit distended bowel or a thickened mesentery. The vascularity of the stoma should be checked carefully when the stoma is pulled through the abdominal wall.

At other times, a primary anastomosis may be performed with proximal diversion. Creation of a loop transverse colostomy or loop or split ileostomy are possible. A number of complications are possible after creation of either type of stoma (51), although we believe that loop ileostomy, in general, is easier to manage (15,16,52,53). It is useful to draw the ileal loop through the abdominal wall with an umbilical tape passed through a window created at the junction of the mesentery and the bowel. A small rod is passed through the mesenteric hole to support the bowel. The ileostomy is matured using a transverse incision encompassing two-thirds of the circumference along the distal limb of the loop just above the skin level. The proximal or functional limb can be everted with interrupted absorbable sutures in standard Brooke fashion.

The incidence of *parastomal hernia* (54–57) is difficult to ascertain from the literature and varies from 0 to 60%. Most long-standing colostomies have an associated asymptomatic fascial defect. The risk of parastomal hernias is higher with colostomies than with ileostomies (58,59) and with stomas brought out lateral to the rectus muscle rather than through the rectus muscle itself. Hernias are associated with a number of other factors, including obesity, steroid intake, suboptimal nutrition, and chronic pulmonary disease (Fig. 21.15). An effective method of repair incorporates mesh: the defect is bridged with mesh and the stoma is brought out through the mesh (Fig. 21.16) (60,61). A colostomy also can be brought out lateral to the mesh (62). Relocation of the stoma to another part of the abdominal wall is another acceptable technique of repair (54).

Stomal retraction usually is attributable to ischemia or excess tension (Figs. 21.17 and 21.18). Inadequate bowel or mesenteric mobilization, obesity (with a thick abdominal wall and foreshortened mesentery), or an emergency procedure with bowel distention or edema

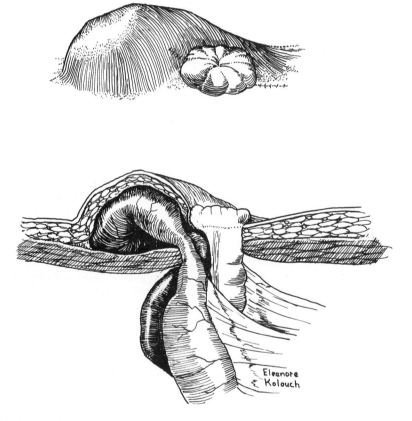

Figure 21.15.   Views of a paracolostomy hernia containing small bowel. External view (upper) and schematic cross-sectional view (bottom). (Reprinted with permission from Bloom GP, Welch JP. Hernias causing bowel obstruction. In: Welch JP, ed. Bowel obstruction. Differential diagnosis and clinical management. Philadelphia: WB Saunders, 1990:241–313) [Ref. 75].

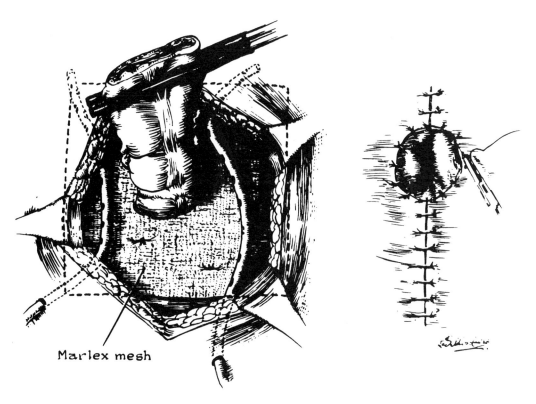

Figure 21.16.   New colostomy stoma brought through mesh after repair of paracolostomy hernia. (Reprinted with permission from Rosin JD, Bonardi RA. Paracolostomy hernia repair with Marlex mesh: a new technique. Dis Colon Rectum 1977;20:299–302.)

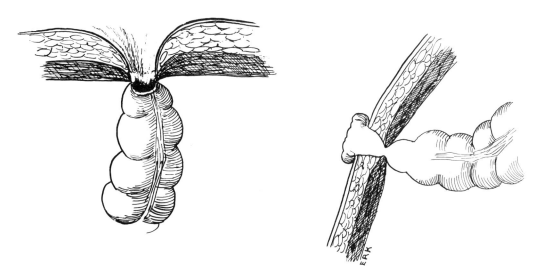

Figure 21.17.   Colostomy complications. On the left is retraction of the stoma; a subfascial stricture is present on the right. (Reprinted with permission from Welch JP. Perioperative techniques and decisions. In: Welch JP, ed. Bowel obstruction. Differential diagnosis and clinical management. Philadelphia: WB Saunders, 1990:499–545) [Ref. 76].

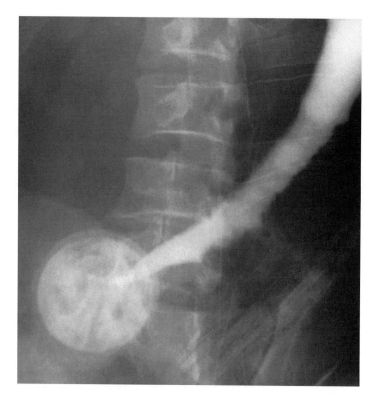

Figure 21.18.   Barium enema following installation of contrast into a stenotic colostomy stoma 3 months after a Hartmann procedure. The stoma had been brought up under tension, and narrowing of the colon leading into the tight stoma is visible.

are associated factors. Sufficient mobilization of the bowel and mesentery are important to lessen tension involving the newly created stoma.

Ischemia of a permanent colostomy created during an elective procedure should be largely avoidable. Mobilization of sufficient mesentery or bowel length should eliminate tension and associated ischemic problems. Before the stoma is created, the bowel should be examined closely for vascularity and signs of diminished perfusion. Marginal or clearly devascularized bowel should be resected, and a healthy segment should be selected for a stoma.

More commonly, a suboptimally perfused stoma results at the end of a difficult and lengthy emergency procedure. Although technical problems should be addressed, other factors, including abdominal distention, diminished peripheral perfusion secondary to shock, vasospasm, and bowel distention with edematous mesentery, contribute to a relative lack of mucosal perfusion. In this setting, a perfect ostomy may not be possible, and a viable, functional stoma is the goal. *At times, despite inadequate perfusion of an end stoma, creation of a loop stoma with intact mesentery will ensure sufficient mucosal blood flow.*

The incidence of *stomal prolapse* (63) varies and depends on the type and location of the stoma. Loop stomas are more prone to prolapse than end stomas, and transverse colostomies prolapse more frequently than sigmoid colostomies or ileostomies. There is a frequent association with parastomal hernias, especially with colostomies created in the presence of intestinal obstruction. It is necessary to make a large fascial and cutaneous aperture for the distended bowel. Gradual decompression of the proximal colon creates a fascial defect that leads to formation of a parastomal hernia with an associated stomal prolapse. The acute prolapse can be dramatic, and surgical excision and formation of a new stoma are necessary. Decreased edema of the stoma has been reported with the application of ordinary sugar to the prolapse (64).

Closure of the stoma also can be associated with a number of complications (65); the early complication rate was 22% in one series of colostomy closures (51).

Anastomotic Strictures

An anastomotic stricture is a narrowing at the anastomosis that occurs at some time during the postoperative period. Usually the stricture is detected with a contrast study or endoscopy, or in the case of a low anastomosis, by digital rectal examination. Symptoms such as constipation, narrowing of the stools, or diarrhea may result from the stricture.

Among the most frequent causes of anastomotic strictures following sigmoid resection for diverticular disease are subclinical anastomotic leaks, inflammatory changes caused by numerous sutures at the anastomosis, or technical complications of stapled low anastomoses using the circular stapler. Technical factors frequently are at fault. The stapled anastomosis should involve at least a 29-mm stapler, and the anastomosis should be free of tension and well vascularized. A two-layer sutured anastomosis is more apt to narrow than a one-layer anastomosis. In a survey of colorectal surgeons, obesity and abscesses frequently were associated, as well as intraoperative "incomplete doughnuts" with stapled anastomoses, and anastomotic leaks or pelvic infections postoperatively (66).

Stricturing of stapled anastomoses is apparent within weeks of the operation. Low strictures can be dilated digitally and higher strictures can be dilated with endoscopic techniques such as balloon dilatation. Other methods, such as introduction of a sigmoidoscope in an attempt to dilate the stricture directly with balloons (67) or stricturotomy with the cautery, papillotomy knife (68), or laser, can risk perforation. Balloons more than 51-French diameter tend to be effective in dilating colonic anastomoses (69). The endo-gastrointestinal anastromosing instrument (GAI) stapler also has been used (70). For few symptomatic patients who do not respond to these measures, resection of the anastomosis should be performed; for the high-risk individual, proximal diversion should be performed individually.

In a group of 178 patients undergoing reanastomosis following Hartmann procedures, 12 patients (6.1%) developed anastomotic strictures; two strictures were associated with anastomotic leaks. All strictures except one were opened using sigmoidoscopic dilatations (71–76).

REFERENCES

1. Kollmorgen CF, Nivatvongs S. Complications in colon and rectal surgery. Early diagnosis and management. Rev Gastroenterol Mex 1996;61:93–99. *A review article discussing the common complications, with 48 references.*
2. Belmonte C, Klas JV, Perez JJ, et al. The Hartmann procedure: first choice or last resort in diverticular disease? Arch Surg 1996;131:612–617. *Describes the surgical treatment of 227 consecutive patients. Of 52 patients with postoperative morbidity, 15 had prolonged ileus and 7 had wound infection.*
3. Daly JM, DeCosse JJ. Complications in surgery of the colon and rectum. Surg Clin North Am 1983;63:1215–1231. *An informative discussion of operative and postoperative complications, with 59 references.*
4. Alanis A, Papanicolaou GK, Tadros RR, et al. Primary resection and anastomosis for treatment of acute diverticulitis. Dis Colon Rectum 1989;32:933–939. *The wound infection rate was 23% after the Hartmann procedure.*
5. Agachan F, Joo JS, Weiss EG, et al. Intraoperative laparoscopic complications. Are we getting better? Dis Colon Rectum 1996;39:S14–S19. *Complication rates decreased from 29% to 7% during the learning period.*
6. Panton ON, Bell GA. Hartmann resection for perforated sigmoid diverticulitis. Dis Colon Rectum 1984;27:253–256. *The most common postoperative complications were wound infection (24%) and intra-abdominal abscess (5.2%).*

7. Tolins SH. Surgical treatment of diverticulitis. Experience at a large municipal hospital. JAMA 1975; 232:830–832. *Twenty-one percent of patients admitted to this New York hospital with diverticulitis were operated on; the operative mortality rate was 22%, related to delayed diagnosis, inadequate surgery, and a high incidence of associated disease.*

8. Rodkey GV, Welch CE. Colonic diverticular disease with surgical treatment. A study of 338 cases. Surg Clin North Am 1974;54:655–674. *An in-depth analysis of this group of patients treated over a decade.*

9. Peel AL, Benyon L, Grace RH. The value of routine preoperative urological assessment in patients undergoing elective surgery for diverticular disease or carcinoma of the large bowel. Br J Surg 1980;67:42–45. *A prospective study of 176 patients; 20 of the 31 patients with an abdominal mass had an abnormal IVP.*

10. Pearse HD, Barry JM, Fuchs EF. Intraoperative consultation for the ureter. Urol Clin North Am 1985;12:423–437. *An excellent description of the various techniques that can be used for repair of the injured ureter. The authors emphasize that one technique will not solve all problems. Operative principles should include repair with viable tissue, anastomosis without tension, adequate drainage, and proper use of stents, proximal diversion, and antibiotics. A well-illustrated review.*

11. Andersson A, Bergdahl L. Urologic complications following abdominoperineal resections. Arch Surg 1976;111:969–971. *Five patients had ureteral injuries. Late results of repair were satisfactory in only two of the five patients.*

12. Fry DE, Milholen L, Harbrecht PJ. Iatrogenic ureteral injury. Arch Surg 1983;118:454–457. *All patients with injuries missed during the primary operation had poor results. Primary reconstruction should not be attempted in the presence of prior pelvic radiotherapy or intra-abdominal infection.*

13. Pollard CW, Nivatvongs S, Rojanasakul A, et al. Carcinoma of the rectum. Profiles of intraoperative and postoperative complications. Dis Colon Rectum 1994;37:866–874. *The overall leak rate for anterior and low anterior (including coloanal) anastomoses was 7%.*

14. Taggert RE. Colorectal anastomosis: factors influencing success. J R Soc Med 1981;74:111–118. *Reduction in blood viscosity by hemodilution may improve the microcirculatory flow to the colorectal anastomosis.*

15. Fasth S, Hulten L, Palselius I. Loop ileostomy — an attractive alternative to a temporary transverse colostomy. Acta Chir Scand 1980;146:203–207. *There were 21 patients having each operation, and the complications were evaluated.*

16. Editorial. Munro I. Colostomy or ileostomy. Lancet 1987;2:82.

17. Foster ME, Lancaster JB, Leaper DJ. Leakage of low rectal anastomosis. An anatomic explanation? Dis Colon Rectum 1984;27:157–158. *In this angiographic study of rectums of cadavers, a midline paucity of vessels was found anteriorly and posteriorly.*

18. Garnjobst W, Hardwick C. Further criteria for anastomosis in diverticulitis of the sigmoid colon. Am J Surg 1970;120:264–269. *In a series of 98 resections for sigmoid diverticulitis, anastomotic complications were most frequent in low anastomoses.*

19. Bokey EL, Chapuis PH, Pheils MT, et al. Elective resection for diverticular disease and carcinoma. Comparison of postoperative morbidity and mortality. Dis Colon Rectum 1981;24:181–182. *Forty-seven patients undergoing elective resection for diverticular disease (excluding complications at surgery such as abscess or fistula) and 106 patients undergoing left colectomy for carcinoma were compared. The mortality and anastomotic leak rates, as well as the wound infection rate, were higher in the diverticular group; there was also a higher percentage of two-stage resections in this group, perhaps suggesting a higher risk for surgery.*

20. Slim K, Pezet D, Riff Y, et al. High morbidity rate after converted laparoscopic surgery. Br J Surg 1995;82:1406–1408. *The results of 65 laparoscopically-assisted colorectal procedures were compared with 225 planned open procedures during the same time period. The anastomotic leak rate was 25% and 8% in the converted and open groups.*

21. Langevin JM, Rothenberger DA, Goldberg SM. Accidental splenic injury during surgical treatment of the colon and rectum. Surg Gynecol Obstet 1984;159:139–144. *The authors describe eight patients with splenic injuries: three patients required splenectomy and the remaining spleens were salvaged with topical hemostatic agents.*

22. Danforth DN Jr, Thorbjarnarson B. Incidental splenectomy: a review of the literature and the New York Hospital experience. Ann Surg 1976;183:124–129. *Most of the splenic lacerations occurred because of excessive manipulation rather than pathologic conditions involving the spleen. Significant morbidity and mortality occurred.*

23. Buntain WL, Lynn HB. Splenorrhaphy: changing concepts for the traumatized spleen. Surgery 1979;86:748–760. *A detailed review of postsplenectomy sepsis and of the techniques of splenic salvage. Well illustrated, with 107 references.*

24. Stolfi VM, Milsom JW, Lavery IC, et al. Newly designed occluder pin for presacral hemorrhage. Dis Colon Rectum 1992;35:166–169. *Discusses a new 7-mm titanium pin for control of presacral hemorrhage.*

25. Nivatvongs S, Fang DT. The use of thumbtacks to stop massive presacral hemorrhage. Dis Colon Rectum 1986;29:589–590. *Two titanium thumbtacks controlled massive presacral hemorrhage.*

26. Cirocco WC, Golub RW. Endoscopic treatment of postoperative hemorrhage from a stapled colorectal anastomosis. Am Surg 1995;61:460–463. *In this review of the literature, 17 of 775 patients (1.8%) bled from stapled colorectal anastomoses postoperatively and required surgery or transfusions. Six patients had endoscopic electrocoagulation.*

27. Harbrecht PJ, Garrison RN, Fry DE. Early urgent relaparotomy. Arch Surg 1984;119:369–374. *A study of 113 patients undergoing early urgent relaparotomy. The most common indications were infection with intact organs, suture line leaks, and dehiscence. Bleeding caused the earliest laparotomies and obstruction caused the latest.*

28. Stewart RM, Page CP, Brender J, et al. The incidence and risk of early postoperative small bowel obstruction. Am J Surg 1987;154:643–647. *A loss of bowel function with distention and pain following advances to a diet was most characteristic of postoperative bowel obstruction.*

29. Quatromoni JC, Rosoff L, Halls JM, et al. Early postoperative small bowel obstruction. Ann Surg 1980;191:72–74. *The usual signs, symptoms and radiographic findings associated with small bowel obstruction were not useful in deciding which patients needed an operation.*

30. Nadrowski L. Paralytic ileus: recent advances in pathophysiology and treatment. Curr Surg 1983;40:260–273. *A review covering pathophysiology, clinical manifestations, and treatment, with 37 references.*

31. Sarr MG, Bulkley GB, Zuidema GD. Preoperative recognition of intestinal strangulation obstruction. Prospective evaluation of diagnostic capability. Am J Surg 1983;145:176–182. *This prospective study showed that even experienced clinical surgeons could not reliably detect ischemic bowel before operation.*

32. Chung CC, Meng WC, Yu SC, et al. A prospective study on the use of water-soluble contrast follow-through radiology in the management of small bowel obstruction. Aust N Z J Surg 1966;66:598–601. *Using 4 hours as a cutoff time was highly predictive of outcome; if the contrast reached the cecum within 4 hours, obstruction was insignificant. The surgeon made the decision to operate on clinical grounds, and he was blinded to the results of the contrast studies.*

33. Hammond JA, Deckers PJ. Postoperative small bowel obstruction. In: Welch JP, ed. Bowel obstruction. Differential diagnosis and clinical management. Philadelphia: WB Saunders, 1990:411–422.

34. Bulkley GB, Zuidema GD, Hamilton SR, et al. Intraoperative determination of small intestinal viability following ischemic injury. Ann Surg 1981;193:628–637. *A prospective, controlled trial of two adjuvant methods (Doppler and fluorescein) compared with standard clinical judgment.*

35. Carter MS, Fantini GA, Sammartano RJ, et al. Qualitative and quantitative fluorescein fluorescence in determining intestinal viability. Am J Surg 1984;147:117–123. *In an experimental study, visual fluorescence was not reliable in assessing intestinal viability, but quantitative fluorometric fluorescence was quite reliable.*

36. Lurie K, Plzak L, Deveney CW. Intra-abdominal abscess in the 1980s. Surg Clin North Am 1987;67:621–632. *A brief review of the available imaging techniques, with discussions of pertinent anatomy, techniques of percutaneous drainage, and comparison of radiologic and surgical approaches.*

37. Baron TH, Morgan DE. Endoscopic transrectal drainage of a diverticular abscess. Gastrointest Endosc 1997;45:84–87. *A sigmoid diverticular abscess was drained by the transrectal approach using an endoscope in a high-risk patient.*

38. Levison MA, Zeigler D. Correlation of APACHE II score, drainage technique and outcome in postoperative intra-abdominal abscess. Surg Gynecol Obstet 1991;172:89–94. *A retrospective study of 91 patients having drainage of postoperative intra-abdominal abscesses. If the APACHE score was 15 or higher, the survival was 8% and 30% after percutaneous drainage and surgery, respectively.*

39. Fry DE, Garrison RN, Heitsch RC, et al. Determinants of death in patients with intra-abdominal abscess. Surgery 1980;88:517–523. *A retrospective study of 143 patients having surgery for intra-abdominal abscess. Factors associated with a fatal outcome included organ failure, lesser sac abscess, positive blood culture, recurrent/persistent/ multiple abscesses, age more than 50, and subhepatic abscess.*

40. Coit DG. Care of the surgical wound. In: Wilmore DW, Brennan MF, Harken AH, et al., eds. American College of Surgeons, Care of the surgical patient. New York: Scientific American, Inc., 1992;VI:7:1–10. *A publication edited by the Committee on Pre- and Postoperative Care, including a detailed algorithm.*

41. Schein M, Saadia R, Freinkel Z, et al. Aggressive treatment of severe diffuse peritonitis: a prospective study. Br J Surg 1988;75:173–176. *A prospective study of 22 patients managed with electively-staged multiple laparotomies. Some abdomens were left open with a mesh covering; the overall mortality rate was 32%.*

42. Van Goor H, Hulsebos RG, Bleichrodt RP. Complications of planned relaparotomy in patients with severe general peritonitis. Eur J Surg 1997;163:61–66. *A study of 24 consecutive patients; 29% of the patients died. Initial control of peritonitis was gained by creation of stomas.*

43. Kourtesis GJ, Williams RA, Wilson SE. Surgical options in acute diverticulitis: value of sigmoid resection in dealing with the septic focus. Aust N Z J Surg 1988;58:955–959. *Six of 78 patients had postoperative wound infections. The least morbidity occurred when sigmoid resection was performed at the initial procedure.*

44. Scheibel JH, Nielsen ML, Wamberg T, et al. Septic complications in colo-rectal surgery after antibiotic bowel prep Acta Chir Scand 1978;144:527–532. *A correlation was found between colonic bacterial concentrations and the degree of contamination in the peritoneal cavity and subcutaneous tissue.*

45. Meissner K, Meiser G. Primary open wound management after emergency laparotomies for conditions associated with bacterial contamination. Reappraisal of a historical tradition. Am J Surg 1984;148:613–617. *In 85 patients with emergency abdominal surgery and bacterial contamination, there were no wound complications with subcutaneous approximation and open skin treatment.*

46. Fagniez P-L, Hay JM, Lacaine F, et al. Abdominal midline incision closure. Multicentric randomized prospective trial of 3,135 patients, comparing continuous vs interrupted polyglycolic acid sutures. Arch Surg 1985;120:1351–1353. *Continuous closure is advocated because it is more economic and expeditious; it had the same incidence of wound dehiscence as interrupted suture closure.*

47. Knight CD, Griffen FD. Abdominal wound closure with a continuous monofilament polypropylene suture. Experience with 1,000 cases. *The wound dehiscence rate was 0.4% and the incisional hernia rate was 0.7%. The suture is useful for dirty wounds and eliminated the need for retention sutures in the authors' practice.*

48. Ellis H, Heddle R. Does the peritoneum need to be closed at laparotomy? Br J Surg 1977;64:733–736. *In a randomized study, the authors show that closure of the peritoneum as a separate layer does not have any clinical benefit.*

49. Poole GV Jr. Mechanical factors in abdominal wound closure: the prevention of fascial dehiscence. Surgery 1985;97:631–639. *A review that details the facets of satisfactory fascial closure, with 111 references.*
50. Wilson SE, Kitts DG, Williams RA. Reoperation for abdominal wound dehiscence. In: McQuarrie DG, Humphrey EW, eds. Reoperative general surgery. St. Louis: Mosby Year Book, 1992: 467–484.
51. Dolan PA, Caldwell FT, Thompson CH, et al. Problems of colostomy closure. Am J Surg 1979;137:188–191. *There was an early 22% complication rate in an analysis of 118 cases.*
52. Chen F, Stuart M. The morbidity of defunctioning stomata. Aust N Z J Surg 1996;66:218–221. *The loop ileostomy was easier to manage and was not associated with a higher complication rate than loop colostomy.*
53. Winkler MJ, Volpe PA. Loop transverse colostomy — the case against. Dis Colon Rectum 1982;25:321–326. *The author favors end colostomy and points out many of the pitfalls of loop transverse colostomy.*
54. Allen-Mersh TG, Thomson JP. Surgical treatment of colostomy complications. Br J Surg 1988;75:416–418. *The most frequent complication was stenosis, followed by paracolostomy, hernia, and prolapse.*
55. Leslie D. The parastomal hernia. Surg Clin North Am 1984;64:407–415. *The author recommends relocating the stoma and repairing the hernia unless there is no other satisfactory site.*
56. Pearl RK. Parastomal hernias. World J Surg 1989;13:569–572. *Approximately 10–20% of patients need repair of these hernias.*
57. MacKeigan JM, Cataldo PA, eds. Intestinal stomas. Principles, techniques, and management. St. Louis: Quality Medical Publishing, Inc., 1993:414.
58. Babcock G, Bivins BA, Sachatello CR. Technical complications of ileostomy. South Med J 1980;73:329–331. *Obese patients had an 80% incidence of complications.*
59. Williams JG, Etherington R, Hayward MW, et al. Paraileostomal hernia: a clinical and radiological study. Br J Surg 1990;77:1355–1357. *The rate of hernia formation was similar whether the stoma emerged through the rectus or lateral to it.*
60. Abdu RA. Repair of paracolostomy hernias with Marlex mesh. Dis Colon Rectum 1982;25:529–531. *A report of five patients with large paracolostomy hernias.*
61. Rosin JD, Bonardi RA. Paracolostomy hernia repair with Marlex mesh: a new technique. Dis Colon Rectum 1977;20:299–302. *A description of this technique in seven patients; no recurrences were seen in follow-up for up to 4 years.*
62. Sugarbaker PH. Peritoneal approach to prosthetic mesh repair of paracolostomy hernia. Am Surg 1985;201:344–346. *Six patients were operated on; no recurrences were seen with 4- to 7-year follow-up.*
63. Chandler JG, Evans BP. Colostomy prolapse. Surgery 1978;84:577–582. *There was an incidence of stomal prolapse of 14% among 491 patients. The mechanism seemed to be a discrepancy between the size of the fascial defect and the less edematous bowel after decompression.*
64. Myers JO, Rothenberger DA. Sugar in the reduction of incarcerated prolapsed bowel. Dis Colon Rectum 1991;34:416–418. *Report of two cases. An irreducible ileostomy prolapse rapidly reduced in size after ordinary table sugar was applied to it.*
65. Khoury DA, Beck DE, Opelka FG, et al. Colostomy closure. Dis Colon Rectum 1996;39:605–609. *In 46 patients, the overall complication rate was 24%.*
66. Luchtefeld MA, Milsom JW, Senagore A, et al. Colorectal anastomotic stenosis. Results of a survey of the ASCRS membership. Dis Colon Rectum 1989;32:733–736. *A series of 123 patients collected in a mail survey. Ninety-three of the stenoses were in the sigmoid colon or rectum, and two-thirds were stapled anastomoses.*
67. Venkatesh KS, Ramanujam PS, McGee S. Hydrostatic balloon dilatation of benign colonic anastomotic strictures. Dis Colon Rectum 1992;35:780–791. *No complications were encountered in 25 patients treated with endoscopic balloon dilatations.*
68. Accordi F, Sogno O, Carniato S, et al. Endoscopic treatment of stenosis following stapler anastomosis. Dis Colon Rectum 1987;30:647–649. *The papillotomy knife was used to cut the stenotic ring at three points.*
69. Kozarek RA. Hydrostatic balloon dilatation of gastrointestinal stenoses: a national survey. Gastrointest Endosc 1986;32:15–19. *A survey that includes 64 patients undergoing hydrostatic dilatation of the colon with a 79% technical success rate and a 56% rate of acute symptomatic improvement. There were three perforations and two serious bleeding incidents. Surgical consultation is recommended before colonic dilatation.*
70. Pagni S, McLaughlin CM. Simple technique for the treatment of strictured colorectal anastomosis. Dis Colon Rectum 1995;38:433–434. *A strictured colorectal anastomosis was opened with the EndoGIA stapler.*
71. Wigmore SJ, Duthie IE, Young EM, et al. Restoration of intestinal continuity following Hartmann's procedure: the Lothian experience 1987–1992. Br J Surg 1995;82:27–30. *During the period from 1987-1992, 345 patients had Hartmann procedures and 178 had later restoration of intestinal continuity. The mortality was 0.6%. The authors discuss the complications of the procedures.*
72. Goligher JC. Surgery of the anus, rectum and colon. 5th ed. London: Baillière Tindal, 1984:909.
73. Welch JP. Operative techniques, decisions, and complications. In: Welch JP, ed. Bowel obstruction. Differential diagnosis and clinical management. Philadelphia: WB Saunders, 1990:423–448.
74. Ferrucci JT, van Sonnenberg E. Intra-abdominal abscess. Radiological diagnosis and treatment. JAMA 1991;246:2728–2733. *A review of the available radiologic techniques, with 50 references.*
75. Bloom GP, Welch JP. Hernias causing bowel obstruction. In: Welch JP, ed. Bowel obstruction. Differential diagnosis and clinical management. Philadelphia: WB Saunders, 1990:241–313.
76. Welch JP. Perioperative techniques and decisions. In: Welch JP, ed. Bowel obstruction. Differential diagnosis and clinical management. Philadelphia: WB Saunders, 1990:499–545.

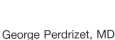

22 Diverticular Disease in the Immunocompromised Patient

George Perdrizet, MD
Cameron Akbari, MD

> **KEY POINTS**
>
> - Immunocompromised patients developing diverticulitis have a complicated course with higher medical failure rates
> - Severity of clinical symptoms diminished (steroid effects)
> - Transplant recipients stop immunosuppressive drugs except steroids perioperatively
> - Higher rates of free perforation
> - Impaired wound healing and risk of anastomotic leakage
> - Increased surgical mortality

ILLUSTRATIVE CASE

A 38-year-old female presented with mild lower abdominal pain and nausea. She had undergone a cadaveric kidney transplant 5 years earlier; her immunosuppression consisted of prednisone, azathioprine, and cyclosporine. On examination, she seemed to be in mild discomfort, afebrile, and with mild left lower abdominal tenderness and no rigidity. The admission white blood cell (WBC) count was 14,500 with no toxic granulations.

She was admitted with a diagnosis of diverticulitis and was started on intravenous antibiotics with only sips of liquids allowed. Her immunosuppression was continued as 15 mg of Solu-medrol daily; azathioprine and cyclosporine were withheld. An abdominal and pelvic computed tomography (CT) scan was suggestive of colonic diverticulitis with no evidence of perforation or abscess.

The patient's pain and tenderness improved, and as her WBC count normalized, she was started again on azathioprine and cyclosporine. Just before discharge, she complained of mild shoulder pain with only minimal abdominal physical findings. A repeat CT scan revealed pneumoperitoneum, and the patient underwent an urgent exploratory laparotomy. Findings included perforation of the distal sigmoid colon without gross feculent peritonitis. The perforated segment was resected and a colostomy and end mucous fistula was created. Perioperative steroid coverage was given as 40 mg of Solu-medrol just before induction, with a quick taper postoperatively to 15 mg of Solu-medrol daily.

The patient's renal function remained stable, and she was started on oral feeds upon return of her bowel function. Azathioprine and cyclosporine were resumed after oral feeding was started, and she was discharged home 14 days postoperatively on prednisone, azathioprine, and cyclosporine. An uncomplicated colostomy closure was performed 6 months later with no untoward effects on graft function.

CASE COMMENTS

Diverticulitis is the most frequent cause of colonic complications developing in renal transplant recipients (1). This patient had minimal pain and physical findings in the presence of a pneumoperitoneum caused by perforation of the sigmoid colon. The case is a good example of the fashion in which symptoms of peritonitis can be diminished in patients taking steroids (2).

With an immunocompetent patient, a primary anastomosis may have been attempted in this situation, because no feculent peritonitis was seen. In this instance, gross peritonitis was probably diminished due to the effect of steroid intake on the inflammatory response (3). Wisely a Hartmann procedure was performed, rather than a primary anastomosis, due to the significant risk of an anastomotic leak.

DISCUSSION

The immunocompromised state implies a dysfunctional immune system, with subsequent predisposition to infection. A second consequence of an impaired immune response is the inhibition of normal wound healing, disruption of fibroblast proliferation, and a relative lack of collagen accumulation. These alterations in the host may be the result of exogenous administration of immunosuppressive agents (e.g., hematologic malignancy, uremia, human immunodeficiency virus [(HIV, hypercortisolism, and malnutrition)].

A classic example of the immunocompromised patient in need of surgical treatment is the patient receiving exogenous corticosteroids. The immunosuppressive effects of this class of drugs are very wide-ranging. The number and function of circulating leukocytes are altered. It is not uncommon to see chronically elevated leukocyte counts in the patient receiving baseline corticosteroid therapy. The steroid-associated leukocytosis is caused by a relative neutrophilia, as a result of increase in bone marrow release and cellular half-life. However, this increase in neutrophil count is offset by a decrease in neutrophil margination and migration.

Concomitantly, there is a decrease in the number of T lymphocytes (predominantly due to lymphoid sequestration) and reduced monocyte and eosinophil counts. T lymphocyte and monocyte-macrophage function is also altered, due to impaired antigen-presenting function, chemotaxis, complement receptor expression, and cytokine secretion (particularly interleukin-1). The sum effect is a diminished immune response.

In addition to its effects on host defense, steroid excess enhances protein breakdown, inhibits fibroblast proliferation, and decreases protein synthesis. This catabolic state leads to a disruption of normal wound healing and a weakening of normal connective tissue. The latter fact partially explains the fragile skin, bone, and bowel often encountered in this patient population.

An additional consequence of the anti-inflammatory properties of steroids is a masking of clinical signs and symptoms of acute disease processes. The clinical presentation of an immunocompromised patient presenting with peritonitis due to colonic perforation is often subtle, which may delay diagnosis and therefore contribute to the excessive morbidity and mortality often observed. *The combination of a reduced host response to infection and delay to definitive treatment leads to a higher mortality in the immunocompromised patient with abdominal infection.* Patients receiving steroid therapy seem to be at a higher risk of dying of abdominal infection than is predicted by APACHE II scores (4).

The immunocompromised host represents a heterogenous and complex spectrum of patients. On one hand, immunosuppression has lead to improved survival in transplant recipients, a better quality of life in patients with autoimmune disease, and major advances against malignancy. Alterations in immune defense have made these patients particularly vulnerable to infection. The care and management of the immunocompromised patient with diverticular disease of the colon, therefore, pose a special challenge to the clinician.

NATURAL HISTORY OF DIVERTICULOSIS IN IMMUNOCOMPROMISED PATIENTS

The underlying pathophysiology of colonic diverticulosis is an altered colonic motility with subsequent exaggerated increases in intraluminal pressure and, thus, a predisposition to mucosal herniation. It is evident, therefore, that colonic diverticulosis is more likely to occur in the setting of increased intraluminal pressure or increased bowel wall weakening. The former implicates the role of dietary fiber, as low residue typically leads to decreased fecal bulk and higher intraluminal pressures. Similar events are noted in patients with constipation and various types of colonic dysmotility.

Although the immunocompromised patient may display greater colonic wall weakening (from exogenous steroid therapy, chemotherapy, or uremia) and constipation (from diabetic colonic paresis or uremia), it is not known whether these patients have a higher incidence of colonic diverticulosis. Barium enema studies have revealed a 45–50% incidence of diverticulosis among patients with renal failure and a 13% incidence in transplant patients (5). It seems, therefore, that uremic patients may have a higher incidence of diverticulosis coli, particularly at a younger age (6), again most likely secondary to decreased tissue strength and chronic constipation. A very high incidence of diverticulosis is seen in patients with polycystic kidney disease (PKD); one study has reported that barium enema documented diverticulosis in 10 of 12 patients with PKD and diverticular perforation in four of these patients (7).

Approximately 15–20% of all patients with colonic diverticulosis will present with clinical evidence of diverticulitis during their lifetime (8). It is unknown whether asymptomatic immunocompromised patients with diverticulosis have a higher predilection to developing acute diverticulitis (5,6). One study noted a 13% incidence (seven patients) of diverticulosis among 55 renal transplant recipients with the subsequent development of severe diverticulitis in four of these seven patients (9). Similar results have not been obtained in other studies of immunocompromised patients with diverticulosis.

Several reports have indicated that immunocompromised patients with acute diverticulitis have a more complicated course when compared with immunocompetent patients (2,6,9–14). Natural history studies have demonstrated that 15–20% of all patients with diverticulitis will require surgical intervention (15). In contrast, two studies have shown that among a total of 50 immunocompromised patients presenting with a single episode of diverticulitis, 33 (66%) patients failed medical therapy (11,12). In addition, mortality rates for immunocompromised patients requiring surgery for diverticulitis is strikingly higher when compared with those of immunocompetent ones (Table 22.1) (16). A number of factors contribute to the higher mortality rates, including delays in diagnosis, extracolonic

Table 22.1.   Surgical Mortality for Immunocompromised Patients with Acute Diverticulitis

Reference	Number of Patients	Number of Deaths	Mortality Rate
Tyau et al, 1991 (11)	23	9	39%
Church et al, 1986 (14)	7	3	42%
Starnes et al, 1985 (5)	25	7	28%
Perkins et al, 1984 (12)	10	1	10%
Sakai et al, 1981 (10)	8	4	50%
Guice et al, 1979 (6)	7	4	57%
Carson et al, 1978 (16)	6	5	83%
Sawyerr et al, 1978 (9)	4	3	75%
Total:	**90**	**36**	**40%**

sepsis due to an inability to localize intra-abdominal infection, higher rates of free perforation, and poor immune responses to infection (2,13,14).

In summary, *the immunocompromised patient does not show a higher predilection toward the development of diverticulosis or a greater likelihood of developing diverticulitis from asymptomatic diverticulosis. However, diverticulitis in this patient population is clearly more complicated*, with higher morbidity, mortality, and need for urgent surgical therapy. Because surgical intervention is required in nearly two-thirds of these patients after a first episode of diverticulitis, it is not known what percentage of patients will develop a second episode after successful medical therapy for a first episode of diverticulitis.

PATHOLOGY

Numerous colonic complications have been reported in the immunocompromised patient, particularly in the transplant recipient, the individual on exogenous corticosteroids, and the renal failure patient. These include pseudomembranous colitis, ischemic colitis, nonobstructing colonic dilatation, stercoral ulceration, cytomegalovirus (CMV) infection, and diverticulitis (9,14,17–20). These conditions are most likely to manifest as fecal peritonitis and free perforation. Abscesses and fistulization may occur, although with lesser frequency than in the nonimmunocompromised population. Absence of abscess formation is due to a reduced inflammatory response and impaired leukocyte migration to the site of perforation. Histologic examination of the colon from patients taking exogenous corticosteroids reveals atrophy of lymphoid aggregates and decreased turnover of mucosal cells, with subsequent thinning of the bowel wall (14). Collagen and polysaccharide deposition is decreased, and fibroblast motility is impaired, which in turn leads to an inability to wall off a localized area of perforation (12,18).

Similar effects on tissue strength and inflammatory response are seen in the uremic patient, with resultant increased risk of free perforation (5,6,18). Uremia also has been shown to predispose patients to intestinal ischemia (18); the combination of localized ischemia, bowel wall weakening, and chronic constipation may lead to a greater likelihood of free perforation from colonic diverticulitis.

DIAGNOSIS

Signs and symptoms of acute colonic diverticulitis in the immunocompromised patient, when present, are similar to those seen in the general population and include left lower quadrant abdominal pain and tenderness, leukocytosis, and fever. A history of constipation (as may be seen in the renal failure patient or transplant recipient) should suggest possible colonic diverticulosis. However, several important features differentiate the immunocompromised patient from the general population.

A far greater proportion of younger renal failure patients (and subsequently renal transplant recipients) develop symptomatic diverticular disease when compared with the nonuremic population (Table 22.2) (5). Failure to recognize this phenomenon may lead to delays in treatment for the younger immunocompromised patient, particularly for the uremic patient, renal transplant recipient, and the patient with PKD. Compounding this problem is the often vague expression of abdominal pain and absence of physical findings, especially in the patient on exogenous corticosteroids.

The anti-inflammatory effect of corticosteroids will typically mask symptoms and signs of peritoneal irritation that are present in the immunocompetent patient (2,14). This masking effect may be attributed to a depressed cellular immune response, a decreased number of circulating lymphocytes, and depressed chemotaxis by circulating monocytes (2). In the absence of infection, many patients on exogenous corticosteroids display a relative leukocytosis secondary to a neutrophilia. Therefore, a leukocytosis in the patient with peritonitis and minimal physical findings is often erroneously attributed to "being on steroids." *A helpful differentiating point is the presence of toxic granulations,* which is specific for sepsis and is not seen in steroid-related leukocytosis.

It seems that the inability to exhibit peritonitis and the paucity of physical findings is related to the dosage of exogenous corticosteroids (2,11,14), with greater delays in diagnosis in patients taking higher doses of these agents. Most patients taking these high doses (greater than 20 mg of prednisone daily) will demonstrate normal bowel function despite fecal peritonitis; often, the only sign or symptom present is the subjective expression of abdominal pain or abdominal distention (2).

Because both free colonic perforation and delay in diagnosis contribute significantly to higher mortality rates complicating colonic diverticulitis (2,5,6,14), further evaluation should be pursued promptly of the immunocompromised patient presenting with abdominal pain. Plain film radiographs may display massive pneumoperitoneum secondary to free perforation of the colon (Fig. 22.1). Although earlier reports have recommended water-soluble contrast enema to study the colon (6,7,12), *contrast-enhanced CT scanning of the abdomen and pelvis has evolved as the primary diagnostic modality.* Findings on CT scan may include mesenteric streaking consistent with contained diverticulitis, pericolonic air, or pneumoperitoneum (Fig. 22.2). Peritoneal lavage can be useful for the uremic patient receiving ambulatory peritoneal dialysis, with Gram's stain and culture

Table 22.2.   Prevalence of Diverticulitis in the Young Immunocompromised Patient

Reference	Population	Total Number of Patients with Disease	Number of Patients <50 Years of Age (%)
Church et al, 1986 (14)	Renal transplant	7	4 (57%)
Starnes et al, 1985 (5)	Renal failure	25	11 (44%)
Guice et al, 1979 (6)	Renal transplant	7	6 (85%)
Carson et al, 1978 (16)	Renal transplant	6	5 (83%)
Sawyerr et al, 1978 (9)	Renal transplant	4	2 (50%)
Total:		**49**	**28 (57%)**

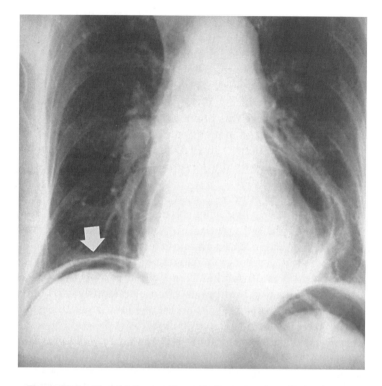

Figure 22.1. Upright chest radiograph shows free intra-abdominal air.

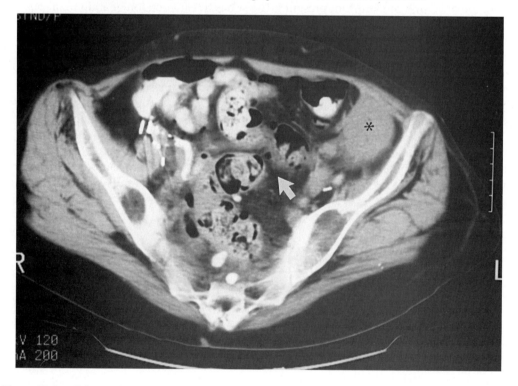

Figure 22.2. Abdominal CT scan demonstrating pneumoperitoneum, extracolonic air in the mesentery (arrow), and kidney allograft (*).

yielding multiple enteric organisms. Diagnostic laparoscopy also may be considered, particularly as an adjunct in the intensive care unit for the critically ill, immunocompromised patient with enteric septicemia.

TREATMENT

Clinical evaluation alone often underestimates the severity of disease in the immunocompromised patient with active diverticulitis. Radiologic studies, especially contrast-enhanced CT scanning, can help determine which patients require urgent surgical therapy. Conversely, clinical and radiographic evaluation together may help predict which patients will respond to medical therapy alone.

Regardless of whether medical or surgical intervention is required for the disease process, several treatment principles should be followed for the immunocompromised patient. Because malnutrition commonly may accompany the immunocompromised state, it should be treated aggressively.

Dosages of immunosuppressive drugs, including corticosteroids, should be altered during treatment for acute diverticulitis. *In the transplant recipient, all immunosuppression should be stopped, except for exogenous corticosteroids,* the latter serving largely to preserve graft function and prevent acute adrenal insufficiency. The perioperative administration of "stress steroids" to the patient receiving chronic corticosteroid therapy has been reviewed recently (21,22). Current recommendations suggest less aggressive therapy than has been advocated in the past for the prevention of acute adrenal insufficiency. *Important considerations in the dosage of perioperative corticosteroid coverage are preoperative corticosteroid dose and severity of surgery* (Table 22.3). In fact, stable renal transplant patients receiving baseline prednisone dosages equaling 5–10 mg daily and undergoing a variety of surgical procedures need not receive additional corticosteroids beyond their usual daily dose (22). In the treatment of colonic perforation, several reports have documented ongoing graft function with only small doses of corticosteroids perioperatively (6,14,16,17).

Because similar organisms are cultured from both immunocompromised and nonimmunocompromised patients with fecal peritonitis, *similar antibiotic regimens may be used with several important caveats.* Nephrotoxic drugs should be avoided in the renal allograft patient. Dosages of antibiotics with renal clearance should be adjusted in uremic individuals. In addition, in the immunocompromised patient with ongoing sepsis despite appropriate treatment, a strong suspicion of possible fungemia and CMV infection should be maintained. Whether to use antifungal prophylaxis for these high-risk patients remains to be established from controlled studies (23).

Table 22.3.   Suggested Peri-operative Glucocorticoid Coverage

Surgical Stress	Total Daily Dose (mg)		
	Intravenous Hydrocortisone	Intravenous Methylprednisolone	Oral Prednisone
Mild (e.g., herniorrhaphy)	25	5	5
Moderate (e.g., colon resection)	50–75	10–15	10–15
Severe (e.g., cardiopulmonary bypass)	100–150	20–30	20–30

Medical Treatment

Although most immunocompromised patients with acute colonic diverticulitis will require urgent surgical intervention, some may be managed with medical therapy alone. This decision is based on the clinical and radiographic findings. Patients with no evidence of extracolonic sepsis or free perforation and CT findings consistent with only mild mesenteric inflammation ("fat-streaking") fall into this category. Treatment is similar to that in the nonimmunocompromised patient (intravenous antibiotics and bowel rest) with the added precautions noted above. Consideration may be given to percutaneous drainage of abscesses when present on CT scan, although the frequency of abscesses is much less than in the general population for reasons cited previously.

If medical therapy is determined to be appropriate, the immunocompromised patient requires very close observation. Worsening abdominal pain or failure to improve should be evaluated with repeat CT scanning. Evidence of worsening disease or a new complication such as perforation or fistula formation is deemed a failure of medical therapy, and surgical intervention should proceed.

Surgical Treatment

Surgical treatment options for acute complications of diverticulitis are similar for both the immunocompromised and immunocompetent patient. For colonic perforation, earlier reports advocated either exteriorization or proximal colostomy and drainage (6,10). More recently, resection with end colostomy has become the procedure of choice (5,12). This has been based on higher reported mortality rates for the traditional three-stage treatment in the general population. Resection and anastomosis has been reported in most series (5,6,11,12,16); however, this cannot be recommended in view of fecal peritonitis and impaired anastomotic healing in the immunocompromised patient. Fistulization also may occur, as either colovesical or colovaginal fistulas. Surgical treatment is identical to that in the immunocompetent patient.

Impaired wound healing is common in these patients. The abdominal wall fascia should be closed precisely. To prevent postoperative evisceration, retention sutures should be considered. Steroid-induced impairment of wound healing is secondary to its anti-inflammatory effects and is, therefore, most detrimental at days 3 through 6 of wound healing. Impaired wound healing from steroid excess can be reversed with supplemental vitamin A in a dose of 25,000 IU daily. Because the skin is allowed to heal by secondary intention in these contaminated cases, contraction and final closure of the wound may take several months in the immunocompromised patient.

Elective Resection

In view of the high mortality associated with acute colonic diverticulitis in the immunocompromised patient, earlier reports recommended routine barium enema examination in potential renal transplant recipients and resection if there was evidence of diverticulosis (9).

However, considering the low frequency of diverticulitis arising from asymptomatic diverticulosis, such practices have been largely abandoned. One exception may be the subgroup of patients with polycystic kidney disease. These patients have a very high frequency of colonic diverticulosis; diverticulitis arises in as many as one-third of patients (7). If elective resection is offered to these patients before renal transplantation, subtotal colectomy with ileoproctostomy is recommended to eliminate any possible future focus of diverticular disease (6).

It is unknown what percentage of immunocompromised patients successfully treated medically for a first episode of acute diverticulitis will develop a second episode. *It is recommended that elective sigmoid resection be performed in the immunocompromised patient with a previous episode of symptomatic diverticulitis (5,16,18,19).*

EDITORIAL COMMENTS

Immunosuppressed patients are a diverse group, with underlying problems such as chronic alcohol abuse, acquired immunodeficiency syndrome (AIDS), or metastatic malignancies. Renal transplant patients are one subset of immunosuppressed patients who have been discussed in particular depth in this chapter and in the surgical literature.

The most important aspects of diverticular disease in the immunocompromised host are the increased likelihood of failure of medical therapy for diverticulitis and the difficulty of detecting peritonitis. Management of these patients with any degree of abdominal pain requires vigilance and repeated radiologic and laboratory evaluation as well. Delayed treatment of peritoneal contamination may prove disastrous. In essence, early surgical intervention must be considered for immunocompromised patients presenting with diverticulitis. Not only may it be difficult to follow patients clinically, but in addition, multiple studies confirm the potential lethality of the disease (3). There also is virtually no scenario in which nonelective surgery should include an anastomosis because of the significant risk of anastomotic leakage. Wound closure must be performed with care because of the risk of dehiscence.

We are in agreement that patients with renal transplants should not undergo "prophylactic" colectomy for diverticulosis (except perhaps those with polycystic kidneys). On the other hand, transplant patients with symptomatic diverticular disease should be considered candidates for colectomy.

SUGGESTED READINGS

1. Tyau ES, Prystowsky JB, Joehl RJ, et al. Acute diverticulitis: a complicated problem in the immunocompromised patient. Arch Surg 1991;126:855–859. *The authors present their experience with acute diverticulitis in 40 immunocompromised patients over a 5-year period. Compared with immunocompetent controls, higher rates of free perforation and a more complicated course were manifest in these patients.*
2. Remine SG, McIlrath DC. Bowel perforation in steroid-treated patients. Ann Surg 1980;192:581–586. *Seventy-nine patients on chronic corticosteroid therapy with associated gastrointestinal perforation were studied. Higher mortality rates were noted in patients taking larger doses of exogenous steroids; greater delays in diagnosis were a principal cause.*
3. Perkins JD, Shield CF, Chang FC, et al. Acute diverticulitis: comparison of treatment in immunocompromised and nonimmunocompromised patients. Am J Surg 1984;148:745–748. *The authors discuss various surgical procedures in the treatment of acute diverticulitis in 10 immunocompromised patients. They conclude that resection with colostomy results in fewer complications in this high-risk group of patients.*
4. Church JM, Fazio VW, Braun WE, et al. Perforation of the colon in renal homograft recipients. Ann Surg 1986;203:69–76. *The authors draw from their own experience at one of the world's foremost institutions specializing in colorectal surgery. In addition, an excellent review of the literature is provided.*
5. Salem M, Tainsh RE, Bromberg J, et al. Perioperative glucocorticoid coverage: a re-assessment 42 years after emergence of a problem. Ann Surg 1994;219:416–425. *This is an excellent review of the historical basis for perioperative glucocorticoid coverage. The authors provide new recommendations for these glucocorticoid-dependent patients who require surgery.*

REFERENCES

1. Soravia C, Baldi A, Kartheuser A, et al. Colonic complications after kidney transplantation. Acta Chir Belg 1995;95:157–161. *Of patients with renal allografts, 0.5% had acute colonic complications; all 12 patients had acute peritonitis (caused by diverticulitis in 75). The use of cyclosporine since 1985 did not reduce the incidence of colonic complications. Includes an extensive literature review with 40 references.*

2. ReMine SG, McIlrath DC. Bowel perforation in steroid-treated patients. Ann Surg 1980;192:581–586. *The mean delay from onset of symptoms to treatment was 8 days in patients taking high-dose corticosteroids (more than 20 mg daily).*

3. Warshaw AL, Welch JP, Ottinger LW. Acute perforation of the colon associated with chronic corticosteroid therapy. Am J Surg 1976;131:442–446. *A clinical study of 13 patients with colonic perforation who were receiving corticosteroids for conditions unrelated to the bowel. Because of few symptoms, delays in treatment and incorrect preoperative diagnoses were frequent.*

4. Bohnen JM, Mustard RA, Schouten BD. Steroids, APACHE II score, and the outcome of abdominal infection. Arch Surg 1994;129:33–38. *Patients receiving steroids have a higher risk of dying of abdominal infection than predicted by APACHE II scores.*

5. Starnes HF, Lazarus JM, Vineyard G. Surgery for diverticulitis in renal failure. Dis Colon Rectum 1985;28:827–831. *Mortality was considerably higher in patients older than 50 years of age.*

6. Guice K, Rattazzi LC, Marchioro TL. Colon perforation in renal transplant patients. Am J Surg 1979;138:43–48. *Seven of 392 patients (1.8%) had perforated colonic diverticulitis following renal transplant.*

7. Scheff RT, Zuckerman G, Harter H, et al. Diverticular disease in patients with chronic renal failure due to polycystic kidney disease. Ann Intern Med 1980;92:202–204. *The authors suggest that patients with chronic renal failure due to polycystic disease have a high incidence of diverticulosis and diverticulitis.*

8. Parks TG. Natural history of diverticular disease of the colon. Clin Gastroenterol 1975;4:53–69. *A comprehensive review of the natural history of diverticular disease in a 233-page monograph on diverticular disease.*

9. Sawyerr OI, Garvin PJ, Codd JE, et al. Colorectal complications of renal allograft transplantation. Arch Surg 1978;113:84-86. *Exclusion from transplant or elective colectomy before transplant is proposed in immunocompromised patients with symptoms of diverticulitis and documented diverticulosis by barium enema.*

10. Sakai L, Daake J, Kaminski DL. Acute perforation of sigmoid diverticula. Am J Surg 1981;142:712–716. *None of the patients on chronic steroids had well-localized perforations.*

11. Tyau ES, Prystowsky JB, Joehl RJ, et al. Acute diverticulitis: A complicated problem in the immunocompromised patient. Arch Surg 1991;126:855–859. *Of 40 immunocompromised patients with acute diverticulitis, 58% underwent surgery with a postoperative mortality of 39%.*

12. Perkins JD, Shield CF, Chang FC, et al. Acute diverticulitis: comparison of treatment in immunocompromised and nonimmunocompromised patients. Am J Surg 1984;184:745–748. *All immunocompromised patients needed surgery; colostomy and resection of the involved segment are recommended.*

13. Corder A. Steroids, non-steroidal anti-inflammatory drugs, and serious septic complications of diverticular disease. BMJ 1987;295:1238. *Extension of sepsis outside the colon was associated with intake of steroids or nonsteroidal anti-inflammatory drugs.*

14. Church JM, Fazio VW, Braun WE, et al. Perforation of the colon in renal homograft recipients. Ann Surg 1986;203:69–76. *Mortality has been lowered by a high clinical index of suspicion, reduction of immunosuppression, antibiotic coverage, and early exteriorization of the perforated colon.*

15. Rodkey GV, Welch CE. Changing patterns in the surgical treatment of diverticular disease. Ann Surg 1984;200:466–478. *Eleven percent of patients seen between 1974 and 1983 were immunosuppressed (chronic alcoholism, cancer chemotherapy or radiotherapy, diabetes, chronic steroid intake, or transplant patients), compared with 3% from 1964–1973.*

16. Carson SD, Krom RA, Uchida K, et al. Colon perforation after kidney transplantation. Ann Surg 1978;188:109–113. *Elective colon resection is recommended before transplantation in patients with symptomatic diverticular disease.*

17. Koneru B, Selby R, O'Hair DP, et al. Nonobstructing colonic dilatation and colon perforations following renal transplantation. Arch Surg 1990;125:610–613. *Nonobstructing colon dilatation was seen in 13 patients 1–13 days after transplantation. Twelve patients had poorly functioning allografts and five of six patients undergoing colonoscopy had resolution of dilation.*

18. Flanigan RC, Reckard CR, Lucas BA. Colonic complications of renal transplantation. J Urol 1988;139:503–506. *Ischemic colitis and diverticulitis were the most common complications in a review of more than 3000 patients.*

19. Benoit G. Moukarzel M, Verdelli G, et al. Gastrointestinal complications in renal transplantation. Transplant Int 1993;6:45–49. *Sixteen percent of renal transplant recipients with colonic complications had a history of diverticula, compared with 3% of those without colonic complications.*

20. Aubia J, Lloveras J, Munne A, et al. Ischemic colitis in chronic uremia. Nephron 1981;29:146–150. *The authors propose that accelerated arterial disease with terminal uremia may predispose to ischemic colitis, along with constipation and intestinal motility disorders.*

21. Salem M, Tainsh RE, Bromberg J, et al. Peri-operative glucocorticoid coverage. A reassessment 42 years after emergence of a problem. Ann Surg 1994;219:416–425. *Maintains that current perioperative glucocorticoid coverage is excessive and gives specific guidelines for dose recommendations.*

22. Bromberg JS, Alfrey EJ, Barker CF, et al. Adrenal suppression and steroid supplementation in renal transplant patients. Transplantation 1991;51:385–390. *Maintains that renal allograft recipients do not need high doses of "stress steroids" to meet the demands of physiologic stress.*

23. Solomkin JS. Pathogenesis and management of candida infection syndromes in non-neutropenic patients. New Horizons 1993;1:202–213. *The gastrointestinal tract is believed to be the primary source of entry for yeast.*

23 Diverticular Disease and the Younger Patient

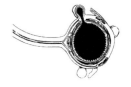

Peter S. Edelstein, MD
Stanley M. Goldberg, MD

KEY POINTS

- Patients 40 years of age or younger:
  - diverticula occur in 6–9%
  - include up to 30% of hospitalized patients with diverticulitis
  - mild diverticulitis diagnosed or cause for hospitalization less than in elderly patients
  - have similar disease presentation as elderly patients (left-sided pseudodiverticula)
- Male predominance may reflect underdiagnosis in females
- Diverticulitis misdiagnosed in 34–59% (especially appendicitis)
- Elective resection recommended after second bout of diverticulitis

INTRODUCTION

The treatment of diverticular disease in younger patients is based on anecdotal experiences and limited retrospective reviews. Therefore, some clinical theories about the disease process become dogma without undergoing serious scrutiny and prospective analysis. Recognizing the paucity of such data, we present the following goals for this chapter: first, to organize and review the available reports concerning diverticular disease in young patients (40 years of age or younger); and second, to identify topics of significant controversy in the literature on this subject. The focus will be on the prevalence of colonic diverticula in patients 40 years of age or younger and on the nature, diagnosis, and treatment of acute diverticulitis and its complications in this younger population.

PREVALENCE OF DIVERTICULA

Most published studies are limited because their analyses include only symptomatic patients who are admitted to the hospital. Such reviews obviously shed little light on the prevalence of asymptomatic colonic diverticula in the general population. Autopsy series, however, provide a more accurate estimate of the prevalence of acquired colonic diverticula. In the United States, diverticula are present in approximately two-thirds of the population by 80 years of age (1–3). Hughes performed autopsies on 200 unselected patients and found colonic diverticula in 9% of patients 50 years of age or younger (4). Lee reported on 1014 consecutive autopsies in Singapore, noting the presence of diverticula in 19 of 293 patients (6.5%) younger than 40 years of age and in 52 of 425 patients (12.2%) younger than 50 years of age (5). These reports, which do not rely on patient symptoms or hospital admissions, suggest that *colonic diverticula are present in 6–9% of the general population who are 40 years of age or younger.*

Although few in number, postmortem analyses provide more information than just prevalence of diverticula. Although Hughes did not focus on younger patients in his 1969 autopsy series, he found that in every age group the diverticula (including cecal) were histologically identical, all being "false" or pseudodiverticula (4). He also noted regarding location and extent of diverticula that "total colonic involvement occurred on the average a decade later than did lesser degrees [of colonic involvement]" (4).

Gender

The relationship between gender and colonic diverticula is confusing because of the differences among groups analyzed. For example, in most studies, researchers evaluate only patients with acute diverticulitis, whereas others include asymptomatic patients. Despite these logistical pitfalls, important conclusions can be drawn. Although in patients older than 40 years of age with acute diverticulitis gender results range from a male predominance in 54% of cases to a female predominance in 66% of cases (6–8), most authors suggest a female:male ratio of 3:2 (9–12). This is in striking contrast to gender analysis in younger patients with diverticulitis, in which men comprise 62–100% of patients in all reports (6–8,11,13,14). In one rare study of young patients that include those with asymptomatic diverticula, Ouriel and Schwartz noted a 1:1 female:male ratio (13). These results suggest that diverticulitis is either a more common occurrence in young men or is simply less diagnosed in young women. The list of differential diagnoses for abdominal pain, leukocytosis, and fever is significantly greater for a young woman, mostly due to obstetric and gynecologic pathologic processes. *The overwhelming male predominance noted in young patients with diverticulitis, which appears to be absent in asymptomatic young patients, may simply reflect an inappropriately low frequency of correctly diagnosing acute diverticulitis in women of reproductive age.*

Ethnicity

The role of ethnicity in the development of diverticular disease in the younger population has been examined to only a small extent. Based on studies of the prevalence of diverticular disease among different geographic and dietary groups, the development of colonic diverticular disease in all ages in the western world has been attributed primarily to environmental rather than genetic factors (9,11). However, some reports have concluded that in American regions in which Hispanics represent a significant portion of the population, an even larger proportion of male Hispanics is represented among young patients with acute diverticulitis (8). Still, these studies again suggest that although Hispanic ethnicity may play a role, environmental factors are more significant in the development of diverticular disease (8).

Comorbid Conditions

Patients 40 years of age or younger in apparent good health who develop acute diverticulitis and its complications do not seem to have any specific associated medical conditions, with one exception: *obesity (mild to morbid) has been noted in as many as 84–97% of patients.* This high percentage is significantly greater than noted in the older patient population (8,10). The pathophysiologic relationship between obesity and diverticulitis is unclear. Clinically, the association is a useful reminder that acute diverticulitis must be included in the differential diagnosis of a young, symptomatic patient, especially one who is overweight.

SYMPTOMATIC DISEASE

Difficulties in Analysis

Numerous reports have been published concerning symptomatic diverticular disease in young patients. Incidence is expressed as a percentage of all cases of symptomatic diverticular disease that occur in younger patients. However, it is important to suggest the possibility that patients of various ages may address minimally symptomatic diverticular disease in different ways. It seems plausible that an otherwise healthy young patient might choose *not* to seek medical attention when mild abdominal pain and low-grade fever develop. Also, the diagnosis of acute diverticulitis in a young patient, particularly a woman of reproductive age, may never be entertained seriously by the physician. With time, the inflammatory process resolves. Finally, even when diagnosed correctly, a mildly symptomatic young patient may be treated on an outpatient basis. An elderly patient, however, is much more likely to suffer from additional medical illnesses and may more quickly seek medical attention when mild symptoms first develop. *The diagnosis of acute diverticulitis in the older patient is more likely to be considered and pursued. Furthermore, due to comorbid conditions plus a limited ability to administer their own care, older individuals are almost always treated as inpatients.* If such speculation is accurate, only a subset of young patients with diverticulitis are symptomatic enough to present, be correctly diagnosed, and require hospital admission. This hospitalized subset would tend to have more severe disease than older patients with diverticulitis, who present and are admitted with a broader range of symptoms and severity of disease. Comparisons between the two age groups could lead to an erroneous conclusion found throughout journal publications and textbooks—in patients 40 years of age or younger, diverticulitis represents a more virulent form of the disease (7–11,13,15). *The actual explanation would be that the disease is no more virulent in the younger population, but fewer young patients with mild symptoms are included in the comparisons* because they are seen less frequently by a physician, are diagnosed correctly, and ultimately are admitted for treatment of acute diverticulitis.

Incidence

With the above scenario in mind, a discussion of symptomatic diverticular disease can begin. In one recent analysis of 248 patients with documented acute diverticulitis admitted to a hospital system in Pennsylvania, 29 patients (11.7%) were younger than 40 years of age (10). Other recent reports have found that younger patients account for an even greater proportion, between 20 and 30%, of all acute diverticulitis cases (6–8). In this younger group, acute diverticulitis occurs most commonly in the fourth decade (8,10). Therefore, whereas colonic diverticula may be present in 6–9% of the young population, *up to 30% of symptomatic patients diagnosed correctly and requiring hospital admission for acute diverticulitis may be 40 years of age or younger.*

Location

The location of the acute inflammatory process in young patients with diverticulitis has been described clearly and extensively. Although some reports examine only young patients with diverticulitis who undergo surgical treatment, their conclusions are similar to those found in studies including nonsurgically treated young patients. Inflamed

Table 23.1.   Sites of Colonic Involvement[a]

Site of Inflammation	Range of Results (%)
Left colon (descending and sigmoid)	80–100
Sigmoid colon (alone)	68–82
Cecum	0–20[b]
Ascending colon	0–3
Transverse colon	0[c]

[a]Data from: Freischlag J, Bennion RS, Thompson JE. Complications of diverticular disease of the colon in young people. Dis Colon Rectum 1986; 29:639–643; Schauer PR, Ramos R, Ghiatas AA, et al. Virulent diverticular disease in young obese men. Am J Surg 1992; 164:443–448; Konvolinka CW. Acute diverticulitis under age forty. Am J Surg 1994; 167:562–565; Ouriel K, Schwartz SI. Diverticular disease in the young patient. Surg Gynecol Obstet 1983;156:1–5; Chodak GW, Rangel DM, Passaro E. Colonic diverticulitis in patients under age 40: need for earlier diagnosis. Am J Surg 1981;141:699–702.
[b]20% rate from a study of only 15 patients.
[c]Single inflamed diverticulum identified in only one study.

diverticula are confined to the left colon (descending and sigmoid) in 80–100% of patients with diverticulitis who are 40 years of age or younger (Table 23.1). As much as eighty percent of cases of acute diverticulitis in younger patients are found solely in the sigmoid colon (8,10). Microscopic examination of inflamed diverticula identified similar histologic features in younger and older patients (10). This percentage is similar to that described in older diverticular patients. These findings support the conclusion that *the etiology, development, anatomic, and pathologic characteristics of colonic diverticula, and the associated inflammatory state, do not differ between younger and older patients.*

Diagnosis

Acute diverticulitis in young patients is initially diagnosed correctly in only 34–59% of cases (7,8,10,13,16). The extremely high frequency of misdiagnosis is in sharp contrast to the 14% misdiagnosis rate for patients with acute diverticulitis who are older than 40 years of age (9). In the younger population, the *most common incorrect initial diagnosis, acute appendicitis, is made in approximately 33–60% of cases.* Pelvic inflammatory disease, gastroenteritis, pancreatitis, intestinal obstruction, cholecystitis, pyelonephritis, and testicular torsion are a few of the numerous other reported misdiagnoses (8,13,16). It is clearly important to determine the reasons for the significantly higher rate of misdiagnosis in younger patients with diverticulitis.

In young, symptomatic patients with diverticulitis, abdominal pain is the most frequent complaint, present in 91–96% of cases. Abdominal tenderness is the most common physical finding, present in 96–100% (8,10,13) (see Table 23.2). Therefore, the frequency and characteristics of the most common symptom and sign of acute diverticulitis are similar in patients younger and older than 40 years of age. Although textbooks always include fever as a presenting sign in the typical older acute diverticulitis patient, the presence or absence of an elevated temperature is actually quite variable in all age groups (9,11,17). In young patients, fever is present 27–90% of the time; most studies report an incidence greater than 50% (10,13,14,16).

Likewise, an increased white blood cell count is a common but by no means ubiquitous sign of diverticulitis in the older patient. Most reviews report an elevated white blood cell count in 66–100% of young patients with diverticulitis (8,10,13,16). A palpable abdominal mass, which may sometimes be detected in the older patient with diverticulitis (9,11,17), is noted in 20–24% of younger patients (10,13,14,16). Other findings, such as diarrhea, are seen occasionally in both younger and older individuals.

In conclusion, in young patients, the presence and frequency of specific symptoms and signs of acute diverticulitis do not differ significantly from those demonstrated in older patients. However, the misdiagnosis rate in these two age groups does differ significantly. One probable explanation is that the diagnosis is rarely entertained initially by the physician examining the young patient. The problem is further compounded in the young female patient, for whom a multitude of possible obstetric and gynecologic causes must be considered. As physicians become more aware of the incidence of the disease, their index of suspicion will rise, accompanied by an increase in the frequency of correctly diagnosed cases of acute diverticulitis in younger patients.

COMPLICATIONS OF DIVERTICULITIS

Difficulties in Analysis and Incidence of Disease

Gordon noted that in the general population, "the frequency with which complications occur in patients with diverticular disease is impossible to determine"(18). It is even more difficult to specifically determine the frequency of complications in younger patients. An estimate of the overall complication rate may be based on the rate of surgical intervention. This approach is not perfect, because some patients with uncomplicated, recurrent inflammatory attacks undergo an operation, whereas other patients with actual diverticular complications are considered too high a risk for surgery. Approximately 20–30% of patients with diverticulitis of all ages require an operation (15,17,18). Unfortunately, results concerning the need for surgical intervention in young patients with diverticulitis are variable and quite confusing and, as illustrated in Table 23.3, can lead to a number of different conclusions. Whether younger patients undergo operations more, less, or equally

Table 23.2.   Sites of Abdominal Tenderness

Site of Tenderness	Range of Results (%)
One or both lower quadrants	94–100
Left lower quadrant alone	40–56
Right lower quadrant alone	0–25

From Schauer PR, Ramos R, Ghiatas AA, et al. Virulent diverticular disease in young obese men. Am J Surg 1992;164:443–448; Konvolinka CW. Acute diverticulitis under age forty. Am J Surg 1994;167:562–565; Ouriel K, Schwartz SI. Diverticular disease in the young patient. Surg Gynecol Obstet 1983;156:1–5; Simonowitz D, Paloyan D. Diverticular disease of the colon in patients under 40 years of age. Am J Gastroenterol 1977;67:69–72; Chodak GW, Rangel DM, Passaro E. Colonic diverticulitis in patients under age 40: need for earlier diagnosis. Am J Surg 1981;141:699–702.

Table 23.3.   Incidence of Surgical Intervention in Younger and Older Diverticulitis Patients

Authors (Reference No.)	<40 Years (%)	>40 Years (%)
Ambrosetti et al (21)	15	33[a]
Simonowitz and Paloyan (14)	30	(no comparison)
Acosta et al (6)	41	54
Schauer et al (8)	48	33
Ouriel and Schwartz (13)	60[b]	(no comparison)
Konvolinka (10)	76	17
Freischlag et al. (7)	88	42[c]

[a]Patients divided into <50 years and >50 years of age.
[b]If patients without complications who underwent elective resection after initial attack are excluded, 50% of young patients in study required surgical intervention. If patients without complications who underwent resection after a second inflammatory attack are also excluded, 35% of young patients in study required surgical intervention.
[c]Patients with diverticular disease managed as outpatients are excluded from analysis.

as frequently as older patients is not clear. Therefore, estimating the frequency of diverticular complications in the younger population based on the incidence of surgical intervention is extremely difficult.

Disease Virulence

Retrospective studies claim that 51–76% of younger patients with diverticulitis require surgery for complications and intractable inflammation; perforation and abscess formation are the leading indications (6,7,10,13). Such results lead a number of authors to conclude that, for young patients, diverticulitis is a more virulent and aggressive disease (7–11,13,15). Younger patients with mildly symptomatic disease, however, may seek medical attention less frequently, receive the correct diagnosis less often, and undergo treatment as inpatients less often than older symptomatic individuals. In fact, one report "focused on patients under the age of 40 years with diverticular disease of the colon who were admitted to the hospital. . . . Patients with diverticular disease managed solely in the outpatient department were excluded" (7). While hospitalized, older patients with diverticulitis would include the minimally, moderately, and severely afflicted, whereas the younger hospitalized patients would all tend to be more ill, representing a smaller proportion of all young patients with diverticulitis. It is likely that a higher percentage of these more seriously ill young inpatients would require surgical intervention.

Therefore, comparisons between two such different hospitalized patient groups are inherently flawed. *The conclusion that acute diverticulitis is more virulent in younger patients is compromised by the exclusion of minimally symptomatic, undiagnosed patients, as well as those treated as outpatients.* In clinical terms, the physician who diagnoses acute diverticulitis in the young patient and determines that the attack is severe enough to warrant hospitalization should be prepared for the possibility that conservative treatment will fail and surgical intervention will be required.

Indications for Resection

In terms of specific complications, Milsom and Singh noted that "obstruction, bleeding, fistula formation, and chronic pain requiring surgery all occur rarely in the younger group" (19). The indications for surgical intervention in patients with these complications should vary little between different age groups, although bleeding may be better tolerated in the otherwise healthy young patient. Likewise, most agree concerning the need for surgical intervention in any patient, young or old, with peritonitis secondary to perforation. However, the treatment of one of the most common complications of acute diverticulitis is more controversial: i.e., a diverticular perforation complicated by abscess formation (Chapter 15). Not all physicians recommend elective resection to every young patient after abscess drainage. The approach to treatment of these abscess patients must address several questions. What is the incidence of a second complication after successful abscess drainage? Are recurrent complications more or less likely to develop in young, healthy patients? Do the risks of surgical intervention outweigh the risks of further diverticular complications? Answers to these pertinent questions would best be determined through prospective, randomized trials. *Presently, after successful percutaneous drainage of an abscess in an otherwise healthy young patient who has experienced one bout of diverticulitis, some physicians first evaluate the colon endoscopically and radiographically.* If the region of colon harboring the suspect diverticulum appears soft, compliant, and limited in length, and assuming there is no previous history of symptoms attributable to diverticular disease, the patient will be followed without performing elective colonic resection (20). *A long or rigid diseased segment may be an indication for elective resection.* By evaluating each young patient individually with endoscopy, and in some cases contrast studies, those whose disease is neither extensive nor severe may be able to avoid a major operation.

INDICATIONS FOR ELECTIVE RESECTION

Another area of disagreement specifically concerning younger patients is the role of elective resection after the first attack of uncomplicated acute diverticulitis. Elective surgical resection in the general population is recommended for patients who have suffered two or more documented attacks of uncomplicated acute diverticulitis (9,11,18). However, numerous authors recommend elective resection for patients 40 years of age or younger after resolution of the initial bout of uncomplicated acute diverticulitis (9–11,13,14,17–19,21). In making such a recommendation, the frequency, morbidity, mortality, and costs of all subsequent attacks (whether or not surgery is required) must be weighed against the morbidity, mortality, and costs when *all* young patients undergo surgery after only one inflammatory attack. Put more simply, is it better to operate on every young patient, even if a significant number would never require surgery, to avoid future bouts of diverticulitis and its complications in a subset of the group?

In 1969, Parks reported on 317 patients of all ages who were successfully treated medically for their first attack of acute diverticulitis. Of these, 78 patients (24.6%) were later readmitted for a second attack, 12 patients (3.8%) were readmitted for a third attack, and five patients (1.6%) were readmitted for a fourth attack. During the first readmission (second attack), six patients (7.7%) died and 20 patients (26%) required surgical treatment (12). In a more recent study, 11 of 40 (28%) medically treated patients younger than 50 years of age suffered subsequent attacks, complications, or surgery during a mean follow-up of 25 months (15). Other studies claim similar results, with 29–55% of medically treated young patients eventually requiring readmission for recurrent attacks and complications, most of these undergoing either elective or emergent surgery (13,14,16,21).

Therefore, it is unclear whether young patients who recover from their first bout of uncomplicated acute diverticulitis are at greater risk for recurrent attacks, complications, and surgery than older patients. However, it is important to note that *minimal to no mortality is reported in young patients who subsequently require surgery for recurrent disease after successful medical treatment of their initial inflammatory attack* (16). Analysis of these studies suggests that at least 45–71% of young patients who recover from their initial attack of acute diverticulitis do not require readmission for an additional inflammatory attack. Furthermore, among those who are subsequently hospitalized, some still do not require surgery. Finally, for the otherwise healthy young patients who do eventually require operations, the mortality associated with the delay in surgical intervention is negligible. *It therefore seems quite reasonable to treat healthy, asymptomatic younger and older patients similarly, recommending elective resection after resolution of the second documented bout of uncomplicated acute diverticulitis.*

SUMMARY

Many publications analyze numerous aspects of diverticular disease in young patients, yielding an enormous variety of results and conclusions. However, upon careful analysis of these reports, a number of important clinical points become evident. First, the location and gross and microscopic anatomy of these diverticula do not differ from those found in the older population. Second, no definite relationship between ethnicity and diverticular disease in the young has been established. Third, obesity (mild to morbid) seems to be the only comorbid condition present in a significant number of these otherwise healthy young patients. Fourth, the apparent male predominance in young patients with diverticulitis may be artifactual, perhaps due to the complexity of diagnosing lower abdominal and pelvic symptoms in young women. Fifth, between 6 and 9% of the population 40 years of age or younger harbors colonic diverticula. Sixth, acute diverticulitis in younger patients is not a rarity. From 11 to 30% of documented cases of acute diverticulitis occur in young patients, especially those in their fourth decade of life.

The criteria for emergent surgical intervention in younger patients should be similar to criteria for the general diverticulitis population. It is possible, however, that different surgical procedures may be used in younger patients due to their overall good health. For example, longer procedures (such as intraoperative lavage and primary anastomosis) may be better tolerated by younger patients than by the more medically fragile older patient population. The extent of resection should not depend on patient age, and the need for resection of the entire sigmoid colon distally is as important for young as for old patients to reduce recurrence. Most diverticulitis complications are dealt with similarly for patients of all ages. The greatest sources of controversy, and important areas of focus both medically and financially, concern: (*a*) those whose diverticular abscesses have resolved after percutaneous drainage; and (*b*) the indications for elective resection in young patients who have undergone successful medical treatment of their first bout of acute diverticulitis. For the former group, treatment must be based on an assessment of the patient and the diseased segment of colon. After catheter drainage of an abscess, a healthy young patient whose disease is limited and whose colon is pliable on endoscopy should not automatically receive a recommendation for elective resection. Similarly, recommending elective resection for all healthy young patients after resolution of the first documented bout of uncomplicated acute diverticulitis does not seem to be indicated. Such an approach may eliminate the medical risks, patient discomfort and inconveniences, and monetary costs associated with an unnecessary operation in approximately one-half to two-thirds of young patients, without placing patients who do require subsequent surgery at significant risk.

EDITORIAL COMMENTS

The authors have made a good case challenging the popular notion that diverticular disease is inherently more virulent in patients younger than 40 years of age (22). The fact that the disease is misdiagnosed frequently in young patients, especially females, is well documented, and many of these patients are treated for other illnesses as outpatients. Young patients hospitalized with diverticular disease tend to have complicated variants only — unlike the hospitalized elderly patients, who have a wider spectrum of disease. This selection bias may account for some misconceptions about sequelae of diverticular disease in young people as a whole.

We agree that it is not necessary to operate on all young patients who have been hospitalized with one attack of diverticulitis. In our own study with a 5- to 9–year follow-up, two-thirds of patients who had been hospitalized with diverticulitis did not require surgery (23). If operations were performed, they were done electively rather than emergently.

Unlike the authors, we generally would operate on the young patient who has had successful percutaneous drainage of an abscess complicating diverticulitis. We believe that there are not ample data supporting conservative treatment of this group, and our bias, considering the seriousness of this complication, is to operate (24).

Perhaps laparoscopy should be used more frequently in these patients, especially if the results of a CT scan are not available. Peritonitis due to appendicitis clearly requires appendectomy, whereas limited diverticulitis (without diffuse peritonitis, feculent peritonitis, etc.) can be treated medically after laparoscopy.

REFERENCES

1. Rodkey GV, Welch CE. Changing patterns in the surgical treatment of diverticular disease. Ann Surg 1984;200:466–478. *Males predominated in the group younger than 50 years of age undergoing surgery for complications of diverticular disease.*
2. Mendeloff AI. Thoughts on the epidemiology of diverticular disease. Clin Gastroenterol 1986;15:855–877. *An interesting discussion of epidemiology, detailing international incidence, etiology, dietary considerations, and clinical studies.*
3. Parks TG. Natural history of diverticular disease of the colon. Clin Gastroenterol 1975;4:53–69. *A review. The author believes that diverticular disease in younger people occurs in an aggressive form.*
4. Hughes LE. Postmortem survey of diverticular disease of the colon. Gut 1969;10:336–351. *Colonic diverticula were seen in 9% of patients younger than 50 years of age in this survey of autopsies of 200 selected patients.*
5. Lee Y-S. Diverticular disease of the large bowel in Singapore. Dis Colon Rectum 1986;29:330–335. *In this autopsy study of 1014 cases of people older than 14 years old, diverticulitis began appearing after the second decade.*
6. Acosta JA, Grebenc ML, Doberneck RC, et al. Colonic diverticular disease in patients 40 years old or younger. Am Surg 1992;58:605–607. *The authors found an increased risk in male patients.*
7. Freischlag J, Bennion RS, Thompson JE. Complications of diverticular disease of the colon in young people. Dis Colon Rectum 1986;29:639–643. *Fifteen of 17 patients younger than 40 years of age with acute diverticulitis had urgent or emergent operations.*
8. Schauer PR, Ramos R, Ghiatas AA, et al. Virulent diverticular disease in young obese men. Am J Surg 1992;164:443–448. *Many of the patients younger than 40 years of age with acute diverticulitis were obese males.*
9. Roberts PL, Veidenheimer MC. Current management of diverticulitis. Adv Surg 1994;27:189–208. *After 40 years of age, the incidence of diverticula increases linearly with age. The authors recommend elective resection for patients younger than 40 years of age with one well-documented episode of diverticulitis.*
10. Konvolinka CW. Acute diverticulitis under age forty. Am J Surg 1994;167:562–565. *Most patients were men in the fourth decade; resection is recommended after the first documented attack.*
11. Schoetz DJ Jr. Uncomplicated diverticulitis. Surg Clin North Am 1993;73:965–974. *Recommends aggressive surgical approach for young patients.*

12. Parks TG. Natural history of diverticular disease of the colon. A review of 521 cases. BMJ 1969;4:639–645. *Diverticular disease was rarely seen in patients younger than 40 years of age.*
13. Ouriel K, Schwartz SI. Diverticular disease in the young patient. Surg Gynecol Obstet 1983;156:1–5. *Forty-five percent of the medically managed patients had a subsequent operation; rehospitalization occurred within an average of 27 months.*
14. Simonowitz D, Paloyan D. Diverticular disease of the colon in patients under 40 years of age. Am J Gastroenterol 1977;67:69–72. *More than two-thirds of these patients had an incorrect admission diagnosis and 30% required surgical treatment.*
15. Ambrosetti P, Robert JH, Witzig J-A, et al. Acute left colonic diverticulitis; a prospective analysis of 226 consecutive cases. Surgery 1994;115:546–550. *Severe diverticulitis was seen by CT in 37% of the patients younger than 50 years of age.*
16. Chodak GW, Rangel DM, Passaro E. Colonic diverticulitis in patients under age 40: need for earlier diagnosis. Am J Surg 1981;141:699–702. *The diagnosis was entertained in only one-third of these patients; barium enema proved to be useful as a diagnostic tool.*
17. Freeman SR, McNally PR. Diverticulitis. Med Clin North Am 1993;77:1149–1167. *A basic review with 64 references.*
18. Gordon PH. Diverticular disease of the colon. In: Gordon PH, Nivatvongs S, eds. Principles and practice of surgery for the colon, rectum, and anus. St. Louis: Quality Medical Publishing, 1992:739–797.
19. Milsom JW, Singh G. Diverticulitis in young patients. Semin Colon Rectal Surg 1990;1:103–108. *Recommends elective resection of affected bowel segment 2–3 months after the first attack of diverticulitis subsides.*
20. Goldberg SM, Rothenberger DA, Wong WD. Personal communication. Minneapolis: University of Minnesota, 1994.
21. Ambrosetti P, Robert JH, Witzig J-A, et al. Acute left colonic diverticulitis in young patients. J Am Coll Surg 1994;179:156–160. *Younger men had severe acute diverticulitis more commonly than older ones, but operative treatment was needed less often during the first episode. Young men had a higher chance of poor secondary outcome after conservative treatment.*
22. Eusebio EB, Eisenberg MM. Natural history of diverticular disease of the colon in young patients. Am J Surg 1973;125:308–311. *A study of 181 patients 40 years of age or younger with diverticular disease. Two-thirds ultimately needed surgery. The authors believed that with longer follow-up even more patients would need operation, and they promoted an aggressive approach.*
23. Vignati PV, Welch JP, Cohen JC. Long-term management of diverticulitis in young patients. Dis Colon Rectum 1995;38:627–629. *A study of 40 patients 50 years of age or younger. Twenty-five percent of patients underwent surgery during the first admission. Two-thirds of the remaining patients did not require surgery during the follow-up period of 4–9 years.*
24. Scully RE, ed. Case records of the Massachusetts General Hospital. Case 27-1992. N Engl J Med 1992;327:40–44. *A good discussion of the presentation, differential diagnosis, and treatment of a 20-year-old patient with sigmoid diverticulitis complicated by pericolonic abscess.*

24 Critical Illness Arising From Diverticular Disease

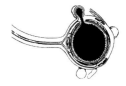

Rocco Orlando, III, MD
Lori L. Fritts, MD

KEY POINTS

- Reasons for ICU admission:
  - unstable with GI bleeding
  - postoperative complication
  - sepsis with diverticulitis
- PEEP the mainstay of treatment for ARDS
- Abdominal compartment syndrome lowers urine output, ease of ventilation
- Patients at risk of malnutrition and translocation of bacteria/endotoxin
- Multiple organ dysfunction cause of death with sepsis

INTRODUCTION

Diverticular disease of the colon is not a common reason for admission to an intensive care unit (ICU). Patients with diverticular disease who require ICU monitoring generally have one of three problems: (*a*) diverticular bleeding resulting in hemodynamic instability; (*b*) a medical complication after surgery for diverticular disease; or (*c*) complications resulting from sepsis associated with acute diverticulitis.

ILLUSTRATIVE CASE

A 48-year-old man presented to a small community hospital 12 hours after the sudden onset of diffuse lower abdominal pain. He had recently noted constipation and mild left lower quadrant discomfort but was otherwise in good health. Past medical history revealed a one pack-per-day smoking history but no evidence of preexisting cardiac or pulmonary disease. Physical examination demonstrated a fever of 102.4°F and marked abdominal tenderness, greatest in the lower abdomen with rebound tenderness. Initial laboratory studies included a hematocrit of 42.5 and a white blood cell count of 17,000 with a left shift. The platelet count was 125,000. Electrolytes, liver and renal chemistries, and coagulation studies were normal. Abdominal and chest radiographs showed free air.

After administration of intravenous fluids and broad-spectrum antibiotics, the patient was brought to the operating room. Laparotomy revealed free perforation of the sigmoid colon with diffuse peritonitis. Sigmoid resection with end colostomy and closure of the distal segment was performed. Intraoperatively, arterial oxygen saturation declined and the anesthesiologist noted that it was increasingly difficult to ventilate the patient. In addition, oliguria persisted despite the administration of 4 liters of crystalloid. The patient was extubated in the operating room but required reintubation in the postanesthesia care unit because of labored breathing and hypoxemia. After reintubation and institution of mechanical ventilation, blood gases on 80% oxygen revealed: pO_2 = 58, pCO_2 = 36, and pH = 7.32. No pulmonary improvement occurred with application of 10 cm of H_2O of positive end-expiratory pressure (PEEP) and urinary output remained poor. Arrangements were made for transfer to a tertiary care facility via air ambulance.

Upon arrival in the surgical intensive care unit (SICU) after transfer, PEEP was increased to 15 cm H_2O and an oximetry pulmonary artery catheter was placed. The cardiac index was 4.6, and pulmonary artery occlusion pressure was 10 mm Hg. Additional fluids were given with continued poor urinary output. During the next 12 hours, 11 liters of fluid was infused to increase filling pressures above 14 mm Hg, but urinary output remained poor despite the use of low-dose dopamine ("renal dose" dopamine = 0.5–2 μg/kg per minute). Hypoxemia was refractory to the application of PEEP at 22 cm H_2O and pulmonary compliance fell to 15. With continued hypoxemia, the patient was switched to high-frequency jet ventilation with improvement in blood gases, permitting a reduction in the FiO_2 to 55%. However, urinary output remained low and marked abdominal distention was noted. Intraperitoneal pressure was measured at 48 mm Hg via a pressure transducer applied to the bladder catheter. With this information, the patient's abdominal incision was reopened at the bedside under anesthesia and a silo was fashioned with an Esmarch latex rubber bandage to reduce intraperitoneal pressure. After this maneuver, pulmonary compliance dropped, oxygenation improved, and urinary output increased. During the next week, mechanical ventilation was gradually weaned. One week after the incision was opened, a secondary closure was performed. The patient improved and was discharged from the hospital 3 weeks later.

CASE COMMENTS

This patient exemplifies the systemic effects of established peritonitis on multiple organ systems. The scenario is typical of individuals with advanced sepsis. He developed advanced pulmonary failure (adult respiratory distress syndrome [ARDS]) that required not only intubation but later PEEP and finally jet ventilation. The abdominal compartment syndrome developed, and to relieve the abnormally high intra-abdominal pressure, it was necessary to reopen the abdominal wound and to fashion a silo. This maneuver allowed the patient to "turn the corner" and wean from the ventilator. This outcome was fortunate because the risks of mortality with multiple system organ dysfunction or failure remain high; advanced age and involvement of several organs have detrimental effects in particular (1–6).

Early operative intervention is vital in the presence of freely perforated peritonitis, especially of the feculent type. This hopefully can prevent the cascade or organ failure that developed in this patient.

DISCUSSION

Of approximately 1000 annual admissions to the Hartford Hospital ICU, 30% are general surgery patients (Fig. 24.1). Among the 300 general surgical patients, 20 have diverticular

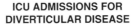

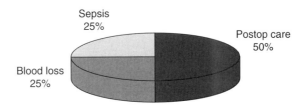

Figure 24.1. Distribution of patients in surgical intensive care at Hartford Hospital.

disease. Of these, 25% are admitted for bleeding, 50% are admitted for postoperative complications, and 25% are admitted for septic complications of acute diverticulitis. Patients with hemorrhage are admitted for hemodynamic instability, often with a reduced threshold for admission in elderly patients with cardiac comorbidity. Patients with bleeding often can be managed safely at lower cost in a surgical step-down or intermediate care unit. *We admit bleeding patients to the ICU only when invasive hemodynamic monitoring is required or when the rate of bleeding requires massive infusion of blood products and intravenous solutions.* The second group of patients who need ICU care includes those who suffer medical complications of surgery for diverticular disease. These complications are most commonly cardiac or pulmonary in nature and are almost always related to preexisting medical conditions. These problems are beyond the scope of this chapter and are well described in textbooks of critical care. The focus of this chapter is on the management of patients with overwhelming infection from acute diverticulitis, usually with perforation or abscess.

Acute Respiratory Failure

Patients with profound intra-abdominal sepsis secondary to perforated diverticulitis occasionally present with the adult respiratory distress syndrome (ARDS) (7–9) (Fig. 24.2). *Bacteremia and endotoxemia result in the elaboration of a cascade of cytokines with broad and diverse systemic effects.* The pulmonary injury associated with this condition is characterized by the development of a pulmonary capillary leak resulting initially in interstitial pulmonary edema. This may progress to alveolar edema with the eventual appearance of arterial hypoxemia. The development of this noncardiogenic pulmonary edema is accompanied by a reduction in pulmonary compliance and a reduction in functional residual capacity of the lung. As a result, these patients exhibit tachypnea, dyspnea, and ultimately cyanosis if the condition is unrecognized. Pulse oximetry reveals a decrease in arterial saturation. Blood gases early in the development of ARDS show a depressed pCO_2 manifesting as an increased minute ventilation but a declining pO_2.

Initial therapy is directed at improving arterial oxygenation with supplemental oxygen. Patients who fail to respond to supplemental oxygen but who are still able to ventilate adequately (as evidenced by a normal or depressed pCO_2) may be managed with continuous positive airway pressure (CPAP) administered by face mask (mask CPAP). These patients require close monitoring for signs of impending respiratory failure. Endotracheal intubation and mechanical ventilation are initiated when signs of respiratory failure develop, including a rising pCO_2, worsening tachypnea and dyspnea, and refractory hypoxemia.

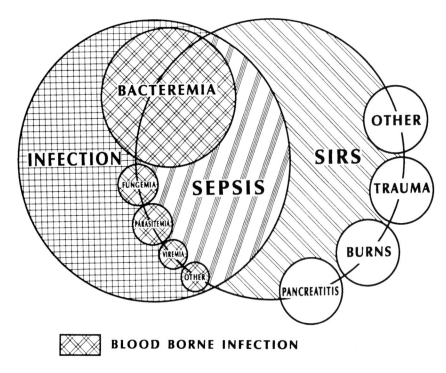

BLOOD BORNE INFECTION

Figure 24.2. Diagram showing the complex relations between the systemic inflammatory response syndrome, sepsis, and infection. (Reprinted with permission from Bone RC, Balk RA, Cerra FB, et al. Definitions for sepsis and organ failure and guidelines for the use of innovative therapies in sepsis. Chest 1992;101:1644–1655.)

The mainstay of treatment of ARDS in this setting is application of PEEP. After endotracheal intubation, mechanical ventilation is instituted with a fraction of inspired oxygen of 0.6 and PEEP of 5. PEEP is increased in increments of 2–3 cm H_2O to achieve an arterial oxygen saturation of greater than 90% at an FiO_2 of 0.4 or less. For patients who are not responsive to application of PEEP in the range of 20–25 cm H_2O, *several options are possible, including application of very high levels of PEEP ("super PEEP"), inverse ratio ventilation, pressure-controlled ventilation, and ultra high-frequency jet ventilation* (10). Although overall mortality is high, satisfactory results have been achieved with all of these techniques. The choice of approach should depend on institutional experience because all of these techniques are fraught with complications including barotrauma, air trapping, hypercarbia, and cardiovascular depression.

There is increasing acceptance that permissive hypercapnia is reasonable as long as arterial oxygen saturation is maintained and severe acidosis is avoided. This may allow a reduction in minute ventilation with its associated barotrauma. Other adjuncts to high levels of pulmonary support include hemodynamic monitoring with a pulmonary artery catheter to detect cardiovascular depression. Continuous mixed venous oximetry is useful in assessing the balance between oxygen supply and demand in these critically ill patients. Increasing levels of pulmonary support may result in improvement in arterial oxygenation but at the expense of cardiac output. The mixed venous oxygen saturation (SVO_2) will alert the clinician to levels of pulmonary support that may require institution of cardiovascular support. Often, transfusion of packed red blood cells will result in improvement in SVO_2 to clinically satisfactory levels. Most patients who exhibit cardiovascular depression from high levels of pulmonary support will respond to administration of intravascular volume, but a small number will require the addition of an inotropic agent such as dobutamine or epinephrine. If there is limited familiarity with these methods of advanced pulmonary support, transfer to a tertiary care center for surgical critical care should be considered.

Abdominal Compartment Syndrome

The illustrative patient at the beginning of this chapter exhibited the abdominal compartment syndrome, an uncommon but treatable complication of abdominal sepsis (11). The condition is characterized by the development of elevated intra-abdominal pressures as a result of massive tissue edema. The syndrome is often associated with sepsis but is also seen in patients with severe trauma who require massive transfusions and volume administration. Retroperitoneal or intra-abdominal hemorrhage from either trauma or conditions such as a ruptured abdominal aortic aneurysm are possible acute etiologies as well. Chronically, the condition may result from ascites, large tumors, or peritoneal dialysis.

Increased abdominal pressure has many physiologic consequences (Table 24.1). Cardiac output is diminished and systemic vascular resistance is increased, putting additional strain on the heart. Venous return is decreased as a result of a decrease in the cross-sectional area of the inferior vena cava and because of increased vascular pooling caudal to the diaphragm. Visceral blood flow is diminished, most importantly to the kidneys. A reduction in glomerular filtration rate occurs as a result of decreased cardiac output and a reduction in the renal perfusion pressure caused by the high intra-abdominal pressure that is transmitted to the kidneys. At moderate elevations of pressure of 15–30 mm Hg, oliguria develops, followed by anuria at higher pressures. The elevation of the hemidiaphragms results in decreased pulmonary compliance, making ventilation progressively more difficult. *The diagnosis of the abdominal compartment syndrome should be suspected when oliguria*

Table 24.1.   Physiologic Consequences of Increased Intra-Abdominal Pressure

	Increased	Decreased	No change
Mean blood pressure	–	–	+
Heart rate	+	–	–
Pulmonary capillary wedge pressure	+	–	–
Peak airway pressure	+	–	–
Central venous pressure	+	–	–
Thoracic, pleural pressure	+	–	–
Inferior vena caval pressure	+	–	–
Renal vein pressure	+	–	–
Systemic vascular resistance	+	–	–
Cardiac output	–	+	–
Venous return	–	+	–
Visceral blood flow	–	+	–
Renal blood flow	–	+	–
Glomerular filtration rate	–	+	–
Abdominal wall compliance	–	+	–

From Schein M, Wittman DH, Aprahamian CC, et al. The abdominal compartment syndrome: the physiological and clinical consequences of elevated intra-abdominal pressure. J Am Coll Surg 1995; 180:745–753.

is observed in a setting of massive abdominal distention that is firm to palpation. The diagnosis is made by measuring the intra-abdominal pressure. This can be performed directly with insertion of an intraperitoneal catheter or cannula but is most easily accomplished by measuring the pressure within the urinary bladder via the Foley catheter. Mild intra-abdominal hypertension is characterized by pressures of 10–20 mm Hg and is generally well tolerated. Moderate elevations of 20–40 mm Hg may be associated with adverse clinical effects, especially when accompanied by hypovolemia, low cardiac output, or respiratory failure. Moderate intra-abdominal hypertension and its concomitant oliguria may respond to volume loading, inotropic support, and increases in mechanical ventilatory support.

Severe intra-abdominal hypertension usually is not responsive to these measures. Decompression of the abdominal cavity is required in these most extreme instances. This results in improvement in cardiac output and an increase in pulmonary compliance. With administration of adequate intravascular volume urinary output is improved.

Decompression involves opening and often extending the midline incision and fashioning a silo out of prosthetic material. *Several instances of cardiovascular collapse have*

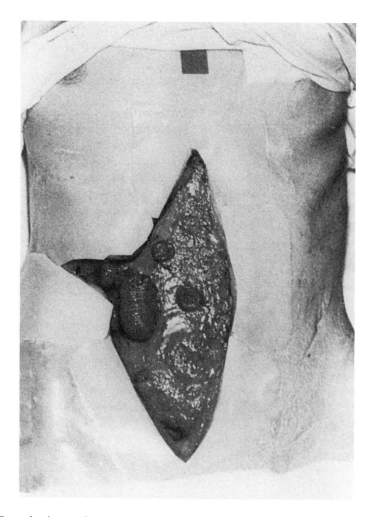

Figure 24.3.   Example of a complex surgical wound in a patient with a history of abdominal sepsis. Note small bowel lying within granulation tissue. (Reprinted with permission from Mughal MM, Bancewicz, Irving MH. "Laparostomy:" a technique for the management of intractable intra-abdominal sepsis. Br J Surg 1986;73:253–295.)

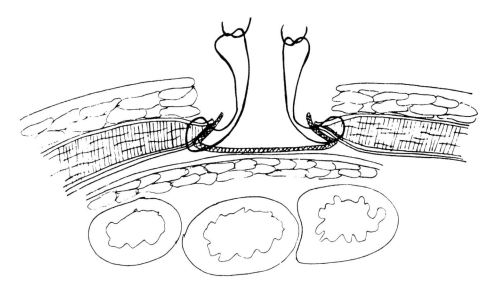

Figure 24.4. Attachment of mesh to fascial edges in open surgical wound. (Reprinted with permission from Wouters DB, Krom RA, Sloof MJ, et al. The use of Marlex mesh in patients with generalized peritonitis and multiple organ system failure. Surg Gynecol Obstet 1983;156:609–614.)

been reported at the time of decompression. This complication can be avoided with a slow release of the pressure at the time of reoperation. A variety of materials have been used for this purpose including Esmarch bandages, Velcro-like devices, sterilized plastic intravenous fluid bags, polypropylene mesh, polytetrafluoroethylene (PTFE) mesh, and absorbable mesh. We favor latex bandages because they are inexpensive and the underlying bowel does not adhere to them. When the patient recovers, the prosthesis is removed and the abdominal wall is closed. Sometimes, a staged approach to closure is helpful by making a tuck in the prosthetic material to effect eventual wound closure. If the patient remains sick for a long enough period of time, fascial closure is not possible. The wound is then managed with closure of the skin only or with placement of absorbable mesh and eventual skin grafting on the bowel. Definitive repair of the fascial defect then is performed in 6–12 months.

These abdominal closure techniques are also useful in the management of patients with generalized or intractable intra-abdominal infection who require open abdominal packing to gain control of their sepsis (12–18) (Figs. 24.3 and 24.4).

MEDIATORS AND CYTOKINES

Patients with diverticulitis who are admitted to the intensive care unit frequently are severely ill with manifestations of overt sepsis. *Sepsis can be defined as the systemic inflammatory response within the setting of known infection.* Clinically, sepsis is marked by alterations in body temperature, accelerated heart rate, increased respiratory rate, and an elevated white blood cell count. Sepsis is considered severe when associated with hypotension and/or end-organ hypoperfusion. *Septic shock is defined as sepsis with hypotension, which is resistant to fluid resuscitation and which often requires vasoactive drug support.* Gram-negative bacteria are frequently associated with diverticular sepsis (19); gram-negative sepsis is the most widely studied form of sepsis and has been the model through which the identity and biologic function of endotoxin and of many cytokines have been elucidated.

Endotoxin is the primary culprit responsible for many of the clinical consequences of gram-negative bacterial infections. Endotoxin is a complex lipopolysaccharide molecule that comprises part of the outer bacterial membrane. Increases in mortality, myocardial depression and the incidence of multiple organ failure during septic shock have been demonstrated when endotoxin is present (20). Survival from gram-negative sepsis is improved in the presence of antibodies to endotoxin (21–23).

The direct effects of endotoxin include activation of complement, the fibrinolytic pathway, polymorphonuclear leukocytes, and macrophages to release cytokines, largely tumor necrosis factor (TNF) and interleukin-1 (IL-1). TNF and IL-1, in turn, amplify the systemic response to endotoxin through stimulation of leukocytes, platelets and endothelial cells leading to release of additional cytokines and related mediators.

Cytokines are messenger molecules produced by endothelial cells at sites of tissue injury and by various cells of the immune system. Cytokines can act locally or systemically, affecting the metabolic response to injury or infection. *If left unchecked, the systemic effects of cytokines can lead to hypotension and subsequent organ dysfunction.* Four polypeptide cytokines that seem to play pivotal roles in the stress response are TNF, IL-1, interferon-gamma (INF gamma), and IL-6.

TNF, which is also known as cachectin, is considered by many investigators to be the primary mediator of the systemic effects of endotoxin. At low circulating levels, TNF is associated with tachycardia, tachypnea, fever, and anorexia; hypotension, organ failure and ultimately death follow higher levels of TNF. TNF is largely produced by macrophages but can also be synthesized by lymphocytes, Kupffer cells, and other cells of the immune system.

IL-1 mediates pathophysiologic changes similar to those of TNF. It has been associated with increased acute-phase hepatic protein synthesis as well as accelerated ACTH, glucocorticoid, and insulin secretion. Albumin synthesis and trace element levels are decreased when IL-1 levels are elevated. The combined effects of IL-1 and TNF often are greater than those of each mediator alone. *INF* is a type II interferon that has been shown to increase the number of TNF receptors on various target cells.

IL-6 has been identified as a major regulator of hepatic acute-phase protein synthesis, highlighting some of the beneficial, preservation-oriented actions of individual cytokines. IL-6 promotes a qualitative alternation in liver protein synthesis such that transport peptide (albumin, transferrin, etc.) production is diminished and acute-phase protein (C-reactive protein, fibrinogen, etc.) production is augmented. Although the exact role of acute-phase proteins remains poorly understood, many act as opsonins, coagulation cofactors, antiproteases, and wound repair factors. IL-6-promoted acute-phase proteins seem to aid in limiting tissue damage, offering a distinct survival advantage (24).

CLINICAL MANIFESTATIONS OF SEPTIC SHOCK

Patients who develop bacterial sepsis may display clinical hallmark features, including altered body temperature, changes in circulating white blood cell populations, changes in cardiac performance, altered vascular tone, and hypercatabolism. Body core temperature represents the balance between heat production and heat dissipation. Increases in core temperature frequently are seen with bacterial infections and may serve as a protective function, because most metabolic reactions occur faster and more efficiently at higher body temperatures. In an effort to localize tissue damage, cytokines promote local vasodilation to facilitate an influx of circulating neutrophils and monocytes into the injured area. Both TNF and IL-2 act locally as white cell chemotactic factors, as well as at the level of the bone marrow, to promote demargination of immature cell forms into the systemic circulation (24).

The hemodynamic changes seen in septic shock are, in part, due to changes in cardiac function. Cardiac output is elevated with an associated rise in heart rate. Interestingly, most patients in septic shock also demonstrate an element of myocardial depression, probably cytokine-mediated. Myocardial compliance diminishes, leading to left ventricular diastolic dysfunction and ultimately biventricular compromise (25–28). Experimental studies have demonstrated that coronary artery blood flow is maintained during myocardial dysfunction, refuting the suggestion that cardiac depression is the result of myocardial ischemia (29). Other investigators have shown that down-regulation of β receptors occurs during septic shock, possibly limiting the effectiveness of endogenous and exogenous catecholamines (30–32).

Disruptions in arterial and venous tone also are seen in septic shock, leading to decreased systemic vascular resistance, venous pooling, and hypotension. Different vascular beds may be variably affected. Factors such as TNF, IL-1, complement activation, prostacyclins, nitric oxide, and endothelial relaxing factor contribute to changes in septic-related vascular tone and permeability. Experimental evidence suggests that α receptor down-regulation occurs as well, perhaps accounting for the relative insensitivity of some patients to vasopressor agents (33).

As systemic and pulmonary vascular permeability increases, tissue edema develops, impeding diffusion of nutrients and oxygen and leading to tissue hypoxia. As tissues are deprived of oxygen, there is a shift toward anaerobic metabolism with accumulation of lactate. The severity of a patient's lactic acidosis is proportional to the oxygen debt. Sustained high levels of lactate are good predictors of mortality; a patient's ability to clear lactic acid correlates with the likelihood of surviving the critical illness or injury (34–36).

Many investigators have observed that patients in septic shock demonstrate hyperdynamic hemodynamics and a rising lactic acid level, despite less than maximal oxygen extraction. No changes in the oxygen dissociation curve are seen, suggesting that suboptimal oxygen extraction follows suboptimal oxygen utilization at the end-organ level (37,38). It has been suggested that suboptimal oxygen delivery and utilization can be explained by regional changes in blood flow distribution, creating circulatory mismatches (39,40). Some studies have shown improved survival from septic shock in patients who achieve elevated levels of systemic oxygen delivery and consumption (41–43).

Hypercatabolism is another hallmark of septic shock. Glucose metabolism is altered as standard stores are depleted rapidly. Gluconeogenesis may be suppressed by changes in splanchnic blood flow. Accelerated lipolysis and skeletal muscle breakdown occur in an effort to produce alternate fuel sources and the amino acids needed for acute-phase protein synthesis. Nitrogen excretion is elevated and negative nitrogen balance develops. Anorexia is frequently seen in association with severe infection and, for patients who are capable of eating, anorexia may contribute to body tissue loss.

As the understanding of critical illness increases and the technology to sustain life improves, fewer patients are dying from initial refractory hypotension, early cardiac failure, or overwhelming infection. *Many patients can now survive the early resuscitation from septic shock; most patients who die following sepsis do so because of subsequent development of multiple organ failure (MOF).* Factors that probably contribute to delayed mortality due to MOF include ongoing hypoperfusion, uncontrolled or occult infection, nosocomial infection, complications arising from drugs or therapies, and ongoing systemic oxygen debt (44–46).

Treatment of patients in septic shock should center around (*a*) adequate resuscitation, (*b*) identification and treatment of underlying infection, and (*c*) limiting mediator-promoted responses and injuries where possible. Fluid administration remains the initial therapy for septic shock and should be guided by cardiac performance, pulmonary artery occlusion pressures, and urine output. Vasopressors and inotropic agents are frequently required as well; the exact timing of when to initiate pharmacologic support and the degree to which drug support should be added remain unclear. The endpoint of resuscitation also is not well defined and frequently is linked to indices of local perfusion, crudely marked by clearance of lactic acidosis.

Antibiotic therapy is essential in the setting of severe infection and should be appropriately tailored to the causative agents(s) when speciation and drug sensitivities are known. Until the causative agent(s) are identified, empiric use of either a broad-spectrum single drug or a multidrug regimen is justified. As the understanding of the roles of endotoxin and cytokines in septic shock increases, effective therapies will undoubtedly modulate these substances. Antibodies to endotoxin and various cytokines will limit the actions of these mediators when they are present. Therapies directed at mediator production, such as cyclooxygenase inhibitors, may block subsequent perpetuation of the systemic inflammatory response. Attention also must be paid to routes of entry for late, occult, and nosocomial infection. The gut is gaining increasing recognition for its role in health and disease states and nutritional support therapies must not only deliver nutrients but also must support gut mucosal integrity.

Early Enteral Nutrition

Patients who are critically ill from acute diverticulitis will have increased energy expenditures, requiring as much as 150% of basal caloric needs in the face of severe infection. Loss of body mass can be considerable even in the early stages of septic illness. In addition to removal or drainage of the source of sepsis, the use of broad-spectrum antibiotics, and the use of organ-specific supportive therapies when needed, *treatment must include aggressive and timely nutritional support.* The hypermetabolism seen with sepsis is largely due to increased catecholamine and cortisol production. Cytokines can potentiate catabolism. As glucose stores are rapidly depleted, there is a shift to proteolysis and lipolysis to mobilize amino acids and fatty acids for use as fuel substrates. Relative insulin resistance develops. Trace elements including magnesium, calcium, potassium, zinc, and iron are depleted as negative nitrogen balance accrues. Gluconeogenesis may deteriorate as septic shock progresses, presumably secondary to visceral hypoperfusion.

While playing an essential role in nutrient absorption, *the gut also can be a source of secondary sepsis in a critically ill patient.* Translocation of bacteria and endotoxin from the intestinal lumen into the mesenteric circulation may occur when the host's immune system is compromised or there is intraluminal stasis, as seen with prolonged ileus. Translocation also may occur because of alteration in gut mucosal permeability. Local visceral ischemia, as seen in shock states, can lead to disruption of the brush border and intercellular tight junctions. Bacteria and their toxic byproducts can then freely access splanchnic lymphatics and ultimately the systemic circulation, initiating as well as potentiating the systemic inflammatory response syndrome (SIRS) (Fig. 24.2). Several studies have demonstrated that infections within specific subsets of patients have been linked with bacterial invasion from the gastrointestinal tract (47–53). Other investigators have demonstrated increased gut permeability in infected burn patients as well as in healthy volunteers who received endotoxin (54). Patient nutrition plans must now address the maintenance of a healthy gut mucosa in addition to the delivery of adequate, biologically available nutrients.

Glutamine is an amino acid that seems to play a crucial role in the metabolism of intestinal mucosa. It is classified as a nonessential amino acid in that it can be synthesized routinely from precursor molecules and does not require dietary intake in nonstressed patients. However, when severe illness or injury has resulted in glutamine depletion or intestinal mucosal disruption, enteral glutamine supplementation has been shown to be beneficial in reducing bacterial translocation (55).

In addition to glutamine delivery, enteral feeding exerts a trophic effect on the microvilli of the small bowel, and villous atrophy can be seen within several days in the setting of bowel rest with or without administration of total parental nutrition (TPN) (56). Addition of glutamine to TPN despite its relative instability in solution only partially reverses this atrophy. *Multiple animal and human studies have documented improved outcomes from severe illness or injury when early enteral feedings were used;* less favorable outcomes were achieved when TPN was used under similar conditions, underscoring the beneficial trophic effects of enterally delivered nutrients (57).

Whenever possible, early enteral feeding should be used, reserving parenteral nutritional support for patients who cannot tolerate enteral formulas or for whom enteral access cannot be obtained. Any patient who requires operative intervention for his/her illness should undergo placement of a transnasal feeding tube or a surgical enterostomy feeding tube at the time of definitive surgical therapy. Critically ill patients who do not require operative intervention should undergo placement of transnasal feeding tubes. For patients in whom a prolonged ileus is anticipated with dependence on TPN for nutritional maintenance, a slow infusion of an elemental enteral formula to bathe the intestinal mucosa may be beneficial in reducing the risk of mucosal atrophy and secondary bacterial translocation.

Immunomodulatory enteral feedings, which are enriched with glutamine, arginine, ω-3 fatty acids, and RNA nucleotides are now available, and as the role of gut immunology in health and in critical illness is better elucidated, enteral formulas will be adjusted accordingly.

SUMMARY

Critical illness such as hemorrhagic or septic shock may result from diverticular disease of the colon, necessitating resuscitation and management of patients within an intensive care setting. Intra-abdominal sepsis, through the effect of endotoxin and cytokine activation, can lead to hemodynamic alterations, metabolic derangements, ARDS, and development of abdominal compartment syndrome with associated organ dysfunction. These complications must be anticipated and treated aggressively when present. Early enteral nutrition is important to maintain gut mucosal integrity and minimize the opportunity for bacterial translocation and secondary sepsis.

EDITORIAL COMMENTS

In addition to summarizing certain aspects of basic science, such as the role of mediators and cytokines involved with sepsis, this chapter highlights current concepts of management of a difficult group of patients, those with septic complications of diverticulitis hospitalized in the intensive care unit setting. Among those at risk for these problems are certain patients who (a) enter the hospital with freely perforated diverticulitis, (b) have large intra-abdominal and/or pelvic abscesses that are not amenable to successful percutaneous drainage, or (c) have extensive peritonitis from a dehisced colonic anastomosis. The problems are magnified in patients who are already immunocompromised at the time of the septic insult. Pulmonary insufficiency and the development of ARDS is a major obstacle to recovery, but other facets of the multiple organ failure picture, such as acute renal failure or acute hepatic failure, can be of great significance as well. Attention to aggressive nutrition, by the enteral route if possible, is emphasized. The comments on the abdominal compartment syndrome are important because this entity is associated with serious, potentially fatal complications if not recognized promptly and treated appropriately by the release of the elevated intra-abdominal pressure. The options in care for the septic wound with possible fistulas and accompanying peritonitis are many; these may tax the ingenuity of the surgeon and the resources of the nursing staff.

Clearly, surgeons must work hand in hand with intensivists to salvage this challenging population of patients. The optimal treatment venue is probably in tertiary care centers, where diagnostic and therapeutic techniques will continue to evolve.

REFERENCES

1. Knaus WA, Wagner DP. Multiple systems organ failure: epidemiology and prognosis. Crit Care Clin 1989;5:221–232. *Despite the underlying etiology, MSOF has a uniform and frequently fatal outcome after it develops.*
2. Beal AL, Cerra FB. Multiple organ failure syndrome in the 1990's: systemic inflammatory response and organ dysfunction. JAMA 1994:271:226–233. *Includes reviews of a number of controlled, prospective studies and examines the metabolic response in the systemic inflammatory response syndrome (SIRS) and the multiple organ dysfunction syndrome (MODS).*
3. Bone RC, Balk RA, Cerra FB, et al. Definitions for sepsis and organ failure and guidelines for the use of innovative therapies in sepsis. Chest 1992;101:1644–1655. *A review of definitions of many conditions encountered in critically ill patients in intensive care units.*
4. Baue AE. Multiple organ failure, multiple organ dysfunction syndrome, and the systemic inflammatory response syndrome: where do we stand? Shock 1994;2:385–397. A review with 148 references. A series of principles useful for preventing these major problems are outlined.
5. American College of Chest Physicians/Society of Critical Care Medicine Consensus Conference. Definitions for sepsis and organ failure and guidelines for the use of innovative therapies in sepsis. Crit Care Med 1992;20:864–874. *A succinct summary article with a list of definitions of key terms such as sepsis or the systemic inflammatory response syndrome.*
6. Appel GB, Neu HC. The nephrotoxicity of antimicrobial agents. N Engl J Med 1977;296:663–670, 722–728. *A detailed review, useful when managing renal failure, with 21 references.*
7. Hudson LD, Milberg JA, Anardi D, et al. Clinical risks for development of acute respiratory distress syndrome. Am J Respir Crit Care Med 1995;151:293–301. *A prospective study of 695 ICU patients meeting criteria for initial risk and followed for development of ARDS.*
8. Demling RH. Adult respiratory distress syndrome. New Horizons 1993;1:388–402. *ARDS from shock and trauma is a critical component of a generalized inflammatory reaction to distant tissue trauma. A review with 80 references.*
9. Norwood SH, Civetta JM. The adult respiratory distress syndrome. Surg Gynecol Obstet 1985;161:497–508. *A collective review with 116 references. Sepsis is one of the most common risk factors; therapy combines increased inspired oxygen tensions, positive end expiratory pressure, and some kind of mechanical ventilation.*
10. Gluck E, Heard S, Patel C, et al. Use of ultra high frequency ventilation in patients with ARDS. Chest 1993;103:1413–1420. *Ninety patients not responding to conventional ventilation were changed to ultra high frequency ventilation with improved respiratory gas exchange and decreased airway pressure variables.*
11. Schein M, Wittman DH, Aprahamian CC, et al. The abdominal compartment syndrome: the physiological and clinical consequences of elevated intra-abdominal pressure. J Am Coll Surg 1995;180:745–753. *An excellent review of pathophysiology and clinical findings, with 84 references.*
12. Chan ST, Esufali ST. Extended indications for polypropylene mesh closure of the abdominal wall. Br J Surg 1986;73:3–6. *The mesh was used in 21 patients who were believed to need further exploration; the mesh allowed free drainage and wound inspection for fistulas or pus.*
13. Hedderich GS, Wexler MJ, McLean AP, et al. The septic abdomen: open management with Marlex mesh with a zipper. Surgery 1986;99:399–407. *Of the 10 patients described, three had fecal peritonitis and one diverticular abscess and dehiscence. The Marlex was removed in an average of 10–12 days, and no fistulas resulted.*
14. Wouters DB, Krom RA, Sloof MJ, et al. The use of Marlex mesh in patients with generalized peritonitis and multiple organ system failure. Surg Gynecol Obstet 1983;156:609–614. *Describes wound closure with mesh in 20 patients with generalized peritonitis. Spontaneous epithelization occurred if the mesh was not removed.*
15. Mughal MM, Bancewicz J, Irving MH: "Laparostomy:" a technique for the management of intractable intra-abdominal sepsis. Br J Surg 1986;73:253–295. *The abdomen was left open to heal by granulation in 18 patients. No patient eviscerated and the median time for wound healing was 10 weeks.*
16. Schein M, Saadia R, Decker GG. The open management of the septic abdomen. Surg Gynecol Obstet 1986;163:587–592. *A review with 50 references. This technique is useful when severe intra-abdominal sepsis is present and multiple abdominal re-explorations are anticipated. Advantages include decreased postoperative pulmonary complications, improved drainage of the peritoneal cavity, and improved protection of the viscera.*
17. Duff JH, Moffat J. Abdominal sepsis managed by leaving the wound open. Surgery 1981;90:774–778. *The abdomen was left completely open in 18 critically ill patients. Seven patients died.*
18. Anderson ED, Mandelbaum DM, Ellison E, et al. Open packing of the peritoneal cavity in generalized bacterial peritonitis. Am J Surg 1983;145:131–135. *The abdomen was packed open in 20 patients with suppurative peritonitis; 60% died, and all deaths but one were due to overwhelming sepsis.*

19. Shatney CH, Lillehei RC. Septic shock associated with operations for colorectal disease. Dis Colon Rectum 1978;21:480–486. *Shock was caused by gram-negative or anaerobic bacteria. Only four patients ultimately survived, and all of this group had treatment early in the course of shock.*

20. Danner RL, Elin RJ, Hosseini J, et al. Endotoxemia in human septic shock. Chest 1991;99:169–175. *Endotoxin levels were measured in patients with shock and elevated endotoxin levels were associated with increased frequency of multisystem organ failure and depression of left ventricular function.*

21. McCabe WR, Kreger B, Johns M. Type-specific and cross-reactive antibodies in gram-negative bacteremia. N Engl J Med 1972;287:261–267. *High titers of antibacterial antigen antibodies were associated with improved survival from sepsis.*

22. Ziegler E, Fisher CJ Jr, Sprung CL. Treatment of gram-negative bacteremia and septic shock with HA-1A human monoclonal antibody against endotoxin. N Engl J Med 1991;324:429–436. *Administration of human monoclonal antibody HA-1A was associated with improved survival from sepsis with documented gram-negative bacteremia as compared with placebo. No benefit of treatment was seen in patients with sepsis but without proven gram-negative bacteremia.*

23. Ziegler EJ, McCurthan JA, Fierer J, et al. Treatment of gram-negative bacteremia and shock with human antiserum and without Escherichia coli. N Engl J Med 1982;307:1225–1230. *Human antiserum to lipopolysaccharide core of endotoxin was associated with decreased mortality from gram-negative bacteremia.*

24. Fong Y, Lowry SF. Cytokines and the cellular response to injury and infection. In: Wilmore DW, Brennan MR, Haller AH, et al, eds. Care of the surgical patient. II. Care in the ICU. New York: Scientific American Medicine, 1996;15:1–21. *A concise summary of the field with 194 references. A useful list of major known cytokines is included.*

25. Ellrodt A, Riedinger M, Kimichi A, et al. Left ventricular performance in septic shock: reversible segmental and global abnormalities. Am Heart J 1985;110:402–409. *Depressed left ventricular function and segmental wall motion abnormalities were demonstrated to occur frequently in septic shock. No differences in left ventricular ejection fraction, stroke work index, or frequency of segmental dysfunction were seen between survivors and nonsurvivors.*

26. Jafris, Lavine S, Field B, et al. Left ventricular diastolic function in sepsis. Crit Care Med 1990;18:709–714. *Diastolic dysfunction and greater reliance on atrial systolic contribution to diastolic filling were documented in patients with sepsis and septic shock.*

27. Ognibene FP, Parker MM, Natanson C, et al. Depressed left ventricular performance: response to volume infusion in patients with sepsis and septic shock. Chest 1988;93:903–910. *Left ventricular stroke work index was decreased after volume administration to critically ill patients.*

28. Parker M, McCarthy K, Ognibene F, et al. Right ventricular dysfunction and dilation similar to left ventricular changes characterize the cardiac depression of septic shock in humans. Chest 1990;97:126–131. *Biventricular depression was present in patients with septic shock. Survivors demonstrated normalization of cardiac performance parameters, whereas nonsurvivors failed to do so.*

29. Cunnion RE, Schaer GL, Parker MM, et al. The coronary circulation in human septic shock. Circulation 1986;73:637–644. *Coronary artery flow was measured in seven patients with septic shock. No differences in coronary artery flow were seen between patients with sepsis and myocardial depression, patients with sepsis but without myocardial depression, and controls.*

30. Archer L, Black M, Hinshaw L. Myocardial failure with altered response to adrenalin in endotoxin shock. Br J Pharmacol 1975;154:145–155. *A working canine heart preparation was used to demonstrate that endotoxin-associated myocardial depression was related to increased left ventricular end-diastolic pressure, and decreased myocardial deficiency.*

31. Nasraway SA, Rackow EC, Astiz ME, et al. Inotropic response to digoxin and dopamine in patients with severe sepsis. Cardiac failure and systemic hypoperfusion. Chest 1989;95:612–615. *Digoxin was found to be a potent inotrope in patients with septic shock.*

32. Romano FD, Jones SB. Characteristics of myocardial B-adrenergic receptors during endotoxicosis in the rat. Am J Physiol 1986;251:R359–R364. *In vivo administration of endotoxin in rats was associated with decreased isoproterenol binding, suggesting alterations in agonist-stimulated coupling or modification of the beta-adrenergic receptor during shock.*

33. McMillan M, Chernow B, Roth B. Hepatic gamma-adrenergic receptor alteration in a rat model of chronic sepsis. Circ Shock 1983;19:185–193. *Decreased numbers of hepatic alpha-1-adrenergic receptors were found in septic rats as compared with control animals, suggesting that pressor-refractory hypotension of septic shock may be due in part to decreased alpha-1 receptors or changes in receptor-agonist coupling.*

34. Bakker J, Coffernils M, Leon M, et al. Blood lactate levels are superior to oxygen-derived variables in predicting outcome in human septic shock. Chest 1991;99:956–962. *Blood lactate levels were found to be more useful prognostic indicators of survival from septic shock than oxygen delivery or oxygen uptake.*

35. Weil MH, Affi A. Experimental and clinical studies in lactate and pyruvate as indication of the severity of circulatory shock. Circulation 1970;41:989–1001. *A Wistar rat model of hemorrhagic shock was used to demonstrate that cumulative oxygen debt and elevated lactate levels correlated inversely to survival. In 142 patients with clinical shock, lactate levels were good predictors of survival from shock.*

36. Falk JL, Rackow EC, Leavy J, et al. Delayed lactate clearance in patients surviving circulation shock. Acute Care 1985;11:212–215. *Lactate clearance is delayed in patients surviving septic shock as compared with other causes for lactic acidosis.*

37. Kalter ES, Carlson RW, Thijs L, et al. Effects of methylprednisolone on hemodynamics, arteriovenous oxygen differences. Crit Care Med 1982;10:662–666. *Methylprednisolone administration to patients with bacteremia and*

shock resulted in increased cardiac output and oxygen delivery but was not associated with changes in oxygen extraction or changes in erythrocyte 2,3,-DPG or hemoglobin affinity for oxygen.

38. Weisel R, Vitto L, Dennis R, et al. Myocardial depression during sepsis. Am J Surg 1977;133:512–521. *A prospective evaluation of cardiac performance in patients with gram-negative and gram-positive bacterial sepsis.*

39. Carroll G, Snyder J. Hyperdynamic severe intravascular sepsis depends on fluid administration in cynomolgus monkey. Am J Physiol 1982;243:R131–R141. *A primate model of septic shock was presented and used to evaluate interactions between cardiac output and tissue oxygen consumption.*

40. Teule GJ, den Hollander W, Bronsveld W, et al. Noninvasive detection of blood volume redistribution in canine endotoxin shock. Circ Shock 1981;8:627–634. *Changes in circulating tagged red cell distribution were found after administration of endotoxin to dogs, suggesting physiologic shunting during endotoxemia-associated shock.*

41. Shoemaker W, Appel P, Knaus H, et al. Prospective trial of supranormal values of survivors as therapeutic goals in high-risk surgical patients. Chest 1988;94:1176–1186. *A two-pronged study that demonstrated reduced complications, reduced duration of overall and ICU hospitalization, reduced duration of mechanical ventilation, and reduced costs when pulmonary artery catheter directed protocols aimed at supernormalization of hemodynamics and oxygen delivery parameters were used.*

42. Tuchschmidt J, Fried J, Astiz M, et al. Elevation of cardiac output and oxygen delivery improves outcome in septic shock. Chest 1992;102:216–220. *Augmentation of cardiac index to 4.5 liters/minute/m² was shown in subsets of patients with septic shock to correlate with improved survival.*

43. Tuchschmidt J, Fried J, Swinney R, et al. Early hemodynamic correlates of survival in patients with septic shock. Crit Care Med 1989;17:719–723. *A retrospective review that highlighted significant differences in cardiac index, oxygen delivery and arterial lactate levels between survivors and nonsurvivors of septic shock.*

44. Bihari D, Smithies M, Gimson A. The effects of vasodilation with prostacycline oxygen delivery and uptake in critically ill patients. N Engl J Med 1987;317:397–402. *Prostacycline infusion was associated with increased oxygen delivery in both survivors and nonsurvivors. Survivors demonstrated reduced oxygen extraction, whereas nonsurvivors demonstrated increased oxygen extraction ratios supporting the presence of large tissue oxygen debts in nonsurvivors.*

45. Fry DE, Pearlsteen L, Fulton RL, et al. Multiple system organ failure: the role of uncontrolled infection. Arch Surg 1980;115:136–140. *A retrospective review of the incidence of multisystem organ failure and predisposing factors in 533 consecutive patients undergoing emergency surgery.*

46. Shoemaker W, Appel P, Knaus H. Tissue oxygen debt as a determinant of lethal and nonlethal postoperative organ failure. Crit Care Med 1988;16:1117–1120. *Tissue oxygen debt was calculated during and after high-risk surgical operations in 98 patients and was highest in the group of patients who subsequently developed multisystem organ failure and died.*

47. Moore FA, Feliciano DV, Andrassy J. Early enteral feeding, compared with parenteral, reduces postoperative septic complications. Ann Surg 1992;216:172–183. *A meta-analysis combining data from eight prospective randomized trials. High-risk surgical patients receiving early enteral nutrition had decreased septic morbidity when compared with patients getting early parenteral nutrition.*

48. Kudst KA, Croce MA, Fabian TC, et al. Enteral versus parenteral feeding. Effects on septic morbidity after blunt and penetrating abdominal trauma. Ann Surg 1992;215:503–513. *There was a significantly decreased incidence of septic morbidity in patients fed enterally, especially in the more severely injured ones.*

49. Chiabelli A, Enzi G, Casadei A. Very early nutrition supplementation in burned patients. Am J Clin Nutr 1990;51:1035–1039. *With very early nutritional support, nitrogen balance became positive in 8.8 ± 4.1 days.*

50. Moore EE, Jones TN. Benefits of immediate jejunostomy feeding after major abdominal trauma — a prospective, randomized study. J Trauma 1986;26:874–881. *Early nutrition seemed to decrease septic complications in critically-injured patients.*

51. Moore FA, Moore EE, Jones TN, et al. TEN versus TPN following major abdominal trauma-reduced septic morbidity. J Trauma 1989;24:916–923. *Early enteral feeding decreased septic complications.*

52. Graham TW, Zadrozny DB, Harrington T. The benefits of early jejunal hyperalimentation in the head-injured patient. Neurosurgery 1989;25:729–735. *Early jejunal hyperalimentation was tolerated despite a quiet abdomen, and infections and length of stay in the intensive care unit were reduced.*

53. Moore EE, Moore FA. Immediate enteral nutrition following multisystem trauma: a decade perspective. J Am Coll Nutr 1991;10:633–648. *A review with 99 references.*

54. Souba W, Austen W. Nutrition and metabolism in surgery. In: Greenfield LJ, Mulholland MW, Oldham KT et al, eds. Scientific principles and practices. Philadelphia: Lippincott-Raven, 1997:42–66.

55. Vander Hulst PR, VanKreel BK, von Meyenfeldt MF, et al. Glutamine and the preservation of gut integrity. Lancet 1993;341:1363. *Parenteral administration of glutamine in humans preserved baseline intestinal permeability and intestinal villus height.*

56. Alverdy J. The effect of nutrition on gastrointestinal barrier function. Semin Respir Infect 1994;9:248–255. *Excellent review of contemporary understanding of the interrelationship between nutrition and gastrointestinal barrier function.*

57. Beyers P, Jeejeebhoy KN.: Enteral and parenteral nutrition. In: Civetta JM, Taylor RW, Kirby RR, eds. Critical care, 3rd ed. Philadelphia: Lippincott-Raven, 1997:457–473.

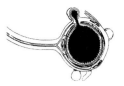

25 Recurrent Diverticulitis Following Resection

Bruce G. Wolff, MD
F. A. Frizelle, MD

KEY POINTS

- Recurrent diverticulitis following resection occurs in 1–10.4%
- Resection rarely necessary (0–3.1%)
- Proximal and distal resection margins of paramount importance
- Workup of recurrent symptoms should include both radiographic/endoscopic evaluation and review of pathologic sections
- Resection may be technically challenging (ureteral stents)
- Resection of previous anastomosis and all remaining sigmoid colon with anastomosis of descending colon to upper rectum mandatory

ILLUSTRATIVE CASE

A 56-year-old male underwent a resection for symptomatic left-sided diverticular disease at an outside hospital. The preoperative barium enema showed extensive diverticular disease (Fig. 25.1). He recovered uneventfully and did well for 18 months. During the next 6 months, the patient experienced three episodes of left lower quadrant pain and fever. He was hospitalized for one of these episodes.

Evaluation at the time of referral was undertaken. A computed tomography (CT) scan of the abdomen and pelvis showed no evidence of abscess. A barium enema was performed and showed a large diverticulum with a small amount of contrast extravasation distal to the anastomosis (Figs. 25.2 and 25.3). It seemed that there was sigmoid colon remaining proximal and distal to the anastomosis. Flexible sigmoidoscopy was performed to evaluate the rectal and colonic mucosa as well as to exclude a carcinoma. Endoscopically, the large diverticulum was noted at 16 cm or just below the anastomosis. In addition, multiple diverticula were visualized 10–15 cm proximal to the anastomosis, and scattered diverticula were seen in the descending colon. As a result of recurrent diverticulitis with remaining sigmoid colon proximal and distal to the anastomosis, reresection was recommended.

At operation, the patient was placed in a combined position and ureteral stents were placed. Mobilization of the colon and rectum was performed. Resection included the distal descending colon, remaining sigmoid colon, and upper rectum. The splenic flexure and rectum were mobilized. Intraoperative endoscopy was used to ensure that the previous anastomosis was included in the resected specimen. A hand-sewn end-to-end anastomosis was completed. The patient recovered uneventfully and is doing well postoperatively.

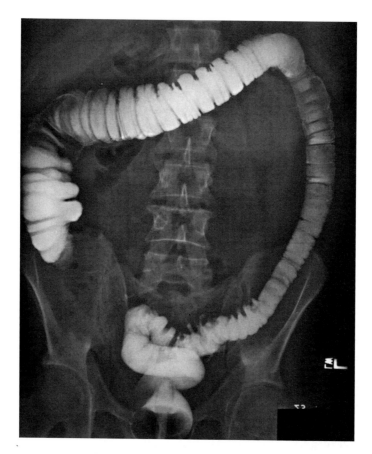

Figure 25.1. Barium enema before first resection for symptomatic diverticular disease. Extensive sigmoid diverticular disease is noted.

CASE COMMENTS

This case presentation highlights certain important features in the management of this vexing problem. Careful preoperative evaluation both by imaging studies and endoscopy are essential. In addition, review of previous pathology slides may provide previously unrecognized information. During the operation, placement of ureteral stents can facilitate identification of the ureters and minimize risk of operative injury. Resection must include the previous anastomosis as well as any remaining sigmoid colon, followed by a descending colon to proximal rectal anastomosis.

INTRODUCTION

Recurrent diverticulitis following resection is an uncommon occurrence. Large series of resections show an incidence between 1% and 10.4% (1–5). Because this is an uncommon problem, large series of recurrent diverticulitis following resection do not exist. The proximal and distal margins of resection are believed to be of particular importance in the pathophysiology of recurrent diverticulitis.

Conditions such as carcinoma or Crohn's disease should be entertained in the differential diagnosis of suspected diverticulitis following previous resection. Initial

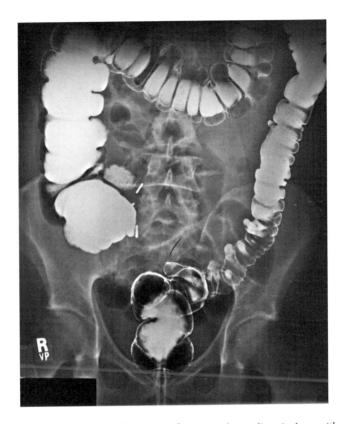

Figure 25.2. Barium enema before second resection showing a large diverticulum with a small amount of contrast extravasation.

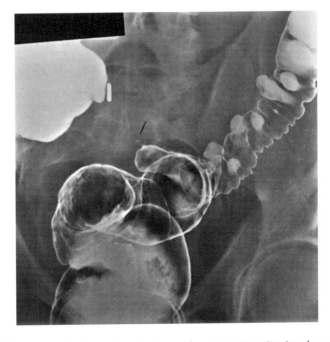

Figure 25.3. Magnified view of the large diverticulum with extravasation distal to the previous anastomosis. Unresected sigmoid colon is seen both proximal and distal to the anastomosis.

diagnostic and treatment measures are the same as those for previously unoperated cases of acute diverticulitis. Reoperation, when indicated, can be technically challenging.

EPIDEMIOLOGY

Considering the progressive nature of diverticulosis and the high incidence of recurrent attacks of diverticulitis in unoperated cases, it may seem surprising that recurrent episodes of diverticulitis are not reported more often following resection. Wychulis et al (6) reported on 136 patients followed for a mean of 9 years after resection and found that 7% suffered pain and 5% recurrent diverticulitis. Benn et al (1) reported on 501 patients undergoing resection and found recurrent symptoms in 52 patients (10.4%); reresection was required in 15 patients (3%). Table 25.1 lists large series of resections with the incidence of recurrent symptoms and reresections.

The time from the primary resection and the development of recurrent diverticulitis has ranged from 1 month to 11.6 years (1). Recurrent symptoms in the immediate postoperative period may be related to an anastomotic complication.

Recurrent symptoms in a patient previously believed to have adequate resection must be investigated thoroughly. Conditions such as Crohn's disease, irritable bowel syndrome, ulcerative colitis, carcinoma, ischemic colitis, and leiomyosarcoma should be considered in the differential diagnosis. *Prior pathology specimens should be rereviewed.* Meyers et al reported an association between diverticular disease and Crohn's disease, particularly in elderly patients (7). The combination is associated with a high incidence of complications such as inflammatory mass, abscess, or fistula due to transmural inflammation within diverticula (Chapter 5). Many patients who have had diverticular disease also may have irritable bowel syndrome, which can present with similar symptoms except for fever and leukocytosis. Colonoscopy with biopsy may aid in differentiating other conditions from recurrent diverticulitis (8).

PROXIMAL RESECTION MARGIN

For patients who are considered for sigmoid resection for diverticular disease, the descending colon is abnormal. The smooth muscle abnormality seen in patients with diverticular disease is not confined to the sigmoid colon but may extend to the descending colon and upper rectum (9). Evidence that the smooth muscle is abnormal is provided by manometric response to balloon distention throughout the descending colon and rectum before and after sigmoid resection (10). However, this does not seem to be clinically significant. Diverticula in the rectum are rare.

Table 25.1.   Incidence of Recurrent Symptoms and Resection Following Sigmoid Resection for Diverticulitis

Author, Year (Reference No.)	Cases	Recurrent Symptoms	Reresection
Bacon and Berkley, 1960 (2)	112	4 (3.6%)	1 (0.89%)
Leigh et al, 1962 (3)	65	3 (4.6%)	2 (3.1%)
Marsh et al, 1975 (4)	100	1 (1%)	0 (0%)
Benn et al, 1986 (1)	501	52 (10.4%)	15 (3%)
Farmakis et al, 1994 (5)	77	2 (2.6%)	0 (0%)

In patients with diverticular disease, intestinal compliance is also abnormal, with an abnormal pressure response to balloon distension compared with controls (11–13). In normal subjects, intraballoon pressures and volumes assume a linear relationship, but in patients with diverticular disease, pressures rapidly plateau to a constant value with increasing balloon volumes. Balloon expansion is associated with pain in patients with diverticular disease at a lower volume and pressure than in controls. The noncompliant colonic wall is due to muscle hypertrophy and intrinsic derangement of collagen fibers in diverticular disease (14). The disordered compliance is also associated with increased elastin between muscle cells in the taeniae coli (15). This lack of compliance and abnormal smooth muscular arrangement is found to extend into the descending colon and upper rectum in patients with diverticular disease.

There seems to be little clinical correlation with these interesting physiologic findings. A Mayo Clinic study reviewed 61 patients who had undergone elective sigmoid resections for diverticular disease and who had barium enema examination before operation, early postoperatively, and at least 5 years later (16). Progression of diverticulosis was noted in nine (14.7%) and was graded as minimal change. Seven patients (11.4%) had signs and symptoms of recurrent diverticulitis, but only three patients demonstrated progression of diverticulosis. It was concluded that resection of all diverticular-bearing colon after sigmoidectomy was not required.

There seems to be no association between either the number of diverticula remaining immediately after resection or appearing on follow-up barium enema and the risk of subsequent development of diverticulitis. On this basis, there seems to be little justification to extend the margin more proximal than the descending colon if all inflamed and indurated colon is resected with the entire sigmoid colon.

DISTAL RESECTION MARGIN

After completing the proximal dissection, the extent of distal resection must be addressed. It is well established that dissection should proceed distally until noninflamed bowel is encountered. It should be soft and pliable without diverticular changes.

The rectosigmoid junction should be identified at the sacral promontory. The approximate junction is confirmed grossly by the convergence of the teniae coli to form a continuous sheet of longitudinal muscle surrounding the rectum. Dissection in the presacral space with mobilization of the upper rectum is frequently required to facilitate resection and anastomosis.

Benn et al (1) reported the effect of the distal margin of resection in a study of 501 resections for diverticular disease. Recurrent diverticulitis developed in 12.5% of patients in whom the distal sigmoid colon had been used as the distal margin compared with 6.7% in whom the rectum was used ($P = .03$). Rates of anastomotic leak and reoperation were not statistically different. In another study, the incidence of recurrent diverticulitis when comparing descending colorectostomies with descending colosigmoidostomies (6.2% versus 22.7%) is even more pronounced. Figure 25.4 summarizes these results graphically (17).

The distal margin of resection should be free of inflammatory changes through soft, pliable rectum. *The use of the distal sigmoid colon for anastomosis is discouraged because it leads to an increased rate of recurrent diverticulitis following resection when compared with the rectum.*

MANAGEMENT

Initial management of the patient who is believed to have recurrent diverticulitis following resection includes resuscitation, if needed, followed by diagnostic studies and

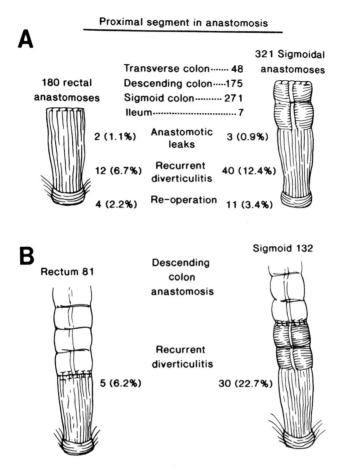

Figure 25.4. **A.,** Level of anastomosis and clinical outcome in 501 patients after sigmoid resection for diverticular disease. **B.,** Incidence of recurrent diverticulitis in the subset of 213 patients who had the entire proximal sigmoid colon removed with anastomosis of the descending colon to the rectum. (Reprinted with permission from Bell AM, Wolff BG. Progression and recurrence after resection for diverticulitis. Semin Colon Rectal Surg 1990;1:99–102.)

treatment. After resuscitation is initiated, diagnostic studies should be obtained, unless emergent operation is indicated based on the physical examination. A CT scan of the abdomen and pelvis is the most important study. Signs of inflammation or abscess formation may be seen, especially in the left lower quadrant and pelvis. A water-soluble contrast radiograph of the colon also may be useful in making an accurate diagnosis if the CT scan is equivocal or negative. Colonoscopy or flexible sigmoidoscopy may be useful, but usually not in the acute setting.

After a diagnosis of recurrent diverticulitis has been established, standard treatment is instituted. This includes bowel rest and intravenous antibiotics, followed by percutaneous drainage if an abscess is identified. An effort is made, if possible, to avoid operation in the acute setting because unprepared bowel and acute inflammation often necessitate a temporary colostomy.

The patients not responding to conservative treatment require surgery. The technique of reoperation is discussed below. The treatment of patients who respond to conservative treatment is more controversial. Options include expectant observation with reoperation if diverticulitis recurs versus elective resection. There are no large series to aid in making this decision. Many of these patients will continue to have problems and eventually will come to reresection. *We advocate an aggressive approach with reresection if there is a documented episode of diverticulitis following a previous resection in all patients medically fit for operation.*

Preoperative Preparation

Having made the decision that the patient would benefit by revisional surgery, arrangements can be made. It is preferable to undertake a reoperation as an elective case; however, this is not always possible. In a complicated case, there may be a need for preoperative drainage of an abscess or clarification of a fistula. The patient should be marked for a left iliac fossa colostomy and a right-sided ileostomy. In addition, we routinely place ureteral stents preoperatively unless the patient is in an immediate life-threatening condition. This maneuver is well tolerated and aids in identification of the ureters, particularly when involved in a mass or abscess cavity.

Position

The patient is placed in the synchronous (combined) position. This allows a third assistant to stand between the patient's legs to aid in retraction. The surgeon also may use this position when mobilizing the splenic flexure or placing an intraluminal stapling device.

Assessment

A long midline incision allows safe exposure and subsequent thorough peritoneal washout. Exploration is performed to assess the extent of diverticular disease and to exclude other conditions. Adhesiolysis is performed. The colon involved by inflammation may be adherent to the lateral pelvic side wall and/or loops of small intestine or may be looped into the pelvis in an inflammatory complex involving the bladder, uterus, or ovaries. An assessment of the extent of the disease is required, but preliminary mobilization usually is necessary to determine the anatomy.

Mobilization

Care must be taken to avoid contaminating the operative field. Contamination from a localized abscess can be minimized by preliminary needle or suction aspiration. *The overriding principle of mobilization of the colon affected by diverticulitis is to start proximally in noninflamed territory to facilitate recognition of the anatomy and to avoid injury to any vital structure* (18). The descending colon is mobilized using cautery along the white line of Toldt, and a plane is developed between the mesocolon and Gerota's fascia. The ureter, gonadal, and iliac vessels are identified.

The previously placed ureteral stent may be rolled under the finger, giving added confirmation of the anatomy. In initial resection with acute inflammation, there usually is an edematous reaction, and additional mobilization can be accomplished safely using blunt dissection. However, this may not be the case in operations for recurrent diverticular disease unless previously undissected planes are entered. With previous surgery or with prior episodes of inflammation and consequent fibrosis, *sharp dissection is usually required.* Attempts to bluntly dissect under these conditions result in seromuscular tears, multiple enterotomies, or damage to retroperitoneal structures.

The splenic flexure should be mobilized. With the patient in reversed Trendelenburg position and tilted to the right, the surgeon should stand between the patient's legs for this mobilization. Retraction of the left costal margin in this position gives excellent exposure. Access to the lesser sac is gained either by elevation of the greater omentum along the bloodless plane of Pauchet or through the gastrocolic omentum. This plane is developed from the midline to the left, to the limit of the lesser sac. Damage to the spleen is avoided by preliminary division of splenic capsule-omental adhesions. The lateral dissection is completed by spreading the fingers under the peritoneal reflection and dividing with cautery. At the limit of dissection from both aspects, the splenic flexure is defined and the remaining attachments are divided between clamps to avoid retraction and hemorrhage.

Extent of Resection

The intestine bearing obvious inflammation should be resected. The proximal margin will be determined by the previous surgery, site of inflammation, and blood supply of the descending colon. *The distal transverse colon is almost always used for anastomosis.* The distal margin should be the rectum at the level of the sacral promontory. However, *it is important to ensure that the previous anastomosis is resected.* The rectum will require mobilization to enable ease of anastomosis. Usually, only posterior dissection is required, but at times, more extensive mobilization may be necessary. All thickened inflamed tissue around the upper rectum should be resected, leaving only pliable, healthy rectum.

Anastomosis

In the presence of gross sepsis, a Hartmann procedure is the preferred operation. When a Hartmann procedure is undertaken, care should be taken with the stoma because there is a possibility that the stoma will be permanent. It may be possible, however, to undertake an anastomosis, either hand-sewn or stapled, depending on ease and personal preference. Closed-suction drains should be placed in the pelvis. A proximal defunctioning colostomy has been popular when there is concern about the anastomosis or sepsis in the operative field. However, because of technical difficulties in creating a temporary loop colostomy with the transverse colon anastomosed to the rectum, a loop ileostomy may be preferred. After the resection and anastomosis have been performed, a thorough lavage and peritoneal toilet are required.

CONCLUSIONS

Recurrent abdominal symptoms following resection for diverticular disease occur in 1–10.4% of cases. Not all of these patients have recurrent diverticulitis. Other conditions such as carcinoma, Crohn's disease, irritable bowel syndrome, chronic ulcerative colitis, and ischemic colitis must be considered in the differential diagnosis. A thorough investigation must be undertaken for patients with recurrent abdominal symptoms, including CT scan, contrast studies, and colonoscopy. Initial management is the same as for primary attacks of acute diverticulitis.

Recurrent diverticulitis may be the result of inadequate previous resection or progression of disease. Reresection for recurrent diverticulitis following previous resection is required in 0–3.1% of cases in collected series. Reresection may be technically demanding, although a permanent colostomy usually is not required. The best method of prevention is adequate initial resection.

EDITORIAL COMMENTS

Recurrent diverticulitis fortunately is an unusual occurrence following sigmoid resection. It usually complicates an inadequate initial resection. Retention of "high pressure" sigmoid colon, most commonly distal to the anastomosis, accounts for most cases. A thorough preoperative evaluation must be performed, including imaging procedures and endoscopy, as well as review of previous diagnostic studies and pathology slides to rule out Crohn's disease or other disease processes. The possibility of rectal diverticulitis is extremely low (19). Reresection must include the previous anastomosis as well as all retained sigmoid colon. Although reoperative colon surgery can be challenging, it can be accomplished quite safely with the use of ureteral stents (20,21) and meticulous attention to the numerous technical details discussed in the rest of this chapter.

REFERENCES

1. Benn PL, Wolff BC, Ilstrup DM. Level of anastomosis and recurrent colonic diverticulitis. Am J Surg 1986;151:269–271. *Removal of the entire distal sigmoid colon with anastomosis to the upper rectum is recommended.*
2. Bacon HE, Berkley JL. The surgical management of diverticulitis of the colon with particular reference to rehabilitation. Arch Surg 1960;80:646–649. *Ninety-seven percent of surviving patients not lost to follow-up are asymptomatic after colon resection for diverticulitis.*
3. Leigh JE, Judd ES, Waugh JM. Diverticulitis of the colon: recurrence after apparently adequate segmental resection. Am J Surg 1962;103:51–54. *Of 65 patients who had undergone resection of diverticulitis, 8% had symptoms of diverticulitis and only two patients required additional surgical therapy.*
4. Marsh J, Liem RKT, Byrd BG, et al. One hundred consecutive operations for diverticulitis of the colon. South Med J 1975;68:133–137. *The mortality was highest after staged procedures. One recurrence occurred during the 2-year follow-up period.*
5. Farmakis N, Judo RG, Keighley MRB. The 5-year natural history of complicated diverticular disease. Br J Surg 1994;81:733–735. *On audit of 300 patients with complicated diverticular disease, interval sigmoid colectomy was recommended to avoid later potential dangerous complications.*
6. Wychulis AR, Beahrs OH, Judd ES. Surgical management of diverticulitis of the colon. Surg Clin North Am 1967;47:961–969. *A review of 152 patients treated surgically: 4% required additional surgery for diverticulitis.*
7. Meyers MA, Alsono DR, Morson BC, et al. Pathogenesis of diverticulitis complicating granulomatous colitis. Gastroenterology 1978;74:24–31. *An evaluation of 21 patients with Crohn's disease who had diverticulosis and resection; 48% had sigmoid diverticulitis confirmed histologically.*
8. Corman MC. Colon and rectal surgery. 3rd ed. Philadelphia: JB Lippincott, 1993.
9. Watters DAK, Smith AN, Eastwood MA, et al. Mechanical properties of the colon: comparison of the features of the African and European colon in vitro. Gut 1985;26:384–392. *Compares mechanical features of the colon in different age groups.*
10. Parks TG. Rectal and colonic studies after resection of the sigmoid for diverticular disease. Gut 1970;11:121–125. *Increased basal rectal activity and response to stretch of colonic muscle is documented after sigmoid resection for diverticular disease.*
11. Parks TG, Connell AM. Motility studies in diverticular disease of the colon. Gut 1969;10:534–542. *The overall activity recorded with miniature balloons was similar under basal conditions and after eating when both normal colons and colons containing diverticula were studied.*
12. Parks TG. Prognosis in diverticular disease of the colon. Proc R Soc Med 1970;63:1262–1263. *A study of 455 patients followed from 1 to 16 years. One-third had surgery initially or subsequently. At the end of the follow-up period 5% had died as a result of diverticular disease.*
13. Eastwood MA, Smith AN. Natural history, clinical features and medical treatment of uncomplicated diverticular disease. In: Allan RN, Keightly MRB, Alexander-Williams J, et al. eds. Inflammatory bowel disease. Edinburgh: Churchill Livingstone, 1997:512–517.
14. Thomson JH, Busuttil A, Eastwood MA, et al. Submucosal collagen changes in the normal colon and in diverticular disease. Int J Colorectal Dis 1987;2:208–213. *Collagen fibers in the left colon become smaller and more tightly packed than those in the right colon with increasing age. The difference was accentuated in diverticular disease.*
15. Whiteway J, Morson BC. Elastosis in diverticular disease of the colon. Gut 1985;26:258–266. *By electron microscopy, the muscle cells were normal in patients with diverticular disease, whereas the elastin content of the taeniae coli was increased more than 200% compared with controls.*
16. Wolff BG, Ready RL, MacCarty RL, et al. Influence of sigmoid resection on progression of diverticular disease of the colon. Dis Colon Rectum 1984;27:645–647. *When surgical resection for diverticulitis is confined to the sigmoid colon, 14.7% of patients will develop new diverticula in the remaining colon and 11.4% will suffer from recurrent diverticulitis.*
17. Bell AM, Wolff BG. Progression and recurrence after resection for diverticulitis. Semin Colon Rectal Surg 1990;1:99–102. *A review covering the principles outlined in the present chapter.*
18. Fozard JBJ, Wolff BG. Mobilization and resection of perforated diverticular disease. Probl Gen Surg 1992;9:739–741. *A discussion of the technical aspects of colectomy in cases of perforated diverticular disease.*
19. Chiu TC, Bailey HR, Hernandez JA Jr. Diverticulitis of the midrectum. Dis Colon Rectum 1983;26:59–60. *Rectal pain caused by a ulcerated midrectal diverticulum was relieved by antibiotic therapy and evacuation of the 3- to 4-cm mass under anesthesia.*
20. Bothwell WN, Bleicher RJ, Dent TL. Prophylactic ureteral catheterization in colon surgery. A five-year review. Dis Colon Rectum 1994;37:330–334. *One-third of the operations described involved complications of diverticular disease.*
21. Kyzer S, Gordon PH. The prophylactic use of ureteral catheters during colorectal operations. Am Surg 1994;60:212–216. *The indication for colectomy in this series was diverticular disease in one-third of the cases. Three of the four ureteral injuries were in patients with diverticulitis.*

26 Complications of Duodenal Diverticula

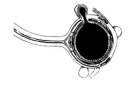

David L. Nahrwold, MD
Jay B. Prystowsky, MD

KEY POINTS
• Solitary, near ampulla
• Second commonest site of diverticula
• Acquired, usually extraluminal
• Most are asymptomatic
• Elderly patients, associated illnesses
• Confused with common disorders
• Complications: inflammation, local compression
• Bile-stained periduodenal phlegmon (perforation)

Duodenal diverticula were first described by Chomel in 1710 (1) and were first demonstrated radiographically in 1913 by Case (2). They are the subject of a number of interesting reports.

ILLUSTRATIVE CASES

Case 1

A 64-year-old man presented with a 2-day history of right flank and abdominal pain. He stated that the onset of pain was rapid and associated with nausea. The pain radiated to the groin. He denied urologic symptoms. His medical history included hypertension, and he had undergone an appendectomy and right inguinal herniorrhaphy in the remote past.

The patient's temperature was 101°F, and physical examination demonstrated right abdominal, flank, and costovertebral angle tenderness. The white blood count was elevated to 27,000 with 21% immature neutrophils.

Evaluation included renal ultrasound and intravenous pyelogram, which were both negative except for bilateral renal cysts. A hepato-iminodiacetic acid (HIDA) scan revealed prompt visualization of the gallbladder and ultrasonography did not show gallstones. An abdominal computed tomography (CT) scan showed "considerable thickening in the second and third portions of the duodenum. In addition, there was some gas posterior to the duodenum and stranding in the retroperitoneum suggesting a perforation of the duodenum."

In light of the findings on CT scan and persisting pain and fever, the patient was explored through an upper midline incision. The right colon and duodenum were mobilized. A diverticulum along the posteromedial aspect of the second portion of the duodenum was found. A gallstone was protruding through the wall of the diverticulum with a small amount of purulent material. The adjacent duodenal wall was significantly inflamed.

The gallstone was removed and the diverticulum excised. The duodenal rent was closed in two layers. An omental patch was placed over the closure as well. Cholecystectomy and intraoperative cholangiogram were performed. Chronic cholecystitis and cholelithiasis were present. The cholangiogram was normal. A closed suction drain was placed near the operative site.

The patient recovered uneventfully and was discharged from the hospital in good condition on the eighth postoperative day.

Case Comments

This patient not only had a perforated diverticulum but also had associated biliary disease. Perforation of a diverticulum by a gallstone is rare (see Table 26.1). Retroperitoneal gas was not present in plain films, and the important diagnostic role of the CT scan is emphasized. Although cholangiography was performed, it would have been useful to have cannulated the common bile duct before excising the diverticulum, unless the location of the papilla was obvious to the operating surgeon when the diverticulum was opened.

Case 2

An 86-year-old woman presented with constipation, weight loss, and anorexia. She denied abdominal pain. She had undergone cholecystectomy 37 years before admission but no other abdominal operations. Other than hypertension, she had no known medical illnesses. She was afebrile and physical examination was unremarkable.

Laboratory evaluations included an elevated alkaline phosphatase (662 units/liter; normal, 30–115), bilirubin (1.8 mg%; normal, 0–1.3), and serum glutamic-pyruvic transaminase (SGOT) (62 units/liter; normal, 0–30). Barium enema was normal. Abdominal CT scan revealed intrahepatic and extrahepatic bile duct dilatation and a "swelling at the ampulla." Endoscopic retrograde cholangiopancreatography (ERCP) was performed, and a duodenal diverticulum was observed. The common bile duct emptied into the duodenum adjacent to the diverticulum. The bile duct was cannulated and cholangiography demonstrated two common bile duct stones. Sphincterotomy and stone extraction were not performed because of the duodenal diverticulum.

Table 26.1.   Etiologies of Perforation of Duodenal Diverticula in 101 Cases

Cause	Percentage
Diverticulitis	57%
Unknown/unspecified	16%
Enterolithiasis	12%
Ulceration	9%
Increased intraluminal pressure	3%
Foreign body	2%
Trauma	1%
Gallstone	1%

From Duarte B, Nagy KK. Perforated duodenal diverticulum. Br J Surg 1992;79:877–881.

The patient underwent common bile duct exploration with stone extraction, completion T-tube cholangiography, and choledochoduodenostomy. Her postoperative course was uncomplicated, and she was discharged from the hospital on the ninth postoperative day.

Case Comments

Although this patient had a duodenal diverticulum and upper abdominal symptoms, the presumed immediate cause of her symptoms was choledocholithiasis. Therefore, treatment of the biliary disease itself was appropriate. The diverticulum may have played some role in the development of the stones, but considering her advanced age, it was unlikely that this would reoccur in her lifetime. Furthermore, excision of the diverticulum would add to the operative risk. Duodenal diverticula should not be excised simply because they are present. Another alternative would have been endoscopic papillotomy if the endoscopist believed the procedure could have been performed safely.

DISCUSSION

The duodenum ranks second behind the colon as the most common site for diverticula in the alimentary tract. Jones and Merendino performed a review of published series of duodenal diverticula through 1960 to determine its incidence (3). In nine autopsy studies (including more than 2,900 postmortem examinations), the incidence ranged from 2.2 to 22%. In 11 radiologic studies (including approximately 90,000 examinations), the incidence ranged from 0.016 to 5% (3). More recently, Chang-Chien prospectively evaluated 1,243 patients who underwent ERCP and observed an incidence of 12% (4). *Duodenal diverticula are rare in patients younger than 40 years of age, and their incidence increases with age. This may account in part for the high incidence of other gastrointestinal diseases characteristic of these patients.* The prevalence is also increasing in Americans. There seems to be no sex predilection.

Classification of duodenal diverticula includes the following:

1. congenital or acquired,
2. true or false,
3. intraluminal or extraluminal, and
4. primary or secondary (5).

True, congenital duodenal diverticula containing all bowel wall layers are rare. *Acquired* diverticula are either *primary* or *secondary,* and they herniate through gaps in the muscular layers. Secondary diverticula are unusual and occur proximal to a stenosis (usually in the first part of the duodenum) due to chronic duodenal ulcer disease. A primary diverticulum has no muscle in its wall and the stoma of the sac varies in diameter from several millimeters to 2–3 cm. They can be found in an intraluminal position but most are extraluminal.

Approximately 90% of duodenal diverticula are solitary and 80% of primary diverticula occur in the retroperitoneum on the medial portion of the second portion of the duodenum within 1.5 cm of the ampulla of Vater (hence termed "peri-Vaterian"), in proximity to or within the substance of the pancreas. Frequently, the common bile duct and pancreatic duct empty directly into the diverticulum. An explanation for the proximity of duodenal diverticula to the ampulla of Vater is that there is a congenital weakness in the duodenal wall at the point at which the common bile and pancreatic ducts enter the duodenal lumen. Also, penetrating blood vessels passing into the mucosa can provide mural weakness facilitating formation of diverticula, analogous to commonly held beliefs regarding the formation of colonic diverticula.

Most patients with duodenal diverticula are asymptomatic. The diagnosis is most commonly made as an incidental finding during upper gastrointestinal radiography or upper endoscopy (Fig. 26.1). ERCP also allows evaluation of the biliary tree and sphincterotomy if indicated. The risk of complications in these patients has not been well defined but seems to be quite low. Whitcomb found that only one of 1064 patients developed a serious complication that necessitated operation (6). Ascribing upper abdominal symptoms to an uncomplicated duodenal diverticulum should be viewed with caution. *Surgical therapy should be reserved for patients with complications or incapacitating symptoms.*

Two main groups of complications are generally recognized, especially those related to increased local compression or to inflammation. Elevated pressure in a poorly emptying diverticulum may produce jaundice, cholangitis, pancreatitis, and rarely, duodenal obstruction. Inflammation can lead to ulceration and subsequently hemorrhage, perforation, abscess formation, and rarely, the formation of internal fistulas (Table 26.2). ERCP is useful to demonstrate the ductal anatomy and to detect stones in the common bile duct or within the diverticulum.

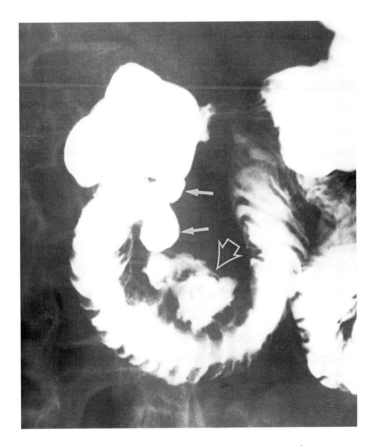

Figure 26.1. Upper gastrointestinal examination of a 56-year-old man with symptoms suggesting acute pancreatitis. Radiographic findings include an inflamed diverticulum (open arrow) with a deformed lumen, ulcerated mucosa, and adjacent thickened duodenal folds due to peridiverticular inflammation. There also is a lobulated periampullary diverticulum (closed arrows). (Reprinted with permission from Gore RM, Ghahremani GG, Kirsch MD, et al. Diverticulitis of the duodenum: clinical and radiological manifestations of seven cases. Am J Gastroenterol 1991;86:981–985.)

Table 26.2.   Serious Complications of Duodenal Diverticula

Torsion
Diverticulitis
  With perforation (8)
  Without perforation
Hemorrhage (11,45)
Duodenocolic fistula (27)
Carcinoma (30)
Duodenal obstruction (foreign body) (22)
Small bowel obstruction (enterolith) (28)
Obstructive jaundice (cholangitis) (14)
Pancreatitis (22)
Torsion
Diarrhea (blind loop syndrome)

Modified after Duarte B, Nagy KK. Perforated duodenal diverticulum. Br J Surg 1992;79:877–881; and Gore RM, Ghahremani GG,
Kirsch MD, et al. Diverticulitis of the duodenum: clinical and
radiological manifestations of seven cases. Am J Gastroenterol
1991;86:981–985.

Lotveit et al described an 85% incidence of biliary calculi in patients with duodenal diverticula (7). Also, in retrospective series, they report an association of duodenal diverticula and pancreatitis. They speculate that duodenal diverticula predispose patients to gallstone formation and gallstone pancreatitis, although it is possible that the two entities are unrelated and the apparent association is merely that diverticula are incidentally found during the evaluation of patients with gallbladder disease. The risk of bacteriocholia with typical intestinal bacteria seems to be increased in the presence of duodenal diverticula, perhaps increasing the risk of developing biliary disease. However, Chang-Chien found no increased incidence of biliary calculi in 153 patients with duodenal diverticula compared with 1090 patients without duodenal diverticula (4).

In general, *the preoperative diagnosis of an inflamed duodenal diverticulum is difficult* in that there is a paucity of specific findings on history and physical examination, plain radiographs, or abdominal sonography. Perforation tends to occur into the retroperitoneum, and only 13 of 100 patients with perforation had radiographic confirmation preoperatively in one review (8). Understandably, the clinician tends to suspect more common diseases such as cholecystitis, duodenal ulcer, or pancreatitis. Upper endoscopy may demonstrate inflammatory changes around the mucosal orifice of the diverticulum. *Abdominal CT scan probably is the most valuable radiographic examination*, because it may demonstrate a thickened diverticular wall, deformity of its lumen, ill-defined haziness of surrounding soft tissues due to dense strands in the adjacent fat, and even extraluminal air or an abscess cavity in cases of perforated diverticulitis (9). CT has improved diagnostic accuracy before surgery considerably (Figs. 26.2 and 26.3).

If a duodenal diverticulum is producing symptoms or complications related to biliary tract obstruction, then cholecystectomy, intraoperative cholangiography, and biliary bypass are indicated. The common bile duct usually is dilated sufficiently to permit choledochoduodenostomy or choledochoenterostomy. As duodenal diverticula are typically in proximity or actually empty into the ampulla of Vater, biliary bypass relieves the obstruction without a direct surgical approach to the diverticulum.

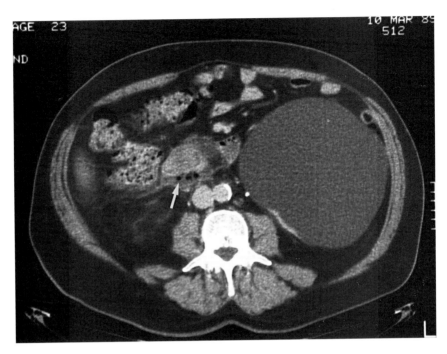

Figure 26.2. Abdominal CT scan of a 47-year-old woman presenting with right flank pain and fever. Radiographic findings include extraluminal air (arrow), thickened duodenal wall, and "stranding" of adjacent perirenal fat, suggestive of perforated duodenal diverticulitis. There is also a large left renal cyst. (Reprinted with permission from Gore RM, Ghahremani GG, Kirsch MD, et al. Diverticulitis of the duodenum: clinical and radiological manifestations of seven cases. Am J Gastroenterol 1991;86:981–985.)

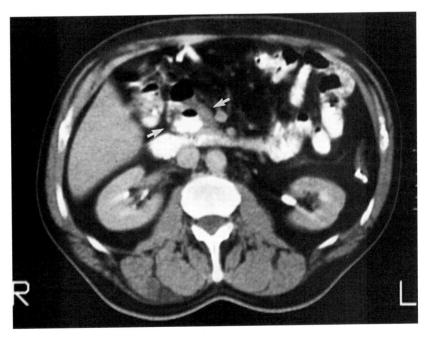

Figure 26.3. Abdominal CT scan demonstrating an abscess (arrows) secondary to a perforated duodenal diverticulum. (Reprinted with permission from Gore RM, Levine MS, Laufer I. Textbook of gastrointestinal radiology. Philadelphia: WB Saunders, 1994:311) [Ref. 51].

Table 26.3.   Management of Major Complications

Bile duct obstruction
  Biliary bypass
Perforation
  Minor inflammation
    Excision, closure if possible
    Cannulate common duct, ampulla
  Marked inflammation
    Patch, inversion
    Duodenojejunostomy
    Pyloric exclusion
    Duodenal diverticulization
Bleeding
  Endoscopy / arteriography
  Ligate bleeding point, excision

After Donald JW. Major complications of small bowel diverticula.
Ann Surg 1979;190:183–188.

If inflammatory complications of a duodenal diverticulum produce perforation or hemorrhage, then a direct surgical approach to the diverticulum may be needed (Table 26.3). Massive bleeding can occur from erosion of a pancreaticoduodenal artery but fortunately is rare (10). If not suspected, a perforated diverticulum may be missed entirely during the operation; there may be minimal evidence of periduodenal fat necrosis, edema, or bile staining (11). *However, the most reliable sign is, in fact, a bile-stained periduodenal phlegmon (12).* During the past 25 years, the postoperative mortality has been 13% when perforation has occurred; this figure probably reflects advanced patient age and a number of associated disorders (8).

Initially, a Kocher maneuver is performed to visualize the posterior and medial aspects of the second portion of the duodenum. Mobilization of the common bile duct and insertion of a soft catheter through a choledochotomy permits palpation of the distal common bile duct and aids in dissection of the diverticulum. The diverticulum can be opened to permit viewing of the papilla. The diverticulum is then excised and the duodenum is closed in two layers. If the catheter or a long-armed T tube are passed into the duodenum, the common duct can be protected from injury as the duodenum is closed. A closed-suction drain may be used if necessary. *Although diverticulectomy is preferred under favorable circumstances (13), it risks development of duodenal or biliary fistulas or pancreatitis (11), and it is best avoided if there is significant inflammation.*

Other procedures have been proposed because of the risk of diverticulectomy. Simple inversion of the diverticulum is possible, although duodenal obstruction or hemorrhage may result. Choledochojejunostomy or choledochoduodenostomy have been complicated by pancreatitis related to intermittent pancreatic duct obstruction by the diverticulum (14), but they are useful if the ampulla enters the dome of the diverticulum in the presence of common duct obstruction (12). A drawback of duodenal diverticulization is the complexity of the procedure. Critchlow et al have proposed duodenojejunostomy, because it accomplishes diversion of the food stream without the risk of excision of a peri-Vaterian diverticulum (14). Lateral duodenostomy with omental patch and gastrostomy have been successful in an 87-year-old patient (12).

SUMMARY

Duodenal diverticula are uncommon anatomic entities that rarely cause complications. The individual surgeon may encounter few or none over a career that require surgical intervention. They are most often solitary and located on the medial aspect of the second portion of the duodenum. Diagnosis typically is incidental to upper endoscopy or upper gastrointestinal radiography. Abdominal CT scan has been reported to be useful in diagnosis of inflamed duodenal diverticula. Complications are related to obstruction or inflammation and surgical therapy should be reserved for patients with complications or incapacitating symptoms. Obstructive complications usually can be treated by biliary bypass without directly approaching the diverticulum. If removal of the diverticulum is necessary, a Kocher maneuver, identification of the distal common bile duct, careful dissection and excision of the diverticulum, and closure of the duodenum in two layers are important components of a direct surgical approach.

EDITORIAL COMMENTS

Anatomically, most duodenal diverticula are acquired and false, situated in an extraluminal location. The occasional congenital diverticulum is either extraluminal or intraluminal. Of great importance, the neck of a duodenal diverticulum tends to lie in the second portion of the duodenum near the ampulla of Vater (Figs. 26.4 and 26.5). Rarely, a diverticulum is situated in the distal duodenum (Fig. 26.6).

Endoscopists encounter duodenal diverticula frequently when performing ERCP. By distorting the choledochoduodenal junction, the diverticulum sometimes complicates access to the papilla, but our colleagues believe that the risk of perforating a diverticulum during papillotomy is low. In a recent study from 16 institutions, periampullary diverticula were considered nonsignificant risk factors during endoscopic sphincterotomy (15).

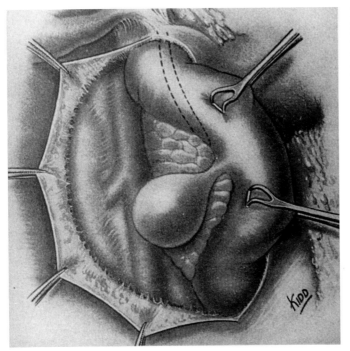

Figure 26.4. Use of the Kocher maneuver to expose a large diverticulum arising from the second portion of the duodenum. The close relation of the diverticulum to the common bile duct and the pancreas must be taken into account, especially in the presence of inflammation. (Reprinted with permission from Ellis H. Diverticula, volvulus, superior mesenteric artery, and foreign bodies. In: Schwartz SI, Ellis H, eds. Maingot's abdominal operations. 9th ed. Norwalk: CT: Appleton and Lange, 1989;1:575–597) [Ref. 50].

Figure 26.5. Operative view of a large diverticulum arising from the second portion of the duodenum. (Reprinted with permission from Chapuis P, Wallace JR. Duodenocolic fistula: an unusual complication of duodenal diverticulum. Dis Colon Rectum 1979;22:318–320.)

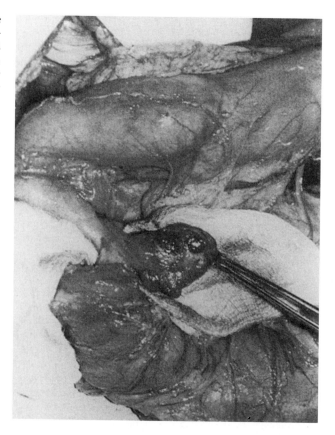

Figure 26.6. Rarely, a diverticulum arises from the distal duodenum. This can be approached through the mesocolon, with care to avoid the right colic artery and the pancreas. The duodenum can also be exposed by mobilization of the right colon, a Kocher maneuver, and division of the ligament of Treitz. (Reprinted with permission from Ellis H. Diverticula, volvulus, superior mesenteric artery, and foreign bodies. In: Schwartz SI, Ellis H, eds. Maingot's abdominal operations. 9th ed. Norwalk, CT: Appleton and Lange, 1989;1:575–597) [Ref. 50].

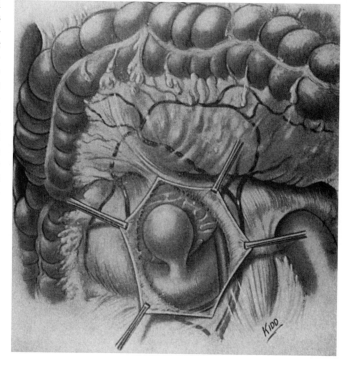

Surgeons, on the other hand, encounter duodenal diverticula as incidental findings when viewing upper gastrointestinal contrast studies. Because the diverticula tend to be asymptomatic or associated with vague symptoms (16,17), they rarely are operated on electively. Instead, operations (including laparoscopic ones) (18) that are as varied as they are complex (19) are performed under emergent or semiemergent conditions for complications such as bleeding, perforation, or intestinal obstruction (20–22). The mortality following perforation still is in the range of 13% (8).

Abdominal pain may be the commonest reason for operating on these patients (23). When the diverticulum is perforated, only one-third of plain films show retroperitoneal or paraduodenal air (8); the most common preoperative diagnoses are cholecystitis and perforated ulcer (8). Recurrent pancreatitis and choledocholithiasis are frequent associations (24), and the risk of bacteriocholia is increased (25). Rare complications have been recorded, including massive bleeding (23), duodenocolic fistula (26,27), enterolith ileus (28,29), and adenocarcinoma (30).

Several points should be made about operations for perforated diverticula. Approximately 100 cases had been reported by 1992 (8). First, it may be difficult to identify the pathology (especially laparoscopically), because the duodenum is situated in a retroperitoneal position (8,31). More than one diverticulum may be present (19). Signs of perforation to look for are retroperitoneal phlegmon, purulence or edema, or bile-staining near the duodenum. How is the diverticulum managed? Usually, it can be excised, but great care must be taken to avoid ampullary/ductal injury (Fig. 26.7). The duodenum can be opened and the ampulla can be palpated during the course of the excision, or the duct can be cannulated from a proximal site (Fig. 26.8) (32–34). If the ampulla is injured, the papilla can be reimplanted or duodenal advancement can be performed over stents

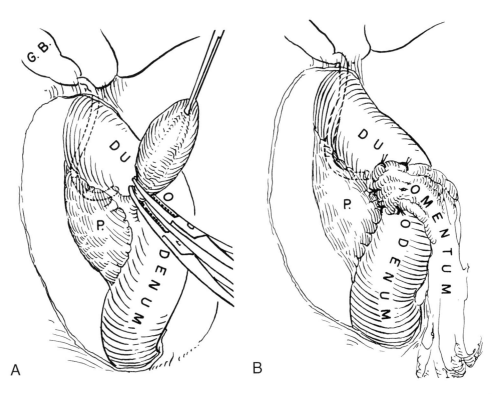

Figure 26.7. Simple excision of a small duodenal diverticulum with clear anatomical landmarks. After the diverticulum is grasped, clamped, and amputated **(A)**; the duodenum is closed in two layers and the suture line can be reinforced by omentum **(B)**. (Reprinted with permission from Welch CE. Surgery of the stomach and duodenum. 5th ed. Chicago: Yearbook Medical Publishers, 1973:106–109.)

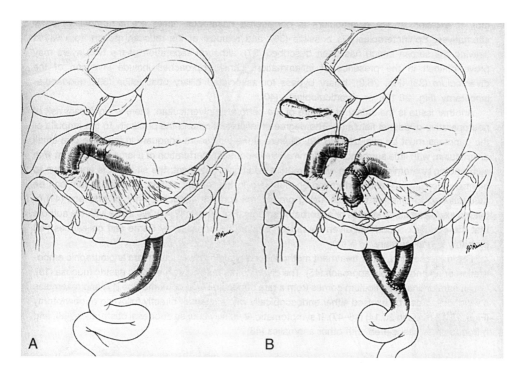

Figure 26.10. Use of duodenojejunostomy. The proposed sites of intestinal division are indicated in **(A)**. Completed duodenojejunostomy is shown in **(B)**. (Reprinted with permission from Critchlow JF, Shapiro MC, Silen W. Duodenojejunostomy for the pancreaticobiliary complications of duodenal diverticula. Ann Surg 1985;202:56–58.)

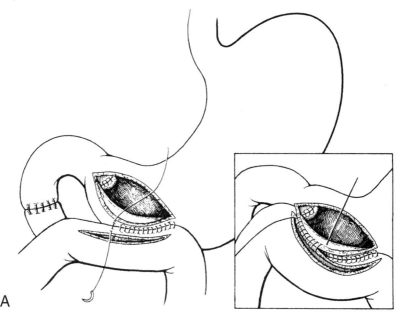

Figure 26.11. **A.,** Pyloric exclusion procedure as used in duodenal trauma. The pylorus has been occluded with nonabsorbable suture material through a gastrotomy. In **(B)**, the proximal duodenum is stapled distal to the pylorus and a gastrojejunostomy is performed. (Reprinted with permission from Asensio JA, Stewart BM, Demetriades D. Duodenum. In: Ivatury RR, Cayten CG. The textbook of penetrating trauma. Baltimore: Williams & Wilkins, 1996:623) [Ref. 52].

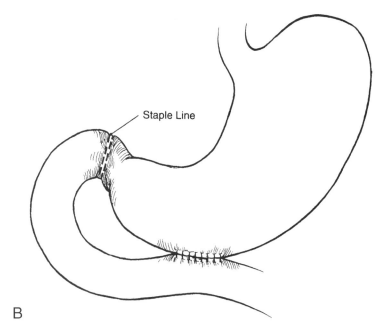

Figure 26.11. *(continued)*

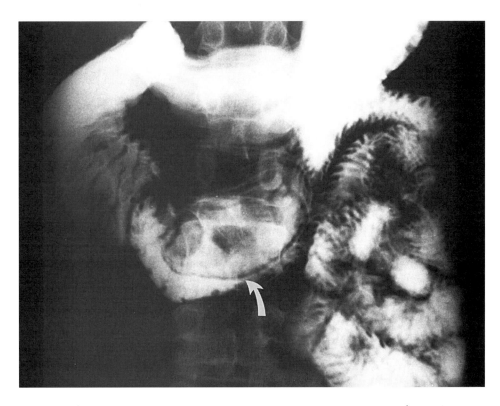

Figure 26.12. Characteristic radiologic appearance of an intraluminal diverticulum of the duodenum (arrow) with a radiolucent "halo."

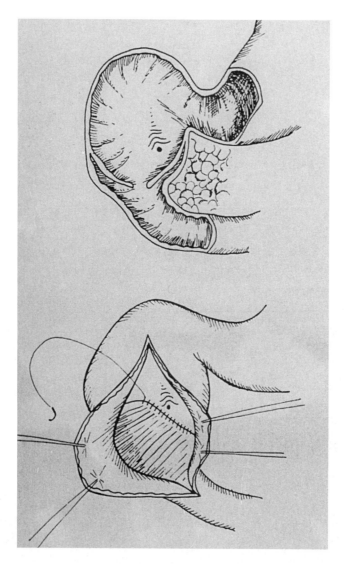

Figure 26.13.   Schematic appearance of an intraluminal diverticulum of the duodenum (top). These rare lesions bulge into the lumen of the duodenum and can cause mechanical obstruction. The saclike diverticulum was excised from the duodenal wall through a radial incision starting in the central ostium; a running suture overlies the resection line (bottom). The ampulla should be avoided carefully. (Reprinted with permission from Soreide JA, Seime S, Soreide O. Intraluminal duodenal diverticulum: case report and update of the literature 1975–1986. Am J Gastroenterol 1988;83:988–991.)

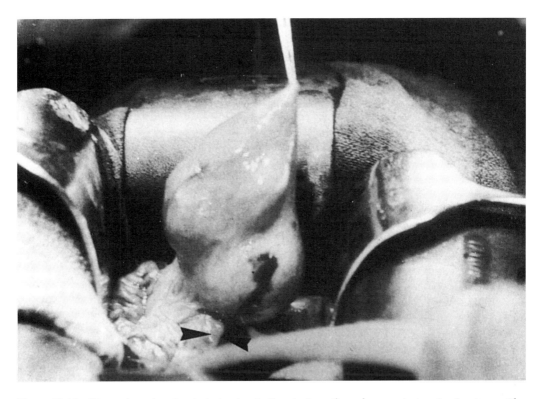

Figure 26.14. View of an intraluminal duodenal diverticulum through an anterior duodenotomy. The diverticulum was excised near its base, carefully avoiding the main papilla (arrowheads). (Reprinted with permission from Willemer S, Dombrowski H, Adler G, et al. Recurrent acute pancreatitis and intraluminal duodenal diverticulum. Pancreas 1992;7:257–261.)

REFERENCES

1. Chomel JBL. L'histoire de l'Academie Royal, Paris. L'Institut de France, Academie des Sciences Gauthiers-Villars, 1910:37.
2. Case JT. Roentgen observations on the duodenum with special reference to lesions beyond the first portion. Am J Roentgenol 1916;3:314–326. *A detailed description of the radiologic anatomy of the duodenum and numerous variations such as duodenal diverticula or dilatation of the ampulla of Vater.*
3. Jones TW, Merendino KA. The perplexing duodenal diverticulum. Surgery 1960;48:1068–1084. *A comprehensive literature review with 87 references.*
4. Chang-Chien CS. Do juxtapapillary diverticula of the duodenum interfere with cannulation at endoscopic retrograde cholangiopancreatography? Gastrointest Endosc 1987;33:298–300. *There was no increased failure rate of cannulation in patients with juxtapapillary diverticula.*
5. Ellis H. Diverticula, volvulus, and ileus. In: Ellis H, Schwartz S, eds. Maingot's abdominal operations. 8th ed. Norwalk, CT: Appleton-Century-Crofts, 1985:643–665.
6. Whitcomb JG. Duodenal diverticulum. A clinical evaluation. Arch Surg 1964;88:275–278. *A study of 1064 patients with duodenal diverticula. Six came to abdominal operation.*
7. Lotveit T, Skar V, Osnes M. Juxtapapillary duodenal diverticula. Endoscopy 1988;20:175–178. *A comprehensive review of juxtapapillary duodenal diverticula. The authors suggest that glucuronidase produced by bacteria may account for the increased incidence of gallstones in these patients.*
8. Duarte B, Nagy KK. Perforated duodenal diverticulum. Br J Surg 1992;79:877–881. *A comprehensive review of the literature since 1969. Forty-one percent of patients had complications following operation, including duodenal fistulas in 20%.*
9. Gore RM, Ghahremani GG, Kirsch MD, et al. Diverticulitis of the duodenum: clinical and radiological manifestations of seven cases. Am J Gastroenterol 1991;86:981–985. *The abdominal CT scan was an essential diagnostic aid in all patients in this series. All patients recovered and five patients were operated on.*
10. Ettman IK, Kongtawng T. Massive gastrointestinal bleeding and perforation of a duodenal diverticulum with co-existing pancreatitis. South Med J 1977;70:761–763. *A fistulous tract from the perforated diverticulum communicated with the pancreas. The bleeding was created by erosion into the pancreaticoduodenal artery.*

11. Neill SA, Thompson NW. The complications of duodenal diverticula and their management. Surg Gynecol Obstet 1965;120:1251–1258. *A detailed discussion of four patients with different major complications attributable to duodenal diverticula.*

12. Scudamore CH, Harrison RC, White TT. Management of duodenal diverticula. Can J Surg 1982;25:311–314. *Fifteen of 104 patients with duodenal diverticula underwent surgery because of significant complications; there were two deaths. Elaborates on the role of ERCP in these patients.*

13. Manny J, Muga M, Eyal Z. The continuing clinical enigma of duodenal diverticulum. Am J Surg 1981;142:596–600. *Forty of 71 patients with duodenal diverticula had serious symptoms and 19 patients were operated on. The best results followed diverticulectomy or bypass procedures.*

14. Critchlow JF, Shapiro MC, Silen W. Duodenojejunostomy for the pancreaticobiliary complications of duodenal diverticula. Ann Surg 1985;202:56–58. *Advocates this procedure based on good results in three patients.*

15. Freeman ML, Nelson DB, Sherman S, et al. Complications of endoscopic biliary sphincterotomy. N Engl J Med 1996;335:909–918. *The 30-day complication rate in 2347 patients in this multi-institutional study was 9.8%. The rate of complications was related to endoscopic technique and to the indication for the procedure rather than to the age or general medical condition of the patients.*

16. Pearce VR. The importance of duodenal diverticula in the elderly. Postgrad Med J 1980;56:777–780. *This study of 39 patients gave evidence that duodenal diverticula are rarely responsible for nutritional deficiencies in the elderly.*

17. Afridi SA, Fichtenbaum CJ, Staubin H. Review of duodenal diverticula. Am J Gastroenterol 1991;86:935–938. *The treatment of each patient must be individualized; coexistent anomalies should be sought before embarking on surgical or endoscopic therapy. Includes 38 references.*

18. Callery MP, Aliperti G, Soper NJ. Laparoscopic duodenal diverticulectomy following hemorrhage. Surg Laparosc Endosc 1994;4:134–138. *The base of the diverticulum was transected with the Endo-GIA stapler.*

19. Cattell RB, Mudge TJ. The surgical significance of duodenal diverticula. N Engl J Med 1952;246:317–324. *A detailed description of this entity, including case reports. The difficulty in selecting surgical cases and the reasons for mortality are described. They recommend removal of less than 5% of diverticula that are identified.*

20. Donald JW. Major complications of small bowel diverticula. Ann Surg 1979;190:183–188. *Includes six detailed case reports and a group of treatment recommendations (Table 3).*

21. Jang LC, Kim SW, Park YH. Symptomatic duodenal diverticulum. World J Surg 1995;19:729–733. *A study of 18 patients with symptomatic diverticula; diverticulectomy is recommended only for significant complications.*

22. Psathakis D, Utschakowski A, Muller G, et al. Clinical significance of duodenal diverticula. J Am Coll Surg 1994;178:257–260. *Four of 50 patients with duodenal diverticula were treated surgically; only six patients had symptoms clearly related to the diverticula. Provides a good discussion of surgical options.*

23. Balkissoon J, Balkissoon B, Lefall LD Jr, et al. Massive upper gastrointestinal bleeding in a patient with a duodenal diverticulum: a case report and review of the literature. J Natl Med Assoc 1992;84:365–367. *Diverticulectomy was done in a patient with persistent upper GI bleeding; the specimen contained dilated blood vessels suggestive of angiodysplasia.*

24. Pinotii HW, Tacla M, Pontes JF, et al. Surgical procedures upon juxta-ampullar duodenal diverticula. Surg Gynecol Obstet 1972;135:11–16. *In this report from Brazil, 18 patients with duodenal diverticula, recurrent pancreatitis and jaundice were treated surgically. A technique of diverticulectomy using eversion of the diverticulum is described. Four of five patients not having diverticulectomy needed reoperation because of new biliary/pancreatic symptoms.*

25. Eggert A, Teichmann W, Wittmann DH. The pathologic implication of duodenal diverticula. Surg Gynecol Obstet 1982;154:62–64. *In a prospective study, patients with duodenal diverticula had a higher incidence of bacteriocholia with intestinal bacteria than others without duodenal diverticula. The rate of bacteriocholia decreased with increasing distance between the papilla and the diverticulum.*

26. Chapuis P, Wallace JR. Duodenocolic fistula: an unusual complication of duodenal diverticulum. Dis Colon Rectum 1979;22:318–320. *Describes two patients with this rare complication.*

27. Yasui K, Tsukagauchi I, Ohara S, et al. Benign duodenocolic fistula due to duodenal diverticulum. Report of two cases. Radiology 1979;130:67–70. *The authors found eight other cases in the literature caused by duodenal diverticula.*

28. Roshkow J, Farman J, Chen CK. Duodenal diverticular enterolith: a rare cause of small bowel obstruction. J Clin Gastroenterol 1988;10:88–91. *This enterolith developed in a patient taking large amounts of Kaopectate.*

29. Yang HK, Fondacaro PF. Enterolith ileus: a rare complication of duodenal diverticula. Am J Gastroenterol 1992;87:1846–1848. *A case report of the 30th example of this clinical entity.*

30. Dennison AR, Watkins RM, Sarr MJ, et al. Adenocarcinoma complicating a duodenal diverticulum. J R Coll Surg Edinb 1987;32:44–46. *According to the authors, this is the third report of this entity.*

31. Desmond AM, Heald RJ. Perforated diverticulum of the duodenum and its treatment. Br J Surg 1968;55:396–397. *The value of gastroenterostomy is emphasized because of the frequency of leakage postoperatively.*

32. Iida F. Transduodenal diverticulectomy. World J Surg 1979;3:103–106. *Transduodenal diverticulectomy was performed on 12 patients without complications.*

33. Scarpa FJ, Sherard S, Scott HW Jr. Surgical management of perforated duodenal diverticula. Am J Surg 1974;128:105–108. *The authors describe surgical techniques used in treating perforated duodenal diverticula.*

34. McSherry CK, Glenn F. Biliary tract obstruction and duodenal diverticula. Surg Gynecol Obstet 1970;130:829–836. *A well-illustrated description of safe excision of duodenal diverticula, using cannulation of the common bile duct as a precaution.*

35. Florence MC, Hart JM, White TT. Ampullary disconnection during the course of biliary and duodenal surgery.

Am J Surg 1981;142:100–105. *Twelve patients are described who had injury or disconnection of the ampulla of Vater. Two had duodenal diverticula, and one had an accidental injury. The authors describe methods of dealing with the complication.*

36. Kaminsky HH, Thompson WR, Davis B. Extended sphincteroplasty for juxtapapillary duodenal diverticulum. Surg Gynecol Obstet 1986;162:280–281. *The simplicity of this technique may allow more aggressive treatment when excision of the diverticulum is dangerous. The possibility of endoscopic treatment is also mentioned.*

37. Slater RB. Duodenal diverticulum treated by excision of mucosal pouch only. Br J Surg 1971;58:198–200. *Describes a technique of removing the mucosal pouch alone, leaving the serosa intact, via a duodenotomy.*

38. Welch CE. Surgery of the stomach and duodenum. 5th ed. Chicago: Yearbook Medical Publishers, 1973:106–109.

39. Gudjonsson H, Gamelli RL, Kaye MD. Symptomatic biliary obstruction associated with juxtapapillary duodenal diverticulum. Dig Dis Sci 1988;33:114–121. *Choledochojejunostomy without resection of the duodenal diverticulum led to relief of symptoms of biliary obstruction.*

40. Trondsen E, Rosseland AR, Bakka AO. Surgical management of duodenal diverticula. Acta Chir Scand 1990;156:383–386. *Diverticuloplasty was performed on five patients, making the diverticular neck so wide that the diverticulum appeared only as a widening of the duodenum. The long-term results were excellent in all cases.*

41. Beech RR, Friesen DL, Shield CF III. Perforated duodenal diverticulum: treatment by tube duodenostomy. Curr Surg 1985;42:462–465. *Tube duodenostomy controlled sepsis caused by a duodenal diverticulum that had perforated 72 hours earlier.*

42. Vaughan GD III, Frazier OH, Graham DY, et al. The use of pyloric exclusion in the management of severe duodenal injuries. Am J Surg 1977;134:785–790. *The authors used temporary pyloric exclusion and gastrojejunostomy to produce "diverticulization" of the duodenum in 75 patients with duodenal trauma. The rate of fistula formation was 5%.*

43. Graham JM, Mattox KL, Vaughan D III, et al. Combined pancreatoduodenal injuries. J Trauma 1979;19:340–346. *Discusses a number of techniques, including temporary pyloric exclusion.*

44. Berne CJ, Donovan AJ, White EJ, et al. Duodenal "diverticulization" for duodenal and pancreatic injury. Am J Surg 1974;127:503–507. *Describes the experience with this operation in 34 patients.*

45. Sim EK, Goh PM, Isaac JR, et al. Endoscopic management of a bleeding duodenal diverticulum. Gastrointest Endosc 1991;37:634. *The side-viewing endoscope visualized the bleeding, which was stabilized before definitive excision.*

46. Abdel-Hafiz AA, Birkett DH, Ahmed MS. Congenital duodenal diverticula: a report of three cases and a review of the literature. Surgery 1988;104:74–77. *A comprehensive review of this entity, including three new cases.*

47. Adams DB. Management of the intraluminal duodenal diverticulum: endoscopy or duodenotomy? Am J Surg 1986;151:524–526. *Report of a single case. The technical aspects are discussed. The intraluminal diverticulum can be excised endoscopically or surgically.*

48. Soreide JA, Seime S, Soreide O. Intraluminal duodenal diverticulum: case report and update of the literature 1975–1986. Am J Gastroenterol 1988;83:988–991. *Surgery is effective treatment for symptomatic patients, although endoscopic incision or excision may also play a role.*

49. Willemer S, Dombrowski H, Adler G, et al. Recurrent acute pancreatitis and intraluminal duodenal diverticulum. Pancreas 1992;7:257–261. *Resection of the diverticulum in this one case led to disappearance of symptoms.*

50. Ellis H. Diverticula, volvulus, superior mesenteric artery, and foreign bodies. In: Schwartz SI, Ellis H, eds. Maingot's abdominal operations. 9th ed. Norwalk, CT: Appleton and Lange, 1989;1:575–597.

51. Gore RM, Levine MS, Laufer I. Textbook of gastrointestinal radiology. Philadelphia: WB Saunders, 1994:311.

52. Asensio JA, Stewart BM, Demetriades D. Duodenum. In: Ivatury RR, Cayten CG. The textbook of penetrating trauma. Baltimore: Williams & Wilkins, 1996:623.

27 Meckel's Diverticulum

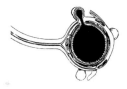

Lawrence Rusin, MD

KEY POINTS

- 2% of population
- 2 feet from ileocecal valve
- Bleeding: age 1 month to 15 years
- Obstruction/inflammation: age older than 15 years
- Diagnosis unexpected preoperatively
- ^{99m}TC-pertechnetate scan for bleeding
- Incidental diverticulectomy in uncomplicated operation

The most common congenital anomaly of the gastrointestinal tract is a Meckel's diverticulum. Histologically, a Meckel's diverticulum is a true diverticulum of the bowel and is composed of all layers of the intestinal wall. In 1598, Hildanus (1) first described the abnormality now known as a Meckel's diverticulum as a pulsion diverticulum of the ileum. Meckel (2,3), a German anatomist, wrote a series of papers from 1809 to 1812 that included anatomic and embryologic studies describing Meckel's diverticulum as a remnant of the embryologic omphalomesenteric duct (4). In 1904, Salzer (5) found ectopic gastric mucosa in a Meckel's diverticulum. Shortly thereafter, in 1907, Deetz (6) identified ulcerations associated with ectopic mucosa.

ILLUSTRATIVE CASE

A 43-year-old male was seen in the emergency department at 11:00 pm complaining of midepigastric bloating and pain radiating to the right upper quadrant. He denied any history of medication use, allergies, or medical illnesses. Physical examination revealed some vague right midabdominal tenderness.

Initial laboratory evaluation included normal complete blood cell count, urinalysis, and liver function studies. However, the serum amylase was slightly elevated. Plain films of the abdomen were normal. A diagnosis of probable biliary colic was made, and he was admitted overnight for observation. Early the next morning, he complained of increasing abdominal pain that had localized in the right lower quadrant. Ultrasonography revealed a normal gallbladder and biliary tree, but fluid was evident in the lower abdomen. A diagnosis of acute appendicitis was made, and he was prepared for operation.

At laparotomy, a normal appendix was found, but cloudy pelvic fluid was identified. The terminal ileum was inspected, and an inflamed Meckel's diverticulum was found adherent to the small bowel mesentery. A limited ileal resection was performed to include the diverticulum.

Postoperatively, the patient had a benign course, and he was discharged on the seventh postoperative day. The final pathologic diagnosis was Meckel's diverticulum with evidence of heterotopic gastric mucosa and peptic ulceration (Fig. 27.1).

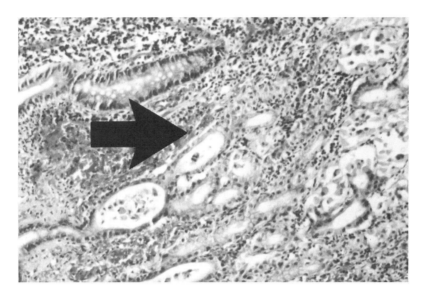

Figure 27.1. The arrow points to gastric mucosa in the Meckel's diverticulum removed from the patient described in the case report.

CASE COMMENTS

The case demonstrates many of the salient points about Meckel's diverticula. Although most symptomatic patients are children, adults may be affected. In adults, inflammation is a common presentation, and the correct preoperative diagnosis rarely is made. Male patients are more likely to have symptomatic disease, and in symptomatic patients, ectopic gastric mucosa is often found.

EMBRYOLOGY

To understand the myriad presentations of a Meckel's diverticulum, it is important to know the embryologic origins of the vitelline or omphalomesenteric duct and its eventual disappearance. The failure of all or part of the vitelline duct to involute gives rise to various types of anomalies, and their frequency is demonstrated in Figure 27.2. Although the term Meckel's diverticulum is entrenched in the literature, a more descriptive term would be anomalies of the vitelline or omphalomesenteric duct.

During the first weeks of embryonic development, the fetus is nourished by the yolk sac. The ventral surface of the entodermal yolk sac forms the dorsal surface of the primordial gut. Between the fourth and fifth week of gestation, the area of communication between the yolk sac and the primordial gut is progressively narrowed, forming the vitelline duct. This narrowing occurs because of the rapid growth of the intestine. As the duct is pinched, it also becomes elongated. By the eighth or ninth week of gestation, the vitelline duct disappears. Biopsies of the duct lining just before this obliteration occurs reveal evidence of primordial crypt formation. In some of the cells, obvious mucous granules are identified. It is from these primordial cells that the heterotopic mucosa found in a Meckel's diverticulum arises (7).

The blood supply to the primordial duct is by paired vitelline arteries, which parallel the omphalomesenteric duct. Normally, these degenerate as the diverticulum degenerates.

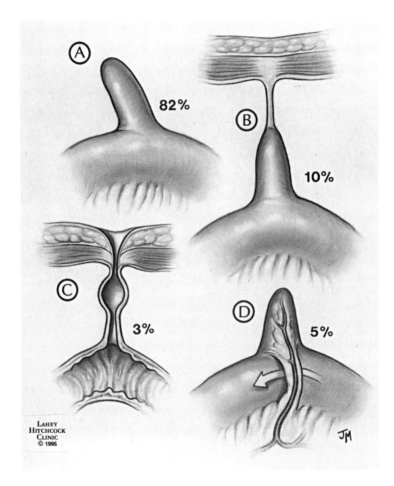

Figure 27.2. **A.**, Classic Meckel's diverticulum. **B.**, Meckel's diverticulum with fibrous band to the umbilicus. **C.**, Umbilical fistula and/or central cyst. **D.**, Mesodiverticular band from persistent left vitelline artery. The percentages reflect the frequency of occurrence. (Reproduced by permission of Lahey Hitchcock Clinic.)

The right vitelline artery persists as part of the superior mesenteric artery, and the left artery normally involutes. Occasionally, the left vitelline artery does not involute and forms a fibrous mesodiverticular band that can cause obstruction.

Simms and Corkery (8) examined the association of Meckel's diverticulum with other congenital anomalies. The incidence of Meckel's diverticulum is increased in children born with major malformations of the umbilicus, alimentary tract, nervous system, and cardiovascular system, in descending order of frequency. Of children with esophageal or anorectal atresia, 10% will have an associated Meckel's diverticulum.

INCIDENCE

The incidence of Meckel's diverticulum in the general population varies from 0.3% to 4.5%, depending on whether the reported series is based on autopsy or clinical findings. *The generally accepted incidence is 2%*, and this percentage is used statistically throughout the medical literature (9,10).

Appendectomy is performed more frequently than procedures involving a Meckel's diverticulum, with a ratio of 55:1 (11). A consecutive series (9) of 1954 appendectomies revealed a 3.2% incidence of Meckel's diverticula. Male patients predominate in symptomatic cases, ranging from 2:1 to 5:1. When all cases of Meckel's diverticula (symptomatic and asymptomatic) are considered, the ratio is less striking. The reason for the male predominance in symptomatic patients is unknown (4,9,11).

Most complications of Meckel's diverticulum occur in patients younger than 25 years of age. In symptomatic ones, 70–80% of diverticula are removed before 40 years of age, but symptomatic disease can and does occur well into the seventh decade of life (4,11).

ANATOMY AND HISTOLOGY

Although so-called Meckel's diverticulum has been described in the jejunum, *98% of all Meckel's diverticula are within 100 cm of the ileocecal valve and are located on the antimesenteric border of the ileum.* When symptomatic Meckel's diverticula are considered, the average distance from the ileocecal valve to the diverticulum is 50–60 cm. Case reports have described Meckel's diverticula measuring 66–100 cm in length, but the average length is 4–5 cm, with a range of 1–10 cm (4,9,10). Diverticula less than 2 cm long are less likely to be symptomatic. The average width is 0.5–4 cm, and *attempts to correlate size with symptoms have been inconsistent.* In general, however, the narrower the diverticulum, the more likely it is to be symptomatic, because 80% of symptomatic patients having a neck 2 cm wide or smaller. Conversely, 80% of the asymptomatic patients also have a diverticulum with a diverticular neck width of 2 cm or less (4).

Heterotopic tissue is noted more commonly in symptomatic than asymptomatic patients and in virtually all infants and children with gastrointestinal bleeding. Of all heterotopic tissue, 85% will be gastric in nature. Pancreatic tissue is the second most common type and often is associated with intussusception (4,9,11) (Tables 27.1 and 27.2). The treatise on Meckel's

Table 27.1.   Anatomic and Histologic Findings in Meckel's Diverticulum

Location	Within 100 cm of ileocecal valve (usually 50–60 cm)
Size	Length: 2–5 cm (<2 cm for asymptomatic patients; >2 cm for symptomatic patients)
Frequency of heterotopic tissue	Symptomatic patients: 34–60% Asymptomatic patients: 9–26%

Table 27.2.   Relative Incidence of Ectopic Tissue in Meckel's Diverticula

Tissue	Percent
Stomach	85
Pancreas	5
Stomach and pancreas	3
Colon	3
Duodenum/jejunum	3
Biliary	1

Adapted with permission from William RS. Management of Meckel's diverticulum. Br J Surg 1981;68:477.

diverticulum by Söderlund (12) included serial microscopic evaluation of 66 resected Meckel's diverticula. In patients with a symptomatic diverticulum associated with heterotopic tissue, the diameter of the heterotopic tissue was 1 cm² or larger. There is no reliable way to detect heterotopic tissue by palpation intraoperatively (9).

COMPLICATIONS

The exact percentage of patients in whom complications develop has been debated. A report (10) based on hospital admissions for clinical disease suggested that complications would develop in 15–25% of patients. Population-based studies suggest the risk to be 4.2–6.4% (13,14). The four broad categories of complications can be described as hemorrhage, diverticulitis, obstruction, and miscellaneous (Table 27.3). *These complications are age-specific, as noted in Table 27.4. Hemorrhage usually occurs in infancy* (after 1 month of age); the peak incidence is at 5 years of age; bleeding is a medical curiosity after 30 years of age. Hemorrhage is rarely life-threatening but often requires transfusion. This self-limited bleeding gives the physician time to perform an adequate workup and to establish a preoperative diagnosis of Meckel's diverticulum.

Intestinal obstruction is the second most common presentation of a Meckel's diverticulum (see Table 27.3) and can result from bands, either congenital or inflammatory, intussusception, and entrapment of a hernia. In the first few months of life, obstruction related to a fibrous

Table 27.3.   Complications of Meckel's Diverticulum Combined Series of 1806 Cases

Complication	No. of Cases	Percentage
Hemorrhage	599	31%
Inflammation	440	25%
Band obstruction	275	16%
Intussusception	201	11%
Hernial entrapment	200	11%
Umbilical sinus or fistula	57	4%
Tumor	34	2%
Total:	1806	100%

Adapted with permission from William RS. Management of Meckel's diverticulum. Br J Surg 1981;68:477.

Table 27.4.   Age-Specific Complications

Age	Complication
<1 month	Obstruction; umbilical drainage
1 month to 15 years	Hemorrhage—peak at 5 years of age
>15 years	Obstruction and inflammation

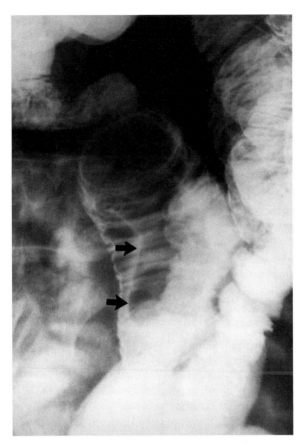

Figure 27.3. An intussuscepting Meckel's diverticulum is seen on an enteroclysis study. Note the coiled spring appearance of the small intestine and the outlined invaginated Meckel's diverticulum.

band from the Meckel's diverticulum to the abdominal wall is the most common presentation. This obstruction is caused by volvulus around the band. Less commonly, a diverticular band from the persistent left vitelline artery can cause obstruction by forming a trap for internal herniation or compression of the ileum. Intussusception occurs because of thickening of the Meckel's diverticulum resulting from low-grade diverticulitis or from pancreatic heterotopic tissue (Fig. 27.3). Tumor masses have also been associated with intussusception.

Diverticulitis with inflammation is a common presentation in adolescents and adults, almost equaling the frequency of obstruction. Appendicitis is most often the preoperative diagnosis in this group of patients (see Illustrative Case); the correct diagnosis rarely is made preoperatively. Often, the pain is more prominent in the midline than in the right lower quadrant. Diverticulitis is caused by foreign bodies, enteroliths, or stasis within the diverticulum (Fig. 27.4). This occurs when the neck of the Meckel's diverticulum is narrow or narrowed by edema from a foreign body or an enterolith. Uncommonly, chronic vague abdominal pain will be caused by chronic peptic ulceration, so-called *dyspepsia Meckelii*. Perforation may be related to peptic ulceration and inflammation.

A Meckel's diverticulum can be entrapped in an inguinal or femoral hernial sac, the so-called Littre's hernia described in 1742 (15). This is probably less common than noted in Table 27.3 because of overreporting of this interesting complication. Obstruction may be a late presentation of a Littre's hernia, because it is a Richter's type of hernia with only the diverticulum trapped in the hernial sac. In this instance, a localized mass and inflammation

Figure 27.4. A long Meckel's diverticulum is outlined with a large enterolith at the apex in a patient who presented with occult blood loss.

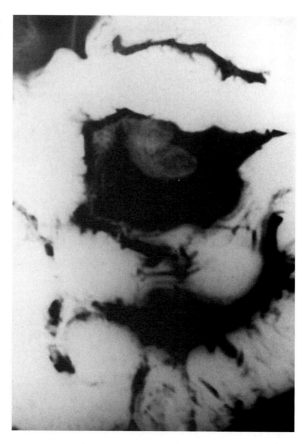

without compromise of the intestinal lumen allow continued passage of intestinal contents. Of these hernias, 50% occur in the inguinal region, 20% are femoral, 20% are umbilical, and 10% are described as miscellaneous (15).

DIAGNOSIS

Meckel's diverticulum should be considered in the differential diagnosis of right lower quadrant pain, bowel obstruction in the virgin abdomen, lower gastrointestinal tract bleeding in children, and cryptogenic bleeding in adults. Unfortunately, *a preoperative diagnosis of Meckel's diverticulum is made rarely* (only 10% of the time in some series) because emergency operation is often necessary. The use of computed tomography in these acute situations could define pathologic conditions in the small bowel in patients who require early intervention.

In a consecutive series of 33 patients with surgically proven Meckel's diverticula reported by Meguid et al (16), the preoperative small bowel series was uniformly unsuccessful in demonstrating the anomaly. Using small bowel enteroclysis, Maglinte et al (17) were able to identify a Meckel's diverticulum in 11 of 13 patients studied, for an 87% sensitivity rate, as demonstrated in Figure 27.5. Occasionally, an invaginated Meckel's diverticulum can be demonstrated on a plain film. *The introduction of* ^{99m}TC-*pertechnetate scanning by Jewett et al (18) in 1970 represented a major advance in the radiologic diagnosis of Meckel's diverticulum, especially in children with bleeding.* The ^{99m}TC-pertechnetate isotope has an infinity for gastric mucosa. Initially, the isotope was believed to be taken up by the parietal cells. Subsequent studies have shown that the isotope accumulates in the surface mucous-secreting cells that line the gastric mucosa. For results of a ^{99m}TC-pertechnetate scan to be positive, at least 1.8 cm^2 of gastric mucosa must be present (8). Figure 27.6 shows a typical technetium scan.

Several techniques have been described to improve the accuracy of the ^{99m}TC-pertechnetate scan. Pretreating patients with pentagastrin, 6 μg/kg subcutaneously, is

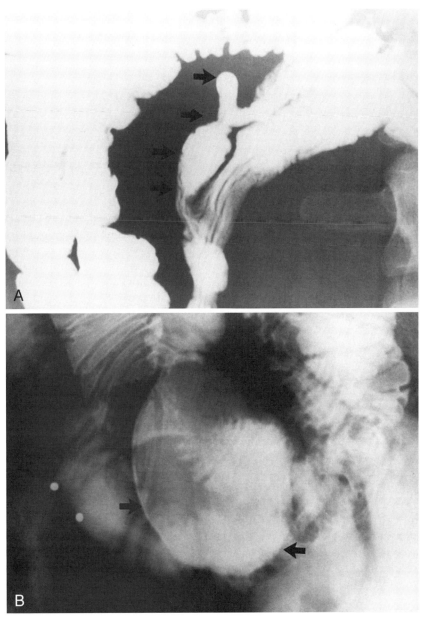

Figure 27.5. **A.,** An anomalous Y-shaped Meckel's diverticulum is shown. **B.,** Typical appearance of a large Meckel's diverticulum discovered on small bowel enteroclysis study.

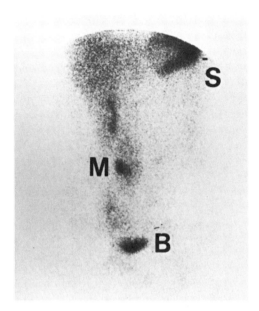

Figure 27.6. Positive Meckel's scan of an adult with recurrent lower gastrointestinal tract bleeding. B, the urinary bladder; M, the Meckel's diverticulum; S, the stomach.

believed to increase the production of mucus and therefore enhance scanning sensitivity. Administration of cimetidine, 300 mg orally four times per day before scanning and 300 mg 1 hour before scanning, results in a more intense blush on the scan. The mechanism of cimetidine enhancement is believed to be the result of blockage of acid secretion and thus better retention of the isotope in the diverticulum. Glucagon also has been used to slow motility and therefore decrease washout of the isotope at the site of the diverticulum (19,20). None of these methods of enhancing the scan for a Meckel's diverticulum have been subjected to rigorous trials.

A retrospective study by Sfakianakis and Conway (21,22) of more than 900 patients found the scan for Meckel's diverticulum to be 85% sensitive and 95% specific. However, most of their patients were children. *When reports of scans for Meckel's diverticulum were stratified for age and only adults were considered, the sensitivity was decreased to 62% and the specificity was 9%* with an accuracy of only 46% (19). The true incidence of false-negative results is difficult to assess but is reported to be 2–50%. False-negative results occur when gastric mucosa is insufficient to concentrate the isotope, when the imaging technique is poor, or when washout caused by rapid bleeding or hypermotility prevents accumulation of the marker. False-positive scans occur in one of the three scans performed in adults. However, in 70% of these false-positive results, other pathologic findings requiring operation were found (19). False-positive results can be caused by benign and malignant tumors, uterine blush, renal cysts or overlapping bladder, arteriovenous malformations, Crohn's disease, intussusception, or enteric duplication. Cooney et al (23) reported 30 positive results in 270 children scanned; false-positive results were reported in 14 instances. In nine children, other pathologic findings were found, but five true false-positive results were reported. The unusually high false-positive rate in children in this study was the result of the use of the scan in children with chronic abdominal pain.

It can be concluded that the ^{99m}TC-*pertechnetate scan is highly useful for children with gastrointestinal tract bleeding but is not useful for patients with vague abdominal pain. For adults with chronic blood loss or recurrent lower gastrointestinal tract bleeding when results of other tests are negative, a* ^{99m}*TC-pertechnetate scan should be considered.* When a Meckel's diverticulum is highly suspected and the initial scan does not indicate the presence of a diverticulum, a repeat scan should be performed with cimetidine or pentagastrin enhancement.

Angiography has proven to be a useful diagnostic and therapeutic tool in lower gastrointestinal tract bleeding in the adult (24). Two characteristic findings can identify a persistent vitelline artery in a bleeding Meckel's diverticulum: an elongated nonbranching artery originates from the distal ileal arteries and the elongated artery ends in a group of small dilated tortuous vessels. As in all angiographic studies, extravasation of dye can be seen in the presence of active bleeding (24).

TREATMENT

A symptomatic Meckel's diverticulum is treated surgically. *The surgeon has two options at laparotomy: resection of the involved ileum or diverticulectomy* with either suture or staple closure of the neck. The neck is closed transversely to the axis of the bowel to prevent narrowing of the lumen. Resection is indicated for induration of the involved bowel segment or free perforation and evidence of surrounding inflammatory reaction of the mesentery.

Intuitively, resection seems to be the procedure of choice in most instances of symptomatic Meckel's diverticulum. Vane et al (25) performed simple diverticulectomy in 41 of 46 pediatric patients operated on for gastrointestinal tract bleeding in whom the bleeding had initially stopped. Bleeding did not recur in this series. In the series of 30 symptomatic patients of Lüdtke et al (11), two-thirds of patients underwent simple resection of the diverticulum. A complicated Meckel's diverticulum can be treated with simple diverticulectomy and removal of any associated adhesions or mesodiverticular bands in appropriate patients.

Most of the controversy surrounding the treatment of patients with a Meckel's diverticulum concerns the appropriate management of the asymptomatic Meckel's diverticulum found incidentally during laparotomy for an unrelated disease process. Historically, the mortality rate associated with resection of a symptomatic Meckel's diverticulum has ranged from 2.5% to 15%; complication rates of 6–30% have been reported (4). Although the mortality rate associated with incidental Meckel's diverticulectomy today is less than 1%, opponents of incidental removal of a Meckel's diverticulum cite a potential morbidity rate of up to 9% as a reason to defer surgery. Many series (13) involving treatment of Meckel's diverticula initially reported that complications were unlikely to occur in the adult.

Soltero and Bill (13) reviewed the incidence of Meckel's diverticula for a 15-year span in the Seattle, WA area, with a population of more than 1,000,000 people. In this time frame, 202 complications of Meckel's diverticula occurred. The authors assumed a 2% incidence of Meckel's diverticulum in this population. The cumulative risk of a complication of Meckel's diverticulum developing was calculated to be 4.2% in children and decreasing to almost 0 in adults older than 60 years of age. Assuming a 1% mortality rate and an 11% morbidity rate in patients with symptomatic Meckel's diverticulum and a 0% mortality rate and 9% morbidity rate in patients with asymptomatic Meckel's diverticulum, they calculated that 400 asymptomatic Meckel's diverticula would have to be removed to save one life. These results, published in 1976, have influenced a generation of surgeons.

An epidemiologic population-based study (14) from Olmsted County, MN and the Mayo Clinic was based on a stable population and an excellent medical record-keeping system. There was a 6.9% risk of developing a complication of a Meckel's diverticulum. Furthermore, this risk was lifelong and extended through the seventh decade of life. Of the 87 patients treated, only one death occurred in the group whose diverticula were removed incidentally. This death was directly related to a complication from an arrhythmia on the tenth postoperative day following a right colectomy. Immediate and long-term complications were also determined. When a Meckel's diverticulum was removed for symptomatic reasons, the operative mortality and morbidity rates were 2% and 12%, respectively, and the risk of long-term postoperative complications was 7%; when an asymptomatic Meckel's diverticulum was removed incidentally, the mortality and morbidity rates were 1% and 2%, respectively, and only a 2% long-term complication rate was noted. The authors (14) concluded that a Meckel's diverticulum should be removed incidentally whenever it can be performed safely.

The report of Matsagas et al (26) concerned 63 patients with a Meckel's diverticulum accumulated over a 15-year period. Of the symptomatic patients, 53% were older than 40 years of age. No deaths occurred in either the symptomatic or asymptomatic groups in this series. Of the 142 patients with symptomatic Meckel's diverticula reported by Söderlund (12), 13 patients (9%) could have had removal of the diverticulum at an earlier operation. No deaths occurred in the group of patients who had an incidental asymptomatic Meckel's diverticulum removed. The morbidity rate was only 2.2%. These results are similar to the results of the population-based study from the Mayo Clinic (14). Other authors (4,11,27) have demonstrated the safety and low morbidity associated with incidental diverticulectomy.

Diverticulectomy of an incidental Meckel's diverticulum is straightforward and secure with current stapling instruments. When indicated, a symptomatic Meckel's diverticulum can be removed using staplers. These instruments can be used either laparoscopically (28,29) or during laparotomy. Laparoscopic exploration of patients with right lower quadrant pain is gaining acceptance. Whenever a normal appendix is found, the distal 100 cm of ileum must be evaluated laparoscopically. Removal of an asymptomatic Meckel's diverticulum using the endoscopic linear stapler is demonstrated in Figure 27.7.

An asymptomatic Meckel's diverticulum found incidentally at laparotomy or laparoscopic exploration should be removed in patients of all age groups. This operation should only be performed when the planned procedure has been completed safely. Prudent clinical judgment is necessary, and *incidental diverticulectomy should not be performed in the presence of sepsis or when the patient's condition is unstable.*

MISCELLANEOUS

Tumors associated with Meckel's diverticula have been the source of numerous case reports. The most common malignant tumors are carcinoids, followed by leiomyosarcomas. In reported series, nearly half of the carcinoid tumors are asymptomatic, but patients may have nonspecific abdominal pain or gastrointestinal bleeding on presentation. Half of the reported carcinoid tumors were not detected at the time of laparotomy and were found only after macroscopic or microscopic pathologic evaluation. Careful appraisal of all incidentally found Meckel's diverticula is warranted, and resection is recommended (30). Carcinoid tumors larger than 5 mm in size have a great tendency to metastasize and should be resected. Malignant tumors tend to be found in patients older than 50 years of age (31). Leiomyosarcomas and adenocarcinomas are treated with

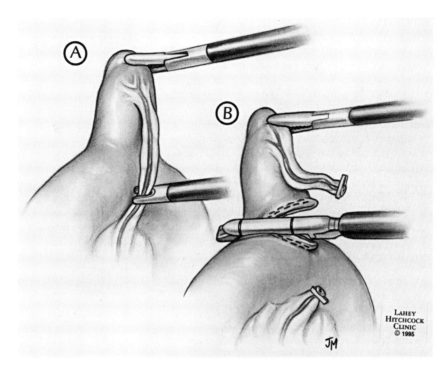

Figure 27.7. Use of the laparoscopic linear stapler to remove a Meckel's diverticulum. A., Division of the aberrant artery supplying the Meckel's diverticulum. **B.**, Division of the diverticulum with the Endo-GIA (Auto-Suture). (Reproduced by permission of Lahey Hitchcock Clinic, Burlington, MA.)

wide surgical resection. Other benign tumors also have been described, including adenomas, fibromas, or leiomyomas.

Anecdotal reports have described an increased prevalence of Meckel's diverticula in patients with Crohn's disease. A retrospective review (32) of 294 consecutive ileocolic resections for Crohn's disease was undertaken at St. Mark's Hospital. Seventeen patients (5.5%) were found to have an associated Meckel's diverticulum, which is two to three times the expected incidence of 2%. None of these patients had heterotopic mucosa in the Meckel's diverticulum. The authors speculated that the Meckel's diverticulum might be a predisposing factor to the development of Crohn's disease.

CONCLUSION

All surgeons operating in the abdomen should be aware of the common complications of Meckel's diverticula: bleeding, obstruction, inflammation. *The type of complication is relatively age-specific*: newborns have obstruction or umbilical drainage, children have bleeding, and the older patient has obstruction or inflammation as predominating symptoms. Symptomatic Meckel's diverticula can occur in any age group through the seventh decade of life.

In the course of abdominal surgery for other disease processes, an asymptomatic, incidentally found Meckel's diverticulum should be removed in both children and adults. This recommendation for removal should be followed only when operation for the symptomatic disease process has been accomplished safely.

EDITORIAL COMMENTS

This chapter examines two major issues: treatment of the complications of Meckel's diverticula and management of incidentally discovered, asymptomatic diverticula.

Symptomatic lesions should be resected in continuity with the adjacent ileum or with simple diverticulectomy. The operation can be performed with the laparoscope and linear stapling device or through a laparotomy incision. The morbidity and mortality rates should be low (e.g., 8.6% and 1.6%, respectively, in combined results of seven reports during the last 20 years [33]).

The approach to asymptomatic diverticula remains controversial. We believe that each of these lesions should be managed individually using good surgical judgment, weighing medical and surgical risks against the incidence of complications of the disease in different age groups. Several recent publications continue to question the value of routine diverticulectomy in asymptomatic patients (33,34). The object of the procedure is to correct the main indication for the operation in the first place, then to approach the diverticulum. Resection of the asymptomatic diverticulum seems the most appropriate in patients younger than 25 years of age: for older patients, the need to resect is less clear (unless ectopic gastric tissue is suspected [35]), and nothing would be recommended for patients older than 70 years of age.

REFERENCES

1. Lichtenstein ME. Meckel's diverticulum. Intestinal obstruction due to invagination and intussusception: peritonitis due to perforation by fish bone. Q Bull Northwestern Univ Med Sch 1941;15:296–300.
2. Meckel JF. Ueber die divertikel am darmkanal. Arch die Physiol 1809;9:421–453.
3. Meckel JF. Handbuch der pathologischen anatomie. Leipzig: CH Reclam, 1812;1.
4. Mackey WC, Dineen P. A fifty year experience with Meckel's diverticulum. Surg Gynecol Obstet 1983;156:56–64. *Seventeen percent of 402 patients had symptoms; the highest risk groups were 40 years of age or younger, male, or had diverticula 2 cm or more in length, containing heterotopic mucosa.*
5. Salzer H. Uber das offene Meckelesche divertikel. Wien Klin Wochenschr 1904;17:614–617.
6. Deetz E. Perforationsperitonitis von einem darmdivertikel mit Magensicleimhautbau ausgenhend. Deutsch Ztsch Chir 1907;88:482–493.
7. Gray SW, Akin JT Jr, Skandalakis JE. Three varieties of congenital diverticulum of the intestine. Surg Clin North Am 1974;54:1371–1377. *Describes Meckel's diverticulum, internal diverticula, and dorsal intestinal diverticula.*
8. Simms MH, Corkery JJ. Meckel's diverticulum: its association with congenital malformation and the significance of atypical morphology. Br J Surg 1980;67:216–219. *The incidence of Meckel's diverticula was increased in children born with certain congenital malformations.*
9. Williams RS. Management of Meckel's diverticulum. Br J Surg 1981;68:477–480. *A concise review with 32 references.*
10. Moses WR. Meckel's diverticulum: report of two unusual cases. N Engl J Med 1947;237:118–122. *A collective review of 1605 cases is included.*
11. Lüdtke F-E, Mende V, Köhler H, et al. Incidence and frequency of complications and management of Meckel's diverticulum. Surg Gynecol Obstet 1989;169:537–542. *The most frequent complications in 84 patients were obstruction and diverticulitis.*
12. Söderlund S. Meckel's diverticulum: a clinical and histologic study. Acta Chir Scand Suppl 1959;248:1–233. *A clinical series of 413 patients, including detailed histologic studies. Numerous references.*
13. Soltero MJ, Bill AH. The natural history of Meckel's diverticulum and its relation to incidental removal: a study of 202 cases of diseased Meckel's diverticulum found in King County, Washington, over a fifteen year period. Am J Surg 1976;132:168–173. *The authors estimate that it would be necessary to remove 800 asymptomatic Meckel's diverticula to save one patient's life from complications of a Meckel's diverticulum.*
14. Cullen JJ, Kelly KA, Moir CR, et al. Surgical management of Meckel's diverticulum: an epidemiologic, population-based study. Ann Surg 1994;220:564–569. *Removal of Meckel's diverticula discovered incidentally at operation is recommended, regardless of age.*
15. Perlman JA, Hoover HC, Safer PK. Femoral hernia with strangulated Meckel's diverticulum (Littre's hernia): case report and review of the literature. Am J Surg 1980;139:286–289. *Because most complications occur in patients younger than 30 years of age, incidental removal of the Meckel's diverticula discovered incidentally at operation in adults is not recommended.*
16. Meguid MM, Wilkinson RH, Canty T, et al. Futility of barium sulfate in diagnosis of bleeding Meckel's diverticulum. Arch Surg 1974;108:361–362. *In a study of infants, the yield of a careful history, physical, and sigmoidoscopy is greater than that following contrast exams.*
17. Maglinte DD, Elmore MF, Isenberg M, et al. Meckel's diverticulum: radiologic demonstration by enteroclysis. Am J Roentgenol 1980;134:925–932. *Demonstrates the value of enteroclysis for detecting Meckel's diverticula in 11 patients.*

18. Jewett TC Jr, Duszynski DO, Allen JE. The visualization of Meckel's diverticulum with ^{99m}TC-pertechnetate. Surgery 1970;68:567–570. *Describes the technique of this method.*
19. Schwartz MJ, Lewis JH. Meckel's diverticulum: pitfalls in scintigraphic detection in the adult. Am J Gastroenterol 1984;79:611–618. *It is suggested that Meckel's scanning be supplemented with small bowel infusion and/or arteriography to improve diagnostic accuracy in adults.*
20. Wilton G, Froelich JW. The "false-negative" Meckel's scan. Clin Nucl Med 1982;7:441–443. *A repeat Meckel's scan proved positive despite a negative initial scan.*
21. Sfakianakis GN, Conway JJ. Detection of ectopic gastric mucosa in Meckel's diverticulum and in other aberrations by scintigraphy. I. Pathophysiology and 10-year clinical experience. J Nucl Med 1981;22:647–654. *The overall sensitivity of Pertechnetate (TC-99m) scintography was 85% over a 10-year period.*
22. Sfakianakis GN, Conway JJ. Detection of ectopic gastric mucosa in Meckel's diverticulum and in other aberrations by scintigraphy. II. Indications and methods — a 10-year experience. J Nucl Med 1981;22:732–738. *The accuracy of this method was greater than 90%.*
23. Cooney DR, Duszynski DO, Camboa E, et al. The abdominal technetium scan (a decade of experience). J Pediatr Surg 1982;17:611–619. *This test should detect 80 to 90% of Meckel's diverticula and accurately exclude Meckel's diverticula in more than 90% of patients.*
24. Routh WD, Lawdahl RB, Lund E, et al. Meckel's diverticula: angiographic diagnosis in patients with non-acute hemorrhage and negative scintigraphy. Pediatr Radiol 1990;20:152–156. *A report of two cases. Meticulous visceral angiography proved diagnostic, even in the absence of focal contrast extravasation.*
25. Vane DW, West KW, Grosfeld JL. Vitelline duct anomalies: experience with 217 childhood cases. Arch Surg 1987;122:542–547. *Elective resection is recommended in asymptomatic young children having laparotomies for other conditions.*
26. Matsagas MI, Fatouros M, Koulouras B, et al. Incidence, complications, and management of Meckel's diverticulum. Arch Surg 1995;130:143–146. *Resection of the unexpected Meckel's diverticulum was done safely, with a low complication rate, despite patient age.*
27. Michas CA, Cohen SE, Wolfman EF Jr. Meckel's diverticulum: should it be excised at operation? Am J Surg 1974;129:682–685. *Recommends incidental Meckel's diverticulectomy if the mortality of the primary operation will not be increased significantly.*
28. Sanders LE. Laparoscopic treatment of Meckel's diverticulum. Surg Endosc 1996;9:724–727. *Describes the use of the laparoscope in treating one case of small bowel obstruction (resected laparoscopically) and one of gastrointestinal bleeding (resected extracorporeally).*
29. Teitelbaum DH, Polley TZ Jr, Obeid F. Laparoscopic diagnosis and excision of Meckel's diverticulum. J Pediatr Surg 1994;29:495–497. *Describes the technical aspects of laparoscopic treatment of two pediatric patients.*
30. Weber JD, McFadden DW. Carcinoid tumors in Meckel's diverticula. J Clin Gastroenterol 1989;11:682–686. *A literature review with 37 references.*
31. Nies C, Zielke A, Hasse C, et al. Carcinoid tumors of Meckel's diverticula: report of two cases and review of the literature. Dis Colon Rectum 1992;35:589–596. *Tumors more than 5 mm have a marked risk of metastasis and aggressive management is recommended.*
32. Andreyev HJ, Owen RA, Thompson I, et al. Association between Meckel's diverticulum and Crohn's disease: a retrospective review. Gut 1994;35:788–790. *Seventeen of 294 consecutive patients having right hemicolectomy for Crohn's disease had Meckel's diverticula.*
33. Peoples JB, Lichtenberger EJ, Dunn MM. Incidental Meckel's diverticulectomy in adults. Surgery 1995;118:649–652. *A retrospective review of 94 patients with Meckel's diverticula included 90 incidental diverticulectomies. Concludes that incidental diverticulectomy should be ended, based on decision analysis (risk of resecting symptomatic diverticula 0.2%).*
34. Kashi SH, Lodge JPA. Meckel's diverticulum: a continuing dilemma? J R Coll Surg Edinb 1995;40:392–394. *Based on a long-term review of 43 cases, incidental diverticulectomy is not recommended.*
35. Bemelman WA, Hugenholtz E, Heij HA, et al. Meckel's diverticulum in Amsterdam: experience in 136 patients. World J Surg 1995;19:734–737. *A retrospective review of 136 patients; 77% of symptoms occurred in patients younger than 30 years of age.*

28 The Atypical Presentations of Diverticulitis

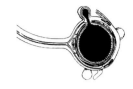

Hiram C. Polk, Jr. MD
Wayne B. Tuckson, MD
Frank B. Miller, MD

> **KEY POINTS**
>
> - Consider diverticulitis when causes for disorders are unclear:
>   - chronic hip, thigh, or knee infections with enteric bacteria
>   - left adnexal masses in middle-aged women
>   - inflammation/necrosis in perineum, genitalia
>   - subcutaneous emphysema of legs, neck, abdominal wall
>   - hepatic abscesses in non-world travelers
>   - skin lesions like pyoderma gangrenosum
> - Useful diagnostic tests:
>   - CT scanning

Diverticulitis can mask as a number of disease processes and the "atypical" presentations are particularly diverse. For many, they are medical curiosities and are anecdotal. However, considering the prevalence of diverticular disease in North America, most physicians could expect to encounter one or more such cases in the course of a career (Table 28.1).

Atypical cases have been described in a variety of ages and disease states. Abscesses complicating perforated diverticulitis can track in a number of directions, into extraperitoneal locations or into other organs. Young patients with diverticulitis are, in a sense, "atypical," but the actual disease presentation in these patients tends to be classic albeit not suspected (see Chapter 23) (1). Certain populations of patients are particularly prone to atypical manifestations of diverticulitis: those immunocompromised by certain diseases, including AIDS or cancer, or by chemotherapeutic and immunosuppressive medications. These individuals usually present with symptoms "typical" of diverticulitis but also may have atypical manifestations, in that the signs of infection and inflammation are not at all clear (2).

ILLUSTRATIVE CASE

A 78-year-old woman had felt ill for 6 weeks but had no specific symptoms. Previous radiographs of a painful left hip were normal. She presented with fever, leukocytosis, and a erythematous, warm mass in the left groin. Incision and drainage showed an 8-cm necrotic cavity filled with pus, which cultured coliform bacteria, including *Bacteroides fragilis*. The patient improved rapidly, but the drain site in the left groin continued to discharge pus for 8 weeks. A barium enema, as part of an extensive and otherwise negative

Table 28.1.   Unusual Extra-Abdominal Presentations

Dermatologic:	Orthopedic:	Vascular:
Pyoderma gangrenosum	Osteomyelitis (35)	Femoral vein thrombosis
	Arthritis	Mesenteric vein thrombosis
Urinary:	**Gynecologic:**	Pylephlebitis
Ureteral obstruction	Colouterine fistula	Colovenous fistula
Coloureteral fistula	Ovarian tumor/abscess	
Soft tissue:	**Genital:**	**Perineal:**
Thigh abscess	Epididymitis	Fournier's gangrene
Necrotizing fasciitis	Pneumoscrotum	Complex anal fistula
	Neurologic:	
	Coloepidural fistula	

imaging workup, showed diverticulosis of the sigmoid colon. A subsequent sinus tract injection from the left groin shows a communication with the sigmoid.

CASE COMMENTS

The goal here is for the surgeon to consider diverticulitis when treating a patient with a recalcitrant lower extremity infection (including subcutaneous emphysema, cellulitis, or abscess) that cultures enteric organisms and is resistant to what seems to be good and sensible local treatment. Radiographs may have shown gas in the subcutaneous tissues of the leg. A computed tomography (CT) scan would also have been useful to demonstrate diverticulitis, although the fistulogram and barium enema have defined the problem in this case. Definitive treatment is needed early, i.e., resection of the diseased bowel with colostomy, together with wide drainage of the abscess. If the process is allowed to progress to the development of emphysema in the leg, the mortality is very high.

One review of the unusual extraperitoneal presentations of diverticulitis (25 cases) showed that the typical patient was an elderly female with hip involvement; other sites included the perineum, scrotum, buttocks, joints, thigh, lower extremities, mediastinum, and neck (3).

DISCUSSION

We will divide atypical complications of diverticulitis arbitrarily into intra-abdominal and extra-abdominal ones.

Intra-Abdominal Complications

Left adnexal masses can be confused with diverticulitis (4). Gynecologists have been surprised to discover that diverticulitis can be the underlying cause of an apparent left adnexal mass. One solution to this problem would be the uniform use of a mechanical bowel preparation on all patients before elective gynecologic surgery, especially for left adnexal masses. Another gynecologic complication is development of a *colouterine fistula* (5,6), much less common than a colovaginal fistula, which is discussed in Chapter 11. Only six colouterine fistulas were found in several large reviews of patients with diverticulitis (1600 in total) (6). The rarity of colouterine fistulas probably is due to the thickness of the uterine wall. Usually, the diagnosis is not made until the time of laparotomy. Most patients have a feculent, purulent, or hemorrhagic vaginal discharge, and dilatation and curettage should be performed because endometrial cancer is in the differential (6). Hysterectomy is favored along with sigmoid resection, especially if necrotizing myositis of the uterus occurs (3).

If the *urinary tract* is considered, colovesical fistulas are well recognized as manifestations of abscesses (Chapter 10) in men and in women who have undergone hysterectomy (7). A rare cause of ureteral obstruction is nonspecific retroperitoneal fibrosis associated with occult diverticulitis (8). Ureterocolic (9) and nephrocolic (10) fistulas have also occurred. Rarely, a colovesical fistula presents in the form of epididymitis (11).

A common "stump the visiting professor" scenario is the presentation of an isolated *hepatic abscess* due to enteric organisms without any antecedent history (Chapter 33) (12).

Unusual *vascular* complications that can lead to hepatic abscesses include pylephlebitis, pneumophlebitis, and a whole variety of changes in the portal venous system (13,14). The inferior mesenteric vein also may be involved specifically by intravasation of barium. Significant intravasation can lead to sudden death (13) (Fig. 28.1). A case of sigmoid-biliary fistula has been reported, probably based on spread in the mesenteric venous system (15).

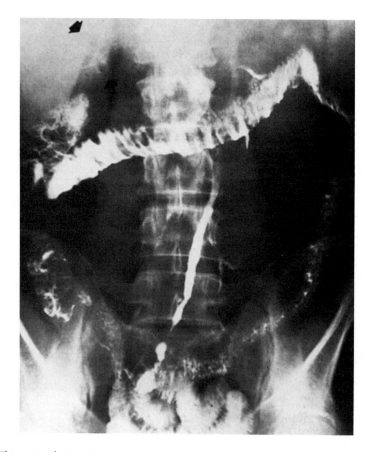

Figure 28.1.   This patient had a colovenous fistula. Postevacuation film shows barium in the inferior mesenteric vein. The patient later died with thrombosis of the portal and splenic veins and multiple liver abscesses. (Reprinted with permission from Smith J, Berk RN, James JO, et al. Unusual fistulae due to colonic diverticulitis. Gastrointest Radiol 1978;2:387–392.)

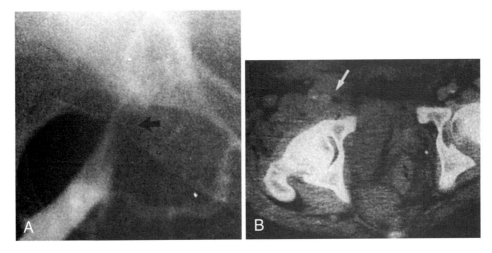

Figure 28.2. **A.,** Unilateral iliofemoral vein thrombosis caused by psoas abscess secondary to sigmoid diverticulitis. Right leg venogram demonstrates the venous thrombosis (arrow) and collateral venous drainage (top). **B.,** A CT scan view at the level of the femoral heads shows inflammation around the right femoral vein (arrow). (Reprinted with permission from Wittram C. Sigmoid diverticulitis presenting as unilateral iliofemoral vein thrombosis. Abdom Imaging 1994;19:257–258.)

When catastrophic aortocolic fistulas occur, the only opportunity for successful intervention may be at the time of the "herald" or premonitory bleeding. This bleeding also may occur in the case of aortoiliac prosthetic grafting, such as for aneurysmal disease or occlusive disease of the aortic bifurcation.

Progressive diverticulitis can have a local effect on the iliac vein, or the patient can present with iliofemoral venous disease (16) (Fig. 28.2). Typically, the patient will have been treated with anticoagulants without response, and the first treating physician will have failed to discover a probable underlying cause.

The clinician frequently is concerned about differentiating diverticulitis from a locally perforated colon cancer (Chapter 4). On the other hand, there are isolated reports in which a colon cancer may actually arise in a colonic diverticulum (17).

Extra-Abdominal

Occasionally, diverticulitis is complicated by *retroperitoneal abscess* formation (18,19); this is not surprising because 75% of sigmoid diverticula are contiguous with the retroperitoneal tissues (3). A particularly obscure manifestation of diverticulitis is the presentation of a persistent inflammatory or infectious lesion in the thigh or knee (see Illustrative Case) (20). The differential diagnosis includes pyomyositis, posttraumatic hematoma, osteomyelitis, malignant tumors of the soft tissue or bone, thrombophlebitis, and localized cellulitis or abscess of the subcutaneous tissue (21). Radiographs of the thigh frequently show collections of gas (Fig. 28.3); the gas tends to be between muscle planes rather than within the muscle (unless there is extensive gas) (22), which is characteristic of gas gangrene (23). Anatomic communication from the pelvis to the upper thigh, and later to the knee, explains the spread of sepsis from the pericolonic area to these distant sites (Fig. 28.4) (Table 28.2) (3,18,19,24). The route of spread to the thigh may be through two main routes: (*a*) by direct extension from the extraperitoneal rectum or (*b*) from the extraperitoneal space through anatomic defects in the abdominal wall, including the psoas muscle, femoral canal,

Figure 28.3. Radiograph shows gas in the leg of a patient with perforated sigmoid diverticulitis. (Reprinted with permission from Haiart DC, Stevenson P, Hartley RC. Leg pain: an uncommon presentation of perforated diverticular disease. J R Coll Surg Edinb 1989;34:17–20.)

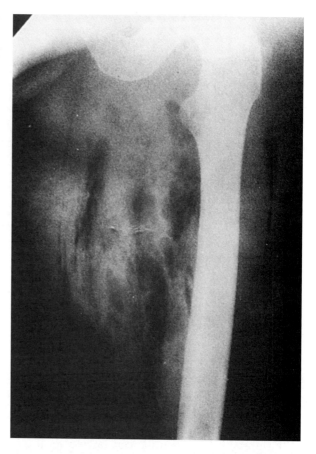

Figure 28.4. The insertions of abdominal and pelvic muscles outside of the pelvis facilitate spread from colonic perforations into the thigh. The pyriformis and obturator internus muscles insert laterally on the greater trochanter of the femur; the iliopsoas muscle group inserts medially on the lesser trochanter. (Reprinted with permission from Meyers MA, Goodman KJ. Pathways of extrapelvic spread of disease: anatomic-radiologic correlation. Am J Roentgenol 1975;125:900–909.)

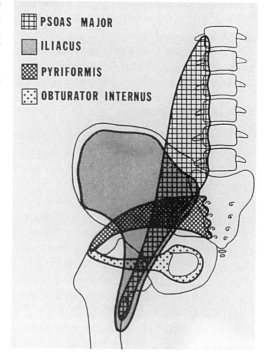

PSOAS MAJOR

ILIACUS

PYRIFORMIS

OBTURATOR INTERNUS

Table 28.2.   Potential Pathways for Retroperitoneal Spread of Infection

- Along nerves, vessels, and genital structures
- Inguinal ring
- Obturator foramen
- Femoral canal
- Psoas muscle fascia
- Denonvilliers' fascia

obturator foramen, and the sacrosciatic notch (21,24). Left-sided thigh abscesses tend to complicate colorectal pathology, and right thigh abscesses may follow appendiceal or small bowel disease (21). The mortality rate was 69% for 13 cases of thigh abscess or emphysema due to perforated diverticular disease (20); aggressive treatment, including fecal diversion, is mandatory if the outcome is to be improved in these patients.

The *external genitalia* occasionally are the site of the earliest manifestations of diverticulitis, and a variety of scrotal inflammations, including scrotal gangrene, may occur (25). Two cases of pneumoscrotum have been seen complicating perforated sigmoid diverticulitis (26). Necrotizing fasciitis of the male genitalia, perineum, and perianal area (Fournier's gangrene) usually is associated with urinary or perirectal infections or local trauma but may complicate intra-abdominal processes such as diverticulitis (27). A high index of suspicion could prove to be lifesaving in this situation because treatment of the unsuspected intra-abdominal process is essential.

Subcutaneous emphysema caused by perforated diverticulitis also has presented in the neck in a patient with minimal lower abdominal symptoms probably masked by analgesics and corticosteroids (28). This rare complication (29) follows escape of retroperitoneal air into the mediastinum and then the neck.

The *nervous system* can be involved by a brain abscess (Fig. 28.5) (30,31), mimicking a primary neoplasm, or by a coloepidural fistula (22).

A *colocutaneous fistula* (22,23,32) raises suspicion of perforated diverticulitis when it is in the left lower quadrant of the abdominal wall, but its presentation in the upper abdomen often confuses clinicians (Fig. 28.6). As soon as one thinks of this possibility, it is fairly easy to clarify, especially with a contrast study of the fistula. Similarly, *pyoderma gangrenosum* and *arthritis* are recognized associations with diverticulitis that need not be directly connected to the inflammatory process (33,34). The clinician may make the mistaken diagnosis of idiopathic inflammatory bowel disease in this setting (up to 50% of patients with pyoderma gangrenosum have inflammatory bowel disease) and submit the patient to prolonged medical therapy with inappropriate medications (33). These extraintestinal symptoms may cease promptly after segmental colonic resection (Fig. 28.7).

This litany of atypical manifestations of diverticulitis is meaningful for the clinician only in the sense that it reminds him or her that the manifestations of the disease are protean. After these entities have been recognized for what they are, the diverticulitis is treated in the sensible and well-thought-out ways discussed elsewhere in this volume.

Figure 28.5. CT scan of head following contrast injection shows a metastatic cerebral abscess complicating sigmoid diverticulitis. (Reprinted with permission from Dixon AR, Holmes JT, Waters A. Intracranial abscess complicating diverticulitis with CT scan mimicking primary glioma. Postgrad Med J 1989; 65:565–567.)

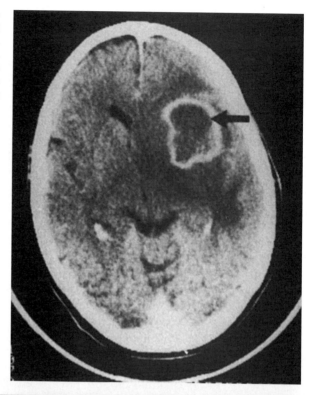

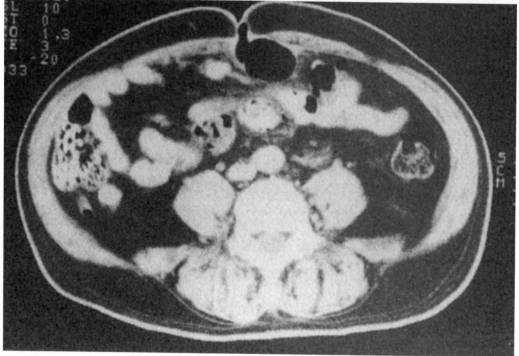

Figure 28.6. Cut from a CT scan shows a cavity that complicated perforated sigmoid diverticulitis and fistulized into the umbilicus.(Reprinted with permission from Pracyk JB, Pollard SG, Calne Sir RY. The development of spontaneous colo-umbilical fistula. Postgrad Med J 1993;69:750–751.)

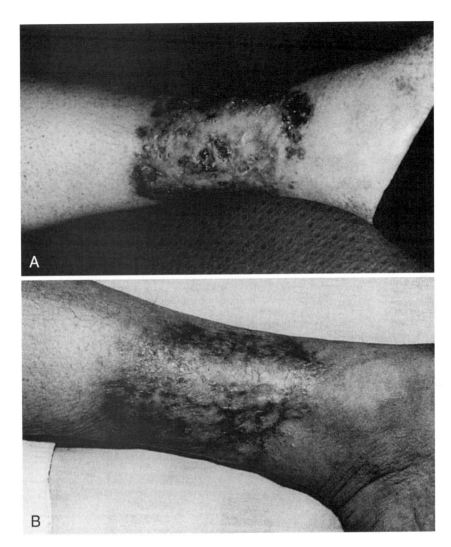

Figure 28.7. **A.,** Pyoderma gangrenosum involving the left ankle in a woman with sigmoid diverticulitis. **B.,** The wound was debrided and 2 weeks after sigmoid resection, complete healing had occurred. (Reprinted with permission from Kurgansky D, Foxwell MM Jr. Pyoderma gangrenosum as a cutaneous manifestation of diverticular disease. South Med J 1993;86:581–584.)

EDITORIAL COMMENTS

The great variety of manifestations of diverticulitis involving many organ systems recounted in this chapter is reminiscent of Crohn's disease or appendicitis. Many of these are extremely rare and the source of case reports and anecdotal experiences. Immunocompromised individuals are at particular risk of developing such complications. For patients with signs of sepsis or unusual abscesses, CT scans provide valuable anatomic information that can direct possible percutaneous drainage. Sigmoid resection is an important part of definitive treatment in most cases. Pathology specimens should be examined carefully for signs of Crohn's disease or other rare infectious diseases involving the colon.

REFERENCES

1. Konvolinka CW. Acute diverticulitis under age 40. Am J Surg 1994;167:562–565. *Most patients in this group were obese males in the fourth decade. Colon resection is recommended after the first attack.*
2. Tyau ES, Prystowsky JB, Joehl RJ, et al. Acute diverticulitis: a complicated problem in the immunocompromised patient. Arch Surg 1991;126:855–859. *Describes 209 patients with diverticulitis, 40 of whom were immunocompromised. The immunocompromised patients had a greater need for surgery, a higher risk of free perforation, and a higher morbidity and mortality.*
3. Ravo B, Khan SA, Ger R, et al. Unusual extraperitoneal presentations of diverticulitis. Am J Gastroenterol 1985;80:346–351. *Examines the anatomic spread of perforated diverticulitis into unusual extraperitoneal locations in a literature review of 25 cases.*
4. Walker JD, Gray LA, Polk HC Jr. Diverticulitis in women: an unappreciated clinical presentation. Ann Surg 1977;1185:402–405. *In a group of 69 patients undergoing surgery for a final diagnosis of diverticular disease, 38% were believed to have a gynecologic disorder because of the presence of a pelvic mass.*
5. Chaikof EL, Cambria RP, Warshaw AL. Colouterine fistula secondary to diverticulitis. Dis Colon Rectum 1985;28:358–360. *Discusses two cases of this rare complication. In one instance, benign colonic mucosa was found in an endometrial curettage.*
6. Huettner PC, Finkler NJ, Welch WR. Colouterine fistula complicating diverticulitis: charcoal challenge test aids in diagnosis. Obstet Gynecol 1992;80:550–552. *Orally administered charcoal passed from the cervical os on the following day, whereas a barium enema did not demonstrate the fistula.*
7. Amin M, Nallinger R, Polk HC Jr. Conservative treatment of selected patients with colovesical fistula due to diverticulitis. Surg Gynecol Obstet 1984;159:442–444. *Nonoperative therapy is possible in selected patients.*
8. Harbrecht PJ, Ahmad W, Fry DE, et al. Occult diverticulitis: a cause of retroperitoneal fibrosis. Dis Colon Rectum 1980;23:255–257. *Granulomatous and fibrotic changes in the mesocolon and retroperitoneum attributed to diverticulitis caused ureteral and colonic obstruction.*
9. Cirocco WC, Priolo SR, Golub RW. Spontaneous ureterocolic fistula: a rare complication of colonic diverticular disease. Am Surg 1994;60:832–835. *The fifth reported case of this disorder, 100% had symptoms of a urinary tract infection and a barium enema demonstrated the fistula 75% of the time.*
10. Underwood JW. An unusual renocolic fistula. J Urol 1977;118:847–848. *Chronic renal disease with atrophied perinephric fat is characteristic.*
11. O'Brien WM, Lynch JH. Epididymitis — an unusual presentation of colovesical fistula — report of a case. Dis Colon Rectum 1988;31:570–572. *This is a rare complication of diverticulitis.*
12. Liebert CW Jr. Hepatic abscess resulting from asymptomatic diverticulitis of the sigmoid colon. South Med J 1981;74:71–73. *A patient with subacute diverticulitis of the colon at laparotomy had a liver abscess and later developed another hepatic abscess, finally succumbing from sepsis.*
13. Juler GL, Dietrich WR, Eisenman JI. Intramesenteric perforation of sigmoid diverticulitis with non-fatal venous intravasation. Am J Surg 1976;132:653–656. *Five of 10 patients in the literature with venous intravasation during barium enema had diverticular disease.*
14. Nordahl DL, Siber FJ, Robbins AH, et al. Non-fatal venous intravasation from the site of diverticulitis during barium enema examination. Am J Dig Dis 1973;18:253–256. *The first reported case of this nonfatal complication of barium enema in a patient with diverticulitis. Discusses other complications of barium enema.*
15. Blanco-Benavides R, Rodriguez-Jerkov J. Sigmoid-biliary fistula: a rare complication of colonic diverticulitis (letter). Am J Gastroenterol 1992;87:810–811. *The first report of this complication probably occurring via the perivenous route.*
16. Wittram C. Sigmoid diverticulitis presenting as unilateral iliofemoral vein thrombosis. Abdom Imaging 1994;19:257–258. *An iliopsoas abscess compressed the iliofemoral vein and inflammation around the femoral vein caused iliofemoral vein thrombosis.*
17. Kricun R, Stasik JJ, Reither RD, et al. Giant colonic diverticulitis. Am J Roentgenol 1980;135:507–512. *Carcinoma arose within a diverticulum in one of the five patients reviewed.*
18. Crepps JT, Welch JP, Orlando R III. Management and outcome of retroperitoneal abscesses. Ann Surg 1987;205:276–281. *A review of 50 cases that emphasizes the occult presentation of these problems and the marked improvement in diagnostic accuracy with CT scanning. High mortality was associated with persistent fever or positive blood cultures within 48 hours of drainage.*
19. Leu S-Y, Leonard MB, Beart RW Jr, et al. Psoas abscess: changing patterns of diagnosis and etiology. Dis Colon Rectum 1986;29:694–698. *Psoas abscess has become primarily a complication of intestinal disorders, especially Crohn's disease.*
20. Haiart DC, Stevenson P, Hartley RC. Leg pain: an uncommon presentation of perforated diverticular disease. J R Coll Surg Edinb 1989;34:17–20. *Describes five patients with perforated diverticulitis where leg or thigh pain was the predominant symptom.*
21. Rotstein OD, Pruett TL, Simmons RL. Thigh abscess: an uncommon presentation of intra-abdominal sepsis. Am J Surg 1986;151:414–418. *Discusses two cases of thigh abscesses complicating intra-abdominal sepsis and reviews 46 cases from the literature. Thirty-nine cases originated in the colorectum (after perforation and abscess formation in the extraperitoneal space), including 10 with diverticulitis and 17 with carcinoma.*
22. Smith J, Berk RN, James JO, et al. Unusual fistulae due to colonic diverticulitis. Gastrointest Radiol 1978;2:387–392. *Includes radiographs of a number of rare fistulas and a comprehensive literature review.*

23. Drabble E, Greatorex RA. Colocutaneous fistula between the sigmoid colon and popliteal fossa in diverticular disease. Br J Surg 1994;81:1659. *This immunocompromised patient died 9 days after a transverse colostomy was performed.*
24. Meyers MA, Goodman KJ. Pathways of extrapelvic spread of disease: anatomic-radiologic correlation. Am J Roentgenol 1975;125:900–909. *An excellent discussion comparing the anatomic routes of spread of subcutaneous emphysema of gastrointestinal origin to radiologic findings.*
25. Klutke CG, Miles BJ, Obeid F. Unusual presentation of sigmoid diverticulitis as an acute scrotum. J Urol 1988;193:380–381. *Retroperitoneal necrotizing fasciitis complicating perforated sigmoid diverticulitis caused acute scrotal inflammation.*
26. Watson HS, Klugo RC, Coffield KS. Pneumoscrotum: report of two cases and review of mechanism of its development. Urology 1992;40:517–521. *Pneumoscrotum may be an early sign of a life-threatening condition or an incidental finding associated with more benign conditions.*
27. Gerber GS, Guss SP, Pielet RW. Fournier's gangrene secondary to intra-abdominal processes. Urology 1994;44:779–782. *Fournier's gangrene arose because of perforated diverticulitis, but the abdominal process was not immediately apparent.*
28. Cappell MS, Marks M. Acute colonic diverticular perforation presenting as left ear pain and facial swelling due to cervical subcutaneous emphysema in a patient administered corticosteroids. Am J Gastroenterol 1992;87:899–902. *Air can track into the mediastinum, along the trachea and esophagus through either Grodinsky's space or the retropharyngeal space to produce cervical subcutaneous emphysema.*
29. Lipsit ER, Lewicki AM. Subcutaneous emphysema of the abdominal wall from diverticulitis with necrotizing fasciitis. Gastrointest Radiol 1979;4:89–92. *Elaborates on the mechanisms of abdominal wall emphysema.*
30. Dixon AR, Holmes JT, Waters A. Intracranial abscess complicating diverticulitis with CT scan mimicking primary glioma. Postgrad Med J 1989;65:565–567. *The patient recovered fully after abscess drainage through a frontal burr hole.*
31. Brewer NS, MacCarty CS, Wellman WE. Brain abscess: a review of recent experience. Ann Intern Med 1975;82:571–576. *One of 60 patients with brain abscess was suspected to have diverticulitis as the etiologic factor.*
32. Pracyk JB, Pollard SG, Calne Sir RY. The development of spontaneous colo-umbilical fistula. Postgrad Med J 1993;69:750–751. *Other causes of spontaneous enteroumbilical fistulas include Crohn's disease and tuberculous peritonitis.*
33. Klein S, Mayer L, Present D, et al. Extraintestinal manifestations in patients with diverticulitis. Ann Intern Med 1988;108:700–702. *Arthritis and pyoderma gangrenosum in three patients with diverticulitis disappeared promptly after colectomy.*
34. Kurgansky D, Foxwell MM Jr. Pyoderma gangrenosum as a cutaneous manifestation of diverticular disease. South Med J 1993;86:581–584. *A case report of an elderly patient with no GI symptoms who had resolution of cutaneous symptoms after colectomy.*
35. McCrea ES, Wagner E. Femoral osteomyelitis secondary to diverticulitis. J Can Assoc Radiol 1981;32:181–182. *A patient with a fistula between the colon and left hip developed septic arthritis and osteomyelitis of the proximal femur.*

29 Acquired Diverticula of the Small Bowel and Appendix

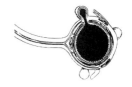

Anthony L. Imbembo, MD

> ### KEY POINTS
> - 75% of jejunoileal diverticula involve proximal jejunum
> - They may be caused by motility disorders
> - Symptoms appear in 50%
> - Enteroclysis best radiologic diagnostic technique
> - Perforation has mortality of 20–40%
> - Massive GI bleeding usually from jejunal diverticula
> - Resection recommended if operating for complications
> - Appendiceal diverticulitis usually involves recurrent episodes without migration of pain
> - Appendectomy recommended if appendiceal diverticula discovered at laparotomy

ILLUSTRATIVE CASES

Case 1

A 60-year-old man was seen in the office complaining of chronic periumbilical pain and bloating exacerbated by eating. He denied gastrointestinal (GI) bleeding or constipation; occasionally, he had episodes of diarrhea. He had been seen in the emergency department 3 weeks earlier with more marked upper abdominal pain. Radiographs at that time had shown a few dilated small-bowel loops. His pain had resolved within a few hours and he was discharged. He had previously undergone an appendectomy.

A subsequent ultrasound showed no gallstones. An upper GI (UGI) series and small bowel series were performed, showing extensive jejunal diverticulosis but no obstruction.

The patient was placed on a low-fiber diet, vitamin supplements, and tetracycline. His chronic complaints diminished markedly, except for occasional "gas cramps" over the ensuing 3 years.

Case Comments

This patient had rather vague abdominal symptoms that probably are related to intestinal dysmotility. The contrast study was diagnostic. In this case, the patient responded well to dietary modifications alone. In some instances, there may be chronic megaloblastic anemia, vitamin B_{12} deficiency, and diarrhea complicating bacterial overgrowth. These complications require treatment with vitamin B_{12} and broad-spectrum antibiotics and, if unresponsive to medical therapy, elective segmental resection.

Case 2

A 72-year-old female presented to the emergency room complaining of severe left upper quadrant abdominal pain radiating to the back. She denied vomiting, weight loss, or GI bleeding. Because of chronic indigestion, she had undergone a recent UGI series and ultrasound of the upper abdomen. The stomach and duodenum were normal, and two small gallstones were floating in a thin-walled gallbladder.

She was nonicteric and afebrile with a normal blood pressure. The abdomen was diffusely tender but not rigid; there was some guarding in the left upper quadrant. Abdominal films were nondiagnostic. The white blood cell count was 15,700 with a marked left shift. Liver function tests, the serum amylase, and a urinalysis were normal.

The following day, the patient's abdominal pain worsened, and her temperature increased to 102°F. A computed tomography (CT) scan showed free air and an upper abdominal mass with some free fluid.

She was taken to the operating room, where a perforated proximal jejunal diverticulum was found on the mesenteric border with surrounding mesenteric thickening. A primary resection and anastomosis were performed, and the abdomen was lavaged with several liters of saline and with antibiotics. She was discharged home 8 days later and did well.

Case Comments

This case shows the rather vague symptoms that characterize some of these cases, unless a major complication occurs. The CT scan proved diagnostic, although an earlier small bowel series would have shown the diverticula. The risk of perforation of small-bowel diverticula is low, and thus "prophylactic" excision is unnecessary. The mesenteric location of the diverticula interferes with their recognition during exploratory laparotomy and makes the actual resection technically more difficult.

Case 3

A 74-year old male developed melanotic stools and weakness at home and was sent by his doctor to the emergency room. The patient's blood pressure was 100/60, and his pulse was 110. He appeared pale and, with sitting, his blood pressure fell to 90/55, with a pulse of 115. He had no history of peptic ulcer disease or alcoholism; diverticulosis had been noted on a screening colonoscopy.

A nasogastric aspirate contained bilious material that was guaiac-negative. The abdomen was soft without palpable masses and there were no stigmata of cirrhosis.

The hematocrit was 24%, white blood cell count was 8,000, blood urea nitrogen (BUN) was 35, creatinine was normal, PT and PTT were normal, and electrolytes, blood sugar, and liver function tests were normal.

The patient was kept n.p.o. for 24 hours, and there was obvious bleeding. The bowel was prepped with GoLYTELY solution, and a colonoscopy was performed. There were several sigmoid diverticula, and some dark fluid was seen in the colon, which seemed to be coming from a site proximal to the ileocecal valve. An upper endoscopy showed minimal gastritis but no evidence of varices, ulcer, or arteriovenous malformations. A bleeding scan was faintly positive in the region of the left upper quadrant, presumably in the proximal small bowel. Several large melanotic stools then developed, and the patient became hypotensive. Angiography was performed after he was resuscitated, but no active bleeding was seen. After transfusion of 5 units of packed cells, the hematocrit was 29%. The patient was taken to the operating room for exploration. Search of the small bowel revealed several jejunal diverticula and the small bowel was filled with blood. The diverticula were resected in a

25-cm segment of jejunum with primary anastomosis. Ulceration was found in one of the diverticula containing a visible vessel. Postoperatively, the patient developed atrial fibrillation but had no additional bleeding and was discharged home 8 days later.

Case Comments

The diagnosis of small-bowel bleeding should be considered in patients with nonconvincing evidence of gastric or colonic sites of hemorrhage. Operation was performed semiurgently on this patient because of recurrent massive rebleeding. If the actual bleeding diverticulum could not be identified in a large group of diverticula, possible options would include blind resection with search for an ulcer in the bowel afterward, on-table enteroscopy through closed or open bowel, or clamping of the small bowel during massive bleeding to identify the source. The diagnosis of small-bowel diverticula had not been established in this case by contrast studies or CT, but the bleeding scan had suggested a possible small-bowel source. In some instances, the bleeding can be treated successfully with arteriography and embolization. Some patients will have persistent bleeding that is not massive; push enteroscopy can be useful to identify slowly bleeding jejunal diverticula, while enteroclysis can demonstrate the diverticula.

DISCUSSION

Diverticula of the small intestine are encountered infrequently. Because such diverticula are often difficult to demonstrate either radiologically or anatomically, their true incidence probably is underestimated. Jejunoileal diverticula have been found in 0.3–4.5% of autopsies and 0.5–2.3% of small intestinal contrast studies (1). Jejunoileal diverticula are seen primarily in late middle age and in elderly patients, probably with no significant gender predominance. Small intestinal diverticula are multiple in approximately 75% of cases. *Approximately three-quarters occur in the proximal jejunum,* followed by the distal jejunum (20%) and the ileum (5%) (2).

When Meckel's diverticulum is excluded, most jejunoileal diverticula are acquired lesions, consisting of herniations of the mucosa and submucosa through the muscularis propria of the intestinal wall. They usually are quite thin-walled, with the muscular layer absent or markedly attenuated. Muscularis is present at the neck of the diverticulum and often is locally hypertrophied. The mucosa and submucosa generally are normal with no evidence of inflammation. When inflammation does occur, it is the jejunal diverticula that are most apt to be involved. Such inflammation may result in extensive adhesion formation or in subserosal dissection of the diverticulum. The walls of inflamed diverticula often are markedly thickened by edema and/or fibrosis.

Jejunal diverticula vary in size from 1 to 10 cm, generally being considerably larger than those occurring in the ileum. Some of the largest diverticula identified occur in the proximal jejunum at the duodenojejunal flexure (3). Most diverticula have a globular appearance, but variants, particularly with larger lesions, include cylindric and lobulated forms. The ostia of jejunal diverticula tend to be relatively large, ranging from several millimeters to 3 cm. The size of the ostium tends to correlate directly with the size of the diverticulum. In the ileum, diverticula range from 0.2 to 1.5 cm and usually have narrow ostia. *Most diverticula are located on the mesenteric aspect of the bowel* and, therefore, protrude between the mesenteric leaves and, potentially, into the retroperitoneum.

Small intestinal diverticula usually contain chyme, which only rarely becomes inspissated due to its liquid consistency. The relatively large size of jejunal diverticular ostia also works against stasis. However, thickened matter and vegetable fibers can be found in large, complicated lesions. Enteroliths, foreign bodies, and parasites all have been reported in diverticula (4).

Pathogenesis

Although the factors contributing to the formation of acquired small intestinal diverticula have not been identified precisely, it generally is believed that pulsion forces combined with a weakened intestinal wall are responsible. The pulsion hypothesis is supported by the absence or attenuation of muscularis propria in the walls of most diverticula and, perhaps, by the increasing incidence with age (5). The factors responsible for weakness of the intestinal wall are largely unknown. It is probable that diverticula develop at points at which the mesenteric vessels penetrate the intestinal wall. It has been suggested that, as with colonic diverticula, pulsion diverticula develop most readily at these points of relative weakness. Acquired diverticula are most often located on the mesenteric aspect of the bowel circumference and occur with greatest frequency in the proximal jejunum. It has been shown that the vasa recti are of greatest diameter in this bowel segment (6). Furthermore, it is possible that the greater diameter of the jejunum results in attenuation of the longitudinal muscle layer, thereby contributing to relative weakness of the bowel wall at this level.

Experimental efforts to create diverticula by subjecting small bowel to sustained elevation of intraluminal pressure have been unsuccessful. Therefore, it has been suggested that localized segments of increased intraluminal pressure develop secondary to motor abnormalities of the small intestine. Herniation of the mucosa adjacent to a blood vessel then occurs secondary to high intraluminal pressure generated by excessive muscular contraction in adjacent segments of intestine (7). The muscular hypertrophy, which is often found adjacent to diverticular ostia, may support this hypothesis. Uncoordinated contractions with episodes of retrograde peristalsis in bowel segments containing diverticula may also be a contributing developmental factor. Acquired small intestinal diverticulosis, especially of the jejunum, may be a heterogeneous disorder caused, in part, by various smooth muscle and myenteric plexus abnormalities. *These abnormalities may result in intestinal dysmotility, which can, in itself, be responsible for symptoms while also contributing to diverticulum formation* (8).

Jejunal diverticulosis occasionally may develop secondary to a systemic disease process. Diseases that have been implicated include systemic sclerosis (scleroderma), rheumatoid arthritis, ulcerative colitis, thyroiditis, and nonviral hepatitis. A number of conditions seem to occur with increased frequency in association with acquired jejunal and ileal diverticula. In one series, the following associations were reported: colonic diverticula (61%), urinary bladder diverticula (20%), and esophageal diverticula (4%). In addition, congenital abnormalities were noted in 29% of patients. The latter included Meckel's diverticulum, hepatic hemangiomas, congenital pyloric stenosis, and malrotation and exstrophy of the bladder (9).

Clinical Manifestations

In the older literature, it was reported that most patients with small intestinal diverticulosis remain asymptomatic. *This has been challenged recently with the overall incidence of symptoms estimated to be approximately 50%* (6). Symptoms may develop secondary to obstruction of the diverticulum. This can result in stasis, bacterial proliferation, diverticular distention, and inflammation. A distended diverticulum can compress the intestinal lumen, causing obstructive symptoms. Obstructive symptoms also may be due to an associated motility disorder, especially in the jejunum. Symptoms secondary to an inflamed jejunal diverticulum may be indistinguishable from those caused by acute pancreatitis, peptic ulcer disease, Crohn's disease, or partial intestinal obstruction. In addition, symptoms of an inflamed ileal diverticulum may mimic acute appendicitis. Inflammation can result in additional complications, including perforation, ulceration, and gastrointestinal hemorrhage, all of which are uncommon.

Abdominal pain seems to occur in 10–30% of patients with jejunal diverticula. In addition, steatorrhea, megaloblastic anemia, and other vitamin-deficiency states have been associated with jejunal diverticulosis. It has been postulated that bacterial overgrowth is responsible, because the latter problems are often alleviated by antibiotics. *Many of the symptoms associated with jejunal diverticulosis may be due to a motility disorder.* Jejunal dyskinesia consists of to-and-fro movements of chyme within affected intestinal segments. This abnormality occurs frequently in segments of jejunum containing diverticula and can explain symptoms of partial intestinal obstruction and the blind-loop syndrome. Typical complaints of patients who are symptomatic from jejunal diverticulosis include crampy abdominal pain, intermittent abdominal distention, steatorrhea, flatulence, weight loss, and fatigue. The blind-loop syndrome is believed to be due to bacterial overgrowth in segments of bowel affected by jejunal dyskinesia. Bacterial overgrowth results in deconjugation of bile acids with resultant steatorrhea and malabsorption of fat-soluble vitamins. True mechanical obstruction can develop secondary to intestinal kinking, volvulus, or direct luminal compression caused by diverticular distention. In summary, the triad of obscure *abdominal pain, megaloblastic anemia, and dilated loops of jejunum should suggest small-bowel diverticulosis* (10). Colicky abdominal pain and borborygmi, in the absence of mechanical causes of obstruction, are consistent with jejunal dyskinesia.

In a recently reported series from the Mayo Clinic, 112 patients with jejunoileal diverticula were identified during a 15-year period (2). In 42% of the patients, the diverticula were considered incidental and the patients were asymptomatic. In the remaining 65 patients, symptoms included chronic abdominal pain (51%), diarrhea (58%), bloating (44%), weight loss (24%), and vomiting (11%). The mean duration of symptoms before a diagnosis was made was 22.5 months (2). *The most common symptom complex was chronic pain and malabsorption caused by bacterial overgrowth (40%).* The complications reported were obstruction (6%), perforation (5%), pseudo-obstruction (5%), gastrointestinal bleeding (2%), and diverticulitis without perforation (0.9%).

Diagnosis

Small intestinal diverticula are most often diagnosed incidentally by radiologic study or at laparotomy. In either case, diverticula can be difficult to demonstrate. The use of nonflocculating barium for radiologic study, along with manual compression of the abdomen and fluoroscopy, is often helpful. Fluoroscopic examination is essential, because contrast may not be retained for long in jejunal diverticula due to their typically wide ostia.

Enteroclysis is probably the most reliable radiologic technique for demonstration of small-bowel diverticula. This is best accomplished following placement of a nasoduodenal tube permitting direct filling of the small intestine. On small-bowel contrast examination, jejunal diverticula usually appear as collections of barium in continuity with the intestinal lumen or, alternatively, as semilunar air-containing shadows. Residual barium seen on delayed films may outline rounded or multiloculated lucencies corresponding to diverticula. Delayed films taken at 24 hours may help demonstrate ileal diverticula because these lesions tend to have narrow ostia and correspondingly slow emptying.

Ileal diverticula may be particularly difficult to demonstrate due to their small size and narrow neck. In addition, the terminal ileum may overlie previously filled loops of small bowel. It generally is believed that antegrade and retrograde barium contrast studies are equally effective in the demonstration of ileal diverticula. Ileal diverticula may have a somewhat different radiologic appearance than jejunal diverticula. Occasionally, three distinct layers may be seen: an upper layer of gas, a middle layer of intestinal contents, and a lower layer of barium contrast.

Small-bowel diverticula also may be difficult to identify at laparotomy. Because these acquired diverticula tend to protrude between the leaves of the mesentery, visualization may be limited. This is particularly true if the diverticula are collapsed. The demonstration of diverticula may be facilitated by milking of intestinal contents.

Selective angiography of the superior mesenteric artery during active bleeding, at a minimal rate of 1.0 mL/minute, may demonstrate findings typical of bleeding jejunal diverticula. These include pooling of contrast as a smooth-walled collection during the arterial and capillary phase, with rapid emptying of contrast into the intestinal lumen during the venous phase (11). Rapid emptying is typical of jejunal diverticula because these lesions tend to have wide ostia.

Under normal circumstances, the UGI tract contains less than 105 bacteria per milliliter. These are largely gram-positive aerobes and facultative anaerobes. Stasis due to jejunal dyskinesia may result in proliferation of bacteria and the blind-loop syndrome. The syndrome may be confirmed by breath test. Excessive bacterial utilization of a $[^{14}C]$ substrate, administered orally, such as $[^{14}C]$ xylose or $[^{14}C]$ cholyglycine, results in increased $[^{14}C]O_2$ production, which is detected by breath analysis (12).

Complications

Significant complications occur in approximately 5–10% of patients with jejunal diverticulosis. Complications of ileal diverticula are extremely rare, consisting primarily of diverticulitis, perforation, or ileal obstruction. *Most complications of jejunal diverticula are secondary to inflammation, stasis, or intestinal dyskinesia.* The blind-loop syndrome can cause megaloblastic anemia, steatorrhea, fat-soluble deficiency states, and hypoproteinemia. Inflammation with resultant ulceration within a diverticulum may cause massive hemorrhage due to erosion into a mesenteric vessel coursing next to the lesion. Inflammation also may result in localized perforation with mesenteric abscess formation or, less frequently, free perforation with generalized peritonitis. Occasionally, asymptomatic pneumoperitoneum has been reported. Jejunal dyskinesia itself can cause a functional nonmechanical small-bowel obstruction. True mechanical obstruction can develop secondary to intestinal kinking, volvulus, intussusception, or luminal compression by a dilated diverticulum. Development of a neoplasm within a small intestinal diverticulum is an exceedingly rare event; lipomas, fibromas, sarcomas, and adenocarcinomas have all been recorded, however.

Perforation and Inflammation

Perforation of small intestinal diverticula carries a mortality as high as 20–40% (5). Perforation may be difficult to recognize at laparotomy because much of the inflammation may be confined between the leaves of the mesentery. The specific preoperative diagnosis of perforated jejunal diverticulum also is difficult to make because the symptoms and signs are indistinguishable from those associated with many other inflammatory conditions, such as perforated peptic ulcer or acute pancreatitis. Similarly, the symptoms and signs associated with perforation/inflammation of an ileal diverticulum may be indistinguishable from those of acute appendicitis, cecal diverticulitis, Crohn's disease, and occasionally, sigmoid diverticulitis. Abdominal films may demonstrate localized or generalized pneumoperitoneum or retroperitoneal and/or intramesenteric air. CT may be helpful in making a precise diagnosis. Suggestive findings on CT include retroperitoneal air and/or intramesenteric air, along with evidence of inflammation such as bowel-wall thickening.

Small intestinal diverticulitis in the absence of perforation is a rare problem (13,14). The relative infrequency of inflammation may be due to the wide ostia of most jejunal diverticula facilitating drainage. Prompt drainage tends to prevent stasis with resultant bacterial proliferation and inflammation. Occasionally, enterolith formation within a diverticulum is responsible for stasis and inflammation. Enteroliths usually consist of bile and/or fatty acids deposited around a foreign body nidus, such as vegetable fiber. The low mineral content of most enteroliths usually precludes radiologic visualization. Another postulated mechanism for diverticular inflammation is retention of intestinal contents because of the paucity of muscle in the diverticular wall. The resultant stasis exposes the mucosa to alkaline duodenal contents, causing inflammation. As inflammation proceeds, the ostium narrows, eventually becoming obstructed. This results in bacterial proliferation, further inflammation, ischemia, and perforation. Perforation almost always occurs at the apex of a diverticulum corresponding to the point most removed from the blood supply (15).

A series of 33 patients with perforated jejunal and ileal diverticula has been reported by Herrington (13). In most of these cases, multiple diverticula were present, and in three cases, there were multiple perforations. The proximal jejunum was the most common site for perforation. Acute diverticulitis caused the perforation in 27 patients, whereas blunt trauma was the cause in four cases and a foreign body was the cause in two cases. The overall mortality was 21%; the correct preoperative diagnosis was made in only three instances. In the four patients with perforation of an ileal diverticulum, three additional complications were noted, namely right lower quadrant abscess, enterovesical fistula, and erosion into the right colic artery with massive gastrointestinal hemorrhage. *At laparotomy, for obscure causes of peritonitis and/or pneumoperitoneum, the small intestine must be examined carefully for diverticula*, possibly using air insufflation of the lumen as an adjunctive technique (5).

Hemorrhage

Massive gastrointestinal hemorrhage is one of the more common major complications of jejunal diverticula, although bleeding from ileal diverticula is extremely rare. Chronic or massive melena is the usual presentation; approximately one-third of patients have no other complaints related to the diverticula (16). Small-bowel diverticula develop at points of penetration of the bowel wall by mesenteric vessels. The diverticular wall is particularly prone to erosion, secondary to inflammation, trauma, or an enterolith, because the muscular layer is absent. Congenital arteriovenous malformations also have been reported as a very rare cause of hemorrhage from a jejunal diverticulum. *Selective angiography is the study of choice for active small intestinal bleeding*, permitting both diagnosis and localization. Despite successful preoperative localization of a bleeding site, it may be difficult to correlate radiologic findings with those at laparotomy.

Obstruction

Obstruction is probably the most common complication of small-bowel diverticula. Acute intestinal obstruction may be nonmechanical due to jejunal dyskinesia (pseudo-obstruction) or mechanical secondary to volvulus, kinking, intussusception, or direct compression of the lumen by a distended diverticulum. Volvulus of a jejunal diverticulum occurs occasionally when a large diverticulum rotates on its base and secondarily obstructs the bowel lumen. As with colonic diverticula, small-bowel diverticulitis may cause fibrotic scarring and resultant stenosis of the lumen. External adhesions also may form secondary to acute inflammation. Such adhesions may be responsible for kinking of the bowel or serve as a fulcrum for volvulus. Volvulus of the intestine in the absence of external adhesions is rare and has been ascribed to the increased weight of the affected segment due to accumulation of intestinal contents in a large diverticulum. Enteroliths or bezoars arising in jejunal diverticula also can cause intestinal obstruction. It has been suggested that intestinal spasm developing around a small enterolith causes the obstruction in some cases. More commonly, enterolith extrusion with obstruction of the lumen at a point distal to the diverticulum has been reported (17).

Management

For patients with proven but asymptomatic jejunal diverticula, no specific treatment is required, although a low-residue diet has been advocated by some to minimize the likelihood of diverticular inspissation. Symptomatic patients should be placed on a small frequent-feeding regimen. In addition, patients may be encouraged to rest in a supine position for 1 hour after meals whenever possible (18). The blind-loop syndrome with associated malabsorption often can be relieved by antibiotics with a spectrum of coverage for enteric organisms, including especially *Bacteroides* and the gram-negative species. Metronidazole or tetracycline may be used, either continuously or intermittently, for this purpose.

Failure to achieve relief of pain or symptoms may warrant consideration of surgical intervention. Surgical intervention is indicated specifically for complications including perforation with peritonitis or retroperitoneal sepsis, massive gastrointestinal hemorrhage, recurrent episodes of hemorrhage, or mechanical intestinal obstruction. *Resection of the involved bowel segment with primary anastomosis is the treatment of choice.* Exploratory diagnostic laparoscopy coupled with laparoscopic-directed small-bowel resection for jejunal diverticulitis with perforation has been reported (19). *Local excision and/or invagination is usually difficult and ill-advised* due to the intramesenteric position of most jejunal diverticula, as well as the presence of peridiverticular inflammation or scarring (5). The criteria for resection when diverticula are found as incidental findings at laparotomy have not been established due to great variability in the natural history of this condition. *In most cases, such incidentally found diverticula should not be resected unless there is evidence of peridiverticular inflammation.*

DIVERTICULAR DISEASE OF THE APPENDIX

Diverticula of the appendix are uncommon; the autopsy incidence is 0.20–0.66%, and the incidence in appendectomy specimens is 0.004–2.1% (20). Radiologic identification of appendiceal diverticula is rare with either retrograde or antegrade barium studies. Diverticula of the appendix are both congenital and acquired, but almost always the latter. Congenital diverticula consist of all layers of the bowel wall and usually are solitary. Acquired diverticula consist of mucosal and submucosal protrusions and frequently are multiple (21). There is associated hypertrophy of the submucosa and muscularis, along with narrowing of the appendiceal lumen. Acquired appendiceal diverticula usually occur in the absence of colonic diverticula (22).

Appendiceal diverticula in the absence of acute inflammation are asymptomatic. Inflammation of a diverticulum is notable for peridiverticular infiltration by neutrophils with spread of the inflammatory process into the periappendiceal fat and connective tissue. The process often culminates in abscess formation. The mucosa of the appendix usually is normal.

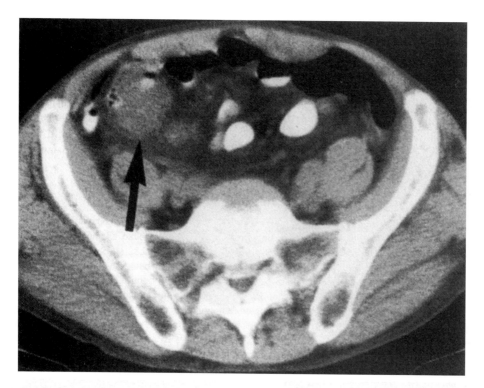

Figure 29.3. CT view of a patient with ileal diverticulitis. There is a mass lesion in the right lower quadrant with surrounding inflammation. (Reprinted with permission from Rosing MA, Amory S. Perforated ileal diverticulitis. An atypical presentation with definitive diagnosis by laparoscopy. Surg Endosc 1995;9:622–624.)

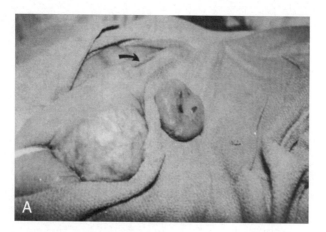

Figure 29.4. A., Operative view of an enterolith that originated in a jejunal diverticulum causing small bowel obstruction. (Reprinted with permission from Lopez PV, Welch JP. Enterolith intestinal obstruction owing to acquired and congenital diverticulosis. Dis Colon Rectum 1991;34:941–944.)   (*cont.*)

are diverticulitis and bleeding (23,26,29,30), but the variety of complications is extensive (31). Diverticula also may facilitate small-bowel obstruction by mechanisms such as volvulus (32) or formation of bezoars or enteroliths (Fig. 29.4) (33). The location of the diverticula near the mesentery may be related to the occasional development of pylephlebitis and liver abscesses (34–36) and the rarity of abdominal wall abscesses (37).

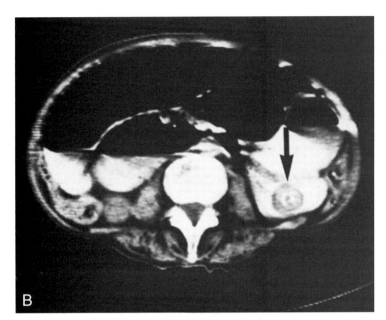

Figure 29.4. (*continued*) **B.,** CT view of an enterolith (arrow) that caused small bowel obstruction. (Reprinted with permission from Welch JP. Obturation obstruction. In: Welch JP, ed. Bowel obstruction. Differential diagnosis and clinical management. Philadelphia: WB Saunders, 1990:378–393.)

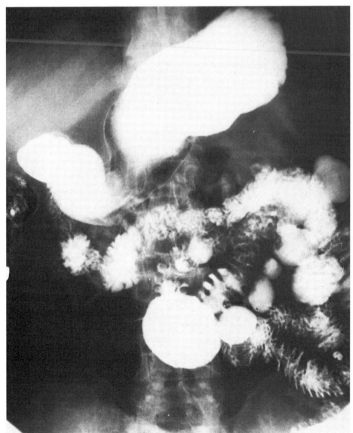

Figure 29.5. Multiple diverticula of differing sizes are present in this view from a small bowel series. (Reprinted with permission from Welch JP. Miscellaneous causes of small bowel obstruction. In: Welch JP, ed. Bowel obstruction. Differential diagnosis and clinical management. Philadelphia: WB Saunders, 1990:449–496.)

Useful "mapping" diagnostic tests for the surgeon include (a) enteroclysis in the elective setting to show the number and location of diverticula and possible other pathologies such as small bowel tumors (barium tends to flow out of the wide ostia during routine small bowel series) (Fig. 29.5) (38,39), and (b) CT scanning for acute complications such as perforation (Fig. 29.6). The abdominal surgeon should consider jejunoileal diverticula, in particular, in certain situations (Table 29.2).

When these patients are operated on, the entire small bowel should be examined, including the mesenteric border (Fig. 29.7). Air distention through a nasogastric tube or milking of fluid and air along the bowel may facilitate identification of diverticula (3,24,25). Diagnostic laparoscopy has been used to facilitate appropriate surgery through a small incision (40). Near the site of perforation, the mesentery is likely to be thickened, containing thickened lymph nodes. We favor resection and anastomosis rather than diverticulectomy (31) for major complications such as bleeding, obstruction, or perforation with surrounding soilage. Only the offending diverticula are removed if a long segment of bowel is involved by diverticula. Unfortunately, the mortality remains high, in the range of 20%, for major complications such as perforation (26). Increased awareness of this condition will be vital in an effort to improve these results.

Appendiceal diverticulitis is also an unusual entity that can be a source of right lower quadrant pain. The pathogenesis is unknown (41), although it has been proposed that false diverticula can develop after perforation of the appendix. It seems to cause a clinical picture distinct from acute appendicitis (42). Appendiceal diverticulitis occurs in an older age group than appendicitis, and the symptoms tend to be more chronic. However, some cases of diverticulitis can lead to peritonitis rapidly (43,44). If a diverticulum of the appendix is seen at surgery, appendectomy should be performed because of the significant risk of appendiceal diverticulitis at a later time.

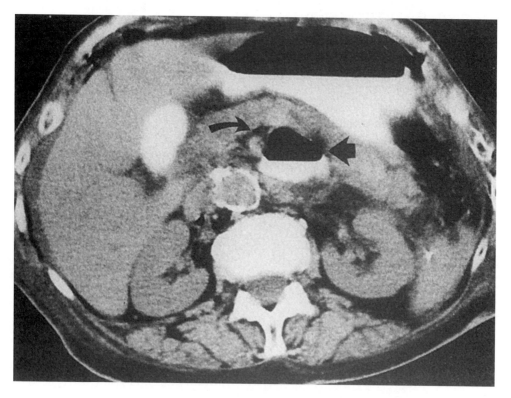

Figure 29.6.   This perforated retropancreatic jejunal diverticulum is partially filled with contrast (arrow). Extraluminal gas can be seen dissecting into the root of the mesentery (curved arrow) and the retroperitoneal fat adjacent to the inferior vena cava and both kidneys. (Reprinted with permission from Hibbeln JF, Gorodetsky AA, Wilber AC. Perforated jejunal diverticulum: CT diagnosis. Abdom Imaging 1995;20:29–30.)

Table 29.2.   Settings in Which Jejunoileal Diverticula Should be Suspected

Unexplained GI bleeding
Unexplained small intestinal obstruction
Unexpected cause of acute abdomen
Chronic abdominal pain
Anemia
Malabsorption

From Longo WW, Vernava AM III. Clinical implications of jejunoileal diverticular disease. Dis Colon Rectum 1992;35:381–388.

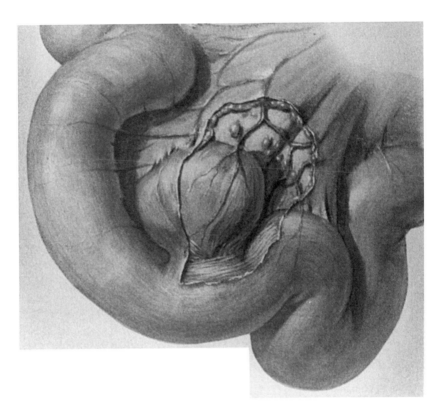

Figure 29.7.   Schematic view of a solitary diverticulum on mesenteric border of small intestine. (Reprinted with permission from Netter FH. The CIBA collection of medical illustrations. Part II: Lower digestive tract. West Caldwell, NJ: CIBA Pharmaceutical Co., 1952;3:129.)

REFERENCES

1. Wilcox RD, Shatney GH. Surgical complications of jejunal diverticula. South Med J 1988;81:1386–1391. *Fifteen percent of a group of 86 patients required surgery for various complications.*
2. Tsiotus GG, Farnell MB, Ilstrup DM. Non-Meckelian jejunal or ileal diverticulosis. Surgery 1994;116:726–732. *This disorder usually is asymptomatic and can be observed. Eleven of 20 patients with acute complications required surgery, with minimal morbidity and one death.*
3. Altemeier WA, Bryan LR, Wulsin JH. The surgical significance of jejunal diverticulosis. Arch Surg 1963;86:732–745. *Jejunal dyskinesia was prominent in 11 of 16 patients with symptomatic jejunal diverticulosis. The authors describe alternative treatment when complete resection of the diverticula is not possible.*

4. Christensen N. Jejunal diverticulosis. Am J Surg 1969;118:612–618. *Treatment with antibiotics may improve absorptive problems and decrease symptoms.*

5. Roses DF, Gouge TH, Scher KS, et al. Perforated diverticula of the jejunum and ileum. Am J Surg 1976;132:649–652. *The four patients reviewed had a more chronic history of abdominal pain.*

6. Brian JE Jr, Stair JM. Noncolonic diverticular disease. Surg Gynecol Obstet 1985;161:189–195. *A review with 46 references. A high incidence of suspicion is recommended to facilitate diagnosis and treatment.*

7. Edwarts HC. Diverticula of the duodenum and jejunum. Lancet 1934;1:169–174. *An interesting illustrated review of anatomic and clinical aspects.*

8. Krishnamorthy S, Kelly MM, Rohrmann CA, et al. Jejunal diverticulosis: a heterogeneous disorder caused by a variety of abnormalities of smooth muscle and myenteric plexus. Gastroenterology 1983;85:538–547. *The authors view the diverticula as one manifestation of an abnormal intestinal wall: the major problem is ineffective or uncoordinated motility.*

9. Benson RE, Dixon CF, Waugh JM. Non-Meckelian diverticula of the jejunum and ileum. Ann Surg 1943;118:337–393. *Describes a number of complications in a review of 122 patients, with 57 references.*

10. Nobles ER Jr. Jejunal diverticula. Arch Surg 1971;102:172–174. *A study of 15 patients. Jejunal diverticulosis can be suggested by the triad of obscure abdominal pain, anemia, and dilated loops of jejunum.*

11. Tisnado J, Konerding KF, Beachley MC, et al. Angiographic diagnosis of a bleeding jejunal diverticulum. Gastrointest Radiol 1979;4:291–293. *Selective arteriography successfully demonstrated a bleeding jejunal diverticulum preoperatively.*

12. Holt PR. The small intestine. Clin Gastroenterol 1985;14:713–723. *A portion of a monograph on gastrointestinal disorders in the elderly with numerous references.*

13. Herrington JL Jr. Perforation of acquired diverticula of the jejunum and ileum: analysis of reported cases. Surgery 1962;51:426–433. *The hospital mortality was 21% in a series of 33 cases.*

14. Sibille A, Willcox R. Jejunal diverticulitis. Am J Gastroenterol 1992;87:655–658. *Enteroclysis is recommended as the best diagnostic test.*

15. Zeifer HD, Goersch H. Duodenal diverticulitis with perforation. Arch Surg 1961;82:746–754. *Reviews a total of 23 cases. Surgical excision is recommended.*

16. Shackelford RT, Marcus WY. Jejunal diverticula: a cause of gastrointestinal hemorrhage: a report of three cases and review of the literature. Ann Surg 1960;151:930–938. *Most patients have multiple acquired diverticula along the mesenteric margin of a proximal jejunal segment.*

17. Lopez PV, Welch JP. Enterolith intestinal obstruction owing to acquired and congenital diverticulosis. Dis Colon Rectum 1991;34:941–944. *Twenty cases of bowel obstruction secondary to jejunal enterolithiasis and five cases secondary to Meckel's enterolithiasis were found in the literature.*

18. Brown JD, Woolverton W, Pearce CW. Jejunal dyskinesia: case report and review of the literature. South Med J 1969;62:1102–1106. *The dyskinetic activity is progressive, and cure can be accomplished with resection of the involved jejunum.*

19. Cross MJ, Synder SK. Laparoscopic-directed small bowel resection for jejunal diverticulitis with perforation. J Laparoendosc Surg 1993;3:47–49. *An 87-year-old patient underwent a successful laparoscopic-assisted small bowel resection.*

20. Lipton S, Estrin J, Glasser I. Diverticular disease of the appendix. Surg Gynecol Obstet 1989;168:13–16. *The authors found a 2% incidence of diverticular disease in a retrospective review of 3343 appendectomies. Diverticulitis usually occurs after the third decade with a long history, few gastrointestinal symptoms and an increased risk of appendiceal perforation.*

21. Collins DC: A study of 50,000 specimens of the human vermiform appendix. Surg Gynecol Obstet 1955;101:437–445. *A detailed pathologic analysis; 1.4% had acquired inflammatory diverticula, and 0.01% true congenital diverticula.*

22. Buffo GC, Clair MR, Bonheim P. Diverticulosis of the vermiform appendix. Gastrointest Radiol 1986;11:108–109. *Appendiceal diverticula tend to be multiple and are rarely associated with complications.*

23. Meagher AP, Porter AJ, Rowland R, et al. Jejunal diverticulosis. Aust N Z J Surg 1993;63:360–366. *A clinical review of 20 cases. Nine were complicated by inflammation or perforation. The diagnosis was delayed in 8 of 10 patients with chronic abdominal pain. The varying pathologic characteristics are detailed.*

24. Longo WW, Vernava AM III. Clinical implications of jejunoileal diverticular disease. Dis Colon Rectum 1992;35:381–388. *A detailed clinical review with 89 references. Resection and primary anastomosis is recommended for symptomatic diverticula that are operated on; a small percentage of patients with chronic abdominal pain may benefit from resection.*

25. Williams RA, Davidson DD, Serota AI, et al. Surgical problems of diverticula of the small intestine. Surg Gynecol Obstet 1981;152:621–626. *The mortality for the six patients having surgery was 50%.*

26. Chendrasekhar A, Timberlake GA. Perforated jejunal diverticula: an analysis of reported cases. Am Surg 1995;61:984–988. *The authors review 22 cases of perforated jejunal diverticula in the literature. Outcome was worsened when there was a longer duration of symptoms prior to operation.*

27. Resnick DJ, Ratych RE, Imbembo AL. Small-intestinal diverticula. In: Shackelford's surgery of the alimentary tract. 4th ed. Philadelphia: WB Saunders, 1996;5:417–445.

28. Krummen DM, Camp LA, Jackson CE. Perforation of terminal ileum diverticulitis: a case report and literature review. Am Surg 1996;62:930–940. *These are located close to the ileocecal valve. Perforation usually is considered to be appendicitis preoperatively.*

29. Palder SB, Frey CB. Jejunal diverticulosis. Arch Surg 1988;123:889–894. *Complications developed in 14 of 47 patients with jejunal diverticulosis.*

30. Ross CB, Richards WO, Bertram PD, et al. Diverticular disease of the jejunum and its complications. Am Surg 1995;56:319–324. *A discussion of four clinical cases and a review of the clinical spectrum of the disorder, with 33 references.*
31. Cools P, Bosmans E, Onsea J, et al. Small bowel diverticulosis. A forgotten diagnosis. Acta Chir Belg 1995;95:261–264. *Presents two case reports and reviews the literature.*
32. Chiu K-W, Changchien C-S, Chuah S-K. Small-bowel diverticulum: is it a risk for small-bowel volvulus? J Clin Gastroenterol 1994;19:176–177. *Small bowel diverticula are an independent risk factor for small bowel volvulus, at least in older people.*
33. Billings PJ, Farrington GH. Small bowel obstruction caused by bezoars from intestinal diverticula. Br J Surg 1987;74:1186. *A report of two cases; more than 20 others are reported in the literature.*
34. Hoover EL, Webb H, Walker C, et al. Perforated jejunal diverticulum with multiple hepatic abscesses. South Med J 1990;83:54–56. *A case report.*
35. Navarro C, Clain DJ, Kondlapoodi P. Perforated diverticulum of the terminal ileum. A previously unreported cause of suppurative pylephlebitis and multiple hepatic abscesses. Dig Dis Sci 1984;29:171–176. *The first report of suppurative pylephlebitis and liver abscess originating in ileal diverticulitis.*
36. Posthuma EF, Bieger R, Kuypers TJ. A rare cause of hepatic abscess: diverticulitis of the ileum. Neth J Med 1993;42:69–72. *A 41-year-old male recovered following drainage of the hepatic abscess and antibiotic therapy.*
37. Alvarez OA, Majia A, Ostrower VS, et al. Jejunal diverticulitis manifesting with abdominal wall abscess. Am J Gastroenterol 1995;90:2060–2062. *A rare case of jejunal diverticulitis associated with fistula formation and an abdominal wall abscess. Because of the location of diverticula at the mesenteric border, perforation usually is associated with intra-abdominal abscesses.*
38. Maglinte DD, Chernish SM, DeWeese R, et al. Acquired jejunoileal diverticular disease: subject review. Radiology 1986;158:577–580. *Of 519 patients having enteroclysis, 12 (2.3%) had small bowel diverticula.*
39. Freimanis M, Plaza-Ponte M. Radiologic diagnosis of jejunal diverticulum. Gastrointest Radiol 1988;13:312–314. *Criteria for the diagnosis of colonic peridiverticular inflammation were applied to the small bowel in a contrast study.*
40. Rosing MA, Amory S. Perforated ileal diverticulitis. An atypical presentation with definitive diagnosis by laparoscopy. Surg Endosc 1995;9:522–524. *A case report. Diagnostic laparoscopy facilitated placement of a small incision over the pathology.*
41. Trollope ML, Lindenauer SM. Diverticulosis of the appendix: a collective review. Dis Colon Rectum 1974;17:200–218. *Only 43 of 1373 appendiceal diverticula reviewed were of the "true" or congenital type. Includes 175 references.*
42. Deschenes L, Couture J, Garnea R. Diverticulitis of the appendix. Report of sixty- one cases. Am J Surg 1971;121:706–709. *Sixty-one cases of acute diverticulitis of the appendix are compared with 61 cases of acute appendicitis chosen at random. Periappendiceal inflammation was more common with diverticulitis, but generalized peritonitis occurred in less than 10% of both groups.*
43. Delikaris P, Teglbjaerg PS, Fisker-Sorensen P, et al. Diverticula of the vermiform appendix. Alternative of clinical presentation and significance. Dis Colon Rectum 1983;26:374–376. *A study of 10 patients with appendiceal diverticular disease seen over 1 year.*
44. Ladin P. Diverticulosis and diverticulitis of the vermiform appendix. A brief review and report of sixteen cases. Arch Surg 1951;62:514–519. *The author speculates that weakening of the wall by infection together with increased intraluminal pressure due to obstruction/secretion leads to development of diverticula in the appendix.*
45. Bloch C, Bryk D. Diverticular disease of the terminal ileum. Mt Sinai J Med 1976;43:122–128. *A discussion of four cases with a number of views from contrast studies.*
46. Hibbeln JF, Gorodetsky AA, Wilber AC. Perforated jejunal diverticulum: CT diagnosis. Abdom Imaging 1995;20:29–30. *Case report of a perforated jejunal diverticulum extending into the retroperitoneum.*
47. Welch JP. Miscellaneous causes of small bowel obstruction. In: Welch JP, ed. Bowel obstruction. Differential diagnosis and clinical management. Philadelphia: WB Saunders, 1990:449–496.
48. Welch JP. Obturation obstruction. In: Welch JP, ed. Bowel obstruction. Differential diagnosis and clinical management. Philadelphia: WB Saunders, 1990:378–393.
49. Netter FH. The CIBA collection of medical illustrations. Part II: Lower digestive tract. West Caldwell, NJ: CIBA Pharmaceutical Co., 1952;3:129.

30 Giant Diverticula of the Colon

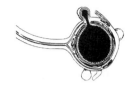

Nilto Carias de Oliveira, MD
John P. Welch, MD

> ## KEY POINTS
> - A rare consequence of diverticular disease
> - Usually involves sigmoid colon in elderly patients
> - Actual mechanisms of formation are unknown
> - Vague symptoms with a soft, mobile abdominal mass
> - Resection and anastomosis preferred

A fascinating complication of diverticular disease is the occasional evolution of a giant diverticulum, also described by terms such as giant air cyst, solitary gas cyst, or pneumocyst of the colon.

ILLUSTRATIVE CASE

A 70-year-old female was seen in a physician's office complaining of mild lower abdominal pain and diarrhea. The pain was steady in nature and had not been progressive in severity. She had noted some irregularity of bowel habits over several months, but no vomiting, gastrointestinal bleeding, or weight loss. She had not taken antibiotics recently. Past operations included a hysterectomy and appendectomy. A 12-cm soft, moderately tender, mobile midabdominal mass was palpable.

Laboratory studies included a hematocrit level of 45%, white cell count of 11,000 with a left shift, a normal urinalysis, sedimentation rate of 45, and normal serum amylase. A plain film showed a radiolucent structure in the lower abdomen (Fig. 30.1).

A Foley catheter was inserted without release of gas or disappearance of the mass effect. Intravenous fluids and antibiotics were started. A computed tomography (CT) scan showed that the cystic structure arose from the sigmoid colon, whereas the kidneys, duodenum, and retroperitoneum were normal. A barium enema was not performed because of the possibility of peritonitis.

After 2 days, the abdominal mass remained but fever and abdominal tenderness abated. The white blood cell count fell to 5000. An oral bowel preparation was started, and the patient was operated on during the fourth hospital day. Ureteral stents were placed before the incision was made. A large cyst involving the sigmoid colon was found, surrounded by omental adhesions and densely adherent to the bladder and transverse mesocolon. Numerous diverticula were present in the sigmoid, but there was no evidence of an abscess

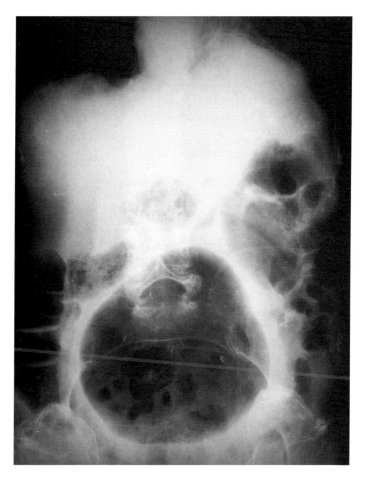

Figure 30.1. Plain film of the abdomen shows a prominent air-filled structure that proved to be a giant sigmoid diverticulum.

or perforation. The mass was resected in continuity with the colon and a primary anastomosis was constructed successfully.

CASE COMMENTS

A number of diagnoses should be considered in a case such as this (Table 30.1). The rarity of giant colonic diverticula also should be kept in mind. A colonic volvulus would not be suspected, considering the appearance of the abdominal film. Any form of biliary disease or duodenal diverticulum is also unlikely, considering the location of the cyst. A duplication cyst, pancreatic pseudocyst, dilated bowel loop, or a bladder disorder must be ruled out.

The CT scan allowed an early diagnosis. This was preferable to a barium enema, because the abdominal tenderness suggested that some form of peritonitis could have been evolving.

Early operation could have been elected. In the absence of generalized peritonitis or pneumoperitoneum, however, it was possible to prepare the bowel for a one-stage resection and anastomosis. As anticipated, the pelvic dissection was difficult because of adhesions to the giant diverticulum; ureteral stents simplified identification of the ureters.

**Table 30.1.   Gas-Filled Abdominal Mass:
Differential Diagnosis**

Giant sigmoid diverticulum
Congenital duplication of colon
Cholecystenteric fistula
Colonic volvulus
Emphysematous cholecystitis
Infected pancreatic pseudocyst
Pneumatosis cystoides intestinalis
Meckel's diverticulum
Intra-abdominal abscess
Giant duodenal diverticulum
Dilated intestinal loop
Gastric dilatation
Tubo-ovarian abscess
Mesenteric cyst

DISCUSSION

Despite the high frequency of diverticular disease in the western world, the development of a giant diverticulum in an individual is highly unlikely. Both sexes are affected equally. Seventy-eight cases were reported in the English literature from 1946 until 1989 [1,2], primarily in elderly patients, averaging 66 years in one review [1]. Only 12% of patients are younger than 50 years of age. The diverticula may be as large as 30–40 cm in diameter [2,3] and are an average of 13 cm in diameter [1]. Two large diverticula may occur concurrently [4]. Some are asymptomatic, found by chance during radiologic or physical examination; others can lead to acute or chronic symptoms. The sigmoid colon is involved almost exclusively, although rare giant diverticula have involved the transverse [5,6] and descending colon [7].

The mechanisms of formation of giant diverticula are speculative. One theory involves a ball-valve mechanism related to fecal material intermittently occluding the neck of the diverticulum. Air may be forced into the diverticulum and become trapped as the intraluminal pressure in the colon increases. Another conceivable mechanism is enlargement of the cyst by gas-producing microorganisms when the neck is obstructed by inflammation or fecal residue. Because some diverticula have wide necks at least 2 cm in diameter [8] (Fig. 30.2), the latter theory, in particular, is not very convincing.

There probably are several pathologic types of giant diverticula; McNutt et al have described three of these [9]. A few lesions are true diverticula containing all three layers of the bowel wall [10,11]. *Most are pseudodiverticula (no muscle wall) that gradually increase in size.* This type of diverticulum is lined by chronic granulation tissue interspersed with colonic mucosa. Another form of diverticulum has an inflammatory wall and does not contain any layers of the colon wall [9]; it could be termed a pseudocyst. *Most giant diverticula (except true diverticula) arise on the antimesenteric border of the bowel.*

Clinical presentations can be acute or chronic. *Classically, patients have vague, chronic abdominal symptoms such as bloating.* Less frequently, symptom complexes are acute, when perforation, torsion, or focal infarction of the cyst occur [11]. *Abdominal pain (85%) and an abdominal mass (71%), usually soft and somewhat mobile, are the commonest associations* [1]. There may be tympany over the cyst [12,13]. Fever, diarrhea, gastrointestinal bleeding, and nausea and vomiting are seen in lesser frequencies. Some patients are asymptomatic [7], without an abdominal mass.

The natural history of these cysts is to enlarge (documented in some patients who have either refused surgery or had sequential radiographs), with potential development of dangerous complications such as perforation or volvulus. However, 13% of the cysts have led to major complications such as free perforation (14), small bowel obstruction (15), volvulus (16), or focal infarction (4). Colon carcinoma has been found in a giant diverticulum (7). Peritoneal irritation may be caused by enlargement of the cyst, and cyst enlargement may occur with defecation (17).

An extremely valuable diagnostic test is the plain film of the abdomen. Virtually all films show a solitary gas-filled cyst (Fig. 30.1), usually in the lower abdomen associated with the sigmoid colon, although the upper abdomen or entire abdomen may be involved (2). An air–fluid level may be present within the lucency, approximately 25% of the time (18). The gas density may disappear, corresponding to disappearance of the palpable mass (19). If a barium enema is performed (Fig. 30.3), approximately 45–65% of the cysts are opacified (1,13,20), and the close relationship of the cyst to the sigmoid colon can be seen. Multiple other diverticula usually are present. *A barium enema or CT scan (Figs. 30.4 and 30.5) usually suffices to differentiate a giant sigmoid diverticulum from the other abnormalities in the radiologic differential diagnosis,* listed in Table 30.1.

These other disorders can be distinguished from giant diverticula in a number of ways. Gas in the bladder is readily voided or emptied by a Foley catheter. Meckel's diverticula tend to occur in the terminal ileum of younger patients, and duodenal diverticula are in a different abdominal location, verified with an upper gastrointestinal series. Intestinal duplications are also seen in younger patients in relation to the mesenteric portion of the bowel, and they tend to involve the ileum rather than the sigmoid. They are elongated in

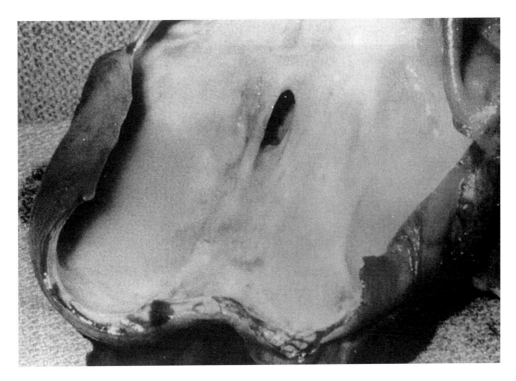

Figure 30.2. A large communication between the colon and a giant diverticulum is shown. (Reprinted with permission from Levi DM, Levi JU, Rogers RI, et al. Giant colonic diverticulum: an unusual manifestation of a common disease. Am J Gastroenterol 1993;88:139–142.)

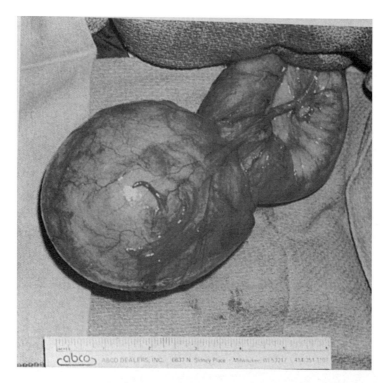

Figure 30.6. Appearance at laparotomy of a giant diverticulum of the sigmoid colon. (Reprinted with permission from Kempczinski RF, Ferruci JT Jr. Giant sigmoid diverticula: a review. Ann Surg 1974;180:864–867.)

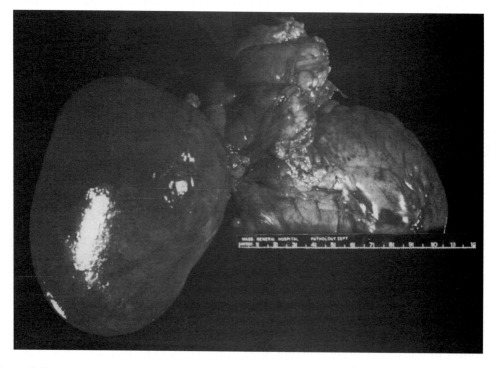

Figure 30.7. A resected specimen of sigmoid colon containing a giant diverticulum. (Reprinted with permission from Ueda P, Hall D. Images in clinical medicine. Giant colonic diverticulum. N Engl J Med 1995;333:228) [Ref. 25].

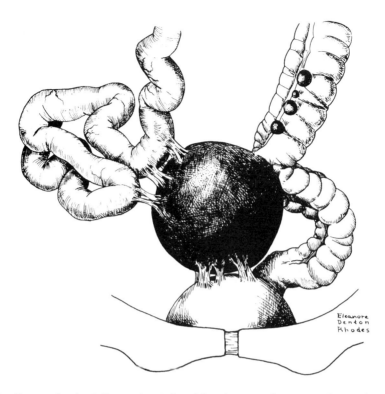

Figure 30.8. Frequently, the inflammation induced by the expanding giant diverticulum leads to dense adherence to surrounding organs such as the bladder or the distal small bowel.

the remaining portions of the cyst wall led to survival of an elderly patient with a huge cyst filling most of the anterior abdomen (2). A simple diverticulectomy usually is not advised because of the wide mouth of the diverticulum and surrounding inflammation (increasing the risk of breakdown of the bowel closure) and the presence of other nearby diverticula. Simple diverticulectomy has been described in a few reports without serious sequelae (6,10), although a postoperative fecal fistula has been seen (22). If there is infarction or perforation (23) of the cyst with established peritoneal contamination, a Hartmann procedure is a useful alternative. Operative deaths are rare, at least in reported cases (1,24), and recurrences have not been reported.

EDITORIAL COMMENTS

Giant diverticula usually arise from the sigmoid colon. This rare diagnosis is suggested by plain radiographs and confirmed by barium enema or CT scan. The treatment of symptomatic lesions should be resection and primary anastomosis. The surgeon should be prepared for the possibility of a difficult resection because of adhesions to adjacent organs and structures. The treatment of asymptomatic incidentally diagnosed giant diverticula is unclear. We recommend elective resection with primary anastomosis, unless the cyst is quite small or the patient is at high risk for elective operation.

REFERENCES

1. Gallagher JJ, Welch JP. Giant diverticula of the sigmoid colon. A review of differential diagnosis and operative management. Arch Surg 1979;114:1079–1083. *Two cases are described, along with a review of 46 others in the literature.*

2. Scerpella PR, Bodensteiner JA. Giant sigmoid diverticula. Report of two cases. Arch Surg 1989;134:1244–1246. *Recommends earlier surgical intervention for these patients.*

3. Mainzer F, Minagi H. Giant sigmoid diverticulum. Am J Roentgenol 1971;113:352–353. *Describes a giant diverticulum in a 38-year-old female.*

4. Kempczinski RF, Ferruci JT Jr. Giant sigmoid diverticula: a review. Ann Surg 1974;180:864–867. *One of two patients had two large cysts on the antimesenteric border of the colon.*

5. Lapeyrie H, Balmes P, Loizon P, et al. Diverticule géant du colon transverse. J Chir 1988;125:717–720. *States that pathogenesis of a giant diverticulum involves progressive increase in size of an ordinary diverticulum.*

6. Wallers KJ. Giant diverticulum arising from the transverse colon of a patient with diverticulosis. Br J Radiol 1985;54:683–684. *The diverticulum was excised at its neck with a smooth postoperative course.*

7. Kricun R, Stasik JJ, Reither RD, et al. Giant colonic diverticulum. Am J Roentgenol 1980;135:507–512. *A report of five patients. One had carcinoma arising within the diverticulum and another had free perforation and peritonitis.*

8. Wetstein L, Camera A, Trillo RA, et al. Giant sigmoidal diverticulum: report of a case and review of the literature. Dis Colon Rectum 1978;21:110–112. *Prophylactic surgical intervention is recommended before complications occur.*

9. McNutt R, Schmitt D, Schulte W. Giant colonic diverticula — three distinct entities: report of a case. Dis Colon Rectum 1988;31:624–628. *The authors followed a giant sigmoid diverticulum over a period of 8 years. Three pathologic types of giant colonic diverticula are described.*

10. Al-Jurf AS, Fougar E. Uncommon features of giant colonic diverticula. Dis Colon Rectum 1983;23:808–813. *Both diverticula in this report were situated outside the sigmoid colon.*

11. Sutorius JD, Bossert JE. Giant sigmoid diverticulum with perforation. Am J Surg 1974;127:745–748. *The first report of a perforation of a giant diverticulum.*

12. Patel D, Diab W. Giant colonic diverticulum. N Y State J Med 1983;83:750–754. *A case report with a good discussion of the differential diagnosis of a rounded radiolucency on the abdominal film.*

13. Levi DM, Levi JU, Rogers RI, et al. Giant colonic diverticulum: an unusual manifestation of a common disease. Am J Gastroenterol 1993;88:139–142. *Recommends resection to alleviate symptoms and avoid complications.*

14. Harris RD, Anderson JE, Wolf EA. Giant air cysts of the sigmoid complicating diverticulitis: report of a case. Dis Colon Rectum 1975;18:418–424. *Detailed review of 31 cases. Emphasizes that most lesions are pseudocysts.*

15. Ona FV, Salamone RP, Mehnert PJ. Giant sigmoid diverticulitis, a cause of partial small bowel obstruction. Am J Gastroenterol 1980;73:350–352. *Small-bowel obstruction is an unusual complication of giant diverticula.*

16. Silberman EL, Thorner MC. Volvulus of giant sigmoid diverticulum. JAMA 1961;177:782–784. *A 15-cm diverticulum twisted on its neck and formed a closed loop obstruction.*

17. Frankenfeld RH, Waters CH, Schepeler TU. Giant air cyst of the abdomen: an unusual manifestation of diverticulitis of the sigmoid: report of a case. Gastroenterology 1959;37:103–106. *The diverticulum inflated to a giant cyst during episodes of straining.*

18. Casas DJ, Tenesa M, Alastrue A, et al. Case report: uncommon radiological and pathological features of giant colonic diverticula. Clin Radiol 1991;44:125–127. *This patient had two giant diverticula on the mesenteric border of the sigmoid colon.*

19. Maresca L, Maresca C, Erikson E. Giant sigmoid diverticulum. Report of a case. Dis Colon Rectum 1981;24:191–195. *Documents growth of the diverticulum over 3 years.*

20. Wetrich RM, Sidhu DS. Giant sigmoid diverticulum. West J Med 1979;128:539–541. *The gas collection in the giant colonic diverticulum was intimately related to the sigmoid colon but did not fill during a barium enema.*

21. Fields SI, Haskell L, Libson E. CT appearance of giant colonic diverticulum. Gastrointest Radiol 1987;12:71–72. *Discusses the value of CT in the diagnosis and evaluation of these lesions.*

22. Ritchie AJ, Carson JG, Humphreys WG. Encysted pneumatocele: a complication of diverticular disease. Br J Surg 1991;78:683. *One patient developed a fecal fistula after local excision of the cystic mass, requiring later sigmoid colectomy.*

23. Ellerbroek CJ, Lu CC. Unusual manifestations of giant colonic diverticulum. Dis Colon Rectum 1984;27:545–547. *Describes two cases, with atypical location, age, and complication by pneumoperitoneum.*

24. Naber A, Sliutz A-M, Freitas H. Giant diverticulum of the sigmoid colon (review). Int J Colorectal Dis 1995;10:168–172. *Reviews reports of 70 patients, with 50 references.*

25. Ueda P, Hall D. Images in clinical medicine. Giant colonic diverticulum. N Engl J Med 1995;333:228.

31 Diverticulitis of the Transverse Colon

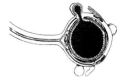

Faek Jamali, MD
John P. Welch, MD

> ### KEY POINTS
>
> - A rare form of colonic diverticulitis
> - Patients average 49 years of age
> - Clinical picture can be variable
> - Appendicitis suspected preoperatively
> - Barium enema and CT scan useful
> - Often confused with carcinoma at operation
> - Usually resection is performed

This chapter reviews an entity that the clinician almost never encounters. Fortunately, the mortality of the disease is not high, and most patients end up under a surgeon's care before irreversible sepsis occurs.

ILLUSTRATIVE CASE

A 58-year-old man presented with a 24-hour history of right upper quadrant abdominal pain and low-grade fever. He complained of anorexia but no fatty food intolerance or vomiting. He denied any changes in bowel or urinary habits, except for two loose bowel movements during the past 24 hours. There was no history of biliary or peptic ulcer disease. He took prednisone (5 mg daily) for asthmatic symptoms.

Vital signs included blood pressure of 140/80, pulse of 90 (regular), and temperature of 100°F by mouth. The patient did not seem to be chronically ill. There was no scleral icterus or adenopathy. The chest was clear. His abdomen was mildly tender in the right upper quadrant with some involuntary guarding extending downward to the level of the umbilicus. No masses were palpable, and there was no marked rigidity or rebound tenderness. The bowel sounds were hypoactive.

The treating clinicians suspected cholecystitis and began administering an intravenous cephalosporin. The hematocrit was 46%, white cell count was 17,000 with a left shift, lactate dehydrogenase (LDH) was 1,200 mg/dL, serum amylase was normal, and liver function tests were otherwise normal. Abdominal films showed no appendicolith, evidence of bowel obstruction, or pneumoperitoneum. However, an abdominal ultrasound showed a normal gallbladder, liver, and kidneys. Although he complained of some abdominal pain, the patient was otherwise stable. A computed tomography (CT) scan was performed soon thereafter, suggesting an inflammatory process involving the hepatic flexure of the colon. Numerous diverticula were present in the colon, and no clear intraluminal mass was present to suggest a neoplasm. A normal appendix was seen in the right lower quadrant. Some free fluid lay in the right paracolic gutter and pelvis, but no collection suggestive of an abscess was seen.

419

Because appendicitis seemed to be ruled out with the possibility of a benign process involving the colon without perforation, additional supportive treatment was elected instead of early laparoscopy or laparotomy. With continued antibiotic infusion, the abdominal tenderness lessened and the fever lysed within 36 hours. A liquid diet was started, and he was discharged on general liquids 2 days later. He had no additional symptoms such as fever, abdominal pain, diarrhea, or weight loss. A colonoscopy 1 month later showed diverticula throughout the colon and no evidence of a mass or inflammatory changes.

CASE COMMENTS

In this case, noninvasive studies were instrumental in making the possible diagnosis of diverticulitis of the transverse colon. Early laparoscopy/laparotomy with possible colectomy were avoided. Of importance, the CT scan visualized a normal appendix in its normal position in the right lower quadrant away from the locus of the abdominal pain; pneumoperitoneum and pericolic abscess were absent as well.

A more aggressive approach would be advised in a number of situations. If the appendix appeared to extend into the inflammatory mass with a visible appendicolith, laparoscopy or laparotomy would be considered; conversely, a phlegmon attributed to appendicitis can be treated expectantly, especially in the absence of an appendicolith. Development of pneumoperitoneum or spreading peritonitis would warrant expeditious laparotomy. A pericolic abscess could be treated percutaneously (if accessible to the interventional radiologist) or by surgery. The approach taken here differs from most published reports in which the inflammatory mass was encountered surgically and resected, because of the suspicion of carcinoma. Because carcinoma of the colon was not seen at the later colonoscopy, subsequent colectomy was unnecessary. Similar non-operative therapies have been recommended for certain patients with right-sided diverticulitis or phlegmons due to appendicitis. The likelihood of a repeat episode of diverticulitis involving the transverse colon probably is low, although this conservative approach is not discussed in literature reports.

DISCUSSION

For the purposes of this discussion, diverticulitis of the transverse colon includes involvement of the hepatic and splenic flexures. The first case was reported by Thompson and Fox in 1944 (1), and less than 20 cases had been recorded by 1979 (2). Presently, approximately 30 cases are documented in the English medical literature. The incidence of transverse colon diverticulitis in the pool of all patients treated surgically for diverticular disease is clearly very low (3); in one series, 3 of 338 patients (0.9%) were affected (4). Autopsy studies suggest that approximately 20% of patients with diverticular disease have involvement of the transverse colon (Fig. 31.1) (5).

There are two morphologic types of transverse colonic diverticula: (*a*) congenital or "true" diverticula, containing all layers of the bowel wall (frequently solitary); or (*b*) acquired pseudodiverticula (through defects in the circular muscle at points of entry of blood vessels), which resemble sigmoid diverticula and are frequently multiple (Fig. 31.2). Giant diverticula also can occur in the transverse colon (6). *More than two-thirds of the cases of diverticulitis of the transverse colon described pathologically have involved single diverticula (7).*

Diverticulitis of the transverse colon is reminiscent of right-sided disease, in which involved diverticula frequently are solitary. Patients tend to be young. *Diverticulitis of the*

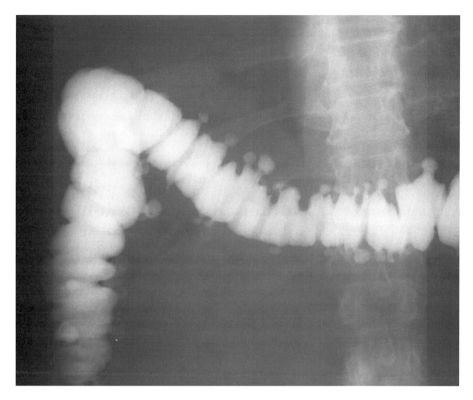

Figure 31.1.   Barium enema view showing a number of diverticula in the transverse colon. There is no evidence of diverticulitis.

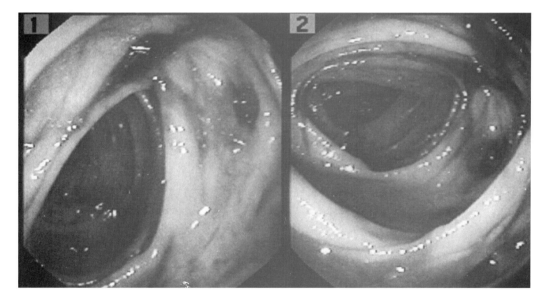

Figure 31.2.   Colonoscopic appearance of diverticula in the midtransverse colon. Multiple diverticula usually are pseudodiverticula lacking a muscular layer at the site of a blood vessel penetrating the bowel wall.

transverse colon affects individuals averaging only 49 years of age, 15–20 years younger than those with sigmoid diverticulitis (7). Most patients are female (8). Diverticulitis of the cecum or ascending colon is much more common, however, and hundreds of cases have been described (see Chapter 32).

The clinical presentation of perforated transverse colon diverticulitis is less "classic" and specific than that of sigmoid diverticulitis; the latter is sometimes coined "left-sided appendicitis." Abdominal pain is the most common symptom, but fever tends to be infrequent (8). *More common disorders usually are suspected by the clinician* (especially when the hepatic flexure region is involved with diverticulitis), including perforated duodenal ulcer, acute cholecystitis, acute pyelonephritis, perforating cancer of the colon, Crohn's disease, or acute appendicitis (Fig. 31.3). Less common diseases to consider include infarction of an appendix epiploica or a psoas abscess. The tip of a long appendix can extend into the right upper quadrant, or a shorter appendix can extend into this area from a high, mobile cecum. In the same fashion, diverticulitis involving a low-lying transverse colon on an elongated mesentery can mimic acute appendicitis (9) or another inflammatory process in the lower abdomen, such as ileitis, Meckel's diverticulitis, or a gynecologic disorder.

Unusual presentations also are possible, including formation of a colocutaneous or internal fistula (10,11) or subcutaneous emphysema of a lower extremity (see Chapter 28) (12). Patients treated with peritoneal dialysis may be at increased risk of developing peritonitis when diverticula are present in the transverse colon (13). Left upper quadrant

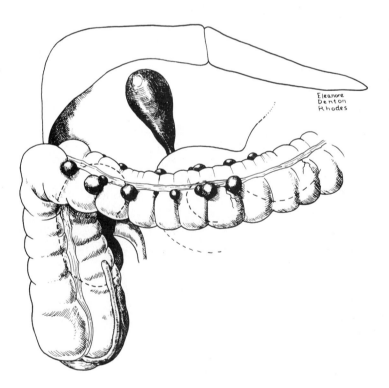

Figure 31.3.   Because diverticulitis of the transverse colon is rare, more common disorders involving adjacent organs must be considered, such as peptic ulcer disease, pyelonephritis, and appendicitis. The tip of an inflamed appendix can reach into the right upper quadrant, whereas the mobile transverse colon can extend into the right lower quadrant.

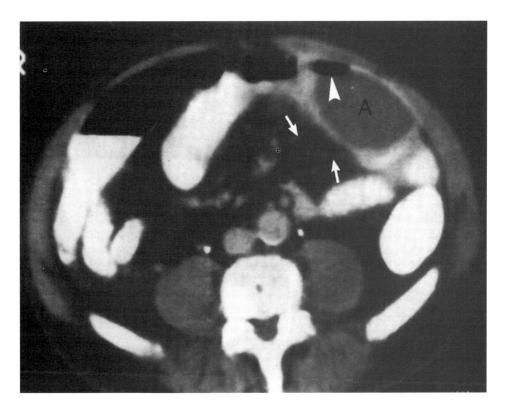

Figure 31.4. CT scan view of diverticulitis of the transverse colon causing a pericolic abscess. There is an air–fluid level (arrowhead) in the abscess **(A)**. The vascularity in the small bowel mesentery is increased (arrows). (Reprinted with permission from Feldberg MAM , Hendriks MJ, Van Waes PFG. Role of CT in diagnosis and management of complications of diverticular disease. Gastrointest Radiol 1985;10:370–377.)

pain caused by diverticulitis can be confused with inflammatory processes in the tail of the pancreas or a splenic abscess. Based on the rarity of this disorder and the nonspecific presenting symptoms, *it is understandable that the preoperative diagnosis is rarely correct in patients undergoing surgery.*

Transverse colon diverticulitis most often masquerades as appendicitis; nine of 20 cases in one literature review were attributed to acute appendicitis (2). Pain, in fact, occurs most frequently in the right lower quadrant, although leakage from the splenic flexure has led to left lower quadrant pain (8). *Patients tend to have a lengthy duration of symptoms,* typically 1–2 weeks or more, rather than a 12- to 48-hour episode following the onset of pain, which is characteristic of acute appendicitis. Upper gastrointestinal symptoms such as nausea and vomiting are more frequent with appendicitis; they may occur if ileus or small bowel obstruction accompanies the diverticulitis. A previous appendectomy should suggest the possibility of transverse colon diverticulitis. Occasionally, an abdominal mass is palpable; its position will depend on the mobility of the transverse colon on its mesentery.

Leukocytosis is present and abdominal films usually do not provide additional clues. Rarely, a fecalith is present in the transverse colon or an air–fluid level is seen within an abscess cavity. If acute appendicitis is not suspected, medical treatment with intravenous fluids and antibiotics, bowel rest, and possible nasogastric suction is preferred for the "stable" patient without peritonitis or hemodynamic instability. *CT scanning has become the examination of choice in most centers* (Fig. 31.4) (14). Although ultrasonography can detect an intra-abdominal abscess or cholecystitis and cholelithiasis, bowel gas will interfere with detection of an abnormality in the wall of the colon or in the pericolic region.

Barium studies are of diagnostic use, showing sites of fistulization and extravasation and helping differentiate benign from malignant disease (Figs. 31.5 and 31.6). Potential risks of barium enema examination include extravasation of barium with the potential to develop barium peritonitis. Resection has been performed successfully despite barium extravasation in literature reports; this may reflect the relative safety of resection and anastomosis when the proximal colon is involved with diverticulitis. A barium enema may (Fig. 31.7) or may not show inflammatory changes (2), which theoretically would be detected with CT.

If there is early resolution of fever and abdominal pain with medical treatment alone, or if the patient is stable with minimal findings of peritonitis, colonoscopy or barium enema /CT scan should be considered to rule out a perforating colon cancer. Colonoscopy also allows biopsy of the colon in the event of other types of colitis. If an abscess is detected by CT, percutaneous drainage allows control of the infection and later elective colon resection (see Chapter 15). More urgent CT scanning or ultrasonography can be performed as in the preceding illustrative case of the patient with peritoneal signs. These studies may give enough diagnostic information to further support medical management.

Conversely, when the patient is clinically unstable, resuscitation and prompt operation should be performed without additional testing. This could include laparotomy preceded by laparoscopy. In many instances, the disease may turn out to be appendicitis and a laparoscopic procedure such as an appendectomy or closure of a perforated ulcer may be possible, depending on the diagnosis. The finding of a normal appendix should prompt

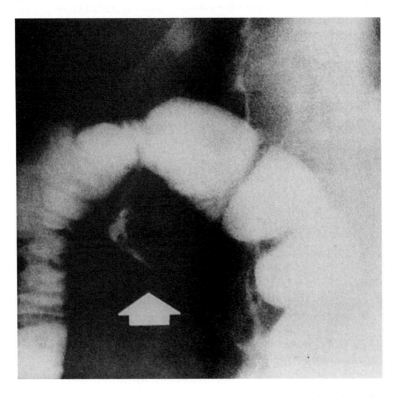

Figure 31.5.   Extravasation of barium (arrow) from perforated diverticulitis at the splenic flexure is visible in this barium enema view. (Reprinted with permission from Peck MD, Villar HV. Perforated diverticulitis of the transverse colon. West J Med 1987;147:81–84.)

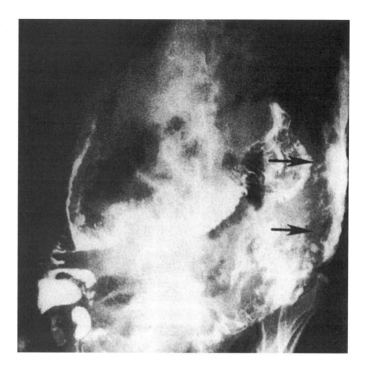

Figure 31.6. Extravasation of barium into the retroperitoneum of the left flank caused by perforated diverticulitis at the splenic flexure. (Reprinted with permission from Peck MD, Villar HV. Perforated diverticulitis of the transverse colon. West J Med 1987;147:81–84.)

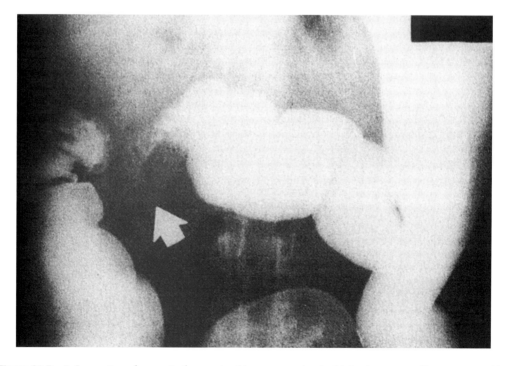

Figure 31.7. Inflammatory changes in the proximal transverse colon in this barium enema film were caused by a perforated colonic diverticulum with a pericolic abscess. (Reprinted with permission from Peck MD, Villar HV. Perforated diverticulitis of the transverse colon. West J Med 1987;147:81–84.)

a more thorough abdominal examination, looking for disorders such as peptic ulcer disease, cholecystitis, enteritis, colon cancer, or colitis.

When inflammation is found involving the transverse colon during laparoscopy, immediate laparotomy and medical treatment (if the patient is stable) are possible alternatives. It would be difficult to identify a carcinoma of the colon definitively with laparoscopy alone; intraoperative colonoscopy would not be feasible because the colon would be unprepped. In the rare event that a single diverticulum is found surrounded by minimal inflammation at laparotomy, a diverticulectomy could be performed with primary closure of the colonic wall. This form of treatment has been quite successful for right-sided diverticulitis (15). In most instances, there will be an inflammatory mass, suggesting colon cancer with localized perforation. For this reason, *the surgeon usually proceeds to colonic resection*, either a segmental one or a right colectomy to include the affected part of the transverse colon. A generous mesenteric resection is favored when the exact diagnosis is in question. With diverticulitis as the splenic flexure, an extended left hemicolectomy is an alternative if extensive diverticulosis is also present in the sigmoid colon (and the patient's history suggests symptomatic sigmoid diverticular disease). The decision whether to perform an anastomosis should rest on the patient's clinical status, the degree of contamination, and the presence or absence of established peritonitis. A significant number of patients reported in the literature have done well after resection and anastomosis, despite perforation of the unprepped transverse colon (3,8), with entry into a pericolonic abscess (8). Deaths have occurred less than 15% of the time in reported cases, usually related to large intra-abdominal abscesses and associated sepsis (8,12,16).

EDITORIAL COMMENTS

Preoperative diagnosis of diverticulitis of the transverse colon requires a high index of clinical suspicion. The disease is discovered most commonly serendipitously during radiologic workup (CT scan). When the appendix is well visualized and there is no free perforation, abscess or overt sepsis, treatment with broad-spectrum antibiotics, and bowel rest should lead to resolution of symptoms. Subsequently, colonoscopy or barium enema should be performed to rule out carcinoma or colitis. If surgery is required in the acute setting, it should consist of resection at the involved segment. The decision to reanastomose the colon should depend on the degree of contamination and the overall condition of the patient.

REFERENCES

1. Thompson GF, Fox PF. Perforated solitary diverticulum of the transverse colon. Am J Surg 1944;66:280–283. *This 35-year-old patient had a freely perforated diverticulum near the hepatic flexure and survived a two-stage procedure.*
2. McClure ET, Welch JP. Acute diverticulitis of the transverse colon with perforation. Report of three cases and review of the literature. Arch Surg 1979;114:1068–1071. *This report summarizes 19 case reports in the English literature. Primary resection was recommended during open laparotomy.*
3. Chughtai SQ, Ackerman NB. Perforated diverticulum of the transverse colon. Am J Surg 1974;127:508–510. *A clinical experience with six patients seen over a 10-year period.*
4. Rodkey GV, Welch CE. Colonic diverticular disease with surgical treatment: a study of 338 cases. Surg Clin North Am 1974;54:655–674. *A comprehensive summary of the surgical approaches over one decade (1964–1973), with 117 references.*
5. Hughes LE. Post mortem survey of diverticular disease of the colon. Gut 1969;10:336–351. *One patient in 200 autopsies had isolated diverticula at the splenic and hepatic flexures. Twenty of 90 patients with diverticula had diverticula both in the transverse colon and in other areas of the colon.*
6. Wallers KJ. Giant diverticulum arising from the transverse colon of a patient with diverticulosis. Br J Radiol 1981;54:683–684. *The diverticulum was suspected to arise from the upper gastrointestinal tract because of its high placement in the abdomen on plain radiographs; the lesion was excised at its neck after late films from a barium follow-through made the diagnosis.*

7. Shperber Y, Halevy A, Oland J, et al. Perforated diverticulitis of the transverse colon. Dis Colon Rectum 1986;29:466–468. *Sixty-three percent of patients in this literature review were suspected to have carcinoma at surgery.*

8. Peck MD, Villar HV. Perforated diverticulitis of the transverse colon. West J Med 1987;147:81–84. *This review summarizes 30 cases of transverse colon diverticulitis in the literature.*

9. Wong JB, Neistadt JS, Winkley JH. Perforated solitary diverticulitis of the transverse colon (letter). Arch Surg 1974;108:249. *A phlegmon was found situated below the umbilicus in the low-lying transverse colon. Appendicitis was suspected preoperatively.*

10. Ghahremani GG, Olsen J. Gastrocolic fistula secondary to diverticulitis of the splenic flexure: report of a case. Dis Colon Rectum 1974;17:98–99. *A pericolic abscess eroded through the gastric wall; the fistula was seen by barium enema.*

11. Rao UP, Venkitzchalam PS, Posner GL, et al. Diverticulitis manifesting as transverse colocutaneous fistula: report of a case and review of literature. Dis Colon Rectum 1980;23:44–48. *The first report of a spontaneous colocutaneous fistula originating in diverticulitis of the transverse colon.*

12. Pickels RF, Karmody AM, Tsapogas MJ, et al. Subcutaneous emphysema of the lower extremity of gastrointestinal origin: report of a case. Dis Colon Rectum 1974;17:98–99. *Prominent symptoms, including erythema of a lower extremity, developed in a patient with diabetes when transverse colonic diverticulitis communicated with a psoas abscess and, subsequently, the groin.*

13. Tranaeus A, Heimburger O, Granqvist S. Diverticular disease of the colon: a risk factor for peritonitis in continuous peritoneal dialysis. Nephrol Dial Transplant 1990;5:141–147. *Peritoneal dialysis patients had an increased risk of developing peritonitis when diverticula were located in the transverse colon as opposed to the sigmoid.*

14. Feldberg MAM , Hendriks MJ, Van Waes PFG. Role of CT in diagnosis and management of complications of diverticular disease. Gastrointest Radiol 1985;10:370–377. *A comprehensive review discussing the anatomic consequences of perforation of different segments of the colon, including the transverse colon. The use of CT in surgical decision-making is also discussed.*

15. Ngoi S, Chia J, Goh MY, et al. Surgical management of right colon diverticulitis. Dis Colon Rectum 1992;35:799–802. *Diverticulectomy or nonoperative treatment were successful in all but 3 of 68 patients.*

16. Vaziri M. Perforated solitary diverticulitis of the transverse colon (letter). Arch Surg 1974;109:588. *This patient developed a large abscess in the posterior aspect of the abdominal wall near the umbilicus. She died 5 weeks after resection.*

32 Cecal Diverticulitis

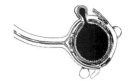

Alan G. Thorsen, MD
Charles A. Ternent, MD

KEY POINTS

- 35–84% of colonic diverticula in the Far East
- 20 years younger than patients with sigmoid diverticulitis
- Most cecal diverticula are false
- Inflammation most common complication — 13%
- Diagnosed preoperatively in 5%
- Nonresection or diverticulectomy for grade I/grade II disease
- Right colectomy for grade III/grade IV disease, failed treatment or possible cancer

ILLUSTRATIVE CASE

A 42-year-old white male complained of a 72-hour history of worsening right lower quadrant pain. He denied nausea, emesis, or diarrhea. His temperature was 38.5°C, pulse was 88, blood pressure was 125/80 mm Hg, and respirations were 12 per minute. Blood work showed a white blood cell (WBC) count of 15,000 and hematocrit of 44%. Urinalysis was normal. Physical examination showed localized rebound tenderness in the right lower quadrant without a palpable mass. Rectal examination showed no masses or tenderness.

Upright and flat abdominal films showed an ileus pattern without free air. An imaging study was obtained in view of the atypical presentation, failure of the pain to migrate from the periumbilical region to the right lower quadrant, and long prodrome for acute appendicitis. A computed tomography (CT) scan of the abdomen showed pericecal inflammation with a 1-cm air- and contrast-filled area anteromedially extending through a thickened cecal wall. The terminal ileum was normal and the appendix seemed to be involved in the process. The preoperative diagnosis was perforated acute appendicitis.

At laparotomy, through a right lower quadrant incision, a normal terminal ileum and appendix were noted. A 4-cm locally perforated anteromedial cecal mass was present. This process was suspicious for a perforated cecal carcinoma. A right hemicolectomy with primary ileotransverse anastomosis was performed through an extended transverse right lower quadrant incision. Histology showed an anteromedially located, inflamed, and perforated false cecal diverticulum, 2 cm from the ileocecal valve. The appendix was normal.

CASE COMMENTS

This is a "classical" presentation of cecal diverticulitis; after the CT scan, the perforated appendicitis was suspected because of the frequency of appendicitis. The exact diagnosis was not clear at laparotomy, and based on the possibility of perforated cecal cancer, right colectomy was chosen. An anastomosis was believed to be safe because there was not widespread peritonitis.

INTRODUCTION

The diagnosis and treatment of cecal diverticulitis was first reported by Potier in 1912 (1). Theories suggest that cecal diverticula may be congenital or acquired through genetic, environmental, and iatrogenic factors. Cecal diverticulitis, by definition, includes inflamed diverticula of the colon caudal to the ileocecal valve. However, cases of diverticulitis of the ascending colon commonly are included in the literature pertaining to cecal diverticulitis. Cecal diverticula can be solitary or multiple and may be associated with other colonic diverticula. They may contain all layers of the bowel wall (true diverticula) or, more commonly, may have an attenuated or absent submucosa and muscularis propria (false diverticula). Large series of cecal diverticulitis emanate from the Orient and Hawaii, where right-sided diverticulosis is predominant (2–8).

Despite advances in imaging techniques and a growing number of documented cases, preoperative and intraoperative diagnosis of cecal diverticulitis may still be difficult. Cecal diverticulitis may present as a projecting fingerlike, inflamed appendage of the large bowel or as a mass hidden within the cecal wall. It is most often found at the time of emergent laparotomy for presumed acute appendicitis. Treatment options at the time of laparotomy include appendectomy combined with either antibiotic therapy or diverticulectomy, as well as right hemicolectomy.

EPIDEMIOLOGY

Cecal and ascending colon diverticula account for 35%, 69%, and 84% of colonic diverticula in Thailand, Singapore, and Japan, respectively (2,9,10). In series from Australia and the West, diverticulosis is mostly localized to the sigmoid colon (11). However, right-sided diverticulitis is not restricted to those of Oriental descent. In Hawaii, 10–16% of cecal diverticulitis occurs in Caucasians (5–13). *Right-sided diverticulitis occurs, on average, at 40 years of age,* whereas left-sided diverticulitis occurs at 59 years of age (2,4,5,12).

The Orient has experienced an increase in diverticular disease of the colon associated with industrialization and adoption of a Westernlike low-fiber diet (2). Nevertheless, *most diverticular disease of the colon in the Orient continues to occur on the right side* (14). This suggests that a genetic role is at least partially responsible for the development of acquired diverticula of the cecum and ascending colon. Some investigators conclude that the anatomic site of diverticula is related to race whereas the prevalence is related to dietary habits (10).

PATHOLOGY

The wall of the intraperitoneal colon is composed of an inner mucosa-muscularis mucosae, submucosa, muscularis propria, and an outer serosa. True diverticula contain all layers of the bowel wall (Fig. 32.1). False diverticula of the colon (Fig. 32.2) are made up of mucosa, muscularis mucosae, and attenuated or totally absent submucosa and muscularis propria (15). Histologic findings in false right-sided diverticular disease vary

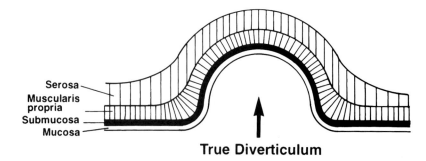

Serosa
Muscularis propria
Submucosa
Mucosa

True Diverticulum

Figure 32.1.   Schematic diagram of a true diverticulum of the colon containing all layers of the bowel wall.

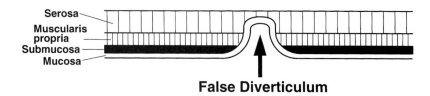

Serosa
Muscularis propria
Submucosa
Mucosa

False Diverticulum

Figure 32.2.   Schematic diagram of a false diverticulum of the colon with mucosa but absent submucosa and muscularis propria.

from a superficial mucosal invagination to full-thickness protrusion through a muscular defect at the site of vasa recta (16). Most cecal diverticula range from 0.2 to 1.5 cm in diameter (11) and are located anteromedially, anterolaterally, and posteriorly in 45%, 38%, and 17% of the cases, respectively (3). Microscopically, the earliest sign of diverticular inflammation is seen within lymphoid aggregates at the apex of the diverticulum. The localized infection can remain at the apex of a projecting diverticulum and can be easily recognized at laparotomy or can dissect along the outer aspect of the muscularis propria to form a hidden type of cecal diverticulitis (17).

Classically, cecal diverticula are believed to contain all layers of the bowel wall and to be wide, solitary, congenital, and located within 2.0 cm of the ileocecal valve (18,19). This description resembles the rare anomaly of an appendix duplex in which a cecal outgrowth forms during the sixth week of human embryologic development and fails to atrophy (20). However, *most cecal diverticula fail to conform to this pattern of a true and solitary entity*. A histologic examination of 39 predominantly right-sided solitary diverticula of the colon found all specimens to be of the false variety (16).

Acquired diverticula may be true or false. Theories on the origin of acquired true cecal diverticula include pulsion, with or without adhesions, and postappendectomy changes of the cecum (9). False cecal diverticula may arise from changes in the intraluminal pressure of the colon. Manometric studies have shown increased intraluminal pressure at rest, postprandially, and after neostigmine administration in the right colon of patients with right-sided diverticulosis (21).

True colonic diverticula containing all layers of the bowel wall (Fig. 32.3) were believed to be a myth when no true diverticula were identified in 200 autopsies that included 24 cecal diverticula (11). However, a recent review of the American literature found true diverticula in 41% of specimens resected for cecal diverticulitis (22). Figure 32.4 shows an attenuated muscularis propria at the apex of a false diverticulum of the colon. Such a false diverticulum may be mistaken as a true diverticulum if apical inflammation destroys the

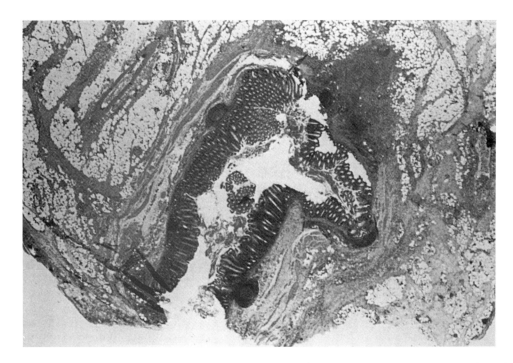

Figure 32.3. Histologic cross-section of cecal diverticulitis with layers of muscularis propria reaching the inflamed apex. This was presented as an inflamed, true cecal diverticulum. (Reprinted with permission from Tan EC, Tung KH, Tan L, et al. Diverticulitis of the cecum and ascending colon in Singapore. J R Coll Surg Edinb 1984;29:373–376.)

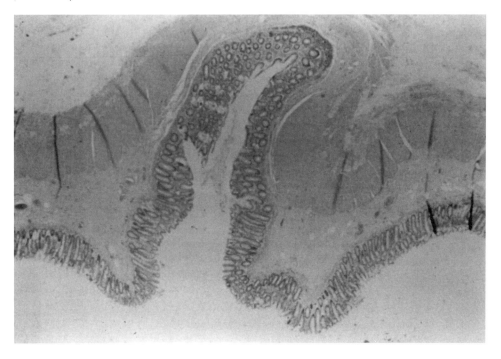

Figure 32.4. Histologic cross-section of a false diverticulum of the colon with mucosa, compressed submucosa, and apically attenuated muscularis propria. (Courtesy of Dr. T. Smyrk, Department of Pathology, Bishop Clarkson Hospital, Omaha, NE.)

areas of attenuated or absent submucosa and muscularis propria. The discrepancy between the number of true and false diverticula of the colon found by autopsy studies without inflammation and those involving specimens of cecal diverticulitis may result from this distortion of the layers of a false diverticulum secondary to inflammation. Thus, *the true cecal diverticulum may be less common than suggested by some studies.*

A study of diverticular disease in Japan showed microscopic thickening of the inner circular and outer longitudinal muscle in segments of colon affected with diverticulosis (14). The increased thickness does not result from hypertrophy or hyperplasia, but from elastosis (17,23). As the taeniae shorten, the redundant bowel forms more haustra. Increased haustration of the colon has been related to a greater number of diverticula. Normally, the muscularis propria is thinnest in the cecum and ascending colon and thickest in the sigmoid colon. This may explain why the muscle abnormality in right-sided diverticular disease has been macroscopically unnoticed in the past. Microscopy of the muscularis propria of the right colon suggests that right-sided diverticulosis, like left-sided disease, is associated with thickening of this muscle layer (14).

NATURAL HISTORY

Inflammation is the most common complication of cecal diverticula and is estimated to occur in 13% of patients with cecal diverticulosis (2,11,12,24). Patients younger than 40 years of age with diverticula of the right side may suffer from diverticulitis more frequently than older patients (2). Data compiled from the literature show an equal distribution of cecal diverticulitis among the sexes (2,4,7,12,19,24–35).

The incidence of diverticulitis has been related to the number of diverticula but not to the location within the colon. Therefore, the greater number of reports of right-sided diverticulitis in the Far East and Hawaii may be due to a greater number of diverticula within the cecum and ascending colon at risk for inflammation (2).

In the continental United States, projecting cecal diverticulitis has been estimated to occur in 1 in 1100 and hidden cecal diverticulitis has been estimated to occur in 1 in 800 laparotomies for an acute abdomen (36). However, another study from the continental United States reported five cases of cecal diverticulitis in 1750 appendectomies (frequency, 1 in 350). All five cases were of the hidden type and presented as a mass mimicking a cecal carcinoma (37). In Kuwait, nine cases of cecal diverticulitis were reported in eight people of Far Eastern nationalities and in one American from among 800 cases of presumed acute appendicitis (frequency, 1 in 90) (38).

Cecal diverticulitis can result from inspissation of feces and obstruction of the diverticular lumen by a fecalith, which is found in 25–49% of the cases (28,32). Carcinomas and polyps can also encroach on the diverticular lumen and instigate inflammation.

Complications of cecal diverticulitis include phlegmon, abscess, perforation, sepsis, fistulization, pylephlebitis, and obstruction. Perforation has been reported in 20% of cases of cecal diverticulitis and carries a mortality as high as 80% when delay in recognition and treatment occurs (12,24,26). Cecal diverticulitis can occur on any aspect of the bowel wall. Perforation can form an intra-abdominal, retrocecal, intramesenteric, or intramural abscess or diffuse peritonitis (29).

DIAGNOSIS

The classic presentation of cecal diverticulitis includes right lower quadrant pain in 86% (duration greater than 24 hours in 73%), nausea in 24%, emesis in 12%, an average WBC count of 12,600 (28), and an average temperature of less than 38.3°C (22). It is associated with an abdominal mass on physical examination in 26–68% of cases (28,39).

Frequently, cecal diverticulitis cannot be differentiated from acute appendicitis by history or physical examination (12). *Acute appendicitis is the preoperative diagnosis in more than two-thirds of cases of cecal diverticulitis.* Only approximately 5% of diverticular inflammation of the cecum is correctly diagnosed preoperatively. However, preoperative diagnosis improves to 16–24% with a greater index of suspicion. *A history of prior appendectomy, similar episodes of right lower quadrant pain in the past, and a previous diagnosis of right-sided diverticulosis may also enhance the ability to make a correct diagnosis preoperatively* (5,13,38).

An American review of 1000 patients operated on for presumed acute appendicitis found two cases of cecal diverticulitis and one case of cecal carcinoma; all three were perforated (40). Finding a normal appendix at laparotomy for acute appendicitis should trigger a careful and methodic abdominal exploration, which should start with mobilization and complete inspection of the cecum. Other considerations in the differential diagnosis of cecal diverticulitis include mesenteric adenitis, Meckel's diverticulitis, perforated duodenal ulcer, infectious and inflammatory colitis, cholecystitis, foreign body perforation, ischemic colitis, pelvic inflammatory disease and other gynecologic pathology, cecal endometriosis, pancreatitis, and left-sided diverticulitis irritating the parietal peritoneum of the right lower quadrant.

The preoperative diagnosis of cecal diverticulitis is not reliable by means of blood work or plain abdominal films. Additional diagnostic studies may be indicated when there are chronic or atypical symptoms of acute appendicitis, when a palpable mass is found on physical examination, or when the appendix is surgically absent (25).

Barium enema has been reported to have a 50% sensitivity for diagnosing cecal diverticulitis (41). Preoperative diagnosis of cecal diverticulitis, using barium enema, was reported in 6 of 30 patients with right lower quadrant pain and a history of appendectomy (28). Barium enema findings in cecal diverticulitis include irregular filling defects, pericecal inflammation, and frank perforation, as well as visualization of cecal diverticula and a normal appendix (Fig. 32.5) (38,41).

Ultrasonography of the right lower quadrant may show uncomplicated cecal diverticulitis as hypoechoic round or oval foci protruding from a segmentally thickened colonic wall. Computed tomographic (CT) findings suggestive of cecal diverticulitis include linear streaky densities in the pericecal fat, bowel wall thickening, and intramural abscess. Abdominal ultrasonography and CT scanning may be complementary to the barium enema study and may allow early diagnosis of cecal diverticulitis in selected cases (Fig. 32.6). However, unless imaging studies show an uncomplicated inflamed cecal diverticulum and a normal appendix, the findings of a thickened bowel wall or pericecal abscess are not diagnostic of cecal diverticulitis (41,42).

Laparoscopy may localize inflammation to the cecum but offers minimal conclusive diagnostic evidence in cases of cecal diverticulitis (26). Similarly, colonoscopy has been shown to have a low diagnostic yield in the setting of acute diverticular inflammation of the colon (43).

Intraoperative diagnosis of cecal diverticulitis is made in 50–89% of cases that are undiagnosed preoperatively (5,25). *Intraoperative findings can vary from an easily recognized inflamed diverticulum to a cecal mass with perforation and diffuse peritonitis. A clinical classification of cecal diverticulitis according to the degree of inflammation and contamination (Fig. 32.7) is helpful to establish a safe and comprehensive treatment plan. Grade I disease represents a locally inflamed, easily identified cecal diverticulum without perforation. Grade II represents an uncomplicated cecal wall mass. Grade III encompasses the previous two*

Figure 32.5.   Barium enema view of 30-year-old man with cecal diverticulitis. The appendix is normal and there is an irregular contour of the posterior cecal wall. There are multiple diverticula of the ascending colon (arrowheads). (Reprinted with permission from Balthazar EJ, Megibow AJ, Gordon RB, et al. Cecal diverticulitis: evaluation with CT. Radiology 1987;162:79–81.)

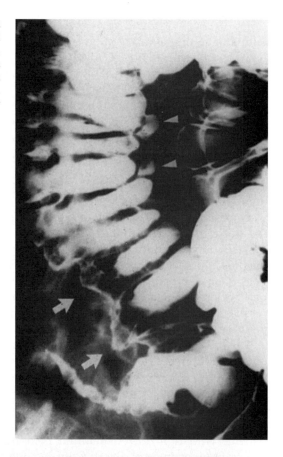

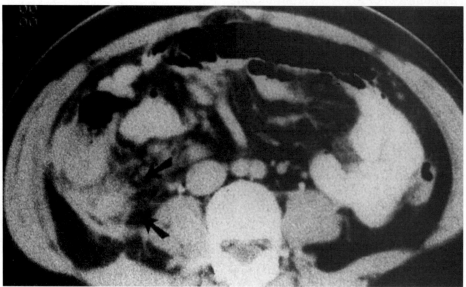

Figure 32.6.   Cecal diverticulitis in same patient as in Figure 32.5 This CT view shows extensive pericecal inflammation (arrows). The inflammatory process, causing thickening and blurring of the adjacent fascial planes, is posterior in location. (Reprinted with permission from Balthazar EJ, Megibow AJ, Gordon RB, et al. Cecal diverticulitis: evaluation with CT. Radiology 1987;162:79–81.)

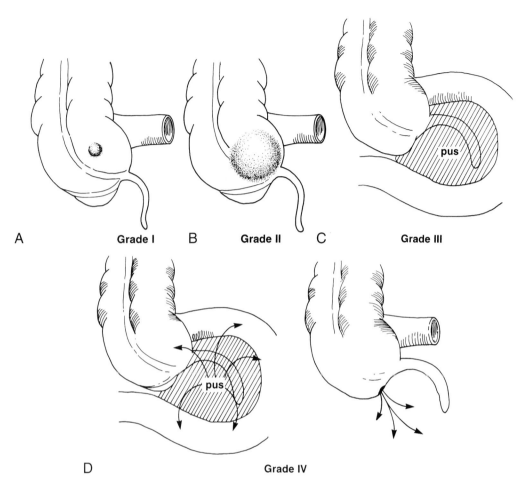

Figure 32.7. Schematic representation of the spectrum of findings in cecal diverticulitis. **A.**, Grade I is an easily recognized projecting inflamed cecal diverticulum. **B.**, Grade II is a cecal mass. **C.**, Grade III encompasses a localized abscess or fistula. **D.**, Grade IV is a free perforation or ruptured abscess with diffuse peritonitis. (Modified from Greaney EM, Snyder WH. Acute diverticulitis of the cecum encountered at emergency surgery. Am J Surg 1957;94:270–281; and Wagner DE, Zollinger RW. Diverticulitis of the cecum and ascending colon. Arch Surg 1961;83:124–131.)

categories complicated by localized abscess or fistula. *Grade IV* cecal diverticulitis is associated with purulent or feculent peritonitis.

A correct intraoperative diagnosis of cecal diverticulitis is likely in grade I disease and less frequently in grade II disease. *Cecal diverticulitis associated with abscess or diffuse peritonitis (grade III or IV) frequently is misdiagnosed as a perforated carcinoma.*

TREATMENT

Since 1912, when Potier (1) described an appendectomy and excision of an inflamed cecal diverticulum, reports have described a wide range of therapeutic options to treat this condition. We believe that the rare case of preoperatively diagnosed uncomplicated cecal diverticulitis is best treated with observation and broad-spectrum antibiotic therapy. The

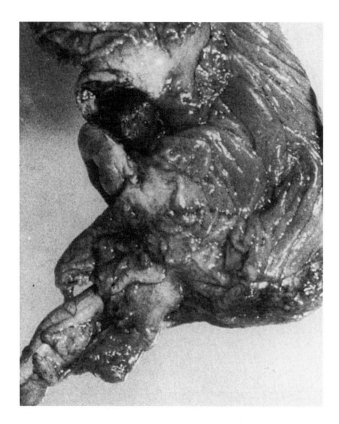

Figure 32.8.   Large, opened cecal diverticulum with a fecalith. (Reprinted with permission from Schuler JG, Bayley J. Diverticulitis of the cecum. Surg Gynecol Obstet 1983;156:743–748.)

indications for surgical intervention in this setting are the same as for left-sided diverticulitis and include recurrence, obstruction, perforation, abscess, and fistula formation (25).

More commonly, the presentation of cecal diverticulitis is similar to that of acute appendicitis, and expedient laparotomy is required. Intraoperatively, the surgeon finds a normal appendix and terminal ileum with various degrees of diverticular and cecal inflammation (Figs. 32.8 and 32.9). Based on a review of 213 cases of right-sided diverticulitis in the literature, a grade I process was identified in 4%, grade II disease was identified in 68%, grade III disease was identified in 22%, and grade IV disease was identified in 1% (2–5,13, 19,24,25,27,28,30–34,36,38,40,41,44,45). At the time of laparotomy, *treatment options for cecal diverticulitis include: (a) appendectomy, nonresection of the diverticulum, and postoperative antibiotic therapy; (b) appendectomy and diverticulectomy; and (c) right hemicolectomy. Appendectomy should accompany nonresection or diverticulectomy, when the base of the appendix is not inflamed, to avoid confusion at a later date.*

In most instances, the scenario is emergent and the finding of cecal diverticulitis is unexpected. The most appropriate treatment must take the severity of disease into account. Figure 32.10 provides an algorithm for the treatment of cecal diverticulitis based on the time of diagnosis and the disease grade. Intraoperative nonresectional therapy of cecal diverticulitis, in a group of 49 patients with grade I–III disease (compiled from the literature) showed 0% and 2% perioperative mortality and morbidity, respectively. Ten

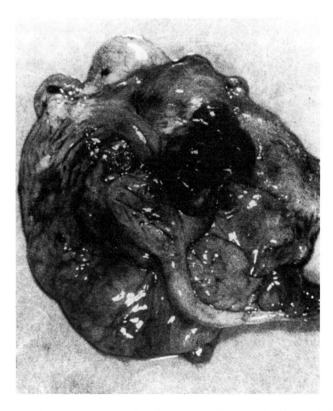

Figure 32.9. Gangrenous diverticulum protruding from cecum. (Reprinted with permission from Schuler JG, Bayley J. Diverticulitis of the cecum. Surg Gynecol Obstet 1983;156:743–748.)

Algorithm for treatment of cecal diverticulitis

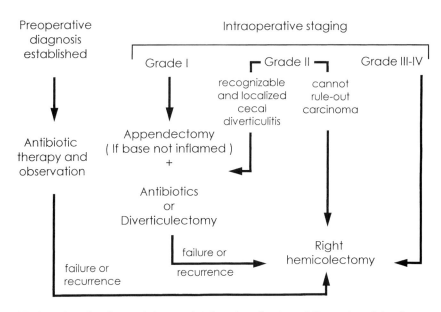

Figure 32.10. Algorithm for cecal diverticulitis based on the time of diagnosis and the disease grade.

percent required a colectomy at an average follow-up of 3.6 years. Failure of nonresectional management of cecal and ascending colon diverticulitis decreased from 10% to 6% when grade III disease was excluded from the analysis (3,5,31,36,41).

Diverticulectomy or wedge resection and appendectomy is an alternative treatment for localized cecal diverticulitis. A TA-55 surgical stapler can be used as long as the resection margins are free of gross inflammation and the remaining ileocecal region is not compromised. A review of 47 cases of grade I–IV cecal and ascending colon diverticulitis treated with diverticulectomy showed 0% and 8% perioperative mortality and morbidity, respectively. Two fecal fistulas and one wound dehiscence resulted when diverticulectomy was applied to grade III and grade IV cecal diverticulitis. One recurrence required a right hemicolectomy 6 months after diverticulectomy (25,28,30–34,36,38,40,44). Nonresection or diverticulectomy for cecal diverticulitis are therapeutic options with comparable morbidity, mortality, and risk of failure requiring right hemicolectomy (Table 32.1). These findings suggest that *nonresection or diverticulectomy is best applied to uncomplicated and recognizable cecal diverticulitis (grade I and possibly grade II).*

At laparotomy, most grade II–IV cecal diverticulitis may be difficult to distinguish from a carcinoma. We avoid cecotomies because of the increased risk of intra-abdominal bacterial contamination and the potential spread of tumor if a carcinoma is found. *When the diagnosis is not clear and localized perforation or abscess is present, we believe that a right hemicolectomy and primary anastomosis are indicated.*

A compiled literature review of 117 cases of grade II–IV right-sided diverticulitis treated with right hemicolectomy between 1950 and 1993 showed 14% perioperative morbidity and 1.6% mortality. One death occurred in a patient with a pericecal abscess and an internal fistula (grade III) who underwent a right hemicolectomy and primary anastomosis. Another death occurred when a free perforation of a cecal diverticulum (grade IV) was treated with resection and diversion (2–5,13,19,24,25,27,32,33,36,38,41,44,45). *Cecal diverticulitis with diffuse peritonitis (grade IV) and an APACHE-II score greater than 15 is treated*

Table 32.1.   Operative Treatment for Cecal Diverticulitis by Grade and Procedure: Summary of Results in the Literature, 1950–1993

Procedure	n	Morbidity (%)	Mortality (%)	Colectomy (%)	Follow-up (Months)
Nonresection/antibiotics					2–120
Grade I	1	0	0	0	
Grade II	44	4	0	4	
Grade III	4	25	0	75	
Grade IV	0	—	—	—	
Diverticulectomy					0–6
Grade I	8	0	0	0	
Grade II	27	0	0	4	
Grade III	11	18	0	0	
Grade IV	1	100	0	0	
Right hemicolectomy					0–36
Grade I	0	—	—	—	
Grade II	47	19	0	—	
Grade III	7	28	14	—	
Grade IV	1	0	100	—	

Data compiled from references 2–5,19,24,25,27,28,30–34,36,38,39,44,45.

optimally by primary resection of the affected area and ileostomy with mucous fistula (46). Other exceptions to primary anastomosis after right hemicolectomy in unprepared bowel may include the presence of one or more risk factors such as diabetes mellitus, steroid dependence, previous abdominal radiation, and chronic renal failure (47).

Treatment of cecal diverticulitis between 1918 and 1947 with simple drainage, diverticulectomy, and right hemicolectomy resulted in 20%, 4%, and 11% mortality, respectively (31). A more recent review of 635 patients with pathologic confirmation of diverticulitis of the cecum and ascending colon between 1958 and 1984 reported 1.7% morbidity and 0.5% mortality for diverticulectomy and 6.7% morbidity and 2.5% mortality for right hemicolectomy (28). Despite improved outcomes in the more recent series, right hemicolectomy still results in a greater morbidity and mortality than diverticulectomy (48,49). However, a lack of prospective randomized trials may result in unjust bias, because colectomy may be used commonly to treat more severe illness than nonresection or local excision.

CONCLUSION

Cecal diverticulitis is an unusual disease process in Western countries that can mimic acute appendicitis preoperatively and cecal carcinoma intraoperatively. In the antibiotic era, morbidity and mortality for emergent right hemicolectomy has declined sharply. Therefore, the continued morbidity of recurrent episodes of cecal diverticulitis and the mortality reported for delays in diagnosis of perforation must be weighed against current operative data. Antibiotic therapy of preoperatively diagnosed uncomplicated cecal diverticulitis is acceptable and parallels the treatment of limited left-sided disease.

Nonresection of an inflamed diverticulum at laparotomy with incidental appendectomy is more controversial. In a review of the world literature, adequate results were noted when nonresectional therapy was used to treat grade I or recognizable grade II disease. Diverticulectomy should be performed only when carcinoma can be ruled out and when the resection margins are free of inflammation, when the ileocecal valve and the vascular supply of the intestine are not compromised by the resection, and when no evidence of perforation, gangrene, or abscess exists.

Cecal diverticulitis is not necessarily self-limited, and recurrences and failures of conservative treatment can be expected. Whenever the diagnosis of cecal carcinoma is suspected or a cecal perforation has ensued, we believe that a right hemicolectomy is the treatment of choice for cecal diverticulitis.

EDITORIAL COMMENTS

Our experience with cecal diverticulitis is similar to that of the author in that diagnosis is usually made intraoperatively. Most patients are explored with the preoperative diagnosis of appendicitis. In our institution, most appendectomies are performed laparoscopically, thereby allowing the diagnosis of cecal diverticulitis to be made with the benefit of minimal access. If the diagnosis is unclear laparoscopically, an open exploration should be performed.

If the degree of inflammation is relatively minimal, we favor nonresectional therapy with antibiotics (together with incidental appendectomy if the cecum at the base of the appendix is uninvolved). Patients responding to this therapy must be evaluated after recovery with colonoscopy to rule out a mass lesion.

Conversely, if the degree of inflammation is severe or if cancer is suspected, a colectomy should be performed. The decision to perform a primary anastomosis depends on the condition of the patient and the degree of contamination at laparotomy. We have seen little if any role for diverticulectomy, especially in this era of diagnostic laparoscopy.

REFERENCES

1. Potier F. Diverticulite et appendicite. Bull Mem Soc Anat Paris 1912;87:29–31.
2. Sugihara K, Muto T, Morioka Y, et al. Diverticular disease of the colon in Japan: a review of 615 cases. Dis Colon Rectum 1984;27:531–537. *Right-sided diverticula were more common in younger patients and in men. Treatment of choice for right-sided diverticulitis was drainage of the inflamed area with incidental appendectomy.*
3. Tan EC, Tung KH, Tan L, et al. Diverticulitis of the cecum and ascending colon in Singapore. J R Coll Surg Edinb 1984;29:373–376. *A series of 40 patients. The average age was 36 years and right hemicolectomy had a higher morbidity than local excision with appendectomy.*
4. Rigler RG, Cherry JW. Diverticulitis of the cecum: preoperative diagnosis. Am Surg 1960;26:405–408. *The author believes that the alert surgeon can make this diagnosis preoperatively if appropriately suspicious and a barium enema is ordered.*
5. Harada RN, Whelan TJ. Surgical management of cecal diverticulitis. Am J Surg 1993;166:666–671. *Appendectomy combined with postoperative antibiotics is an effective method for treating cecal diverticulitis if no abscess is present and carcinoma can be ruled out.*
6. Ngoi SS, Chia J, Goh MY, et al. Surgical management of right colon diverticulitis. Dis Colon Rectum 1992;35:799–802. *Only 3 of 68 patients operated on had colonic resection when a malignancy could not be excluded.*
7. Wada M, Kikuchi Y, Doy M. Uncomplicated acute diverticulitis of the cecum and ascending colon: sonographic findings in 18 patients. Am J Radiol 1990;155:283–287. *The authors concluded that characteristic findings included a hypoechoic round or oval focus protruding from a segmentally thickened colonic wall.*
8. Burgess CM. Diverticulitis of the cecum. Am J Surg 1940;50:108–111. *Reviews five cases and states that the disease tends to subside spontaneously.*
9. Vajrabukka T, Saksornghai K, Jimakorn P. Diverticular disease of the colon in a Far Eastern community. Dis Colon Rectum 1980;23:151–154. *Solitary cecal diverticula accounted for approximately one-fourth of all diverticula of the colon.*
10. Chia JG, Wide CC, Ngoi SS, et al. Trends of diverticular disease of the large bowel in a newly developed country. Dis Colon Rectum 1991;34:498–501. *The prevalence of diverticular disease was 20% in 524 consecutive barium enemas in Singapore.*
11. Hughes LE. Postmortem survey of diverticular disease of the colon. Gut 1969;10:336–351. *A study of 200 autopsies. Twelve percent of the colons had cecal diverticula; all were "false," and none were involved by recent or old inflammation. More than half were associated with diverticula elsewhere in the colon.*
12. Miangalorra CJ. Diverticulitis of the right colon. Ann Surg 1961;153:861–870. *The difficulty of making the diagnosis of right-sided diverticulitis is emphasized.*
13. Arrington P, Judd CS. Cecal diverticulitis. Am J Surg 1981;142:56–59. *A report of 33 cases from Hawaii.*
14. Murayama N, Baba S, Kodaira S, et al. An aetiological study of diverticulosis of the right colon. Aust N Z J Surg 1981;51:420–425. *Suggests that similar mechanisms may lead to diverticulosis of the right and left colon.*
15. Crawford JM. The gastrointestinal tract. In: Cotran RS, Kumar V, Robbin SL, Schoen FJ, eds. Pathologic basis of disease. Philadelphia: WB Saunders, 1994:755–829.
16. Lee YS. Diverticular disease of the large bowel in Singapore: an autopsy survey. Dis Colon Rectum 1986;29:330–335. *In 1400 consecutive autopsies of patients older than 14 years of age, diverticulosis was seen in 19%.*
17. Morson BC. The large intestine. In: Wright GP, St Clair Symmers W, eds. Systemic pathology. New York: Churchill Livingstone, 1979:1100–1151.
18. Lauridsen J, Ross FP. Acute diverticulitis of the cecum. Arch Surg 1952;64:320–330. *Recommends local excision in operative cases.*
19. Langdon A. Solitary diverticulitis of the right colon. Can J Surg 1982;25:579–581. *A mass with a pericolic abscess could not be differentiated from carcinoma.*
20. Waugh TR. Appendix vermiformis duplex. Arch Surg 1941;42:311–320. *Reviews 16 cases of "double appendix" and the embryologic explanations.*
21. Sugihara K, Muto T, Morioka Y. Motility study in right-sided diverticular disease of the colon. Gut 1983;24:1130–1134. *Intraluminal pressure was studied with a catheter-tip transducer introduced through a colonoscope. High intraluminal pressure and abnormal motility in the ascending colon may be related to development of right-sided diverticular disease.*
22. Graham SM, Ballantyne GH. Cecal diverticulitis: a review of the American experience. Dis Colon Rectum 1987;30:821–826. *Describes two types of cecal diverticulitis. Two-thirds present as an inflamed projection from the cecal wall and the rest present as an indurated phlegmon difficult to distinguish from cecal cancer.*
23. Whiteway J, Morson BC. Pathology of the aging-diverticular disease. Clin Gastroenterol 1985;14:829–846. *Discusses a progressive elastosis occurring in the teniae coli with age, along with contracture of the teniae and normal muscle cells.*
24. Canver CC, Freier DT. Management of cecal diverticulitis. Am J Gastroenterol 1986;81:1104–1106. *Describes a patient with 6- to 7-cm posterior cecal mass.*
25. Schmidt PJ, Bennion RS, Thompson JE. Cecal diverticulitis: a continuing diagnostic dilemma. World J Surg 1991;15:367–371. *In three patients, the inflamed diverticulum was left in situ at the initial procedure; all had later excision (one urgently for sepsis).*
26. Luoma A, Nagy A. Cecal diverticulitis. Can J Surg 1989;32:283–286. *Cecal diverticulitis accounted for 0.2% of procedures performed for the acute abdomen.*

27. Scully RE, Mark EJ, McNeely WF, et al. Case records of the Massachusetts General Hospital. N Engl J Med 1987;317:432–440. *A discussion of a case of cecal diverticulitis with ligneous perityphlitis.*

28. Sardi A, Gokli A, Singer JA. Diverticular disease of the cecum and ascending colon: a review of 881 cases. Am Surg 1987;53:41–45. *The diagnosis was correct at operation in only 59%. The overall mortality was 2.5%.*

29. Schuler JG, Bayley J. Diverticulitis of the cecum. Surg Gynecol Obstet 1983;156:743–748. *Treatment may be simplified with more awareness of the diagnosis. Local resection is preferred unless the diagnosis is in doubt or when local resection or invagination could jeopardize the ileocecal valve or the blood supply to the cecum.*

30. McFee AS, Sutton PG, Ramos R. Diverticulitis of the right colon. Dis Colon Rectum 1982;25:254–256. *Barium enema was not a helpful diagnostic aid. Open cecotomy is not recommended to establish the diagnosis.*

31. Anderson L. Acute diverticulitis of the cecum. Study of ninety-nine surgical cases. Surgery 1947;22:479–488. *The average age was 40 years, and 84% of the surgeons believed that acute appendicitis was the preoperative diagnosis. Because barium enema is best avoided in suspected acute appendicitis, the ability to make the correct diagnosis is limited.*

32. Vaughn AM, Narsete EM. Diverticulitis of the cecum. Arch Surg 1952;65:763–769. *Reviews 118 cases from the literature with four additional cases. The diagnosis cannot be distinguished clinically from acute appendicitis.*

33. Kaufman Z, Shpitz B, Reina A, et al. Cecal diverticulitis presented as a cecal tumor. Am Surg 1990;56:675–677. *If a "cecal mass" can be separated from the cecal wall, diverticulectomy or wedge resection of the cecal wall can be performed successfully.*

34. Mariani G, Tedoli M, Dina R, et al. Solitary diverticulum of the cecum and right colon. Report of six cases. Dis Colon Rectum 1987;30:626–629. *Intraoperative misdiagnosis occurs in 28–42%. Use of intraoperative colonoscopy or frozen tissue sections is suggested to avoid unnecessary colectomy.*

35. Cutajar CL. Solitary cecal diverticula. Dis Colon Rectum 1978;21:627–629. *Describes three cases. Drainage of the inflamed area and postoperative antibiotic coverage is recommended.*

36. Greaney EM, Snyder WH. Acute diverticulitis of the cecum encountered at emergency surgery. Am J Surg 1957;94:270–281. *Fourteen cases of cecal diverticulitis were seen during 6781 emergency abdominal procedures. Includes a literature review, case reports and 60 references.*

37. Kovalcik PJ, Simstein NL, Cross GH. Ileocecal masses discovered unexpectedly at surgery for appendicitis. Am Surg 1978;44:279–281. *Emphasizes the relative safety of right colectomy in unprepared bowel.*

38. Al-Hilaly MA, Razzaq HA, El-Saffiti JI, et al. Solitary cecal diverticulitis: recognition and management. Acta Chir Scand 1989;155:475–478. *Recognition of solitary cecal diverticulitis required surgical experience to avoid more radical procedures.*

39. Schapira A, Leichtling JJ, Wolf BS, et al. Diverticulitis of the cecum and right colon. clinical and radiographic features. Am J Dig Dis 1958;3:351–359. *Reviews 18 cases and recommends conservative nonoperative and operative management.*

40. Lewis FR, Holcroft JW, Boey J, et al. Appendicitis: a critical review of diagnosis and treatment in 1000 cases. Arch Surg 1975;110:677–682. *The negative appendectomy rate was 20% in 1000 cases. There were two perforated cecal diverticula, two cases of cecitis, and one nonperforated cecal ulcer.*

41. Balthazar EJ, Megibow AJ, Gordon RB, et al. Cecal diverticulitis: evaluation with CT. Radiology 1987;162:79–81. *CT is a sensitive method to detect cecal diverticulitis; describes characteristic findings in seven patients.*

42. Crist DW, Fishman EK, Scatarige JC, et al. Acute diverticulitis of the cecum and ascending colon diagnosed by computed tomography. Surg Gynecol Obstet 1988;166:99–101. *CT proved useful in early diagnosis of seven patients. Five patients had perforated diverticulitis with abscess formation.*

43. Dean AC, Newell JP. Colonoscopy in the differential diagnosis of carcinoma from diverticulitis of the sigmoid colon. Br J Surg 1973;60:633–635. *Colonoscopy failed to examine the diseased segment in 17 of 36 patients with possible carcinoma in a segment of diverticular disease discovered by barium enema.*

44. Pierce W, Rosato FE, Rolling EF. Acute diverticulitis of the ileocecal region: diagnosis and management. Am Surg 1971;37:408–412. *One of the five patients discussed had an abscess entered during a colectomy; the procedure was complicated by development of a pelvic abscess.*

45. Mittal VK, Cortez JA, Olson AM. Solitary perforated diverticulum of the ascending colon. Dis Colon Rectum 1981;24:47–49. *Describes two cases of this rare entity.*

46. Nespoli A, Ravizzini C, Trivella M, et al. The choice of surgical procedure for peritonitis due to colonic perforation. Arch Surg 1993;128:814–818. *The mortality rate is related to the severity of peritonitis, accurately measured by the Acute Physiology and Chronic Health Evaluation (APACHE) II score and the Mannheim Peritonitis Index (MPI).*

47. Arnspiger RC, Helling TS. An evaluation of results of colon anastomosis in prepared and unprepared bowel. J Clin Gastroenterol 1988;10:638–641. *Concludes that primary anastomosis of the unprepared right colon would be expected to lead to similar results as with prepared bowel in the absence of risk factors (steroid dependence, diabetes mellitus, chronic renal failure, previous radiation, or peritonitis).*

48. Wagner DE, Zollinger RW. Diverticulitis of the cecum and ascending colon. Arch Surg 1961;83:124–131. *Reviews 327 literature cases and adds 18 new ones. The preoperative diagnosis was correct in 5%. The disease is divided into six gross pathologic types on which operative procedures are based.*

49. Fischer MG, Farkas AM. Diverticulitis of the cecum and ascending colon. Dis Colon Rectum 1984;27:454–458. *Hemicolectomy often can be avoided when the condition is recognized intra-operatively. Palpation through the bowel wall may identify the crater produced by the perforation.*

Table 33.1.   Organisms Isolated from Percutaneously Drained Liver Abscesses

	n (%)
Single organism	9 (53)
Multiple organisms	8 (47)
Gram negative rods (*Escherichia coli, Klebsiella*)	6
Streptococcus faecalis	2
Other streptococci	5
Anaerobes	6
Staphylococcus aureus	1
Aspergillus fumigatum	1
Entamoeba histolytica	1

From Wong KP. Percutaneous drainage of pyogenic liver abscesses. World J Surg 1990;14:492–497.

Incidence of Etiologies of Hepatic Abscesses

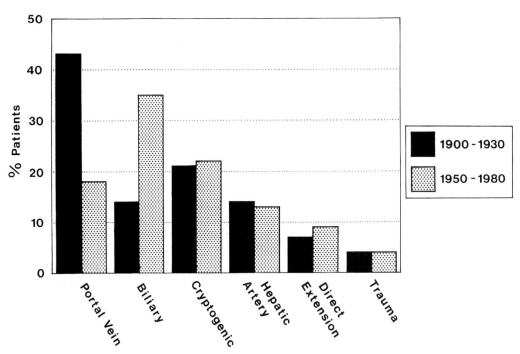

(From Pitt HA, Liver Abscess. In Zuidema GD and Turcotte JG [eds.], Shackelford's Surgery of the Alimentary Tract, Vol.4 [3rd. ed.]. Philadelphia: W. B. Saunders, 1991.)

Figure 33.1.   Differing incidences of the causes of pyogenic liver abscesses, when comparing the years 1900–1930 and 1950–1980. (Reprinted with permission from Pitt HA. Liver abscess. In: Zuidema GD, Turcotte JG, eds. Shackelford's surgery of the alimentary tract. Philadelphia: WB Saunders, 1996;3:541–563.)

abscess coming from the portal system (43% of all cases), and portal sepsis was the commonest cause of abscess. Biliary disease is now the single most common cause of abscess. Appendicitis rarely causes liver abscess today (0–2% of cases). *During the last 20 years, diverticular disease has become the most common source of liver abscess from a portal origin.*

CLINICAL PRESENTATION

The clinical presentation of hepatic abscess complicating diverticulitis is the same as that following other causes, together with the clinical signs of diverticulitis. The clinical diagnosis of liver abscess has been notoriously difficult to establish. There may be a wide spectrum of symptom severity. Table 33.2 illustrates the frequency of presenting signs and symptoms. Most patients will have a fever, leukocytosis, abdominal pain, and mild elevation of liver function tests (LFTs). They may be jaundiced and, in severe cases, exhibit signs of septic shock. *Because of the vague presenting signs and symptoms, a very high index of suspicion is necessary to make a timely diagnosis.*

DIAGNOSTIC EVALUATION

Laboratory data for liver abscess are nonspecific. Leukocytosis and mild elevation of the LFTs occur in most patients. These data are suggestive of, but not specific for, the presence of a liver abscess. Radiologic evaluation can be quite helpful. A plain abdominal radiograph may reveal air in the biliary tree or portal vein or an air–fluid level in an abscess cavity in 10–20% of patients (4). Elevation of the right hemidiaphragm, a right pleural effusion, and atelectasis may be seen on a chest radiograph. Ultrasound will accurately diagnose a liver abscess in 85–95% of patients. In addition, CT is an excellent diagnostic tool. *A CT scan is considered to be the diagnostic test of choice with a sensitivity of 95–100%* (1,4). CT scan and ultrasound are helpful not only to make the diagnosis but also to monitor therapy. This is true regardless of what interventions are performed (5). Other diagnostic modalities are available but have disadvantages. Radioisotope scanning is noninvasive, but the sensitivity is only 75%. Hepatic arteriography is very sensitive but invasive, with attendant risks. Endoscopic retrograde cholangiopancreatography (ERCP) is specific but not sensitive and is most useful in diagnosing abscesses secondary to a biliary source (6).

Table 33.2.   Frequency of Presenting Signs and Symptoms

Symptom or Sign	Frequency (%)
Fever	90
Anorexia	72
Abdominal pain	55
Rigors	53
Tender right upper quadrant	49
Nausea/vomiting	47
Weight loss	47
Malaise	45
Hepatomegaly	38
Jaundice	21

From Srivastava ED, Mayberry JF. Pyogenic liver abscess: a review of etiology, diagnosis and intervention. Dig Dis 1990;8:287–293.

TREATMENT OPTIONS

Liver abscess represents a life-threatening infection. *The hallmark of therapy is high-dose broad-spectrum antibiotics and adequate drainage*. Depending on the patient and the etiology, size, and location of the abscess, drainage can be performed percutaneously or by an open procedure. The use of CT and ultrasound-guided drainage has been shown in a number of studies to be safe and successful most of the time (2,7). Currently, there is no clear consensus regarding treatment for pyogenic liver abscesses. To date, a randomized trial comparing the effectiveness of percutaneous and open drainage procedures has not been published. Because of the changing trends in etiologies, retrospective studies are of little help in guiding current therapy. Authors generally agree that *treatment should be individualized*. The critical factors that affect treatment are the etiology of the abscess, the number and size of the abscess(es), the location of the abscess(es), the presence of loculations, and the overall condition of the patient. In general, *percutaneous drainage is ideal for patients who have a single, small- to moderate-sized unilocular abscess when the identified source of the abscess has been treated (7,8). Open drainage is ideal when the decision to proceed with laparotomy has been made or when there are multiple loculated abscesses. Open drainage is also indicated after failure of treatment by percutaneous drainage (8)*.

Laparoscopic drainage of liver abscess has been described recently, but success, complication rates, and long term follow-up of this technique are unknown (9). With laparoscopic guidance, drains are placed into the abscess using the Seldinger technique. This may become a useful adjunct to patients who have lesions inaccessible to percutaneous technique. Until some experience is gained in this technique, it should be used with caution by experienced laparoscopists.

In liver abscess secondary to diverticulitis, the first decision to be made is whether operative intervention is required to treat the inflammatory process involving the sigmoid colon. If medical treatment or percutaneous drainage of an associated pericolic abscess is entertained, then the liver abscess can be evaluated for percutaneous drainage. If a laparotomy is planned, open drainage of the abscess can be performed at the time of the procedure. One might argue that the presence of a liver abscess is an indication to proceed with colectomy. However, therapy must be individualized. For example, with a frail, elderly patient who is clinically stable, a trial of antibiotics and percutaneous drainage of the liver may be reasonable.

OUTCOME

Historically, pyogenic liver abscess, like other sources of intra-abdominal sepsis, has been treated by open drainage. In the pre-antibiotic era, mortality rates were quite high. Ochsner et al reported a 77% mortality in the largest series collected (10). With the introduction of antibiotics and more aggressive and sophisticated care, the mortality has decreased to 11–33% (1,6,7). The mortality rate has not changed significantly during the last 30 years.

There has been, however, *an increase in the number of immunosuppressed patients during the last 30 years*. This has most likely had a profound effect on the mortality rate in clinical series. In one series that studied immunosuppression in relationship to outcome, five of eight patients (62.5%) in the immunosuppressed group died, as compared with 1 of 16 patients (6.25%) in the nonimmunosuppressed group (1). *Other identified risk factors for mortality are underlying malignancy, the presence of multiple organisms, and the presence of hepatic dysfunction (6)*.

EDITORIAL COMMENTS

The authors have given a concise review of pyogenic liver abscesses as they present today. Interest in pylephlebitis and liver abscess was fueled by the classic paper of Ochsner et al (10), which clearly demonstrated the pathophysiology as it related to appendicitis (Figs. 33.2 through 33.5). Similar mechanisms apply for diverticulitis, and other colonic diseases such as cancer or Crohn's disease (15,16), although the process may originate in veins adjacent to either the right or left colon. Although diverticulitis seems to be the most common portal source of pyogenic liver abscess, actual reports are limited (11–13,17–31). Reviews by Lin (24) and Liebert (19) cite other case reports; 52 cases were found in the literature by 1981 (19). Because of the emphasis on biliary disease as the most frequent causes of pyogenic liver abscesses, gastrointestinal sources may be overlooked in the course of the workup (23). Furthermore, some cases of cryptogenic pyogenic abscess actually may relate to silent diverticular disease (20).

We agree that CT scans are particularly valuable to visualize not only the liver abscesses (Figs. 33.6 and 33.7), or portal-venous gas (32), but the inflammatory process in the colon. Ultrasound is also useful diagnostically. Barium enema and sigmoidoscopy should be performed, especially if there are gastrointestinal (GI) complaints. Multiple anaerobic organisms in the abscess suggest a GI source, whereas *Escherichia coli* suggests a biliary origin (23).

Because liver abscess is a life-threatening disease, it takes priority in the planning of treatment. Fortunately, as long as the patient does not have multiple abscesses in both lobes of the liver, percutaneous drainage has emerged as a highly successful treatment.

We believe that initial nonoperative therapy can be highly beneficial in the overall management. First, when successful, percutaneous drainage reverses the septic course and allows the patient to

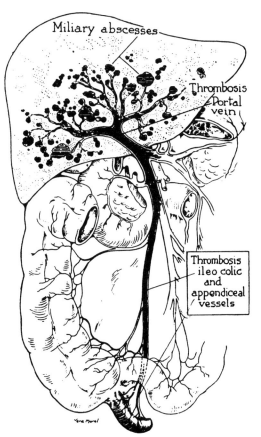

Figure 33.2. Mechanism of spread of infection from the appendix to the liver with pylephlebitis. (Reprinted with permission from Ochsner A, DeBakey M, Murray S. Pyogenic abscess of the liver. II. An analysis of forty-seven cases with review of the literature. Am J Surg 1938;11:292–319.)

Figure 33.3. Photomicrograph of a large mesenteric vein occluded by a septic thrombus (×25). The patient had acute diverticulitis. (Reprinted with permission from Scully RE, Galabini JJ, McNeely BU, eds. Case records of the Massachusetts General Hospital. N Engl J Med 1977; 296:1051–1057) [Ref. 11].

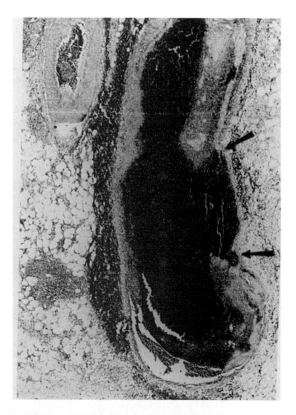

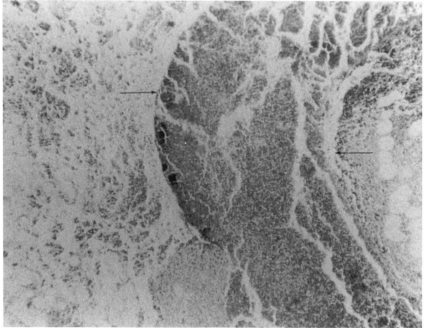

Figure 33.4. Photomicrograph of mesenteric vein containing exudate in the lumen, in a case of mesenteric pylephlebitis. (Reprinted with permission from Navarro C, Clain DJ, Kondlapoodi P. Perforated diverticulum of the terminal ileum. A previously unreported cause of suppurative pylephlebitis and multiple hepatic abscesses. Dig Dis Sci 1984;29:171–177) [Ref. 12].

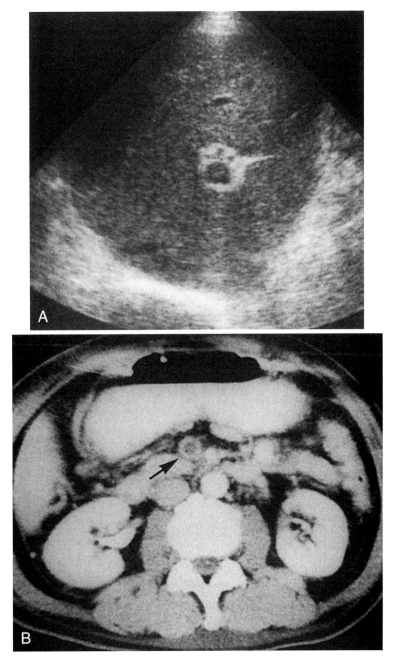

Figure 33.5. **A.**, Abdominal ultrasonogram shows a thrombus in the portal vein at the porta hepatis. The patient had pylephlebitis associated with cecal diverticulitis. **B.**, Intravenous contrast-enhanced CT scan in the same patient. The "ring pattern" of portal vein thrombosis is seen (arrow). (Reprinted with permission from Perez-Cruet M, Grable E, Drapkin MS, et al. Pylephlebitis associated with diverticulitis. South Med J 1993;86:578–580) [Ref. 13].

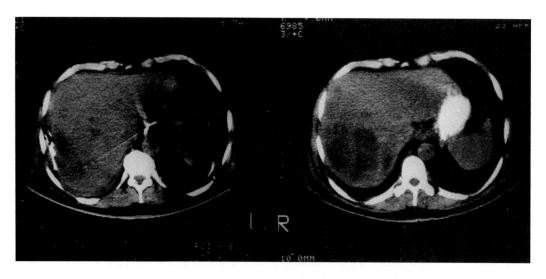

Figure 33.6. CT view of solitary pyogenic abscess involving the right hepatic lobe.

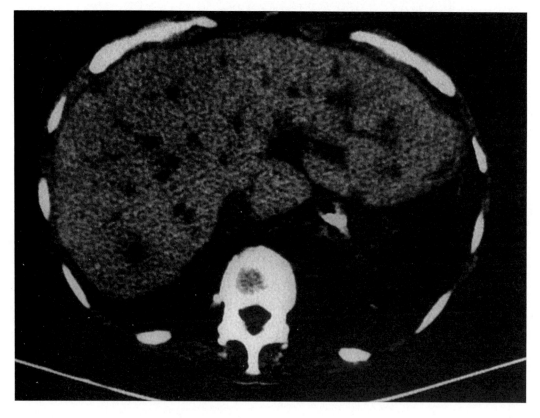

Figure 33.7. CT view of liver containing multiple pyogenic abscesses. (Reprinted with permission from Vukmir RB. Pyogenic hepatic abscess. Am Fam Physician 1993;47:1435–1441) [Ref. 14].

"get healthy" (33). Furthermore, the concomitant use of broad-spectrum antibiotic therapy (34), perhaps supplemented by anticoagulants (26), also treats the primary problem, sigmoid diverticulitis, many times allowing for the ultimate performance of a single-stage resection. Finally, if indicated at the time of percutaneous drainage of the liver abscess, a diverticular abscess also can be drained, thereby increasing the likelihood of avoiding a staged resection with temporary colostomy.

It must be remembered, however, that if initial percutaneous drainage of a liver abscess fails or if the patient has peritonitis, prompt surgical intervention must be performed, considering the severity of the disease and the need for adequate drainage. Patients on steroids or with ascites also may need open drainage (35).

In the open approach, the liver is exposed through a generous midline or subcostal incision. Use of intraoperative ultrasound will facilitate accurate localization and drainage of the abscess(es), although adhesions and deep abscesses may complicate this technique (36). After the primary source of the infection has been dealt with by colectomy, for example (37), the abscess cavity can be broken into after needle aspiration. Multiple soft drains are placed into the cavity, and irrigation and sinograms can be performed through these postoperatively. Multiple microscopic abscesses do not require formal drainage. The rare case of hepatic resection of necrotic liver with liver abscess usually follows long-term biliary obstruction (4).

REFERENCES

1. Hanson N, Vargish T. Pyogenic hepatic abscess: a case for open drainage. Am Surg 1993;59:219–222. *Recommends percutaneous drainage alone only for selected patients.*
2. Wong KP. Percutaneous drainage of pyogenic liver abscesses. World J Surg 1990;14:492–497. *Percutaneous drainage was successful in 18 of 21 patients. There were two deaths.*
3. Pitt HA. Liver abscess. In: Zuidema GD, Turcotte JG, eds. Shackelford's surgery of the alimentary tract. Philadelphia: WB Saunders, 1996;3:541–563.
4. Pitt HA. Surgical management of hepatic abscesses. World J Surg 1990;14:498–504. *A review of amebic and pyogenic liver abscesses. Surgical drainage has advantages at times, using ultrasound of the best drainage site and access to the biliary tree for cholangiography and drainage.*
5. Buchman TG, Zuidema GD. The role of computerized tomographic scanning in the surgical management of pyogenic hepatic abscess. Surg Gynecol Obstet 1981;153:1–9. *CT is the diagnostic study of choice and it is useful to monitor surgically drained abscesses.*
6. Srivastava ED, Mayberry JF. Pyogenic liver abscess: a review of etiology, diagnosis and intervention. Dig Dis 1990;8:287–293. *Reviews reported series from 1970–1987; with 54 references.*
7. Gyorffy EK, Frey CF, Silva J Jr, et al. Pyogenic liver abscess. Diagnostic and therapeutic strategies. Ann Surg 1987;206:699–705. *A study of 26 patients assessing rapid diagnosis and percutaneous drainage. The overall mortality was 11.5%.*
8. Clark RA, Towbin R. Abscess drainage with CT and ultrasound guidance. Radiol Clin North Am 1983;21:445–459. *Discusses technique of catheter drainage and roles of CT and ultrasound in detecting abscesses.*
9. Cappucino H, Campanile F, Knecht J. Laparoscopic-guided drainage of hepatic abscess. Surg Laparosc Endosc 1994;4:234–237. *Report of successful drainage of a liver abscess with laparoscopic guidance.*
10. Ochsner A, DeBakey M, Murray S. Pyogenic abscess of the liver. II. An analysis of forty-seven cases with review of the literature. Am J Surg 1938;11:292–319. *A classic early review of the disease entity with more than 200 references.*
11. Scully RE, Galabini JJ, McNeely BU, eds. Case records of the Massachusetts General Hospital. N Engl J Med 1977;296:1051–1057. *A well-illustrated discussion of pylephlebitis.*
12. Navarro C, Clain DJ, Kondlapoodi P. Perforated diverticulum of the terminal ileum. A previously unreported cause of suppurative pylephlebitis and multiple hepatic abscesses. Dig Dis Sci 1984;29:171–177. *The patient died of gram-negative sepsis from this unusual source.*
13. Perez-Cruet M, Grable E, Drapkin MS, et al. Pylephlebitis associated with diverticulitis. South Med J 1993;86:578–580. *The two reported cases involved diverticulitis of the right colon.*
14. Vukmir RB. Pyogenic hepatic abscess. Am Fam Physician 1993;47:1435–1441. *A review of the radiographic findings of pyogenic hepatic abscess.*
15. Teitz S, Guidetti-Sharon A, Monor H, et al. Pyogenic liver abscess: warning indicator of the silent colonic cancer. Dis Colon Rectum 1995;38:1220–1223. *Colon cancer is a rare cause of pyogenic liver abscess.*
16. Greenstein AJ, Sachar DB, Goldofsky LE, et al. Pyogenic liver abscess in Crohn's disease. Q J Med 1985;56:505–518. *Discusses a total of 13 cases, eight of which involved propagation via the portal vein.*
17. Kramer SE, Rubinson W. Acquired suppurative diverticulitis with pylephlebitis and metastatic suppuration in the liver. Surg Gynecol Obstet 1926;42:540–542. *One of the first reports of liver abscess and pylephlebitis complicating diverticulitis.*

18. Niemann H, Wintzer G. Leberabszebildung als erstmanifestation einer gedeckt perforierten sigmadiverticulitis. Leber Magen Dar 1995;25:35–37. *Case report of a patient with occult sigmoid diverticulitis who developed a solitary abscess in the right hepatic lobe.*

19. Liebert CW Jr. Hepatic abscess resulting from asymptomatic diverticulitis of the sigmoid colon. South Med J 1981;74:71–73. *In this case report, the patient died of sepsis with the involved sigmoid still in place, having had drainage of two liver abscesses and diverting colostomy.*

20. Shaldon C. Portal pyemia. Br J Surg 1958;45:357–360. *One of the larger individual series of liver abscesses attributed to diverticulitis, including five patients with sigmoid diverticulitis. Only one patient was asymptomatic from the colonic disease.*

21. Wallack MK, Brown AS, Austrian R, et al. Pyogenic liver abscess secondary to asymptomatic sigmoid diverticulitis. Ann Surg 1976;184:241–243. *A single case report with reference to previous literature reports.*

22. Waxman BP, Cavanagh LL, Nayman J: Suppurative pylephlebitis and multiple hepatic abscesses with silent colonic diverticulitis. Med J Aust 1979;2:376–378. *The patient developed multiple intrahepatic and extrahepatic abscesses.*

23. Cohen JL, Martin M, Rossi RL, et al. Liver abscess. The need for complete gastrointestinal evaluation. *Seven of 20 patients with pyogenic liver abscess had a GI source, including diverticulitis (three patients), Crohn's disease (two patients), appendicitis (one patient), and colon cancer (one patient).*

24. Lin C-S. Suppurative pylephlebitis and liver abscess complicating colonic diverticulitis: report of two cases and review of the literature. Mt Sinai J Med 1973;40:48–55. *The most complete review on the subject with 28 references.*

25. Graham GA, Berstein RB, Gronner AT. Gas in the portal and inferior mesenteric veins caused by diverticulitis of the sigmoid colon. Radiology 1975;114:601–602. *A rare report of survival after the development of portal-venous gas complicating sigmoid diverticulitis.*

26. Plemmons RM, Dooley DP, Longfield RN. Septic thrombophlebitis of the portal vein (pylephlebitis): diagnosis and management in the modern era. Clin Infect Dis 1995;21:1114–1120. *Six of 19 reviewed cases were precipitated by acute diverticulitis; five of the six patients died.*

27. Duffy FJ Jr, Millan MT, Schoetz DJ Jr. Suppurative pylephlebitis and pylethrombosis: the role of anticoagulation. Am Surg 1995;61:1041–1044. *Anticoagulation may have been responsible for resolving the episode when it was added to antibiotic therapy.*

28. Sridharan GV, Wilkinson SP, Primrose WR. Pyogenic liver abscess in the elderly. Age Ageing 1990;19:199–203. *Four of 17 patients had colonic diverticulitis.*

29. Seeto RK, Rockey DC. Pyogenic liver abscess. Changes in etiology, management, and outcome. Medicine 1996;75: 99–113. *Sixteen of the 142 patients in this study had pylephlebitis, including five with diverticulitis.*

30. Posthuma EF, Bieger R, Kuypers TJ. A rare cause of a hepatic abscess: diverticulitis of the ileum. Neth J Med 1993;42:69–82. *The second report of liver abscesses caused by ileal diverticulitis.*

31. Hoover EL, Webb H, Walker C, et al. Perforated jejunal diverticulum with multiple hepatic abscesses. South Med J 1990;83:54–56. *The first reported case of perforated jejunal diverticulitis, pylephlebitis, and liver abscesses.*

32. Haak HR, Kooymans-Coutinho MF, Teeffelen ME, et al. Portal venous gas in a patient with diverticulitis. Hepatogastroenterology 1990;37:528–529. *A patient with a diverticular abscess involving the sigmoid colon with portal venous gas seen by CT scan survived after sigmoid resection and antibiotic therapy.*

33. Giorgio A, Tarantino L, Mariniello N, et al. Pyogenic liver abscesses: 13 years of experience in percutaneous needle aspiration with US guidance. Radiology 1996;195:122–124. *Cure was achieved with percutaneous needle aspiration (rather than prolonged catheter drainage) in 98%.*

34. Sakata K, Hirai K, Itano S, et al. Evaluation of treatments for liver abscess: significance of intra-arterial antibiotic injection therapy. Clin Ther 1994;16:446–457. *Intra-arterial antibiotic therapy may be effective for some patients in whom intravenous therapy is ineffective.*

35. Huang C-J, Pitt HA, Lipsett PA, et al. Pyogenic hepatic abscess. Changing trends over 42 years. Ann Surg 1996;223:600–609. *A study of 233 patients over a 42-year period compares trends in the 1950–1972 interval with the years 1973–1993. In the latter period, the incidence was higher, and the overall mortality decreased from 65% to 31%.*

36. Stain SC, Yellin AE, Donovan AJ, et al. Pyogenic liver abscess. Modern treatment. Arch Surg 1991;126:991–996. *Two of 54 patients had diverticulitis, and 20 had cryptogenic causes.*

37. Robert JH, Mirescu D, Ambrosetti P, et al. Critical review of the treatment of pyogenic hepatic abscess. Surg Gynecol Obstet 1992;174:97–102. *Control of the primary disease process is critical in determining survival.*

INDEX

References in italics denote figures; those followed by "t" denote tables

Abdominal compartment syndrome
  abdominal closure techniques, *334–335*
  abdominal pressure increases, physiologic conse-
      quences of, 333, 333t
  characteristics of, 333
  decompression for, 334–335
  diagnosis of, 333–334
Abdominal mass, gas-filled, differential diagnosis,
      412t
Abdominal pain
  algorithm for assessing, *38*
  case study presentation, 33–34
  characteristics of, based on type of diverticular
      disease, 36, 37t
  clinical presentation
    in acute diverticulitis, 34–35
    in giant colonic diverticulum, 412
    in ischemic colitis *vs.* diverticulitis, 48
    in jejunoileal diverticular disease, 398
    in symptomatic diverticulosis, 34–35
    in young patients with diverticular disease,
        322, 323t
  computed tomography scan to determine, 36
  differential diagnosis, 36
  diverticular inflammation and, *35*, 35–36
  due to small bowel obstruction, (*see* Small bowel
      obstruction)
  duodenal diverticula and, 361
  editorial comments regarding, 40–41
  irritable bowel syndrome
    abdominal pain associated with, 37t
    differential diagnosis, 36, 41t
  localizing, methods for, 35
  neuronal pathways of, 34–35
  objective signs of presence of, 36, 38
  stimuli for eliciting, 35
Abscess
  diverticular
    case studies of, 206–208
    characteristics of, 208
    computed tomographic imaging of, 208, *212*
    description of, 221
    formation of, 208
    incidence of, 208
    onset of, 296
    pericolic, 211
    postoperative, 296, 298
    resections, 219–220

sites for, *298*
  treatment of
    cost analysis, 220
    laparoscopy, 253
    medications, 209
    mortality and morbidity associated with,
        210t
    on-table lavage, 210
    percutaneous drainage
      contraindications, 211
      CT-scan-guided
        catheter placement, 213, *215*
        collapse of abscess cavity, 218, *219*
        complications of, 219
        drainage routes, 215, *216–218*
        failure of, 219
        indications, 211, *212*
        needle guidance, 213, *214*
        patient preparation, 213
        success rates, 218
        transgluteal drainage, 215, *216–218*
      description of, 210–211
      ultrasound-guided, 218
    resection procedures
      progression to, from percutaneous drain-
          age, 221
      single-stage, 209
      three-stage, 209
      two-stage, 209
  hepatic
    appendicitis infection, *447–449*
    secondary to diverticulitis
      bacterial migration to, 443
      case study of, 442–443
      clinical presentation of, 445
      computed tomographic imaging of, 445, *450*
      description of, *386*, 386–387
      diagnostic evaluation, 445
      epidemiology of, 443, 445
      etiology of, 443–445, *444*, 444t
      outcome, 446
      signs and symptoms, 445, 445t
      treatment options
        description of, 446
        nonoperative, 446–447, 451
        operative approach, 446, 451
        percutaneous drainage
          description of, 446
          failure of, immediate surgical attention
              in event of, 451
  postoperative intra-abdominal, 296, 298, *298*

453

Acute diverticulitis
  with abscess, (*see* Abscess, diverticular)
  diagnostic modalities for
    barium enema, 57
    computed tomography, 59, *62*, 69
    endoscopy, 57, *61*
    transabdominal ultrasonography, 61–62
  differential diagnosis
    with colon cancer, 57
    with ischemic colitis, 47
  in immunocompromised patient, (*see* Immuno-
        compromised patient)
  operative pathologic classification, 237t
  perforated, (*see also* Sigmoid diverticulitis,
        perforated)
    classification of, 226
    description of, 226
    host response based on, 226
  progression of uncomplicated diverticulosis to, 2
  sigmoid, (*see* Sigmoid diverticulitis)
  small bowel obstruction associated with, (*see*
        Small bowel obstruction)
  in young patients, (*see* Young patients, diverticu-
        lar disease in)
Adult respiratory distress syndrome
  description of, 331
  mortality of, 332
  positive end-expiratory pressure for, 330
  treatment of, 331–332
Age, patient, diverticular disease and, correlation
      between, 2, 95, 175
Ampulla of Vater, proximity of duodenal diver-
      ticula to, 354–355, *359–360*
Anastomosis, (*see also* One-stage resection and
      anastomosis)
  hand-sewn, *178, 179*
  for recurrent diverticulitis, 350
Anastomotic leak
  computed tomographic diagnosis of, 290, *291*
  diverting loop ileostomy, 290
  in giant colonic diverticula, 415
  hemorrhoidal vessels and, 290–291
  incidence of, 288
  predisposing factors, 289
  signs and symptoms of, 288–289
Anastomotic stricture, 305
Angiography
  clinical uses
    jejunal diverticula, 399
    for localization of diverticular bleeding, 82–83,
        84, 85
    Meckel's diverticulum, 379
  complications of, 85
Aortic surgery, ischemic colitis after, 49–50
Appendiceal diverticular disease
  acquired *vs.* congenital, 401
  age of onset, 402, 406
  asymptomatic, 401
  description of, 122, 406
  incidence of, 401
  perforation, 402
  radiographic evaluation of, 122, *124*
  surgical removal, 402, 406
Appendicitis
  differential diagnosis of
    with cecal diverticulitis, 433

  with transverse colon diverticulitis, 423
  pyogenic liver abscess infection associated with,
      447–449
ARDS, (*see* Adult respiratory distress syndrome)
Arthritis, diverticulitis presentation and, 389
Atypical presentations, of diverticulitis
  description of, 384
  extra-abdominal
    arthritis, 389
    colocutaneous fistula, 389, *390*
    description of, 385t
    external genitalia, 389
    infectious lesion in thigh or knee, 384–385,
        387–389, *388*
    nervous system, 389, *390*
    pyoderma gangrenosum, 389, *391*
    retroperitoneal abscess formation,
        387–388, *388*
  intra-abdominal
    colouterine fistula, 385–386
    hepatic abscess, *386*, 386–387, (*see also* Hepatic
        abscess)
    left adnexal masses, 385
    perforated colon cancer, 387, (*see also* Colon
        cancer)
  types of, 385t

Barium enema
  air-contrast, 85
  diagnostic use
    cecal diverticulitis, 433, *434*
    colon cancer *vs.* diverticulitis, 56–57, *58–60*
    diverticular bleeding source, 85–86
    diverticular stricture, 196–197, *197*
    giant colonic diverticula, 413, *414*
    jejunal diverticula, 398
    recurrent diverticulitis, *345*
    small bowel obstruction, *147*
    transverse colon diverticulitis, *421*, 424,
        424–425
  mesenteric angiography and, 86
  sigmoid diverticular disease, *39–40*
  vs. sigmoidoscopy, 58
Barium peritonitis, 65
Bleeding, diverticular
  case study of, 76–77
  clinical approaches to, 91
  colorectal neoplasm and, differential diagnosis, 9
  description of, 9
  evaluation of, 78–79
  fluid resuscitation for, 79
  intensive care unit attention for, 331
  pathogenesis of, *77*, 77–78
  sources, diagnosis of
    angiography, 82–83, *84*, 85
    barium studies, 85–86
    endoscopy, *80*, 80–81
    nuclear medicine approaches, 81–82, *82*, 83t
    physical findings, 79
    rigid sigmoidoscopy, 79
  spontaneous resolution of, 87
  treatment of
    colonoscopy, 86, *90*, 91
    embolization, 87
    surgery
      exploratory celiotomy prior to, 88–89

indications for, 87–88, 176
  nonbleeding diverticula, 89
  operative decision, 88
  segmental colonic resection, 89, 89t
  subtotal colectomy, 88, 89, 89t
  vasopressin, 86–87
Blind-loop syndrome
  causes of, 398
  complications of, 398
  treatment of, 401
Bowel dysfunction, differential diagnosis, 41t

Cancer
  diverticular stricture and, biopsy to rule out,
      197–198
  perforated colon, and diverticulitis
    concomitant presentation, 64
    differential diagnosis
      case study, 55–56
      diagnostic tests for
        computed tomography, 59–60, 62–63, 113
        contrast enemas, 56–57, 58–60
        endoluminal ultrasonography, 63
        magnetic resonance imaging, 63
        plain films, 56
        radionuclide scans, 63–64
        sigmoidoscopy, 57–58
        transabdominal ultrasonography, 57–58
Carbohydrates, refining of, and diverticulosis, 3
Carcinoid tumors, associated with Meckel's diver-
      ticulum, 380–381
Carcinoma, (see Cancer)
Cecum
  diverticulitis
    acquired, 430
    acute appendicitis and, differential
        diagnosis, 433
    carcinoma and, misdiagnosis, 435, 438
    cases study of, 428–429
    classification of, based on inflammation and
        contamination, 433, 435, 435
    clinical presentation, 429, 432–433
    complications, 432
    diagnosis of
      barium enema, 433, 434
      computed tomography, 433, 434
      intraoperative, 433, 435, 435
      laparoscopy, 433
      preoperative, 433
      ultrasonography, 433
    with diffuse peritonitis, treatment of, 438–439
    epidemiology of, 429
    ethnic predilection, 429
    false, 430, 431
    historical descriptions of, 429
    incidence of, 432
    inflammation associated with, 432
    morphologic types of, 429
    natural history of, 432
    pathology, 429, 430
    right-sided, 429
    treatment
      algorithm for, 437
      based on grade and procedure, 438t
      diverticulectomy, 438
      hemicolectomy, 438–439

  intraoperative presentation, 436, 436–437
  mortality rates, 439
  nonresectional methods, 436, 438
  of preoperative uncomplicated cases,
      435–436
  surgical options, 436
  true, 429–430, 431
perforation of, associated with large bowel ob-
    struction caused by colonic strictures,
    201–202
radiographic evaluation
  approaches to, 117
  computed tomography, 123
surgical treatment, 203
Coincident diverticular disease
  case studies of, 174–175
  and colon cancer, 64
  and Crohn's disease, 72, 74
  description of, 174
  elective resection, indications for, 176
  found during treatment for other procedure, de-
      cisions whether to resect
    colonic surgery
      elective, 177, 178, 179
      emergent, 176–177
    noncolonic surgery
      elective, 176
      emergent, 176
Colocutaneous fistula, diverticulitis presentation
    and, 389, 390
Colon, (see also specific segment)
  arterial blood supply to, 4
  diverticular disease of, radiographic evaluation
    computed tomography
      abscesses, 120
      advantages of, 113–114
      colon cancer determinations, 113
      diagnostic findings, 109, 113, 118–120
      factors that limit sensitivity of, 113
      fistula formation, 119
      vs. contrast enema, 109
    contrast enema
      advantages of, 108
      characteristic findings, 105, 107
      with computed tomography, 106
      diagnostic criteria, 107–108, 109–117
      indications for, 106
      limitations of, 108
      water-soluble, 106–107
    magnetic resonance imaging, 116
    nuclear imaging, 117, 121
    plain radiography, 104, 105–106
    sonography
      diagnostic findings, 114, 116, 121
      disadvantages of, 116
  giant diverticula of, (see Giant colonic
      diverticulum)
  intraoperative lavage, (see Intraoperative colonic
      lavage)
  muscular changes in, 4
  segmentation of, 42
  strictures of
    biopsies to rule out cancer, 197–198
    case studies, 194–195
    causes of, 196
    colonic, 196

Colon—*Continued*
   diagnosis of
      barium enema, 196–197, *197*
      colonoscopy, *195,* 197–198, *198*
      illustration of, *199*
      incidence of, 196
      large bowel obstruction findings, 196, 200–201,
         200–203
   treatment of
      nonsurgical, 198–199
      surgical, 198, 200
Colon cancer, perforated, and diverticulitis
   concomitant presentation, 64
   differential diagnosis
      case study, 55–56
      diagnostic tests for
         computed tomography, 59–60, *62–63,* 113
         contrast enemas, 56–57, *58–60*
         endoluminal ultrasonography, 63
         magnetic resonance imaging, 63
         plain films, 56
         radionuclide scans, 63–64
         sigmoidoscopy, 57–58
         transabdominal ultrasonography, 57–58
Colonoscopy
   diagnostic uses
      colon cancer *vs.* diverticulitis, 57–58
      diverticular bleeding
         diagnosis of, *80,* 80–81
         treatment of, 89, *90,* 91
      diverticular stricture, 197–198, *198*
      ischemic colitis, 48
      transverse colon diverticulitis, 424
   failure rate of, 58
Colorectal neoplasm, diverticular bleeding and,
      differential diagnosis, 9
Colouterine fistula
   description of, 385
   signs and symptoms of, 386
Colovaginal fistulas
   case study, 167
   clinical examination of, 170t
   clinical studies, 169
   description of, 167–168
   etiology of, 169t
   hysterectomy and, 168
   incidence of, 167–168
   pathogenesis of, 168–169
   radiographic evaluation, 170
   sigmoidoscopy of, 169
   surgical management of
      approaches, 170
      complications, 171t
      one-stage approach, 170–171, 171t, *172*
   symptoms of, 169t, 173
Colovesical fistulas
   barium enema of, *152, 155*
   bladder defects, 162–163
   case studies of, 151–156
   computed tomographic evaluation of,
      153–154, 158
   etiology of, 156t
   gender predilection, 157
   historical descriptions of, 156
   laparoscopic diagnosis of, 164
   nonoperative management, 164

   pathogenesis of, 156–157
   patient evaluation of, 157t
   surgical management of
      in Crohn's disease, 162
      description of, 164
      indications for, 158
      operative principles, 159, *160–162*
      preoperative stenting, 158–159
      procedures, 159t
      technique, 159–163
   symptoms associated with, 156t, 157
   urologic symptoms, 157
Complicated diverticulosis
   outcomes, studies of, 3
   prognosis for, 3
Complications, surgical
   anastomotic leak
      computed tomographic diagnosis of, 290, *291*
      diverting loop ileostomy, 290
      hemorrhoidal vessels and, 290–291
      incidence of, 288
      predisposing factors, 289
      signs and symptoms of, 288–289
   case studies that illustrate, 285–287
   perioperative bleeding
      anastomosis, 293
      presacral venous plexus, 292
      splenic injury, 291, *292–293*
   postoperative intra-abdominal abscess, 296,
      298, *298*
   postoperative monitoring, 287
   postoperative small bowel obstruction
      exploratory laparotomy, 296, *297*
      gangrenous, *295*
      incidence of, 293
      management of, 296
      mechanical
         description of, 293, *294*
         illustration of, *296*
      paralytic ileus, 293, 294t
      strangulation, 293–294, *295*
   risk factors for, 287
   stomal
      parastomal hernia, 302, *303*
      preventive measures, 301
      prolapse, 304–305
      retraction, 302, *303–304*
   ureteral injuries
      common site for, 288
      preventive measures, 288
      ureteral blood supply, *289*
      ureteral stents, 288
   wound contamination
      bacterial pathogens, 299
      classification of, 299t
      in elective procedures, 299
      in emergency procedures, 299
      risk factors, 299
      signs and symptoms of, 299
      treatment of, 300
   wound dehiscence, *300,* 300–301
Computed tomography
   advantages of, 6
   concomitant testing methods, 6
   with contrast agents
      for colon diverticulosis, 106

for differential diagnosis of colon cancer *vs.* diverticulitis, 59, *62*
for diverticulosis in immunocompromised patient, 313, *314*
diagnostic uses
abscess, 208, *212*
acute diverticulitis, 59, 69
cecal diverticulitis, *123*, 433, *434*
giant colonic diverticula, 413, *414–415*
hepatic abscess, 445, *450*
ischemic colitis, 51, *53*
for localization of abdominal pain, 36
malignant diverticulitis, 186, *187–188*
small bowel diverticula, 406, *406*
transverse colon diverticulitis, *423*, 423–424
percutaneous drainage guided by, for diverticular abscess
catheter placement, 213, *215*
collapse of abscess cavity, 218, *219*
complications of, 219
drainage routes, 215, *216–218*
failure of, 219
indications, 211, *212*
needle guidance, 213, *214*
patient preparation, 213
success rates, 218
transgluteal drainage, 215, *216–218*
Contrast agents, computed tomography use with
for colon diverticulosis, 106
for differential diagnosis of colon cancer *vs.* diverticulitis, 59, *62*
for diverticulosis in immunocompromised patient, 313, *314*
Contrast enema
barium, (*see* Barium enema)
diagnostic use
colon cancer and diverticulitis
concomitant presentation, 57
differential diagnosis, 56–57
diverticular disease of colon
advantages of, 108
characteristic findings, 105, *107*
with computed tomography, 106
diagnostic criteria, 107–108, *109–117*
indications for, 106
limitations, 108
water-soluble, 106–107
malignant diverticulitis, 184, *184–186*
vs. computed tomography, 69–70
Corticosteroids, use by immunocompromised patients
effect on diagnosis of diverticular disease, 310–311
immunosuppressive effects of, 310
peritonitis diagnosis and, 313
wound healing impairments and, 316
Critical illness, from diverticular disease
abdominal compartment syndrome
abdominal closure techniques, *334–335*
abdominal pressure increases, physiologic consequences of, 333, 333t
characteristics of, 333
decompression for, 334–335
diagnosis of, 333–334
adult respiratory distress syndrome
description of, 331

mortality of, 332
treatment of, 331–332
case study to illustrate, 329–330
diverticular bleeding, 331
sepsis
adult respiratory distress syndrome associated with, (*see* Adult respiratory distress syndrome)
clinical features of, 335
definition of, 335
effect on intestinal anastomosis, 275
gut as secondary source of, 338
septic shock
clinical manifestations of, 336–338
definition of, 335
hypercatabolism and, 337
mortality from multiple organ failure, 337
treatment of
antibiotics, 338
description of, 337–338
early enteral nutrition, 338–339
Crohn's disease
case study of, 67
clinical findings, 68
colocutaneous fistula associated with, 69, 107
colovesical fistulas and, 156–157, 162
and diverticulitis
concomitant presentation, 72, 74
differential diagnosis
age of onset, 68
clinical manifestations, 68–69
description of, 68
diagnostic modalities
barium enema, 69
endoscopy, 69
editorial comments regarding, 72–74
effect on treatment, 74
fistulas, 69
laparoscopic findings, 70–71
operative findings, 70–71
pathology, 71–72
patient history, 73t
perianal disease, 68–69
physical findings, 73t
postoperative differences, 71
radiologic features, 69–70, 70t
granulomas associated with, 71–72, *73*
Meckel's diverticula in, 381
pathologic findings associated with, 71–72
treatment of, 70–71
CT, (*see* Computed tomography)
Cytokines
description of, 336
physiologic effects, 336
types of, 336

Dehiscence, wound, *300*, 300–301
Differential diagnosis
of diverticulitis
with Crohn's disease
age of onset, 68
clinical manifestations, 68–69
description of, 68
diagnostic modalities
barium enema, 69
endoscopy, 69

Differential diagnosis—*Continued*
  editorial comments regarding, 72–74
  effect on treatment, 74
  fistulas, 69
  laparoscopic findings, 70–71
  operative findings, 70–71
  pathology, 71–72
  patient history, 73t
  perianal disease, 68–69
  physical findings, 73t
  postoperative differences, 71
  radiologic features, 69–70, 70t
  with ischemic colitis
    abdominal pain, 48
    case studies of, 44–46
    clinical presentations, 47
    description of, 46–47
    physical examination, 48
  with perforated colon cancer, (*see* Colon
      cancer)
  of diverticulosis
    with abdominal pain, 37t
      case study of, 33–34
      diagnostic evaluations, 36
      localization of, 35
      pain etiology, 34–35
    with irritable bowel syndrome
      abdominal pain associated with, 37t
      differential diagnosis, 36, 41t
      treatment of, 41
Diverticular bleeding
  case study of, 76–77
  clinical approaches to, 91
  colorectal neoplasm and, differential
      diagnosis, 9
  description of, 9
  evaluation of, 78–79
  fluid resuscitation for, 79
  pathogenesis of, 77, 77–78
  sources, diagnosis of
    angiography, 82–83, *84, 85*
    barium studies, 85–86
    endoscopy, 80, *80–81*
    nuclear medicine approaches, 81–82, *82,* 83t
    physical findings, 79
    rigid sigmoidoscopy, 79
  spontaneous resolution of, 87
  treatment of
    colonoscopy, 86, *90,* 91
    embolization, 87
    surgery
      exploratory celiotomy prior to, 88–89
      indications for, 87–88, 176
      nonbleeding diverticula, 89
      operative decision, 88
      segmental colonic resection, 89, 89t
      subtotal colectomy, *88,* 89, 89t
    vasopressin, 86–87
Diverticular disease, (*see also* Diverticulitis; Diver-
      ticulosis)
  anatomic and pathologic studies
    history of, 7t
    illustration of, 3–5, *4–6*
  classification of, 4, 7t
  concomitant presentation, (*see* Coincident diver-
      ticular disease)

in conjunction with other abdominal
      conditions, (*see* Coincident di-
      verticular disease)
critical illness from, (*see* Critical illness)
diagnostic modalities
  computed tomography, (*see* Computed
      tomography)
  early types of, 5–6
findings associated with, 40–41
gender predilection, 175, 320
historical descriptions of, 1, 3–4
laboratory evaluation, 21–22
natural history of, 2–3
patient age and, 2, 95, 175
patient populations, 1–2, 2t
prevalence of, 103
prognosis, 2–3
surgical treatment
  complications
    illustration of, *15*
    risk factors for, 19t
  considerations for, 275
  developments in, 9t
  early types of, 9
  historical trends, 10t
  indications, 12t, 17t
  intracolonic bypass, 15
  laparoscopic colectomy, 15
  mortality associated with, 12t
  one-stage resections
    description of, 10, 12
    illustration of, *17–18*
  options for, 20t
  surgical series, 11t
  three-stage resections
    description of, 10
    illustration of, *13–14*
  types of, 20t
  trends in, 10t
  two-stage resection, 20t
    Hartmann procedure, (*see* Hartmann
        procedure)
  terminology commonly used, 7t
  Welch's approach to, 20–24
  in younger patients, (*see* Young patients, diver-
      ticular disease in)
Diverticular stricture, (*see* Stricture)
Diverticulectomy
  clinical uses of
    cecal diverticulitis, 438
    giant colonic diverticula, 417
    Meckel's diverticulum, 380
  risks associated with, 358
Diverticulitis
  acute, (*see* Acute diverticulitis)
  atypical presentations
    case study of, 384–385
    description of, 384
    extra-abdominal
      arthritis, 389
      colocutaneous fistula, 389, *390*
      description of, 385t
      external genitalia, 389
      infectious lesion in thigh or knee, 384–385,
          387–389, *388*
      nervous system, 389, *390*

pyoderma gangrenosum, 389, *391*
retroperitoneal abscess formation, 387–388, *388*
intra-abdominal
colouterine fistula, 385–386
hepatic abscess, *386*, 386–387
left adnexal masses, 385
perforated colon cancer, 387
types of, 385t
with bladder/vaginal involvement, abdominal pain associated with, 37t
case studies of, 102–103
cecal, (*see* Cecum, diverticulitis)
with free perforation, abdominal pain associated with, 37t, (*see also* Perforated sigmoid diverticulitis)
malignant, (*see* Malignant diverticulitis)
in Meckel's diverticulum, 375
medical treatment, 6, 8–9
and peridiverticular abscess, abdominal pain associated with, 37t
recurrent, after resection, (*see* Recurrent diverticulitis)
subacute, (*see* Subacute diverticulitis)
surgical complications of, (*see* Complications, surgical)
Diverticulosis
complicated
outcomes, studies of, 3
prognosis for, 3
differential diagnosis of, (*see* Differential diagnosis, of diverticulosis)
in immunocompromised patient, natural history of, 311–312
symptomatic, abdominal pain associated with, 37t
uncomplicated
laparoscopic use, 253
outpatient treatment, 23–24
progression to acute diverticulitis, 2
treatment approaches, 23–24
Diverticulum
in colon cancer *vs.* diverticulitis, 57
colonoscopic presentation of, *38*
duodenal, (*see* Duodenal diverticula)
formation
common sites of, 5, *8*
mechanism of, 5
giant colonic, (*see* Giant colonic diverticula)
right-sided, 77
bleeding associated with, 77
cecal, 429
in sigmoid colon, illustration of, *5–6*
signs and symptoms of, 34
Diverting transverse colostomy, for malignant diverticulitis, 187, 189
Drainage, of abscess, (*see* Percutaneous drainage)
Duodenal diverticula
abdominal pain and, 361
anatomic sites for
distal duodenum, *360*
near the ampulla of Vater, 354–355, *359–360*
asymptomatic presentation, 355
case study of, 352–354, 353t
classification of, 354

complications
biliary calculi, 356
biliary tract obstruction, 356
description of, 124, 355, 356t
illustration of, *357*
Kocher maneuver for, 358, *359*
management of, 358t
description of, 124
diagnosis of, 355, *356*
"giant" variant of, 126, *127–128*
illustration of, *125*
incidence of, 354
intraluminal, treatment of, 363, *365–367*
pathologic processes that mimic, 126
perforated
closure of, 363, *364*
description of, 358
duodenojejunostomy, 358, 363, *364*
signs of, 361
simple excision of, 362, *362–363*
simple inversion for, 363, *363*
radiographic evaluation of, 124, 126, *127–128*
radiologic evaluation of, 356
Duodenojejunostomy, for perforated duodenal diverticula, 358, 363, *364*

Ectopic gastric mucosa, in Meckel's diverticulum, 129, *132–134*
Elective resection
for coincident diverticular disease, 177, *178*, 179
for giant colonic diverticula, 415–417, *416–417*
in immunocompromised patients, 316–317
laparoscopic
anastomosis, 258, *258*
description of, 253
instruments, 254–255
mesenteric division, 256, *257*
mobilization, 255–256, *256*
operating room setup, 254, *255*
patient positioning, 254, *255*
resection, 256, *257*
specimen extraction, 258
trocar placement, 254–255, *255*
in young patients, 325–326
Embolization, for diverticular bleeding, 87
Endoscopic retrograde cholangiopancreatography
for duodenal diverticula
case study use of, 353–354
diagnostic use, 355
for hepatic abscess, 445
Endoscopy
clinical uses
acute diverticulitis, 57, 61
colovesical fistula, 155
Crohn's disease and diverticulitis, differential diagnosis, 69
diverticular bleeding, source of, *80*, 80–81
perforated colon cancer, 57–58
colonoscopy, (*see* Colonoscopy)
sigmoidoscopy, (*see* Sigmoidoscopy)
Endotoxin
description of, 336
physiologic effects, 336
Enema, (*see* Barium enema; Contrast enema)
Enteral nutrition, for septic shock, 338–339

Enteroclysis studies
    for Meckel's diverticulum, 129, *132, 134*
    for small bowel diverticula, 398, *405, 406*
Enteroliths
    composition of, 400
    illustration of, *404–405*
    small bowel obstruction and, 401
ERCP, (*see* Endoscopic retrograde cholangio-
            pancreatography, for duodenal
            diverticula)

Fecal diversion procedures
    for abscess, 210
    for colonic strictures, *203*
Fecal peritonitis, accompanying perforated sigmoid
            diverticulitis
    Hinchey classification system, 233, *233,* 280
    pathologic stages of, 233, *233*
    pneumoperitoneum associated with, 230, *231*
    purulent material, 230, *231*
    surgical treatment of
        case studies, 223–224, *224*
        Coloshield, 233, *235,* 236
        contraindications for, 227, 229
        description of, 224
        Hartmann procedure
            advantages of, 230
            description of, 226
            illustration of, *233–235*
        historical approach to, 224–226
        incidence of, 227
        literature reviews, 227, 228t, 236, 236t
        mortality rates, 227, 228t
        one-stage approach
            arguments against, 229–230
            arguments for, 229
        on-table lavage, 233
        preoperative irrigation and "walling off" of
                    purulent material and fibrinous de-
                    bris, 230, *232*
        three-stage approach, problems associated
                    with, 225–226
Fiber diet, (*see* High-fiber diet)
Fistulas
    colocutaneous, diverticulitis presentation and,
            389, *390*
    in colon diverticulosis, radiographic criteria for,
            107, *109, 113*
    colovaginal
        case study, 167
        clinical examination of, 170t
        clinical studies, 169
        description of, 167–168
        etiology of, 169t
        hysterectomy and, 168
        incidence of, 167–168
        pathogenesis of, 168–169
        radiographic evaluation, 170
        sigmoidoscopy of, 169
        surgical management of
            approaches, 170
            complications, 171t
            one-stage approach, 170–171, 171t, *172*
        symptoms of, 169t, 173
    colovesical
        barium enema of, *152, 155*
        bladder defects, 162–163

case studies of, 151–156
computed tomographic evaluation of,
        153–154, 158
etiology of, 156t
gender predilection, 157
historical descriptions of, 156
laparoscopic diagnosis of, 164
nonoperative management, 164
pathogenesis of, 156–157
patient evaluation of, 157t
surgical management of
    in Crohn's disease, 162
    description of, 164
    indications for, 158
    operative principles, 159, *160–162*
    preoperative stenting, 158–159
    procedures, 159t
    technique, 159–163
symptoms associated with, 156t, 157
urologic symptoms, 157

Giant colonic diverticulum
    case study of, 410–411, *411*
    causes of, 122
    characteristics of, 122
    clinical presentation, 412
    diagnostic studies
        barium enema, 413, *414*
        computed tomography, 413, *414–415*
        plain film, 413, *413*
    differential diagnosis, 413, 415
    elective resection of, 415–417, *416–417*
    mechanism of formation, 412, *413*
    natural history of, 413
    prevalence of, 412
    pseudocyst, 412
    pseudotypes, 412
    radiographic evaluation of, 122, 124, *125*
    true, 412
Glutamine
    description of, 338–339
    effect on bacterial translocation, 339
Gram-negative bacteria, 335–336
Granulomas, in Crohn's disease, 71–72, *73*

Hartmann procedure, 71
    anastomotic stricture after, 305
    clinical uses
        malignant diverticulitis, 187, 189
        perforated sigmoid diverticulitis with
                    generalized purulent or fecal
                    peritonitis
            advantages of, 230
            description of, 226
            illustration of, *233–235*
        recurrent diverticulitis, 350
        severe subacute diverticulitis, 247–248
    colostomy
        creation of, 264
        permanent, 263
    considerations for hemorrhoidal artery, *271*
    description of, 12
    guidelines for, 270–272, *271*
    history of, 263
    illustration of, *18–20*
    Lahey clinic experience, 280
    laparoscopic closure of

description of, 258–259
  patient positioning, 259
  postoperative care, 260
  procedure, 259
  trocar placement, *259*
preoperative considerations, 263
procedure, 263–264
reanastomosis
  case study of, 262
  difficulties associated with, 269
  illustration of, *266–269*
  laparoscopic, 270
  patient positioning, 265
  procedure, 265–266, *266–269*
  rectum mobilization, 265
  stapler passage, 269
  timing of, 264–265
rectum considerations
  mobilization from sacral hollow, contraindications for, 264
  stump, 264
stent placement, 263
wound infection rate, 299
Hematochezia
  bleeding sources, 78
  description of, 77
  management of, 78
Hemorrhage, diverticular, (*see* Diverticular bleeding)
Hepatic abscess
  appendicitis infection, *447–449*
  secondary to diverticulitis
    bacterial migration to, 443
    case study of, 442–443
    clinical presentation of, 445
    computed tomographic imaging of, 445, *450*
    description of, *386*, 386–387
    diagnostic evaluation, 445
    epidemiology of, 443, 445
    etiology of, 443–445, *444*, 444t
    outcome, 446
    signs and symptoms, 445, 445t
    treatment options
      description of, 446
      nonoperative, 446–447, 451
      operative approach, 446, 451
      percutaneous drainage
        description of, 446
        failure of, immediate surgical attention in event of, 451
High-fiber diet
  benefits of, 9
  diverticular disease reductions and, 34

Ileal diverticula
  complications of, 399
  diagnosis of, 398–399
  perforated, 400
  terminal, 402, *404*
Immunocompromised patient, diverticular diseases in
  abscess in, percutaneous drainage contraindications, 211
  case study of, 309–310
  description of, 310
  diagnosis
    description of, 312–313

exogenous corticosteroid use, effects of
  description of, 310
  dosage adjustments, 315
  masking of clinical signs and symptoms, 313
  modalities, 313, *314*
immune response impairments, effects of, 310
natural history, 311–312
pathology, 312
severity of, 312
surgical mortality, 312t
treatment of
  elective resection, 316–317
  medical approaches, 316
  principles, 315
  surgical approaches, 316
in younger patient, 313
Inflammatory bowel disease, (*see* Crohn's disease)
Intensive care unit admissions, for diverticular disease, (*see* Critical illness)
Intestine, (*see* Large bowel; Small bowel)
Intra-abdominal sepsis, (*see* Sepsis, intra-abdominal)
Intracolonic bypass, 15
Intraluminal pressure, of small bowel
  experiments to create diverticula, 397
  motor abnormality effects, 397
Intraoperative colonic lavage
  advantages of, 276
  case study of, 274
  description of, 274–275
  history of, 276
  Lahey clinical experience, 280t—281t, 280–282
  procedure, 276, *276–279*
Intravenous pyelogram, for recurrent sigmoid diverticulitis, 97–98
Intussusception, in Meckel's diverticulum, 375, *375*
Irritable bowel syndrome
  abdominal pain associated with, 37t
  differential diagnosis, 36, 41t
  treatment of, 41
Ischemic colitis
  acute, differential diagnosis of, 48
  after aortic surgery, 49–50
  classification of
    gangrenous, 47
    nongangrenous, 47
  clinical deterioration despite therapy, 49
  definition of, 44
  diagnosis of, 47–48
  forms of, 47
  imaging of
    colonoscopy, 48
    computed tomography, 51, *53*
    endoscopy, 51, *52*
    studies, 48
  laparoscopic diagnosis of, 51
  pathogenesis of, 46–47
  shock-associated, 49
  signs and symptoms of, 50–51
  sites commonly affected, 47
  spectrum of, 46–47
  "spontaneous" episodes of, 46
  total, 50
  treatment of
    approaches, 49–50
    deterioration despite, 49

Ischemic colitis—*Continued*
  vs. diverticulitis, differential diagnosis of
    abdominal pain, 48
    case studies of, 44–46
    clinical presentations, 47
    description of, 46–47
    physical examination, 48
IVP, (*see* Intravenous pyelogram)

Jejunoileal diverticular disease
  abdominal pain associated with, 398
  age of onset, 396
  bleeding associated with, selective angiography
    of, 399
  characteristics of, 396–397
  clinical manifestations, 397–398
  complications, 126, 399, 402t
  diagnosis of, 398–399, *405–406, 406*
  dyskinesia, 400
  extravasation, 126, *131*
  gender predilection, 126
  hemorrhage associated with, 400
  illustration of, *129–130, 403*
  incidence of, 396
  indications of, 407t
  inflammation in, 400
  motility disorders, 398
  pathogenesis of, 397
  perforated, 399–400
  radiographic evaluation of, 126, *131*
  and scleroderma, 126, *130*
  systemic diseases that can cause, 397

Kocher maneuver, 358, *359*

Laparoscopy
  case study of, 251–252
  colectomy, description of, 15, *22*
  contraindications, 252–253
  description of, 252
  diagnostic uses, 253
    cecal diverticulitis, 433
    hepatic abscess drainage, 446
    ischemic colitis, 51
    transverse colon diverticulitis, 424, 426
  elective sigmoid resection
    anastomosis, 258, *258*
    description of, 253
    instruments, 254–255
    mesenteric division, 256, *257*
    mobilization, 255–256, *256*
    operating room setup, 254, *255*
    patient positioning, 254, *255*
    resection, 256, *257*
    specimen extraction, 258
    trocar placement, 254–255, *255*
  Hartmann closure using
    description of, 258–259
    patient positioning, 259
    postoperative care, 260
    procedure, 259
    trocar placement, *259*
  indications, 252–253
  for ischemic colitis, 51
  for recurrent sigmoid diverticulitis, 98–99
  for small bowel diverticula, 399

Laparotomy
  cecal diverticulitis, 436, *436–437*
  diverticular abscess, 219
Large bowel obstruction
  laparoscopic contraindications, 253
  from stricture formation
    description of, 199, 200–201
    illustration of, *201–202*
    surgical approaches, 201, *203*
Lavage, on-table
  clinical uses
    abscess, 210
    colonic strictures, 201
    description of, 282t
    perforated sigmoid diverticulitis with general-
      ized purulent or fecal peritonitis, 233
  intraoperative colonic
    advantages of, 276
    case study of, 274
    description of, 274–275
    history of, 276
    Lahey clinical experience, 280t—281t, 280–282
    procedure, 276, *276–279*
Left adnexal masses, diverticulitis and, 385
Littre's hernia, 375
Liver abscess, (*see* Hepatic abscess)
Longitudinal myotomy
  description of, 12
  illustration of, *21*
Loop ileostomy
  clinical uses
    for large bowel obstruction caused by colonic
      strictures, 201, *203*
    for subacute diverticulitis, 247
  collapse of, 304–305
  creation of, to prevent stomal problems, 301–302
  diverting, for anastomotic leak, 290
  vs. diverting transverse colostomy, for malignant
    diverticulitis, 192
Lower gastrointestinal bleeding, (*see also* Diverticu-
    lar bleeding)
  algorithm for, *78*
  causes of, 78
  diagnosis of
    using angiography, 82–83, *84,* 85
    using colonoscopy, 80–81
Luminal narrowing
  in colon cancer, 57
  in diverticulitis, 57

Magnetic resonance imaging, applications of, 63
Malignant diverticulitis
  anastomotic failure, 190, *190*
  case studies of, 181–183
  clinical features, 184
  description of, 181
  edematous tissue, *189*
  granulomatous colitis and, similarities
    between, 192
  imaging of
    computed tomography, 186, *187–188*
    contrast enema, 184, *184–186*
  incidence of, 184
  inflammation associated with, 181
  management of
    diverting transverse colostomy

description of, 187
vs. loop ileostomy, 192
Hartmann procedure, 187, 189
operative findings, 186–187
preoperative preparation, 186
principles of, 191–192
pathology, 189–190, *189–191*
phlegmonous inflammation, 181, 191
symptoms of, 184
Meckel's diverticulum
anatomic findings, 373t, 373–374
asymptomatic, treatment of, 379–380, 382
bowel obstruction associated with, 130, *133*
case study of, 370–371, *371*
characteristics of, 129
complications, 374t
age-specific nature of, 374t
classification of, 374
diverticulitis, 375
entrapment, 375–376
hemorrhage, 374
intestinal obstruction, 374–375, *375*
in Crohn's disease, 381
diagnosis of
angiography, 379
preoperative, 376
technetium-99m pertechnetate scanning,
376–379, *377–378*
diagnostic findings, 130
differential diagnosis, 376
ectopic gastric mucosa associated with, 129,
132–134
embryology of, 371–372, *372*
enteroclysis studies, 129, *132*, 134
giant colonic diverticulum and, differential diagnosis, 413
histologic findings, 373t, 373–374
historical descriptions of, 370
illustration of, *372*
incidence of, 372–373
radiographic evaluation of, 129–130, *134*
sites of, 373
symptomatic, treatment of, 379–380
treatment of, 379–380
tumors associated with, 380–381
Mediators, 335–336
Mesenteric angiography
for localization of diverticular bleeding, 82–83,
84, 85
reviews of, 85t
Mesentery
border, examination of, 406, *407*
computed tomographic evaluation of, 59–60
MRI, (*see* Magnetic resonance imaging)

Neoplasm, (*see* Cancer)
Nonsteroidal anti-inflammatory drugs
diverticulitis and, 2
effect on diverticular bleeding, 79
NSAIDs, (*see* Nonsteroidal anti-inflammatory
drugs)
Nuclear medicine
clinical uses, diverticular disease of the colon,
117, *121*
radionuclide scans
description of, 63–64

for small bowel obstruction, 141, *142*
using technetium-99 sulfur colloid, 81
using technetium-labeled red blood cells,
81–82
using technetium-99m pertechnetate scanning,
376–379, *377–378*

Obstruction
large bowel
laparoscopic contraindications, 253
from stricture formation
description of, 199, 200–201
illustration of, *201–202*
surgical approaches, 201, *203*
small bowel, accompanying colonic diverticular
disease
adherence concerns, 143, 146, *147*
case studies of, 138–140, *139*
cause of, 146
intestinal decompression for, 141, 143, 149
ischemia, 143, 146
laparoscopic contraindications, 253
management of, 141
operative decisions in, factors that
influence, 141
radiographic evaluation, 146, *147–148*
radionuclide studies, 141, *142*
schematic illustration of, *146*
surgical management, 143–144, *144–145*
suspected, approaches for, 141
symptoms of, 141
Ogilvie's syndrome, *202*
One-stage resection and anastomosis
advantages of, 275
illustration of, *17–18*
in immunocompromised patients, 316
indications
abscess, 209
colovesical fistulas, 159t
small bowel diverticular disease, 401, 406
subacute diverticulitis, 246–248
transverse colon diverticulitis, 426
intraoperative colonic lavage with, (*see* Intraoperative colonic lavage)
problems associated with, 10, 12
types of, 20t
On-table lavage
clinical uses
abscess, 210
colonic strictures, 201
description of, 282t
intraoperative colonic
advantages of, 276
case study of, 274
description of, 274–275
history of, 276
Lahey clinical experience, 280t—281t,
280–282
procedure, 276, *276–279*
for perforated sigmoid diverticulitis with
generalized purulent or fecal peritonitis, 233

Pain, (*see also* Abdominal pain)
transmission pathways, 34
Panendoscopy, 80

Paraileostomy hernia, strangulation obstruction and, *295*
Paralytic ileus, postoperative
  causes of, 294t
  description of, 293
Parastomal hernia, 302, *303*
Percutaneous drainage
  for diverticular abscess
    contraindications, 211
    CT-scan-guided
      catheter placement, 213, *215*
      collapse of abscess cavity, 218, *219*
      complications of, 219
      drainage routes, 215, *216–218*
      failure of, 219
      indications, 211, *212*
      needle guidance, 213, *214*
      patient preparation, 213
      success rates, 218
      transgluteal drainage, 215, *216–218*
    description of, 210–211
    ultrasound-guided, 218
  for hepatic abscess, 446
Perforated duodenal diverticula
  closure of, 363, *364*
  description of, 358
  duodenojejunostomy, 358, 363, *364*
  signs of, 361
  simple excision of, 362, *362–363*
  simple inversion for, 363, *363*
Perforated ileum diverticula, 400
Perforated jejunoileal diverticula, 399–400
Perforated sigmoid diverticulitis, with generalized purulent or fecal peritonitis
  complications, 287
  Hinchey classification system, 233, *233*, 280
  pathologic stages of, 233, *233*
  pneumoperitoneum associated with, 230, *231*
  purulent material, 230, *231*
  surgical treatment of
    case studies, 223–224, *224*
    Coloshield, 233, *235*, 236
    description of, 224
    fecal contamination contraindications for, 227, 229
    Hartmann procedure
      advantages of, 230
      description of, 226
      illustration of, *233–235*
    historical approach to, 224–226
    incidence of, 227
    literature reviews, 227, 228t, 236, 236t
    mortality rates, 227, 228t
    one-stage approach
      arguments against, 229–230
      arguments for, 229
    on-table lavage, 233
    preoperative irrigation and "walling off" of purulent material and fibrinous debris, 230, *232*
    three-stage approach, problems associated with, 225–226
Peritonitis, purulent or fecal, accompanying perforated sigmoid diverticulitis
  Hinchey classification system, 233, *233*, 280

pathologic stages of, 233, *233*
pneumoperitoneum associated with, 230, *231*
purulent material, 230, *231*
surgical treatment of
  case studies, 223–224, *224*
  Coloshield, 233, *235*, 236
  description of, 224
  fecal contamination contraindications for, 227, 229
  Hartmann procedure
    advantages of, 230
    description of, 226
    illustration of, *233–235*
  historical approach to, 224–226
  incidence of, 227
  literature reviews, 227, 228t, 236, 236t
  mortality rates, 227, 228t
  one-stage approach
    arguments against, 229–230
    arguments for, 229
  on-table lavage, 233
  preoperative irrigation and "walling off" of purulent material and fibrinous debris, 230, *232*
  three-stage approach, problems associated with, 225–226
Plain film, diagnostic use
  colon cancer *vs.* diverticulitis, 56
  colon diverticulitis, 104, *105–106*
  diverticulosis in immunocompromised patient, 313, *314*
  giant colonic diverticula, 122, 124, *125*, 413, *413*
Pneumoperitoneum
  associated with perforated sigmoid diverticulitis, 230, *231*
  computed tomographic imaging of, *314*
  plain radiographic evaluation of, 104
Pseudodiverticula
  giant colonic types, 412
  pathogenesis of, 34
  in young patients, 34
Purulent peritonitis, accompanying perforated sigmoid diverticulitis
  Hinchey classification system, 233, *233*, 280
  pathologic stages of, 233, *233*
  pneumoperitoneum associated with, 230, *231*
  purulent material, 230, *231*
  surgical treatment of
    case studies, 223–224, *224*
    Coloshield, 233, *235*, 236
    description of, 224
    fecal contamination contraindications for, 227, 229
    Hartmann procedure
      advantages of, 230
      description of, 226
      illustration of, *233–235*
    historical approach to, 224–226
    incidence of, 227
    literature reviews, 227, 228t, 236, 236t
    mortality rates, 227, 228t
    one-stage approach
      arguments against, 229–230
      arguments for, 229
    on-table lavage, 233

preoperative irrigation and "walling off" of purulent material and fibrinous debris, 230, *232*
three-stage approach, problems associated with, 225–226
Pyoderma gangrenosum, diverticulitis presentation and, 389, *391*

Radionuclide scans
description of, 63–64
for small bowel obstruction, 141, *142*
using technetium-99 sulfur colloid, 81
using technetium-labeled red blood cells, 81–82
using technetium-99m pertechnetate scanning, 376–379, *377–378*
Reanastomosis, after Hartmann procedure
case study of, 262
difficulties associated with, 269
illustration of, *266–269*
laparoscopic, 270
patient positioning, 265
procedure, 265–266, *266–269*
rectum mobilization, 265
stapler passage, 269
timing of, 264–265
Rectal ischemia, after peripheral vascular procedures, 54
Rectum, arterial blood supply to, *4*
Recurrent diverticulitis, after resection
case study of, 343–344, *344–345*
differential diagnosis, 344, 346
distal margin and, 347
epidemiology of, 346, 346t
incidence of, 344
management of
conservation, 348
reresection
anastomosis, 350
assessment, 349
contamination considerations, 349
description of, 348–349
extent of, 350
mobilization, 349–350
patient positioning, 349
preoperative preparation, 349
proximal margin and, 346–347
Recurrent sigmoid diverticulitis
case study, 95
diagnostic evaluation
flexible endoscopy with barium enema, 96, *97*
intravenous pyelogram, 97–98
rigid proctosigmoidoscopy, 96
differential diagnosis, 99–100
indications for resection, 95
rates of, 100
surgery for
bowel resection amount, questions regarding, 99
laparoscopy *vs.* open colectomy, 99–100
patient preparation, 98
postoperative management, 99
preoperative intravenous pyelogram, 97
procedure, 98–99
Renal transplant patients, diverticular disease in
treatment considerations, 315
in younger patients, 313, 313t

Resection
with anastomosis, (*see* One-stage resection and anastomosis)
distal margin, 347, *348*
laparoscopic sigmoid
anastomosis, 258, *258*
description of, 253
instruments, 254–255
mesenteric division, 256, *257*
mobilization, 255–256, *256*
operating room setup, 254, *255*
patient positioning, 254, *255*
resection, 256, *257*
specimen extraction, 258
trocar placement, 254–255, *255*
proximal margin, 346–347
recurrent diverticulitis after
case study of, 343–344, *344–345*
differential diagnosis, 344, 346
distal margin and, 347
epidemiology of, 346, 346t
incidence of, 344
management of
conservation, 348
reresection
anastomosis, 350
assessment, 349
contamination considerations, 349
description of, 348–349
extent of, 350
mobilization, 349–350
patient positioning, 349
preoperative preparation, 349
proximal margin and, 346–347

Segmental colonic resection
advantages of, 275
for diverticular bleeding, 89, 89t
Sepsis, intra-abdominal
abdominal compartment syndrome, (*see* Abdominal compartment syndrome)
adult respiratory distress syndrome associated with, (*see* Adult respiratory distress syndrome)
clinical features of, 335
definition of, 335
effect on intestinal anastomosis, 275
gut as secondary source of, 338
Septic shock
clinical manifestations of, 336–338
definition of, 335
hypercatabolism and, 337
mortality from multiple organ failure, 337
treatment of
antibiotics, 338
description of, 337–338
early enteral nutrition, 338–339
Short-chain fatty acids, 265
Sigmoid diverticulitis
illustration of, *41*
malignant, (*see* Malignant diverticulitis)
perforated, with generalized purulent or fecal peritonitis
Hinchey classification system, 233, *233*
pathologic stages of, 233, *233*
pneumoperitoneum associated with, 230, *231*

Sigmoid diverticulitis—*Continued*
　purulent material, 230, *231*
　surgical treatment of
　　case studies, 223–224, *224*
　　Coloshield, 233, *235*, 236
　　description of, 224
　　fecal contamination contraindications for,
　　　227, 229
　　Hartmann procedure, (*see also* Hartmann
　　　procedure)
　　　advantages of, 230
　　　description of, 226
　　　illustration of, *233–235*
　　historical approach to, 224–226
　　incidence of, 227
　　literature reviews, 227, 228t, 236, 236t
　　mortality rates, 227, 228t
　　one-stage approach
　　　arguments against, 229–230
　　　arguments for, 229
　　on-table lavage, 233
　　preoperative irrigation and "walling off" of
　　　purulent material and fibrinous de-
　　　bris, 230, *232*
　　three-stage approach, problems associated
　　　with, 225–226
　recurrent
　　case study, 95
　　diagnostic evaluation
　　　flexible endoscopy with barium enema,
　　　　96, *97*
　　　intravenous pyelogram, 97–98
　　　rigid proctosigmoidoscopy, 96
　　differential diagnosis, 99–100
　　indications for resection, 95
　　rates of, 100
　　surgery for
　　　bowel resection amount, questions regard-
　　　　ing, 99
　　　laparoscopy *vs.* open colectomy, 99–100
　　　patient preparation, 98
　　　postoperative management, 99
　　　preoperative intravenous pyelogram, 97
　　　procedure, 98–99
　signs and symptoms of, 21
　small bowel obstruction, (*see* Small bowel ob-
　　struction)
Sigmoidoscopy, for differential diagnosis of colon
　　cancer and diverticulitis, 57–58, *61*
Single-stage resection, (*see* One-stage resection and
　　anastomosis)
SIRS, (*see* Systemic inflammatory response syn-
　　drome)
Small bowel diverticular disease
　case studies of, 394–396
　characteristics of, 396–397
　clinical manifestations, 397–398
　complications, 398–399
　diagnosis of, 398–399
　diagnostic laparoscopy for, 406
　duodenal
　　complications of, 124
　　description of, 124
　　"giant" variant of, 126, *127–128*
　　illustration of, *125*
　　pathologic processes that mimic, 126

　　radiographic evaluation of, 124, 126, *127–128*
　　hemorrhage associated with, 400
　　incidental, treatment considerations, 401
　　inflammation associated with, 400
　jejunoileal
　　abdominal pain associated with, 398
　　age of onset, 396
　　bleeding associated with, selective angiogra-
　　　phy of, 399
　　characteristics of, 396–397
　　clinical manifestations, 397–398
　　complications, 126, 399, 402t
　　diagnosis of, 398–399, *405–406*, 406
　　dyskinesia, 400
　　extravasation, 126, *131*
　　gender predilection, 126
　　hemorrhage associated with, 400
　　illustration of, *129–130*, *403*
　　incidence of, 396
　　inflammation in, 400
　　motility disorders, 398
　　pathogenesis of, 397
　　perforated, 399–400
　　radiographic evaluation of, 126, *131*
　　systemic diseases that can cause, 397
　management of, 401
　Meckel's diverticulum, (*see* Meckel's diverticu-
　　lum)
　obstruction associated with, 400–401, 404
　pathogenesis of, 397
　perforation, 399–400
　resection with primary anastomosis for, 401, 406
Small bowel obstruction
　accompanying colonic diverticular disease
　　adherence concerns, 143, 146, *147*
　　case studies of, 138–140, *139*
　　cause of, 146
　　intestinal decompression for, 141, 143, 149
　　ischemia, 143, 146
　　laparoscopic contraindications, 253
　　management of, 141
　　operative decisions in, factors that
　　　influence, 141
　　radiographic evaluation, 146, *147–148*
　　radionuclide studies, 141, *142*
　　schematic illustration of, *146*
　　surgical management, 143–144, *144–145*
　　suspected, approaches for, 141
　　symptoms of, 141
　postoperative
　　exploratory laparotomy, 296, *297*
　　gangrenous, *295*
　　incidence of, 293
　　management of, 296
　　mechanical
　　　description of, 293, *294*
　　　illustration of, *296*
　　paralytic ileus, 293, 294t
　　strangulation, 293–294, *295*
Splenic injury, bleeding associated with, 291,
　　292–293
Stoma
　construction of, 301
　loop ileostomy, (*see* Loop ileostomy)
　postoperative problems
　　parastomal hernia, 302, *303*

preventive measures, 301
prolapse, 304–305
retraction, 302, *303–304*
Stricture
  anastomotic, 305
  colonic
    biopsies to rule out cancer, 197–198
    case studies, 194–195
    causes of, 196
    diagnosis of
      barium enema, 196–197, *197*
      colonoscopy, *195*, 197–198, *198*
    illustration of, *199*
    incidence of, 196
    large bowel obstruction findings, 196, 200–201,
      200–203
    treatment of
      nonsurgical, 198–199
      surgical, 198, 200
Subacute diverticulitis
  case study of, 242–243
  clinical presentation of, 243–244
  diagnosis of, 244
  radiologic evaluation of, 245
  "smoldering" inflammation associated with, 242–
    243, *248*
  treatment of
    medical, 244–245
    surgical
      indications, 245
      preoperative preparation, 245 246
      resection and anastomosis
        procedure, 246–247
        questions regarding efficacy of, 247–248
Surgery, *(see specific procedure)*
Surgical complications
  anastomotic leak
    computed tomographic diagnosis of, 290, *291*
    diverting loop ileostomy, 290
    hemorrhoidal vessels and, 290–291
    incidence of, 288
    predisposing factors, 289
    signs and symptoms of, 288–289
  case studies that illustrate, 285–287
  perioperative bleeding
    anastomosis, 293
    presacral venous plexus, 292
    splenic injury, 291, *292–293*
  postoperative intra-abdominal abscess, 296,
    298, *298*
  postoperative monitoring, 287
  postoperative small bowel obstruction
    exploratory laparotomy, 296, *297*
    gangrenous, *295*
    incidence of, 293
    management of, 296
    mechanical
      description of, 293, *294*
      illustration of, *296*
    paralytic ileus, 293, 294t
    strangulation, 293–294, *295*
  risk factors for, 287
  stomal
    parastomal hernia, 302, *303*
    preventive measures, 301
    prolapse, 304–305

retraction, 302, *303–304*
  ureteral injuries
    common site for, 288
    preventive measures, 288
    ureteral blood supply, *289*
    ureteral stents, 288
  wound contamination
    bacterial pathogens, 299
    classification of, 299t
    in elective procedures, 299
    in emergency procedures, 299
    risk factors, 299
    signs and symptoms of, 299
    treatment of, 300
  wound dehiscence, *300*, 300–301
Systemic inflammatory response syndrome, 338

Taeniae, 4
Tc-rbc, *(see* Technetium-labeled red blood cells)
Tc-SC, *(see* Technetium-99 sulfur colloid)
Technetium-99 sulfur colloid, for localization of
    diverticular bleeding, 81
Technetium-labeled red blood cells, for localization
    of diverticular bleeding, 81–82
Technetium-99m pertechnetate scanning, for
    Meckel's diverticulum, 376–379,
    377–378
Three-stage approach
  description of, 10
  illustration of, *13–14*
  indications
    abscess, 209
    colovesical fistulas, 159t
    perforated sigmoid diverticulitis with general-
      ized peritonitis, 225–226
  types of, 20t
TNF, *(see* Tumor necrosis factor)
Transabdominal ultrasonography
  acute diverticulitis diagnosis using, 61–62
  differential diagnosis for colon cancer *vs.* compli-
    cated diverticulitis, 62
Transverse colon, diverticulitis of
  appendicitis and, 423
  atypical presentations, 422–423
  carcinoma and, 426
  case study of, 419–420
  clinical presentation of, 422
  computed tomographic imaging of, 423, 423–424
  differential diagnosis, 422, *422*
  emergent treatment, 424, 426
  incidence of, 420
  inflammation associated with, 426
  morphologic types of, 420, *421*
  resection and primary anastomosis for, 426
Transverse myotomies, 12, *21*
Tumor necrosis factor, 336
Two-stage resections
  for abscess, 209
  for colovesical fistulas, 159t
  Hartmann procedure, *(see* Hartmann procedure)
  types of, 20t

Ulcerative colitis, description of, 68
Ultrasonography
  endoluminal, for colon cancer *vs.* complicated
    diverticulitis, 63

Ultrasonography—*Continued*
    transabdominal, acute diverticulitis diagnosis
        using, 61–62
Uncomplicated diverticulosis
    laparoscopic use, 253
    outpatient treatment, 23–24
    progression to acute diverticulitis, 2
    treatment approaches, 23–24
Ureteral injuries
    common site for, 288
    preventive measures, 288
    ureteral blood supply, *289*
    ureteral stents, 288
USG, (*see* Transabdominal ultrasonography)

Vaginography, for colovaginal fistulas, 170
Vasopressin, for diverticular bleeding
    complications, 86–87
    success rates, 86–87
    transcatheter infusion, 86

Water-soluble contrast enema, diagnostic use, colon
        cancer *vs.* diverticulitis, 56–57
Wound
    contamination
        bacterial pathogens, 299
        classification of, 299t
        in elective procedures, 299
        in emergency procedures, 299
        risk factors, 299
        signs and symptoms of, 299

    treatment of, 300
    dehiscence, *300,* 300–301
    impaired healing, in immunocompromised pa-
        tient, 316

Young patients (40 years or less), diverticular
        disease in
    comorbid conditions, 320–321
    complications of
        analysis difficulties, 323–324
        disease virulence, 324
        incidence, 323–324
        resection indications, 325
    elective resection, questions regarding necessity
        of, 325–326
    ethnicity and, 320
    gender predilection, 320
    prevalence of, 34, 319–320
    surgical intervention
        emergent, questions regarding necessity
            of, 326
        incidence of, 323, 324t
    symptomatic
        analysis of, difficulties associated with, 321
        diagnosis of, 322–323
        incidence of, 321
        location of, 321–322, 322t
        signs and symptoms of, 322, 323t
    vs. older patients
        disease virulence, 324
        hospitalization, 321